MEDICAL RADIOLOGY

Radiation Oncology

J. J. Lu · J. S. Cooper · A. W. M. Lee (Eds.)

Nasopharyngeal Cancer

Multidisciplinary Management

With Contributions by

R. R. Allison · I. Ayan · K. B. Tan · S. Cao · A. T. C. Chan · C.-J. Chen · Y.-C. Chien
V. F. H. Chong · D. T. Chua · J. S. Cooper · B. S. Glisson · B. C. Goh · V. Grégoire · Y. Guo
W.-L. Hsu · L. Kong · Q.-T. Le · A. W. M. Lee · N. Lee · J.-C. Lin · S. Lin · S. S. Lo · P.-J. Lou
J. J. Lu · B. B.Y. Ma · J. Ma · C. K. Ong · B. O'Sullivan · R. Ove · E. Ozyar · T. C. Putti ·
K. S. Loh · I. W. K. Tham · K.-B. Tam J. Wee · W. I. Wei · E. Yu · M.-S. Zeng · Y.-X. Zeng

Foreword by

L.W. Brady, H.-P. Heilmann, M. Molls, and C. Nieder

With 84 Figures in 117 Separate Illustrations, 52 in Color and 51 Tables

Springer

JIADE J. LU, MD, MBA
Associate Professor and Consultant
Department of Radiation Oncology
National University Cancer Institute of Singapore
National University Health System
National University of Singapore
5 Lower Kent Ridge Road
Singapore 119074
Republic of Singapore
and
Distinguished Clinical Professor
Fudan University Shanghai Cancer Center
270 Dong An Road
Shanghai 200232
P.R. China

JAY S. COOPER, MD
Professor and Chairman
Department of Radiation Oncology
Maimonides Cancer Center
6300 Eighth Avenue
Brooklyn, NY 11220
USA

ANNE W.M. LEE, MD
Department of Clinical Oncology
Pamela Youde Nethersole Eastern Hospital
3 Lok Man Road
Chai Wan
Hong Kong SAR
P.R. China

MEDICAL RADIOLOGY · Diagnostic Imaging and Radiation Oncology
Series Editors:
A. L. Baert · L. W. Brady · H.-P. Heilmann · M. Knauth · M. Molls · C. Nieder · K. Sartor

Continuation of Handbuch der medizinischen Radiologie
Encyclopedia of Medical Radiology

ISBN: 978-3-642-26116-9 ISBN 978-3-540-92810-2 (eBook)

DOI: 10.1007/978-3-540-92810-2

Springer Heidelberg Dordrecht London New York

Medical Radiology · Diagnostic Imaging and Radiation Oncology ISSN 0942-5373

Softcover reprint of the hardcover 1st edition 2010

Cover design: Publishing Services Teichmann, 69256 Mauer, Germany

Printed on acid-free paper

9 8 7 6 5 4 3 2 1

Springer is part of Springer Science+Business Media (www.springer.com)

Foreword

Carcinomas of the nasopharynx represent a relatively uncommon disease process in Western countries, but are more frequently diagnosed as a head and neck malignancy in Southeast Asia. Most of these tumors are epithelial in origin. The nonkeratinizing, poorly or undifferentiated squamous cell carcinomas are the more commonly diagnosed pathologies in Asia, accounting for almost 95% of all cases. However, 75% of cases are World Health Organization Type 1 in North America, whereas those in Southeast Asia are Types 2 and 3. Radiation therapy is the primary treatment for nasopharyngeal carcinomas, and since these tumors tend to present with regional metastasis, combined chemotherapy and radiation therapy is commonly pursued. This is particularly appropriate in patients who have locally advanced disease.

This book, edited by Lu, Cooper, and Lee, discusses the recommendations for diagnosis and staging procedures for nasopharyngeal cancer, staging systems and prognostic factors, and management using radiation therapy for early-stage disease and combined treatment modalities with radiation and cytotoxic chemotherapy for more advanced disease. The supporting scientific evidence clearly indicates that these are the appropriate approaches for the treatment of carcinomas of the nasopharynx.

The volume also deals in detail with techniques of radiation therapy, including intensity-modulated radiation therapy, and outlines appropriate follow-up care and surveillance for those individuals who survive.

Even though nasopharyngeal cancer represents a relatively uncommon tumor in the Western world, it is a common tumor in Southeast Asia and the book by Lu, Cooper, and Lee constitutes a landmark volume identifying the appropriate approaches for the management of this disease process.

PA, USA — Luther W. Brady
Hamburg, Germany — Hans-Peter Heilmann
Münich, Germany — Michael Molls
Bodø, Norway — Carsten Nieder

Preface

Nasopharyngeal cancer is a unique type of head and neck malignancy. Essentially unresectable because of proximity to the skull base, nasopharyngeal cancer historically had been treated by radiation therapy alone. Although cure rates for early-stage disease have been relatively good, the substantially worse outcome for locoregionally advanced disease and the not insubstantial risk of disseminated disease clearly indicated that a more effective therapeutic strategy was needed for more advanced tumors.

The use of concurrent chemotherapy with radiation therapy, popularized by the landmark Intergroup trial (INT0099), has significantly improved the outcome of advanced nasopharyngeal cancers. This trial can be therefore viewed not only as a proof of principal, but also as a starting point for the refinement of chemotherapy-enhanced radiation therapy in the management of this disease, a quest that continues to the present time.

Similarly, technical advances in radiation therapy, particularly the development of intensity modulated radiation therapy (IMRT) and image guided radiation therapy (IGRT), have also improved our abilities to place the radiation dose precisely in three-dimensional space, ensuring adequate coverage of the gross tumor and clinical target volumes while simultaneously sparing normal tissues. As the anatomic location of the nasopharynx is in close proximity to critical organs at risk, appropriate beam shaping and placement previously had been (at times insurmountable) challenges for the radiation oncologist.

However, as occurs in any rapidly evolving field, numerous unanswered questions and controversies remain. The optimal schedule, timing, and specific chemotherapy regimen (both concurrent and adjuvant) are still unknown. The delineation of ideal target volumes for IMRT is both an opportunity and a challenge for radiation oncologists who are specialized in the management of this malignancy. Similarly, recent developments in molecular biotechnology herald the prospect of better diagnosis and/or individualized treatment of the disease. Yet, the practicing physician cannot wait for these answers and must make crucial decisions on his/her patients' behalf today, based on the information available. Clearly, with all these opportunities and challenges, sound understanding of the updated current knowledge of nasopharyngeal cancer is essential.

Hence, we initiated this international collaborative effort to provide a comprehensive review of all key knowledge practicing physicians currently need to know about the management of nasopharyngeal cancer, arranged in four sections. The first part of the book (Chaps. 1–9) discusses the biologic concepts: epidemiology/etiology, pathogenesis, clinically pertinent molecular biology, clinical presentation, diagnosis, and staging. The second part (Chaps. 10–17) details the current concepts of definitive (often multidisciplinary) therapy for nondisseminated nasopharyngeal carcinoma. Critical analyses of the clinical trials that form the basis of currently available evidence-based medicine, current state-of-the art treatment strategies, and novel approaches that promise further improvements in outcome are explained in the chapters of this section. In the third section (Chaps. 18–21), management of more desperate situations, failure after initial treatment, and palliation of distant metastasis are discussed. Patients' long-term quality of life after treatment (Chap. 22), the fortunately rare occurrence of nasopharyngeal cancer in early life, and the staging of the disease (Chap. 24) are reviewed as well. We consider that such an arrangement not only provides appropriate coverage of the core of knowledge and discussions that are crucial to clinical management of nasopharyngeal carcinoma, but also facilitates a structural and systemic way of studying and understanding this knowledge.

We greatly appreciate the expertise and authoritative contributions of all of the included authors, each reflecting their dedication to improve the outcome of care of future patients. Consequently, we have intentionally allowed the authors to address some of the same key issues in different chapters to provide different perspectives of unresolved issues. In the end, the success of this publication must be measured primarily by how well we elicit ideas and provoke thoughts for future research in the clinical management of nasopharyngeal carcinoma.

Singapore
NY, USA
Hong Kong SAR, P.R. China

Jiade J. Lu
Jay S. Cooper
Anne W. M Lee

Contents

The Epidemiology of Nasopharyngeal Carcinoma

1

JUN MA and SUMEI CAO

CONTENTS

1.1 Introduction

Nasopharyngeal carcinoma (NPC) is a malignant tumor of nasopharyngeal epithelium. It is the main type in nasopharyngeal malignant tumors in both endemic areas and regions with low incidence. Epidemiological studies in NPC with the focus on etiology and biological behavior of the disease were strongly encouraged as a result of the International Union against Cancer (UICC) Symposium on Cancer of Nasopharynx held in Singapore in 1964 (MUIR et al. 1967), and investigations in the past four decades have produced many important findings in those aspects. NPC has unique epidemiological features, including obvious regional, racial, and familial aggregation. The aim of this chapter is to detail the incidence and distribution of NPC, as well as risk factors of the development of the disease.

1.2 Regional and Spatial Distribution

Nasopharyngeal cancer is a type of tumor with extremely unbalanced endemic distribution. It can be seen in many countries and areas of the five continents. However, the incidence of NPC is lower than $1/10^5$ in most areas. High-incidence areas are centralized in the southern part of China (including Hongkong). The highest incidence is found in Guangdong province, and the incidence in male can reach 20–50/100000. According to the data of International Agency for Research on Cancer (IARC), approximately 80,000 cases of NPC were newly diagnosed worldwide in 2002, and about 50,000 cases deceased, with Chinese accounting for 40%. Intermediate rates were seen in local inhabitants of

JUN MA, MD
SUMEI CAO, MD
Department of Radiation Oncology, Cancer Center of Sun Yat-sen University, 651 Dongfeng Road, East, Guangzhou, Guangdong 510060, P.R. China

Table 1.1. Incidence of nasopharyngeal carcinoma (NPC) in some cancer registries of five continents in 1998–2002 (N, 1/10[5])

Region and population	Age-standard-incidence rate	
	Male	Female
China		
China, Zhongshan	26.9	10.1
China, Guangzhou	22.2	9.8
China, Hong Kong	17.8	6.7
China, Shanghai	4.1	1.5
China, Nangang District, Harbin City	1.1	0.5
Southeast Asia		
Malaysia, Sarawak	15.0	6.5
Malaysia, Penang	9.3	3.3
Singapore	11.0	3.6
Singapore: Chinese	12.8	4.1
Singapore: Indian	1.8	0.1
Singapore: Malay	5.5	2.0
Philippines, Manila	5.8	2.4
Thailand, Chiang Mai	3.9	1.5
Thailand, Songkhla	2.7	0.9
Thailand, Lampang	2.5	1.5
USA		
USA, Hawaii: Chinese	9.9	1.1
USA, Hawaii: Filipino	3.3	1.3
USA, Hawaii: Hawaiian	2.0	0.2
USA, San Francisco: Chinese	8.1	4.0
USA, San Francisco: Filipino	3.1	1.0
USA, Los Angeles: Chinese	6.0	1.9
USA, Los Angeles: Filipino	3.8	0.8
Middle East/North Africa		
Algeria, Setif	5.4	1.7
Tunisia, Sousse	4.6	1.9
Uganda, Kyadondo	2.3	1.3
Kuwait: Kuwaitis	1.7	0.8
Europe		
Austria	0.4	0.2
Finland	0.3	0.1
Arctic		
Canada, Northwest Territories	4.3	1.3
USA, Alaska	1.5	0.9

Southeast Asia, Eskimos from the Arctic area, and inhabitants from North Africa and the Middle East (Table 1.1) (Parkin et al. 1992, 2002; Waterhouse et al. 1982; Muir et al. 1987).

There is prominent difference in the incidence of NPC between the Northern and Southern parts of China. High-incidence areas are centralized in five Southern provinces (Guangdong, Guangxi, Hunan, Fujian, Jiangxi). The incidence is highest in Guangdong province, so NPC is also called "Canton tumor." Within Guangdong province, the Pearl River delta and Xijiang River basin, especially Zhaoqing, Foshan, and Guangzhou, form a high-incidence core region.

1.3 Gender and Age Distribution

The incidence of NPC is higher in males than that in females, and the ratio is 2–3:1 (Parkin et al. 1992, 2002; Waterhouse et al. 1982; Muir et al. 1987). The predominance in male gender is observed in both endemic and low-incidence areas. However, the distribution of the age of patients diagnosed with NPC differs substantially in areas with various incidences. In low-incidence areas, the incidence of NPC is increased with age, while in the endemic areas, the incidence is increased obviously after 30-years, peaked at 40–59-years, and decreased thereafter (Zong et al. 1983). It has also been reported that in low- to medium-incidence area, the incidence of NPC has a relatively small peak among adolescents and young adults (Burt et al. 1992).

1.4 Racial Distribution

The incidence of NPC is highest in Xanthoderm, then in Melanoderm, and lowest in Caucasian. High-incidence areas are mostly habitations of Xanthoderm, such as Southern China, Hong Kong, and Southeast Asia. Eskimos in the Arctic area also belong to Xanthoderm.

In the same area, the incidence of NPC is different between different races. For example, the incidence is twofold higher in people speaking Cantonese than in people speaking other dialects, such as Hakka, Hokkien, and Chiu Chau (Li et al. 1985). Even after immigrating to other countries in Southeast Asia, the incidence in Cantonese speaking people is still twofolds higher than in other people from Southern China (Lee et al. 1988). In the United States, the incidence is highest in Chinese people living abroad, then in Filipinos, Japanese, black people, Spaniards, and lowest in white people (Burt et al. 1992).

Migrant epidemiological data showed that people from high-incidence areas of Southern China still kept high incidence even after they immigrate to America, Australia, Malaysia, or Japan (Parkin et al. 2002; Armstrong et al. 1979; Mccredie et al. 1999). Similarly, the incidence of NPC in immigrants and their offsprings from North Africa, where the incidence was relatively high, was still higher than local inhabitants after they immigrated to Israel, a low-incidence area (Parkin and Iscovich 1997). However, the incidence in second and third generation of immigrants was decreased to only half of that before immigration (Warnakulasuriya et al. 1999). On the contrary, the incidence of NPC in Caucasian who were born in China or Philippines is obviously increased, when compared with those born in North America, (Buell 1973) and the incidence in French who were born in North Africa was also obviously higher than that in inhabitants from Southern France (Jeannel et al. 1993).

The results of migrant epidemiology suggest that both genetic factors and environmental factors may play an important role in the pathogenesis of NPC. In addition, the distribution of pathological type is also different in different races. Ninety percent of the NPC in Southern China, Hong Kong, Taiwan, and Singapore are undifferentiated or differentiated nonkeratinizing Carcinoma (Zong et al. 1983). While in nonendemic areas, keratinizing squamous cell carcinoma is predominant, it is concluded that the etiological factors may be different in high- and low-incidence areas (Vaughan et al. 1996).

1.5 Familial Aggregation

NPC is a disease with obvious familial aggregation. There have been reports of high-incidence families in high-, medium-, and low-incidence areas. Furthermore, the ratio of cancer family history in high-incidence areas is higher than that in low-incidence areas. For example, the ratio of NPC family history reported in Hong Kong (Yu et al. 1986) and Guangzhou of China (Yu et al. 1990) is 7.2% and 5.9%, respectively. In Greenland, 27% of the patients with NPC have cancer family history, and most are NPC (Albeck et al. 1993). In the city of Shanghai in eastern China, a medium incidence area, the ratio of NPC family history is 1.85% (Yuan et al. 2000). In cancer family, most patients with NPC are first-degree relatives of the probands. The incidence in first-degree relatives of the patients with NPC is 4–10-folds of that in control population. The reason for familial aggregation of NPC may be similar hereditary susceptibility or living environment of the family members. Complex segregation analysis on NPC family in Southern China shows that NPC belongs to multigenic hereditary tumor (Jia et al. 2005).

1.6 Time Tendency

Recently published data demonstrated that the incidence of newly diagnosed NPC has been decreased in certain high-incidence areas. For example, the incidence and mortality of NPC has clearly decreased in Hong Kong from 1970s, in Taiwan from 1980s, and in Singapore from 1990s. The decreased incidence in Chinese people living in North America was also obvious. However, obvious ascending tendency has been observed in a few areas or populations such as Malay people living in Singapore (Wang et al. 2004). The incidence of NPC was stable or slightly increased in

Table 1.2. Comparison between the average annual age-standardized (world population) incidence rates of nasopharyngeal cancer (per 100,000 person-years) in Hong Kong and Sihui City, Guangdong, China

Period	Average annual incidence			
	Hong Kong Chinese		Sihui City of Guangdong, China	
	Male	Female	Male	Female
1973–1977	32.9	14.4		
1978–1982	30.0	12.9	28.1	12.3
1983–1987	28.5	11.2	28.7	14.8
1988–1992	24.3	9.5	28.7	13.4
1993–1997	21.5	8.3	28.0	11.8
1998–2002	17.8	6.7	30.9	13.0

endemic areas of Southern China including Guangdong and Guangxi provinces (JIA et al. 2006) (Table 1.2).

The change in epidemiologic tendency of NPC in these areas may be related with the change in exposure of corresponding population to risk factors. It is generally considered that changes in smoking, consumption of pickled food, and immigration may have great influences on the incidence in Hong Kong, Singapore, and Taiwan. Epidemiologic studies found that smoking was the main reason for keratinizing squamous cell carcinoma, while it had little relationship with nonkeratinizing squamous cell carcinoma. Further investigations found that the decrease of incidence in Hong Kong and North America was due to the decrease of keratinizing squamous cell carcinoma, while the incidence of nonkeratinizing squamous cell carcinoma kept stable (JIA et al. 2006; SUN et al. 2005; TSE et al. 2006). The decrease in smoking frequency in these areas may account for the decrease in incidence of NPC.

In the past 30 years, rapid economy development has been observed in high-incidence areas of NPC in Southern China, such as Guangdong and Guangxi. The eating and living habit has greatly changed. However, the stable incidence rate of NPC in these endemic areas indicate that the risk factors seem unchanged, as more than 90% of NPC cases belong to nonkeratinizing carcinoma.

1.7 Risk Factors

1.7.1 Epstein–Barr Virus

Antibodies to Epstein–Barr virus (EBV) were detected in the serum of patients with NPC by OLD et al. in 1966 (OLD et al. 1966). Subsequent studies showed that the level of anti-EBV antibodies was significantly increased in NPC from different races and areas, compared with the control. Viral DNA can be detected in the nucleus of epitheliums using in situ hybridization technique, while it was not obvious in infiltrating lymphocytes.

In prospective population studies, it was found that increased IgA antibody to Epstein–Barr (EB) viral capsid antigen (VCA) and neutral antibody to EBV DNAse were specific markers of NPC in high-incidence area, since they can effectively predict the development of NPC. For example, CHIEN et al. (2001) found that risk factor of people in Taiwan who were positive for both of the above. For example, in population studies, CHIEN et al. found that elevated IgA antibody against VCA and EBV DNAse are highly specific markers for NPC cases in Taiwan area, predicting a 32.8-fold (95% CI: 7.3-147.2) increase for those with both markers positive. Recently, JI et al. conformed that there was a window phase of about 3 years from seropositivity of EBV to the development of NPC (JI et al. 2007).

Although globally most people were infected by EBV, only a small portion of them developed NPC, which meant that the genesis of NPC was multifactorial. Currently, it was confirmed that many factors can result in the activation of EBV, such as environmental carcinogens and/or immune deficiency (FRIBORG et al. 2007; STOWE et al. 2001). It is still unclear about the mechanism for EBV entrance into epithelial tissue. The pathogenesis in NPC is detailed in Chap. 2.

1.7.2 Salty Fish and Pickled Food

One of the most potent and confirmed risk factors for NPC is salty fish consumption. Fish and other food that conserved in salt are heavily consumed in Southern China and areas with moderate risk factors for NPC such as Southeast Asia and North Africa. These foods contain a known carcinogen N-nitrosamine and its precursor. In different populations, the relative risk for developing NPC in people who eat salty fish on daily basis after adulthood was estimated to be 1.8–7.5, compared with those who did not or only eat a little salty fish (YU et al. 1989; LEE et al. 1994). In addition, the relative risk for developing NPC in people who eat salty fish on daily or weekly basis during weaning period or infancy was estimated to be 1.1–37.7, compared with those who never eat or only eat a little salty fish (YU 1991). On the contrary, eating more fresh fruits and vegetables can reduce the risk of NPC by 30%–50%, which may be due to the effect of antioxidant and antinitrosamine components in Vitamin C and E. However, evidences on the relationship of salty fish and pickled food with NPC from perspective studies are still lacking.

1.7.3 Smoking and Drinking

Results from a number of prospective epidemiological studies revealed that chronic smoking was a risk factor for NPC. In addition, the development of NPC depended on the severity of smoking measured by pack-year. In general, risk of NPC in smokers was 2–6-fold of that in nonsmokers (Friborg et al. 2007; Hsu et al. 2009). The risk of NPC potentially induced by cigarette smoking was lower than the risk for lung cancer or squamous cell carcinoma of the larynx. However, smoking was the main risk factor for squamous cell carcinoma NPC, while its association with undifferentiated or nonkeratinizing NPC has not been demonstrated (Vaughan et al. 1996). This finding indicated that the decrease in morbidity of NPC in North America and Hongkong might result from reduced smoking frequency. Smoking-induced NPC was less significant than lung cancer or laryngeal cancer, which may be due to the lower sensitivity of nasopharyngeal epitheliums to carcinogens in tobaccos than epitheliums in other regions, or the lower content of tobaccos in pharynx nasalis than the respiratory tract.

Most studies performed in China and the United States showed that alcohol drinking was unrelated to the development of NPC. Results from a perspective study performed in Singapore also confirmed this viewpoint (Friborg et al. 2007). However, the results were not completely consistent, since positive results were found at least in two case control studies (Vaughan et al. 1996; Nam et al. 1992). The inconsistency may be caused by experimental design, susceptibility of different people, and other confounding factors.

1.7.4 Effect of Hereditary Susceptibility

The epidemic features of NPC suggested that genetic factors contribute a lot to the genesis and development of NPC. Many investigations have focused on the possible pathogenic effect of human leucocyte antigen (HLA), which is involved in the presentation of foreign antigens, including viral polypeptide, so as to facilitate their directive lysis by immune system. Since EBV can be found in almost all patients with the disease, the risk factor for NPC may be increased in individuals who inherited HLA allele with weaker presenting ability of EBV antigen. On the contrary, the risk factor for NPC was relatively low in individuals who inherited HLA allele with effective presenting ability of EBV antigen (Hildesheim et al. 2002). It was reported currently that HLA-A2-Bw46 and B17 can increase the risk factor for NPC by 2–3-fold. HLA-A11, B13, and A2 can reduce the risk factor for NPC by 1/3–1/2.

Epidemiologic studies also determined the correlation between polymorphism of some genes with the risk of NPC, including homozygous variant derived from cytochrome P4502E1 (CYP2E1), null allele of glutathion S-transferase M1 (GSTM1), (Kongruttanachok et al. 2001; Hildesheim et al. 1995; Nazar-Stewart et al. 1999) T cell receptor polymorphism (TCR), poly immunoglobulin receptor (PIGR), candidate tumor suppressing gene GX6, DNA repair gene hOGG1, and XRCC1. The relative risk was estimated to be 2.0–5.0. CYP2E1 and GSTM1 are involved in the metabolism of nitrosamine and cigarette smoke, respectively. Their etiological effects may be different because of the difference in environment; in other words, they may have different biological interaction with environmental factors, such as salty fish and smoking.

Studies on chromosomal abnormality, heterozygote deficiency, and gene expression, as well as main NPC susceptible sites on No.4 chromosome found by whole genome scanning in familial study performed in Southern China also provided potential opportunities to determine NPC susceptible genes (Feng et al. 2002).

1.7.5 Traditional Chinese Medicine

In certain epidemiological studies performed in Southeast Asia and Southern China, use of traditional Chinese medicine has been associated with an increase in NPC by 2–4-fold (Zheng et al. 1994; Hildesheim et al. 1992). Certain plants and medicinal materials in Chinese traditional medicine can induce the activation of latent EBV. Such features can be attributed to tetradecanoylphorbol acetate (TPA)-like substances in plants and earth. TPA-like substances, in combination with N-butyrate, a product of anoxybiontic bacteria found in pharynx nasalis, can induce the synthesis of EBV antigen in mice, increase EBV-mediated B cell transformation, and promote the genesis of NPC (Tang et al. 1988).

1.7.6 Professional Exposure

Formaldehyde is a well-known carcinogen that can induce carcinoma of nasal cavity in rodents. Meta analysis on more than 30 epidemiological studies showed that exposure to formaldehyde was significantly associated with the genesis of NPC, and a dose-response relationship was demonstrated (Partanen 1993). In 1995, formaldehyde was suggested to be an etiological factor for NPC by IARC.

Middle-sized (5–10 μm) dust particles are easily absorbed to pharynx nasalis. Several epidemiological studies have found that the risk factor for NPC was increased in people exposed in wood dust, and it was dependent on exposure time and dose (Luce et al. 2002). In addition, the risk factor for NPC was reported to be increased in people exposed to extreme temperature and work environment with combustibles. However, the exposure ratio for these professional exposures was relatively low in most endemic areas, so it cannot be confirmed whether these factors are independently important in the high incidence in these areas.

1.7.7 Chronic Upper Respiratory Disease

Most epidemiological studies showed that the risk for NPC was increased by about twofold in people with chronic ear, nose, throat, and upper respiratory disease (Zheng et al. 1994). It may be due to the conversion of nitrate to nitrite by bacteria present in these regions, since nitrite is the component of carcinogen *N*-nitroso.

1.7.8 Trace Element

Nickel is one of the carcinogens to human. Surveys performed in high-incidence areas found that the content of nickel in rice, drinking water, and hair of local inhabitants was significantly higher than that in low-incidence areas. In high-incidence areas, nickel content in NPC patients was also higher than in healthy population. Epidemiological surveys also found that trace elements zinc and cadmium were positively related with the genesis of NPC, while magnesium, calcium, and strontium were negatively related (Bolviken et al. 1997).

1.8 Summary

NPC is a disease with unique epidemiological features. The distribution of the disease demonstrates a clear regional, racial, and gender prevalence. The incidence of the disease is relatively high among local inhabitants of Southern China, Southeast Asia, Eskimos from the Arctic area, and inhabitants from North Africa and the Middle East, with the highest incidence found in Guangdong province of China, and the incidence in male reaching 20–50/10^5. NPC is associated with a number of risk factors. It appears that individuals with hereditary susceptibility were infected by EBV in the early period of life, then EBV was activated under the synthetic action of multiple environmental factors, and eventually NPC was developed. In addition to EBV, other environmental factors such as trace elements and dietary habits may be associated with the initiation and development of the disease. However, changes in lifestyle in the past several decades in Southern China had little association with the etiology of NPC. Further epidemiological investigations will be needed to detect the changes in the trend of NPC and the underlying risk factors, so that prevention and/or early detection of the disease can be realized.

References

Albeck H, et al (1993) Familial clusters of nasopharyngeal carcinoma and salivary gland carcinomas in Greenland natives. Cancer 72(1):196–200

Armstrong RW, et al (1979) Incidence of nasopharyngeal carcinoma in Malaysia, 1968–1977. Br J Cancer 40(4):557–567

Bolviken B, Flaten TP, Zheng C (1997) Relations between nasopharyngeal carcinoma and magnesium and other alkaline earth elements in soils in China. Med Hypotheses 48(1):21–25

Buell P (1973) Race and place in the etiology of nasopharyngeal cancer: a study based on California death certificates. Int J Cancer 11(2):268–272

Burt RD, Vaughan TL, McKnight B (1992) Descriptive epidemiology and survival analysis of nasopharyngeal carcinoma in the United States. Int J Cancer 52(4):549–556

Chien YC, et al (2001) Serologic markers of Epstein-Barr virus infection and nasopharyngeal carcinoma in Taiwanese men. N Engl J Med 345(26):1877–1882

Feng BJ, et al (2002) Genome-wide scan for familial nasopharyngeal carcinoma reveals evidence of linkage to chromosome 4. Nat Genet 31(4):395–399

Friborg JT, et al (2007) A prospective study of tobacco and alcohol use as risk factors for pharyngeal carcinomas in Singapore Chinese. Cancer 109(6):1183–1191

Hildesheim A, et al (1992) Herbal medicine use, Epstein-Barr virus, and risk of nasopharyngeal carcinoma. Cancer Res 52(11):3048–3051

Hildesheim A, et al (1995) Cytochrome P4502E1 genetic polymorphisms and risk of nasopharyngeal carcinoma: results

from a case-control study conducted in Taiwan. Cancer Epidemiol Biomarkers Prev 4(6):607–610
Hildesheim A, et al (2002) Association of HLA class I and II alleles and extended haplotypes with nasopharyngeal carcinoma in Taiwan. J Natl Cancer Inst 94(23):1780–1789
Hsu WL, et al (2009) Independent effect of EBV and cigarette smoking on nasopharyngeal carcinoma: a 20-year follow-up study on 9,622 males without family history in Taiwan. Cancer Epidemiol Biomarkers Prev 18(4):1218–1226
Jeannel D, et al (1993) Increased risk of nasopharyngeal carcinoma among males of French origin born in Maghreb (north Africa). Int J Cancer 54(4):536–539
Jia WH, et al (2005) Complex segregation analysis of nasopharyngeal carcinoma in Guangdong, China: evidence for a multifactorial mode of inheritance (complex segregation analysis of NPC in China). Eur J Hum Genet 13(2):248–252
Jia WH, et al (2006) Trends in incidence and mortality of nasopharyngeal carcinoma over a 20–25 year period (1978/1983–2002) in Sihui and Cangwu counties in southern China. BMC Cancer 6:178
Ji MF, et al (2007) Sustained elevation of Epstein-Barr virus antibody levels preceding clinical onset of nasopharyngeal carcinoma. Br J Cancer 96(4):623–630
Kongruttanachok N, et al (2001) Cytochrome P450 2E1 polymorphism and nasopharyngeal carcinoma development in Thailand: a correlative study. BMC Cancer 1:4
Lee HP, et al (1988) Recent trends in cancer incidence among Singapore Chinese. Int J Cancer 42(2):159–166
Lee HP, et al (1994) Preserved foods and nasopharyngeal carcinoma: a case-control study among Singapore Chinese. Int J Cancer 59(5):585–590
Li CC, Yu MC, Henderson BE (1985) Some epidemiologic observations of nasopharyngeal carcinoma in Guangdong, People's Republic of China. Natl Cancer Inst Monogr 69:49–52
Luce D, et al (2002) Sinonasal cancer and occupational exposures: a pooled analysis of 12 case-control studies. Cancer Causes Control 13(2):147–157
McCredie M, Williams S, Coates M (1999) Cancer mortality in East and Southeast Asian migrants to New South Wales, Australia, 1975–1995. Br J Cancer 79(7–8):1277–1282
Muir C, Waterhouse J, Mack T, et al (eds) (1987) Cancer incidence in five continents, vol. V. IARC scientific publications, Lyon, IARC
Muir CS, Shanmugaratnam K (eds) (1967) Cancer of the nasopharynx. UICC Monograph Series, No.1. Munksgaard, Copenhagen
Nam JM, McLaughlin JK, Blot WJ (1992) Cigarette smoking, alcohol, and nasopharyngeal carcinoma: a case-control study among U.S. whites. J Natl Cancer Inst 84(8):619–622
Nazar-Stewart V, et al (1999) Glutathione S-transferase M1 and susceptibility to nasopharyngeal carcinoma. Cancer Epidemiol Biomarkers Prev 8(6):547–551
Old LJ, et al (1966) Precipitating antibody in human serum to an antigen present in cultured Burkitt's lymphoma cells. Proc Natl Acad Sci U S A 56(6):1699–1704
Parkin DM, Muir CS, Whelan SL, et al (eds) (1992) Cancer incidence in five continents Vol VI. IARC Scientific Publication, Lyon, IARC
Parkin DM, Whelan SL, et al (eds) (2002) Cancer incidence in five continents, vol. VIII. IARC scientific publications, Lyon, IARC
Parkin DM, Iscovich J (1997) Risk of cancer in migrants and their descendants in Israel: II. Carcinomas and germ-cell tumours. Int J Cancer 70(6):654–660
Partanen T (1993) Formaldehyde exposure and respiratory cancer-a meta-analysis of the epidemiologic evidence. Scand J Work Environ Health 19(1):8–15
Stowe RP, Pierson DL, Barrett AD (2001) Elevated stress hormone levels relate to Epstein-Barr virus reactivation in astronauts. Psychosom Med 63(6):891–895
Sun LM, et al (2005) Trends in the incidence rates of nasopharyngeal carcinoma among Chinese Americans living in Los Angeles County and the San Francisco metropolitan area, 1992–2002. Am J Epidemiol 162(12):1174–1178
Tang WP, et al (1988) Wikstroemia indica promotes development of nasopharyngeal carcinoma in rats initiated by dinitrosopiperazine. J Cancer Res Clin Oncol 114(4): 429–431
Tse LA, et al (2006) Incidence rate trends of histological subtypes of nasopharyngeal carcinoma in Hong Kong. Br J Cancer 95(9):1269–1273
Vaughan TL, et al (1996) Nasopharyngeal cancer in a low-risk population: defining risk factors by histological type. Cancer Epidemiol Biomarkers Prev 5(8):587–593
Wang H, Seow A, Lee HP (2004) Trends in cancer incidence among Singapore Malays: a low-risk population. Ann Acad Med Singapore 33(1):57–62
Warnakulasuriya KA, et al (1999) Cancer of mouth, pharynx and nasopharynx in Asian and Chinese immigrants resident in Thames regions. Oral Oncol 35(5):471–475
Waterhouse J, Muir C, Mack T, et al (eds) (1982) Cancer incidence in five continents, vol. IV. IARC scientific publications, Lyon
Yuan JM, et al (2000) Non-dietary risk factors for nasopharyngeal carcinoma in Shanghai, China. Int J Cancer 85(3): 364–369
Yu MC (1991) Nasopharyngeal carcinoma: epidemiology and dietary factors. IARC Sci Publ (105):39–47
Yu MC, et al (1986) Cantonese-style salted fish as a cause of nasopharyngeal carcinoma: report of a case-control study in Hong Kong. Cancer Res 46(2):956–961
Yu MC, et al (1990) Occupational and other non-dietary risk factors for nasopharyngeal carcinoma in Guangzhou, China. Int J Cancer 45(6):1033–1039
Yu MC, Huang TB, Henderson BE (1989) Diet and nasopharyngeal carcinoma: a case-control study in Guangzhou, China. Int J Cancer 43(6):1077–1082
Zheng YM, et al (1994) Environmental and dietary risk factors for nasopharyngeal carcinoma: a case-control study in Zangwu County, Guangxi, China. Br J Cancer 69(3): 508–514
Zong YS, et al (1983) Histopathologic types and incidence of malignant nasopharyngeal tumors in Zhongshan County. Chin Med J 96(7):511–516

Pathogenesis and Etiology of Nasopharyngeal Carcinoma

2

Mu-Sheng Zeng and Yi-Xin Zeng

CONTENTS

Mu-Sheng Zeng, PhD, MD
State Key Laboratory of Oncology in Southern China, Cancer Center of Sun Yat-sen University, 651 Dongfeng Road East, Guagnzhou 510060, P.R. China
Yi-Xin Zeng, MD
Cancer Center of Sun Yat-sen University, 651 East Dongfeng Road, Yuexiu District Guangzhou, Guangdong 510060, P.R. China

2.1 Introduction

Nasopharyngeal carcinoma (NPC) is a squamous cell carcinoma (SCC) that usually develops around the ostium of the Eustachian tube in the lateral wall of the nasopharynx (Sham et al. 1990). This disease was initially reported in 1901 and characterized clinically in 1922 (Wei et al. 2005). NPC is a disease with a remarkable geographic and racial distribution worldwide. This is a rare human malignancy with an incidence below 1/100,000 populations per year in Caucasians from North America and other Western countries. In contrast, the highest incidence is noted in the Southern Chinese population of Guangdong, Inuits of Alaska, and native Greenlanders (Chou et al. 2008; Parkin et al. 1992); particularly, among the Cantonese who inhabit the central region of Guangdong Province in Southern China, the incidence is 15–25 cases per 100,000. NPC is also called the "Canton tumor" in Guangdong Province (Hepeng 2008; Yu et al. 2002). Southern Chinese migrants, irrespective of their country of migration, also exhibit high rates of NPC (Yu et al. 2002), but the rate of NPC among ethnic Chinese born in North America is considerably lower than those born in China (Buell 1974). An intermediate incidence has been reported in Alaskan Eskimos and in the Mediterranean basin (North Africa, Southern Italy, Greece, and Turkey), ranging from 15 to 20 cases per 100,000 persons (Chan et al. 2002). Independence of race–ethnicity, the rates of NPC in men are two to three folds higher than those in women for most populations (Yu et al. 2002). Overall, NPC can occur in all age groups, but has a bimodal age distribution. The incidence peaks at 50–60 years of age, and a small peak is observed during late childhood (Jeyakumar et al. 2006).

The distinct difference in the incidence among geographic and population area implies that both environmental factors and genetic susceptibility play roles in the development of NPC (Lo et al. 2004). The early age incidence peak noted among Southern Chinese may suggest that exposure to the putative carcinogens occur very early in life (Yu et al. 2002). Epidemiological studies have linked childhood intake of locally consumed preserved foods to NPC development in all four groups of populations exhibiting increased risk of NPC – Chinese, natives of Southeast Asia, natives of Arctic region, and Arabs of North Africa (Yu et al. 2002). Moreover, environmental factors may also accelerate to the development of NPC. For example, exposure to smoke or chemical pollutants, including trace elements (e.g., nickle), have been reported to be associated with the development of NPC (Wu et al. 1986; Yu et al. 1981). Therefore, the development and progression of NPC disease is multifactorial with geographic areas, genetics, diet, and environmental exposure.

2.2 Histological Subtypes of NPC

The World Health Organization (WHO) classifies NPC into three histopathological types based on the degree of differentiation. Type 1, SCC, is seen in 5%–10% of cases of NPC and is characterized by well-differentiated cells that produce keratin and demonstrated the presence of intracellular bridges when observed under the electron microscope. Type 2, nonkeratinizing squamous carcinoma, varies in cell differentiation (from mature to anaplastic cells) but does not produce keratin. Type 3 or undifferentiated NPC constitutes the bulk of the tumors seen in patients with NPC, is also nonkeratinizing, but is less differentiated, with highly variable cell types (clear cell, spindle cell, anaplastic) (Shanmugaratnam 1978).

Types 2 and 3 NPC are Epstein–Barr virus (EBV) associated and have better prognoses than type 1; EBV infection is generally absent in type 1, especially in nonendemic areas (Marks et al. 1998). However, more recent data suggest that almost all NPC tumors in the endemic areas, regardless of histologic subtype, have comorbid EBV infections, which is a strong evidence for EBV as the etiology of NPC (Vasef et al. 1997). Undifferentiated NPC or type 3 was frequently characterized as lymphoepithelioma owing to the heavy infiltration of the primary tumor with lymphocytes. In endemic areas such as Southern China, WHO Type 3 accounts for more than 97%, while keratinizing SCC is more common in the Western countries (up to 75%) (Marks et al. 1998). There is no uniform morphological characteristic of NPC-affected tissues; thus, diagnosis of undifferentiated NPC is usually based on the location of the tumor in the nasopharynx and the presence of EBV transcripts in the tumor cells (Gullo et al. 2008). Clonal EBV genome is present in the early preinvasive dysplastic lesion or carcinoma in situ, illuminating that the development of malignant invasive tumor drop behind the infection of EBV (Pathmanathan et al. 1995). This close association with EBV is what makes NPC unique from other head and neck cancers.

2.3 Etiologies and Pathogenesis

In endemic regions, NPC presents as a complex disease caused by an interaction of the oncogenic gammaherpesvirus EBV chronic infection, environmental, and genetic factors, in a multistep carcinogenic process. The highest incidence of NPC in Southern Chinese strongly indicates that both genetic susceptibility and environmental factors contribute to the tumorigenesis of NPC in its development and progression. In addition, a small population of cells sharing properties of normal stem cells (NSC) within tumor has been suggested to be involved in the etiology of NPC. This chapter will focus mainly on three major etiological factors including genetic, environmental, and viral factors.

2.3.1 Genetic Factors

While nasopharyngeal carcinoma is a rare malignancy in most parts of the world, it is one of the most common cancers in Southeast Asia including areas such as Southern China, Hong Kong, Singapore, Malaysia, and Taiwan. The reported incidence in these countries ranges from 10 to 53 cases per 100,000 persons. The incidence is also high among Eskimos in Alaska and Greenland and in Tunisians, ranging from 15 to 20 cases per 100,000 persons (Chan et al. 2002). Familial clustering of NPC has been widely observed in both the Chinese population (Jia et al. 2004; Zeng et al. 2002), and non-Chinese patient cohort (Levine et al. 1992). The familial risk of NPC is among the highest of any malignancy (Suarez et al. 2006). The described relative risk of NPC in first-degree relatives is about 8.0 (Friborg et al. 2005). The high risk of NPC to Cantonese population and the people with familial NPC history suggest that genetically determined susceptibility may play an important role in the etiology of NPC.

An important characteristic of familial cancers is the early age onset of NPC (Zeng et al. 2002). Several linkage analyses studies suggested the association of susceptibility human leukocyte antigen (HLA) haplotypes with NPC development. Most studies conducted among the Chinese population demonstrated an increased risk of NPC for individuals with HLA-A2. A recent study detected a consistent association between NPC and the prevalent Chinese HLA-A2 subtype (HLA-A*0207), but not the prevalent Caucasian subtype (HLA-A*0201) (Hildesheim et al. 2002). The HLA types of AW19, BW46, and B17 have also been reported to be associated with an increased risk, whereas HLA-A11 is associated with a decreased risk (Liebowitz 1994). Significant complex multiple chromosome aberrations are often demonstrated in NPC, as well as in other solid tumors. The finding of translocation, amplification, and deletion of 3p, 5p, and 3q indicates that a minimal region of breakpoints is possible for contributing to NPC (Shih-Hsin Wu 2006; Tjia et al. 2005). Breakpoints have been frequently observed in 1p11–31, 3p12–21, 3q25, 5q31, 11q13, 12q13, and Xq25 (Lo et al. 1997). Inactivation of tumor suppressor genes on 3p, 9p, 11q, 13q, 14q, and 16q and alteration of oncogenes on chromosomes 8 and 12 are important in the development of NPC (Hui et al. 1999; Lo et al. 2000). A recent study provides evidence for the linkage of NPC to chromosome 3p and a fine map of NPC susceptibility locus to a 13.6cM region on 3p21.31–21.2 (Xiong et al. 2004). These results are in agreement with several previous studies that suggest that the deletion of chromosomes 3p is a common genetic event in NPC (Deng et al. 1998; Lo et al. 2000). Many tumor suppressor candidate genes such as *CACNA2D2*, *DLC1*, *FUS1*, *H37*, *HYAL1*, *RASSF1A*, *SEMA3B*, and *SEMA3F* and tumor susceptibility genes such as *hMLH1* have been isolated from the region (Xiong et al. 2004). These studies indicate that genes in the 3p21 may play a critical role in tumorigenesis of familial NPC.

Some studies suggested that genetic polymorphisms in genes that metabolize carcinogens are associated with NPC susceptibility. Cytochrome P450 2E1 (CYP2E1) is one of the cytochrome P450s and is responsible for the metabolic activation of nitrosamines and the related carcinogens. Case-control studies have shown a strong association of the variant form of CYP2E1 (c2 allele) with increased risk of this disease in Chinese populations (Hildesheim et al. 1997; Hildesheim et al. 1995). Other nitrosamine metabolizing genes, such as Cytochrome *P450 2A6* (*CYP2A6*), have also been suggested to play a role in NPC susceptibility (Tiwawech et al. 2006). Phase II detoxification enzyme, glutathione *S*-transferase M1 (GSTM1), was found to be a synergistic risk factor for NPC (Friborg et al. 2007; Nazar-Stewart et al. 1999). The association of other DNA repair genes with NPC susceptibility has also been implied. While a reduced risk for NPC was observed with polymorphism of the *XRCC1* gene (Arg280His), polymorphism of the *hOGG1* gene (Ser326Cys) was shown to be associated with an increased risk for NPC in the Taiwan population (Cho et al. 2003).

2.3.2 Environmental Factors

A large number of case-control studies conducted in diverse populations (Cantonese, other Southern Chinese, Northern Chinese, and Thais) residing in different parts of Asia and North America have confirmed that Cantonese-style salted fish and other preserved foods containing large amounts of nitrosodimethyamine (NDMA), *N*-nitrospyrrolidene (NPYR), and *N*-nitrospiperidine (NPIP) may be carcinogenic factors for NPC (Armstrong et al. 1998; Ning et al. 1990; Sriamporn et al. 1992; Yu et al. 1988; Yuan et al. 2000). Earlier age at exposure in salted fish has been shown to a high risk of NPC in Southern Chinese (Yu et al. 2002). In animal studies, nasal and nasopharyngeal tumors could be induced in rats by feeding them Chinese salted fish (Ning et al. 1990; Yu et al. 1988). Moreover, cigarette smoking and occupational exposure to formaldehyde and wood dust are recognized risk factors as well (Yu et al. 2002). Several studies conducted in high- and low-risk populations during the past decade have obviously implicated the nasopharynx as a tobacco-susceptible cancer site (Yu et al. 2002). Ever smokers exhibit a roughly 30%–100% excess risk relative to life-long nonsmokers (Yuan et al. 2000). Formaldehyde is a recognized nasal cavity carcinogen in rodents. Smoke particles from incomplete combustion of coal, wood, and other materials are also of the size and weight to be deposited mostly in the nasopharynx (Armstrong et al. 2000). The use of certain Chinese medicinal herbs has been suggested to increase the risk for NPC by reactivating EBV infection in the host (Zeng et al. 1994).

2.3.3 Epstein–Barr Virus

It was in 1966 when Old et al. first discovered the relationship between EBV and NPC, using in situ hybridization and the anticomplement immunofluorescent (ACIF) assay (Old et al. 1966). Subsequent studies by others demonstrated the expression of EBV latent genes – Epstein-Barr virus nuclear antigen (EBNA), latent membrane protein-1 (LMP-1), LMP-2, and EBV-encoded small RNAs (EBER) – in NPC cells (Baumforth et al. 1999) confirming the infection of tumor cells by EBV. Intriguingly, expression of EBV early antigen (EA) is positively correlated with the consumption of salted and preserved food, suggesting that development of EBV-positive NPC could be related to dietary habits (Shao et al. 1988), and provides another link to the epidemiological studies with NPC. Approximately 90% of the adult population undifferentiated nasopharyngeal carcinomas (UNPC) all over the world are EBV-positive by serology. In most NPC patients, higher EBV antibody titers, especially of IgA EBV-associated cancer, are observed. So, measuring patients' EBV-specific IgA antibodies is a useful method in screening for early detection of NPC (Cohen 2000). EBV infection is an early, possibly initiating event in the development of nasopharyngeal carcinoma (Pathmanathan et al. 1995). A current hypothesis proposes that EBV plays a critical role in transforming nasopharyngeal epithelial cells into invasive cancer (Lo et al. 2004). Wu et al. (2003) found that EBV-positive tumors grew faster than EBV-negative tumors, and also had clonal EBV terminal repeat sequences. Preinvasive lesions of the nasopharynx are infected with EBV. Since EBV infection indeed precedes clonal expansion of malignant cells (Raab-Traub et al. 1986), EBV is thought to contribute, at least in part, to the overall pathogenesis of NPC. Many studies have demonstrated that UNPC are invariably EBV-positive, regardless of geographical origin (Niedobitek et al. 1991; Weiss et al. 1989).

2.3.3.1 EBV Structure

In 1964, EBV was identified in tumor tissue from a patient who had African Burkitt lymphoma, a fatal malignancy of the B lymphocyte (Epstein et al. 1964). EBV is a γ-herpes virus (Wan et al. 2004) present in over 90% of adults worldwide. It is a member of the *Lymphocryptovirus* genus – viruses that are closely related members of herpesvirus family. The EBV genome is large exceeding 172 kb pairs of linear double-stranded DNA, as in other herpesviruses, the molecule is divided into unique, internal repeat, and terminal repeat domains. EBV was the first herpesvirus to have its genome completely cloned and sequenced (Baer et al. 1984). During growth transformation, the virus does not replicate and produce progeny virions, but rather is replicated by the host DNA polymerase as an extra chromosomal episome (Raab-Traub 2002).

2.3.3.2 EBV Infection in NPC

EBV was the first human virus identified to be associated with human cancers, including lymphomas as well as epithelial tumors (Epstein et al. 1966). The association between EBV infection and NPC is well documented and particularly close with EBV genome present in virtually all NPC cells. Primary EBV infection normally occurs in early childhood, is usually asymptomatic, and results in life-long virus persistence, but when exposure is delayed until adolescence, infection mononucleosis often ensues provoking an infection during early adulthood. EBV has a strong tropism for human lymphocytes and for the epithelium of the upper respiratory tract, where it can remain latent (Borza et al. 2002). This virus has been associated with different neoplastic diseases, like polyclonal B lymphoproliferation in immunosuppressed patients, Burkitt lymphoma, or Hodgkin's disease (Niedobitek et al. 1994). However, the tumor showing the strongest worldwide association with EBV is nasopharyngeal carcinoma (Liebowitz 1994; Pathmanathan et al. 1995). Elevated titers of IgA antibody to EBV viral capsid antigen (VCA) are usually found in patients with NPC. The rise in IgA titers to these antigens can be noticed before the development of UNPC and correlates with tumor burden, remission, and recurrence (Mazeron 1996; Zheng et al. 1994). Therefore, this method of measuring patients' EBV-specific IgA antibodies is useful in screening for early detection of NPC (Cohen 2000).

In almost all cases of EBV infection, the oropharynx is the primary site of infection, as well as the site of viral replication. EBV infects primary resting B lymphocytes to establish a latent infection and yield proliferating, growth-transformed B cells in vitro. In vitro studies demonstrate that EBV infects and potentially activates B cells by binding to the type 2 complement receptor (CR2, or CD21), the putative EBV receptor (Baumforth et al. 1999). Hence, EBV appears to home to the oropharynx, and more specifically, the B cells within the oropharynx. The strain B95-8 can be found in EBV-positive cell lines such as Raji, Namalwa, and CA 46 (Chang et al. 1990). These cell lines are all of B-lymphocyte lineage. This strain has been used as a benchmark to check for EBV positively in NPC.

In vitro, EBV infects resting human B lymphocytes and transforms them into lymphoblastoid cell lines (LCLs), a process that is termed growth transformation and a hallmark of this virus (Altmann et al. 2005). *vBcl-2* genes are essential for the initial evasion of apoptosis in cells in vivo in which the virus establishes a latent infection or causes cellular transformation or both (Altmann et al. 2005). In vivo and in vitro EBV's latent state is characterized by the absence of virus synthesis and maintenance of the viral genome as plasmids in the infected cell. EBV genome delivery to the nucleus as a key rate-limiting step in B-cell transformation, and highlights the remarkable efficiency with which a single virus genome, having reached the nucleus, then drives the transformation program (Shannon-Lowe et al. 2005). NK cell activation by DCs can limit primary EBV infection in tonsils until adaptive immunity establishes immune control of this persistent and oncogenic human pathogen (Strowig et al. 2008).

Four different models have been proposed to explain the transition of EBV from the latent reservoir of infection in blood-borne B lymphocytes to sites of productive replication in oral epithelium. Model 1 proposes that B lymphocytes carrying latent EBV infection migrate from the blood to the epithelium, where the EBV reactivates and infects adjacent epithelial cells (Imai et al. 1998); Model 2 proposes that EBV virions produced by B lymphocytes in the oral submucosa bind submucosal EBV-specific dimeric immunoglobulin A (IgA) and enter basal oral epithelial cells by endocytosis via the polymeric Ig receptor (Sixbey et al. 1992); Model 3 proposes that EBV virions produced by B lymphocytes in oral lymphoid tissues gain access to and infect middle- and upper-layer oral epithelial cells as a result of microscopic traumatic epithelial injury (Niedobitek 2000); Model 4 proposes that blood-borne pre-LC are latently infected with EBV and that oral epithelium cells are likely to be LC harbor EBV infection that can reactivate into productive EBV replication (Walling et al. 2007). However, the process of EBV entry into keratinocytes and NPC cells is more complex, as both keratinocytes and NPC cells express only low levels of CR2 receptor (Billaud et al. 1989). In addition, the relevance of serological tests for EBV infection in predicting the occurrence of NPC is presently still unclear.

2.3.3.3
EBV Subtype in NPC

EBV ubiquitously infects more than 95% of adult population worldwide, but NPC is an endemic disease. One possibility is that there are malignancy-associated EBV subtypes, which are prevalent in NPC endemic area. The first full-length sequence analysis of an NPC-derived EBV strain from a patient with NPC in Guangdong, China, has been analyzed. This EBV strain was termed GD1 (Guangdong strain 1). Compared with prototypical strain B95.8, there are many sequence variations in GD1 when compared with 43 deletion sites, 44 insertion sites, and 1,413 point mutations. The selected GD1 mutations detected with high frequency in Cantonese NPC patients suggest that GD1 is highly representative of the EBV strains isolated from NPC patients in Guangdong, China, an area with the highest incidence of NPC in the world (Zeng et al. 2005).

EBV can be classified as type 1 (A) and type 2 (B) based on sequence divergence in EBNA2, 3A, 3B, and 3C genes (Adldinger et al. 1985; Sample et al. 1990). Type 1 EBV contains an extra *Bam*HI site in the *Bam*HI F region ("f" variant) and loss of a *Bam*HI site at the *Bam*HI W//I boundary ("c" variant) (Bouzid et al. 1998; Lo et al. 2007; Lung et al. 1991). Type 1 EBV is more prevalent in most Southern Chinese patients with NPC or other head and neck tumor patients, while Type 2 EBV or the coexistence of type 1 and 2 EBV are seen only occasionally (Abdel-Hamid et al. 1992; Chen et al. 1992; Choi et al. 1993; Sung et al. 1998; Zimber et al. 1986). But an early report stated that type 2 virus occurs mainly in Africa, and that type 1 is distributed widely in the world (Young et al. 1987). It was found that "f" variant might have an association with the development and/or maintenance of NPC among Southern Chinese (Lung et al. 1991). More evidence showed that these types were just related with EBV geographical distribution (Sandvej et al. 1997). An *Xho*I restriction site loss and a 30 bp deletion within the *LMP1* gene define an EBV strain that is associated with increased tumorigenicity or with disease among particular geographical populations (Li et al. 1996; Sandvej et al. 1997; Trivedi et al. 1994). However, these notions have recently been challenged by the fact that virus with a deleted version of LMP1 is present in the general population in endemic regions, which can also be found in nonendemic areas within Asia (Itakura et al. 1996) and in Western countries (Sandvej et al. 1997). Moreover, it has been shown that the *LMP1* gene from nonendemic Russian NPC harbors a nondeleted version of *LMP1*, whereas the gene with a deletion can be found in healthy subjects from the same area (Hahn et al. 2001). According to *LMP1* C-terminal variants, Edwards et al. (1999) have defined EBV into at least seven substrains: Ch1, Ch2, Med, Ch3, Alaskan, NC, and B95.8. They found among Asian isolates, the Ch1 and B95.8 strains were in normal specimens and the Ch1 and Ch2 strains in NPC. They also found Ch1 strain prevalent in the NPC patients from areas of endemicity and nonendemicity (Edwards et al. 1999). It was also proved the Cantonese population is susceptible to the predominant Ch1 strain in the nasopharyngeal carcinoma endemic region of China, but its relationship with the host remains to be characterized further (Li et al. unpublished data). EBNA-1 can also be classified into five subtypes: P-ala, P-thr, V-val, V-leu, and V-pro based on the polymorphism of amino acids at position 487 (Bhatia et al. 1996; Gutierrez et al. 1997; Snudden et al. 1995), which has been associated with geographical location or disease status (Imai et al. 1998; Zhang et al. 2004). *LMP1* is an EBV oncogene expressed frequently in EBV-associated malignancies (Eliopoulos et al. 1997; Kilger et al. 1998; Wang et al. 1985). A new typing standard based on 155849nt in RPMS1 of EBV may represent a specific EBV subtype (A type) in the NPC endemic region, and could serve as a valuable indicator for a high risk of NPC in Southern China (Li et al., unpublished data).

2.3.3.4
EBV Expression in NPC

In nonkeratinizing NPCs, the virus is detectable in almost all cancer cells, where it is present as a monoclonal episome (Niedobitek et al. 1996; Raab-Traub et al. 1986). Moreover, monoclonal viral genomes have also been detected in *in situ* NPCs (Pathmanathan et al. 1995). Expression of the viral genome in nonkeratinizing NPC has been studied extensively. During latency, up to 11 viral genes are expressed that encode up to nine proteins and EBV infection in NPC is classified as latency type II, which is characterized by expression of the EBERs, EBNA1, LMP1, LMP2A, and the Bam H1 A transcripts, despite LMP1 is only expressed in up to approximately 65% of nasopharyngeal carcinoma tumors (Niedobitek et al. 2000; Young et al. 2000). While remaining latent, EBV can induce RNA and protein production. Recent evidence demonstrated the association of distinct lytic promoter sequence variation with NPC in Southern Chinese and suggested the participation of a lytic-latent switch of EBV in NPC carcinogenesis (Tong et al. 2003).

In NPC cells, the virus is in the form of episome and not integrated into the host genome. *LMP1* and *BARF1* have profound effects on cellular gene expression and may contribute to EBV-mediated tumorigenesis. In vitro, *LMP1* expression in epithelial cells can induce or upregulate the expression of intercellular adhesion molecule 1 (ICAM-1), CD40, and cytokines such as interleukin 6 (IL-6) and IL-8 (Dawson et al. 1990; Eliopoulos et al. 1997). Expression of *LMP1* in immortalized nasopharyngeal epithelial cells induces an array of genes involved in growth stimulation, enhanced survival, and increased invasive potentials (Lo et al. 2004). Blocking the important signaling activities of *LMP1* abrogates transformation and testifies to the importance of such events in the transformation process (Murray et al. 2000). *BARF1* is able to immortalize primate epithelial cells and enhance growth rate of the transfected cells (Wei et al. 1997). A family of rightward transcripts from the *Bam*HI A region was initially identified in cDNA libraries from NPC where they are abundantly and consistently expressed (Gilligan et al. 1991).

2.3.3.5
The Role of EBV in the Pathogenesis of NPC

Biology of EBV Infection

Approximately 90% of the adult population throughout the world is EBV-positive by serology (Lo et al. 2004). After primary infection at early age, persistent EBV latent infection is found in some resting B cells, but has not been detected in the nasopharyngeal epithelia of healthy individuals (Babcock et al. 1998; Tao et al. 1995). However, EBV infection has been demonstrated *in situ* carcinomas of the nasopharynx, which are presumed precursor lesions of NPC (Niedobitek et al. 1996). These findings seem to suggest that EBV infection takes place before invasive growth begins, but probably does not represent the first step in the pathogenesis of NPC. The EBV latent proteins include the six nuclear antigens (EBNAs 1, 2, 3A, 3B and 3C, and EBNA-LP) and the three latent membrane proteins (LMPs 1, 2A, 2B). EBNA-LP is transcribed from variable numbers of repetitive exons. LMP2A and LMP2B are composed of multiple exons located on either side of the terminal repeats (TR) region, which is formed during the circularization of the linear DNA to produce the viral episome. EBER1 and EBER2 are highly transcribed nonpolyadenylated RNAs and their transcription is a consistent feature of latent EBV infection. A pivotal biologic property of the virus is the ability to alter B-lymphocyte growth in vitro, leading to permanent growth transformation.

EBV entering in B lymphocytes is mainly mediated by binding of the major viral envelope glycoprotein, gp350/220 (gp350), to CD21 receptor on the surface of B cells (Nemerow et al. 1987), and through the binding of a second glycoprotein, gp42, to HLA class II molecules as a coreceptor (Borza et al. 2002). EBV encodes more than 100 genes, at least ten genes are for EBV replication, and viral genes include three integral membrane proteins. Apart from latent membrane proteins 1, 2A, and 2B (LMP) and six EBNAs (EBNA1, 2, 3A,3B, 3C, and EBNA-LP), two small untranslated EBV RNAs (EBERs) (Rickinson 2002; Rowe 2001; Roy et al. 2004; Smith 2001) are also encoded by EBV. These viral proteins profit to cell immortalization and malignant transformation by various signaling mechanisms. For example, *LMP1* encoded by EBV is a membrane protein that activates multiple signaling pathways and transcription factors, including nuclear factor-kappaB (NF-κB). NF-κB activation is necessary for Hodgkin/Reed-Sternberg (HRS) cells to proliferate and inhibit apoptosis (Bargou et al. 1997). Furthermore, activation of NF-κB is essential for B-cell immortalization by EBV and *LMP1*-mediated transformation of fibroblasts (He et al. 2000). To understand the pathogenic properties of EBV in NPC, the state of EBV infection and viral gene expression have been determined in biopsy samples of NPC (Raab-Traub 2002).

The EBV-Encoded Nuclear Antigens

Cells infected EBV express a group of nuclear proteins, which influence both viral and cellular transcription. EBNA1 is expressed in all transformed lymphoid cell lines and EBV-associated tumors. This protein is required for the replication and maintenance of the episomal EBV genome through binding to the plasmid origin of viral replication, OriP. EBNA1 can also interact with certain viral promoters as a transcriptional transactivator and has been shown to upregulate the LMP1 promoter (Lin et al. 2002). Humme et al. has reported that EBNA1 does not have a crucial function in in vitro B-cell transformation beyond the maintenance of the viral genome by Gene-knockout method (Humme et al. 2003). EBNA2 is an acidic phosphoprotein, which transcriptionally activates both cellular and viral genes, thus upregulating the expression of certain B-cell antigens, CD21 and CD23, as well as LMP1 and LMP2 (Lin et al. 2002). Two types of EBNA2 have been identified, encoded by divergent DNA sequences, EBNA2A or 2B, that distinguish two types of EBV, EBV1 or 2 (Dambaugh et al. 1984). The three members of the EBNA3 family, EBNA3A, 3B, and 3C, all appear to have a common origin and encode hydrophilic nuclear proteins, which contain heptads repeats of leucine, isoleucine, or valine that can act as dimerization domains (Lin et al. 2002). The EBNA2 and 3 proteins are the major targets of cytotoxic T-lymphocytes that eliminate latently infected, growth-transformed B-cells (Murray et al. 1992). EBNA-LP is encoded by the leader of each of the EBNA mRNAs and encodes a protein of variable size depending on the number of BamHI W repeats contained by a particular EBV isolate (Lin et al. 2002). A role for EBNA-LP in enhancing EBNA2-mediated transcriptional activation has been proposed (Lin et al. 2002).

The EBV-Encoded Latent Membrane Proteins

LMP1 is an integral membrane protein with oncogenic potential encoded by the *BNLF-1* gene (also called *LMP1* gene) of EBV (Hudson et al. 1985), and is the first EBV latent gene found to transform established rodent cell lines and alter the phenotype of both lymphoid and epithelial cells (Martin et al. 1993; Moorthy et al. 1993; Wang et al. 1985). LMP1 is often present in nasopharyngeal carcinomas and was detected in preinvasive lesions of the nasopharynx (Pathmanathan et al. 1995).

EBV-encoded LMP1, expressed in most of NPC, has been suggested to have an important role in the pathogenesis and development of NPC and its expression correlates with poor prognosis (Gullo et al. 2008). The high percentage of detection of LMP1 in

NPC samples, independent of histological type or tumor location (Burgos 2005), supports a role for EBV in the pathogenesis of different types of NPC, where LMP1 overexpression could be an important factor in the development of the disease. LMP1 is an integral membrane protein containing a cytoplasmic amino terminus, six transmembrane domains, and a long cytoplasmic carboxy terminal portion (Raab-Traub 2002). LMP1 functions as a constitutively active tumor necrosis factor receptor (TNFR), activating a number of signaling pathways in a ligand-independent manner (Eliopoulos et al. 1997; Kilger et al. 1998). Functionally, LMP1 resembles CD40 – another member of the TNFR superfamily – and can partially substitute for CD40 in vivo, providing both growth and differentiation signals to B cells (Uchida et al. 1999). The two distinct functional domains, C-terminal activation regions 1 and 2 (CTAR1 and CTAR2), have been identified within the cytoplasmic carboxy terminus of LMP1, which both can activate the NF-κB transcription factor (Liebowitz et al. 1992). The consequences of NF-κB activation are numerous and include the upregulation of antiapoptotic gene products. These roles suggest that LMP1 is, directly or indirectly, a key modulator of the apoptosis process. Expression of LMP1 plays an essential role in immortalization of human B cells through the activation of a number of cellular signaling pathways, including NFκB, JNK, JAK/STAT, p38/MAP, and Ras/MAPK (Young et al. 2004). In human epithelial cells, LMP1 alters many functional properties that may involve in tumor progression and invasions.

Unlike LMP1, the LMP2 protein is not essential for B-cell transformation in vitro (Longnecker et al. 1992). However, the constant expression of this viral gene in EBV-carrying memory B cells from healthy individuals indicates that LMP2 may play an important role in mediating virus persistence (Babcock et al. 1998). The LMP2 proteins are encoded by highly spliced mRNAs that contain exons located at both ends of the linear EBV genome (Laux et al. 1988). LMP2A and 2B are the two forms of LMP2. The LMP2A protein contains a unique 119-amino acid N-terminal cytoplasmic tail that is absent from LMP2B. LMP2A is shown to inhibit the switch from latency to lytic EBV replication induced by BCR triggering (Longnecker 2000). This effect has been related to the ability of LMP2A to interfere with BCR signaling and possibly plays a major role in mediating EBV persistence in the infected host (Dolcetti et al. 2003). It has been approved that the interaction of epithelial cells with extracellular matrix proteins triggers LMP2A phosphorylation, indicating that this EBV protein is involved in signaling pathways activated by cell adhesion (Scholle et al. 1999). Ectopic expression of LMP2A in a human keratinocyte cell line resulted in enhanced proliferation, clonogenicity in soft agar, and inhibition of differentiation (Dolcetti et al. 2003). LMP2B might function by increasing the spacing between LMP2A N-terminals, causing the release of the Src and Syk protein tyrosine kinases and restoring BCR signal transduction (Baumforth et al. 1999).

The EBV-Encoded Noncoding RNAs

Viral microRNAs (miRNAs) were first shown to exist following the cloning of small RNAs from a B cell line latently infected with EBV (Pfeffer et al. 2004). A recently appreciated property of EBV is that it encodes about 30 mature miRNAs from 20 pre-miRNAs, which, given the size of its genome (approximately 165 kb), represents a 1,000-fold enrichment of this class of genes relative to those in its human host (Cai et al. 2006; Grundhoff et al. 2006; Landgraf et al. 2007; Pfeffer et al. 2004). EBV's miRNAs have been detected by Northern blotting or cloning (Cai et al. 2006; Grundhoff et al. 2006; Landgraf et al. 2007; Pfeffer et al. 2004). Among these, BART7, 10, and 12 have been most frequently detected and BART15 and 20–5p rarely or not at all (Cai et al. 2006; Edwards et al. 2008; Grundhoff et al. 2006; Kim Do et al. 2007; Lo et al. 2007). A recent report has shown that by using quantitative, stem-loop, real-time PCR to measure the expression of EBV's miRNAs and found them to differ nearly 50- and 25-fold among all tested cell lines and among EBV-positive Burkitt's lymphomas, respectively (Pratt et al. 2009). There is little or no increased expression of its miRNAs when EBV's lytic cycle is induced (Pratt et al. 2009). EBV does not regulate its productive cycle by altering the levels of its miRNAs exception to BART2 (Barth et al. 2008).

EBV encodes multiple miRNAs from two primary transcripts, the BHRF1 and the BARTs. The expression of BHRF1 miRNAs is dependent on the type of viral latency, whereas the BART miRNAs are expressed in cells during all forms of latency (Pratt et al. 2009). EBV was found to encode five miRNAs clustered within two genomic regions. miR-BHRF1–1, 2, and 3 are located within the untranslated region (UTR) of BHRF1, an antiapoptosis Bcl-2 homolog. miR-BHRF1–1 is located within the 5′UTR with miR-BHRF1–2 and 3 encoded within the 3′UTR.

miR-BART-1 and 2 are located within intronic regions of the BART family of transcripts, which are extensively spliced. The BART family of transcripts has been suggested to encode a number of proteins, although it remains to be convincingly demonstrated that these proteins are expressed during viral infection (Smith et al. 2000). Subsequent investigation identified a further 22 EBV miRNAs not identified in the original study, due to a large deletion in the B95–8 strain used for the initial cloning strategy (Cai et al. 2006; Grundhoff et al. 2006). Three miRNAs encoded within the BART region, miRBART16, miR-BART17–5p, and miR-BART1–5p, have since been shown to target sequences within the 3′UTR of the viral latent membrane protein 1 (LMP1) following the transient transfection of an LMP1 expression plasmid and various BART-derived miRNAs (Lo et al. 2007). In latent infection, EBV also expresses at least 14 BART miRNAs, which are encoded by a genomic region, which also encodes the noncoding BamHI A rightward transcripts (BARTs) (Cai et al. 2005; Grundhoff et al. 2006; Pfeffer et al. 2004). Seven of EBV's microRNAs are closely related to microRNAs of an EBV-related monkey virus (*Rhesus lymphocryptovirus*) and provide a first example of miRNA conservation within the herpesvirus family (Cai et al. 2006).

EBV may also use cellular miRNAs to regulate gene expression. There are at least two cellular miRNAs with pleiotropic cellular effects that may be induced by EBV proteins. LMP1 activates the promoter for mir-146a, a cellular miRNA, which downregulates a large number of interferon-responsive genes (Lo et al. 2007). Thus, EBV may cooperate a cellular miRNA pathway involved in modulating the interferon response to enhance EBV replication in vivo. miR-155 is a cellular miRNA derived from BIC, a noncoding RNA whose expression is upregulated in a variety of B cell malignancies including diffuse large B cell lymphomas, CLL, and Hodgkin's lymphoma (Eis et al. 2005; Fulci et al. 2007; Kluiver et al. 2005). Consistent with an important role for miR-155 in B cell malignancy, transgenic mice carrying an miR-155 transgene develop B cell lymphomas (Costinean et al. 2006). This indicates that EBV induces cell miRNAs with effects on immune responses and oncogenesis.

The most abundant RNAs in EBV-infected cells are small nuclear EBER RNAs that are present at approximately 10^5 copies per cells but are not necessary for lymphocyte transformation (Arrand et al. 1982; Swaminathan et al. 1991). EBER1 and EBER2 have 167 and 172 nucleotides, respectively. The EBERs are expressed in many of the malignancies linked to EBV and presumably contribute in some way to the maintenance of latency in vivo (Raab-Traub 2002). The evolutionary conservation of EBERs among primate homologs of EBV and their ubiquitous expression suggests that they play a critical role in EBV biology, such as apoptosis, lymphomagenesis, cell transformation, and some genes expression (Swaminathan 2008).

In nasopharyngeal carcinoma cells, the EBER2 promoter was stronger than the H1 and U6 promoters in shRNA synthesis, leading to more effective knockdown of the target genes. The EBER promoters fundamentally different from those of H1 and U6 can be used to drive the intracellular expression of shRNAs for effective silencing of target genes in mammalian cells and particularly in EBV-infected cells (Choy et al. 2008).

2.4 NPC Stem Cells

In normal organs, stem cells are defined as a subset of cells with the capacity of self-renewal to maintain the stem cell reservoir and of differentiation to generate various types of cells in the tissue. By self-renewal, stem cells divide symmetrically and perpetuate themselves by generating daughter cells with identical stem cell abilities of parent. By differentiation, stem cells give rise to a hierarchy of limitedly proliferative but functional mature cells. This model was first established in hematopoietic system, in which a small number of donor cells identified with stem cell characteristics can reconstitute the bone marrow by transplantation. After that, tissue-specific stem cells were isolated from multiple organs including lung, skin, liver, and brain. The stem population principally stays quiescent in specialized niches under physiological conditions while actively entering a proliferation state and differentiating in response to specific stimuli. The balance of self-renewal and differentiation is accurately orchestrated to maintain the tissue homeostasis. Zhang and coworkers first described the identification of stem-like cells in normal mouse nasopharyngeal epithelium with the well-established label-retaining cell (LRC) approach, which is based on the evidence that stem cells are able to retain nucleoside analog including bromodeoxyuridine (BrdU) (Tumbar et al. 2004; Zeng et al. 2007). In mouse nasopharyngeal stratified squamous epithelia, less than 3% of cells were long-term BrdU LRCs, of which 64.12% localized in the basal layer and 35.88% were in the superbasal layer. Besides, approximately 12% of LRCs were recruited into cell cycle progression, demonstrated by double-label with BrdU and 3H-TdR. These findings suggested the existence of stem cells in normal nasopharynx.

Borrowed from the view of NSCs, cancer stem cells (CSC) are proposed to be a small population of cells within the tumors, which are capable of self-renewal and generating heterogeneous progeny to constitute the tumor bulk. The idea of CSC is not new but has received increasing attention and enthusiasm in the fields of oncology. This enthusiasm is justified by the identification and characterization of rare tumor-initiating cells analogous to NSCs within hematopoietic malignancy and solid tumors including those of breast, lung, colon, and brain. Several lines of evidence support the existence of CSCs in NPC. First, LRCs were also found in the mouse NPC xenografts in addition to normal mouse pharynx, with a similar percentage of less than 0.5% in mouse xenografts generated by three human NPC cell lines. Second, Wang and coworkers isolated side population (SP) cells fitting the criteria of CSCs from human NPC cell lines by using a cell-permeable DNA-specific bisbenzimidazole dye Hoechst 33342 and further investigated biological characteristics of SP cells including proliferation, self-renewal, and tumor-initiation. In one of the poorly differentiated NPC cell line CNE-2, SP cells accounted for less than 3% of the whole population. After being sorted in vitro, SP cells showed more extensive proliferative potential and generated significantly more clones than non-SP cells. In addition, SP cells can give rise to non-SP cells, whereas non-SP cells were unlikely able to generate SP cells. Furthermore, increased resistance to conventional therapies including chemotherapy and radiotherapy was observed in SP cells. More importantly, in vivo assays revealed that SP and non-SP cells were different in the ability to initiated tumors. Ten thousand SP cells were sufficient to form tumors while 200,000 non-SP cells were required (Friborg et al. 2007).

If the hypothesis is proved to be true about the existence of stem cells in normal nasopharynx and NPC, it will open a new frontier for exploring the oncogensis, progression, and treatment-resistance of NPC. This concept challenges the more traditional view about tumor development, by which tumor cells are assumed equal as for tumorigenesis, and the heterogeneity of tumor evolves from random mutations or an environmental selection progress. Whereas CSC hypothesis proposes that tumor is initiated and maintained by a minority of tumor cells and the heterogeneity of tumor comes from the aberrant "differentiation" of these cells.

Cancer stem cell hypothesis sheds much light on the origin of NPC. Self-renewal is crucial in stemness of CSCs. If the CSC proliferates but fails to self-renew, the CSC pool will be inevitably exhausted. In consideration of the observed similarities between CSCs and its normal counterpart in terms of self-renewal and cell surface markers, it is reasonable to assume that CSCs origin from a mutated NMS, which escapes from proliferation control but spare the self-renewal. Actually, several lines of evidences indicate that this may be the case. For example, Kim et al. 2005 isolated putative bronchioalveolar stem cells (BASC) from mouse lung. Oncogenic *K-ras* was found to activate the expansion of BASCs and transform these cells into adenocarcinoma precursors. Moreover, PTEN deletion in mouse hematopoietic stem cells has been suggested to result in a myeloproliferative disorder and followed by acute T-lymphoblastic leukemia (Guo et al. 2008). Besides, there is another possibility that a restricted progenitor or terminally differentiated cell, which experiences a serial of mutations and acquires the ability of self-renewal, gives rise to the subset of tumor cells with some features of NMSs. Actually, many pathways important for the maintenance of NMSs are found disregulated in a variety of cancers. For example, *Bmi*-1, a member of Polycomb group (PcG) genes, is required for the maintenance and self-renewal of embryonic and somatic stem cells. In the context of NPC, *Bmi*-1 is found highly expressed in both nasopharyngeal carcinoma cell lines as well as NPC samples, which is negatively related to the prognosis of NPC patients. Experimentally, overexpression of *Bmi*-1 sufficiently immortalizes normal nasopharyngeal epithelial cells by induction of telomerase reverse transcriptase activity and inhibition of p16 (Ink 4a) expression (Song et al. 2006).

2.5 Molecular Alterations

The genetic, environmental, and viral causative factors, either acting alone or in combination, would lead to multiple genetic and epigenetic alterations (Lo et al. 2004). The development of NPC involves accumulation of multiple genetic and epigenetic changes leading to the evolution of clonal cell population that possesses growth advantages over other cells (Lo and Huang 2002). By comparative genomic hybridization (CGH) analyses, a large number of primary NPC have recently been examined for the gain and loss of genetic material in the genome, including gain at chromosome 1q, 3q, 8q, 12 and loss at 3p, 9p, 11q, and 14q (Chen et al. 1999; Chien et al. 2001; Fang et al. 2001). The highest frequencies of allelic loss were found on 3p (75%) and 9p (87.0%). Using array-based CGH, frequent amplifications were detected for several oncogene loci, including MYCL1 at 1p34.3 (66.7%), TERC at 3q26.3 (46.7%), ESR at 6q25.1 (46.7%), and PIK3CA at 3q26.3 (40%) (Hui et al. 2002). Loss of heterozygosity analysis (LOH) on 9q, 11q, 13q, and 14q was found in over 50%% of the NPC samples (Lo and Huang 2002). The most frequent LOH were observed at chromosome 3p, 9p, and 14q, which is in agreement with the CGH-based findings. In addition, some karyotyping-based studies have been performed on NPC, where many structural and numerical alterations found on 1p, 3p, 3q, 5q, 9p, 12, 11q, 13q, 14q, 16q, and X (Bernheim et al. 1993; Chang et al. 1989; Hui et al. 1998; Lin et al. 1993; Zhang et al. 1982). Among these alterations, deletion of 3p and gain of 3q are the most frequent events (Lo et al. 1997; Lo and Huang 2002). A recent spectral karyotyping (SKY) analysis on NPC cell lines confirmed most of the abnormalities identified previously by CGH and LOH and illustrated additional breakpoints on a number of apparently balanced chromosomes, including 3p21, 3q26, 5q31, 6p21-p25, 7p14-p22, and 8q22 (Wong et al. 2003).

Genes located on chromosomes 9p21 (p14, p16) and 3p21.3 (RASSF1A) were found to be defective owing to deletion or promoter hypermethylation (Kwong et al. 2002; Lo et al. 1996). Frequent promoter hypermethylation of cancer genes is an important feature of NPC (Lo et al. 2004). The tumor suppressor properties of p16 and RASSF1A have also been demonstrated in NPC cells (Chow et al. 2004; Wang et al. 1999). Induction of epigenetic alterations of cellular genes was proposed as one of the mechanisms for enhancing the transformation of nasopharyngeal epithelial cells by EBV infection (Lo and Huang 2002).

In NPC cells, the apoptosis process may be interfered by multiple genetic changes. Overexpression of Bcl-2 and inactivation of p53 pathway is believed to be the major mechanisms for the reduction in apoptosis in this cancer (Lo and Huang 2002). Bcl-2 product has a high degree of homology with BHRF-1, an open reading frame product in the EBV genome (Cleary et al. 1986) that disturbs epithelial cell differentiation (Dawson et al. 1995). The high prevalence of Bcl-2 detected in NPC is consistent with the frequent immunoreactivity of this oncoprotein exhibited by the basal layer cells of nasopharyngeal normal mucosa, at the same time that Bcl-2 protein produces a significant extension of cell survival may be considered a key event either in cell transformation or in tumor growth (Korsmeyer 1992). EBV can use viral proteins influence the expression of Bcl-2, as LMP1 (Burgos 2005). However, studies on the value of p53 in NPC are controversial; some studies showed that p53 protein accumulation may be a common event in carcinogenesis (Niedobitek et al. 1993; Niedobitek et al. 1994; Sakai et al. 1992), but in the last few years strong evidence indicates the low incidence in p53 modifications in this cancer (Kouvidou et al. 1997; Nasrin et al. 1994; Niemhom et al. 2000; Spruck et al. 1992; Sun et al. 1992). To reveal the tumorigenesis pathway, several studies have examined the early events in NPC development. Some reports have demonstrated clonal proliferation, overexpression of Bcl-2, telomerase activation, and EBV infection in the precancerous lesions (Chang et al. 2000; Jiang et al. 1996; Pathmanathan et al. 1995; Sheu et al. 1997).

From the view of tumor development, emerging data suggest that several pathways essential in development, such as Sonic hedgehog and Wnt/β-catenin, disregulated in CSCs. In NPC, Smo is activated in SP cells and the resistance of SP cells to radiotherapy is partially reversed by cyclopamine, which blocks SHH signaling pathway through binding to Smo (Friborg et al. 2007). Gene expression profiling indicated that multiple components of Wnt/β-catenin pathway were upregulated (Zeng et al. 2007). EBV latent membrane protein 2A (LMP2A) and epigenetic inactivation of Wnt inhibitory factor 1 were suggested to contribute to the aberrant activation of Wnt/β-catenin pathway (Chan et al. 2007; Morrison et al. 2005). These data indicate that Wnt/β-catenin pathway may play an important role in the tumorigenesis and progression of NPC.

2.6 Summary

The geographically constrained distribution of EBV-associated NPC in Southeast Asian populations suggests that both viral and host genetics may influence disease risk (Gullo et al. 2008). NPC undergoes a multistep carcinogenesis. The consistent expression of specific viral genes and the detection of latent membrane protein in every cell in NPC samples and in premalignant lesions suggest that these viral gene products contribute to the abnormal proliferation, as they may serve as specific tumor markers and targets for novel therapy strategies (Lo et al. 2004). Moreover, the induction of EBV replication in latently infected cells is being evaluated as a therapeutic approach to stop malignant cell proliferation (Ambinder et al. 1999). The high frequencies of epigenetic alterations in this cancer suggest the potential application of novel inhibitors targeting DNA methylation and histone acetylation. Additionally, the identification of cancer stem cells in NPC provides important insight into understanding NPC biology and may also help develop new strategies to fight NPC more efficiently, which will ultimately improve the prognosis of NPC patients.

References

Abdel-Hamid M, Chen JJ, Constantine N, et al (1992) EBV strain variation: geographical distribution and relation to disease state. Virology 190(1):168–175

Adldinger HK, Delius H, Freese UK, et al (1985) A putative transforming gene of Jijoye virus differs from that of Epstein–Barr virus prototypes. Virology 141(2):221–234

Altmann M, Hammerschmidt W (2005) Epstein–Barr virus provides a new paradigm: a requirement for the immediate inhibition of apoptosis. PLoS Biol 3(12):e404

Ambinder RF, Robertson KD, Tao Q (1999) DNA methylation and the Epstein–Barr virus. Semin Cancer Biol 9(5):369–375

Armstrong RW, Imrey PB, Lye MS, et al (1998) Nasopharyngeal carcinoma in Malaysian Chinese: salted fish and other dietary exposures. Int J Cancer 77(2):228–235

Armstrong RW, Imrey PB, Lye MS, et al (2000) Nasopharyngeal carcinoma in Malaysian Chinese: occupational exposures to particles, formaldehyde and heat. Int J epidemiol 29(6):991–998

Arrand JR, Rymo L (1982) Characterization of the major Epstein–Barr virus-specific RNA in Burkitt lymphoma-derived cells. J Virol 41(2):376–389

Babcock GJ, Decker LL, Volk M, et al (1998) EBV persistence in memory B cells in vivo. Immunity 9(3):395–404

Baer R, Bankier AT, Biggin MD, et al (1984) DNA sequence and expression of the B95-8 Epstein–Barr virus genome. Nature 310(5974):207–211

Bargou RC, Emmerich F, Krappmann D, et al (1997) Constitutive nuclear factor-kappaB-RelA activation is required for proliferation and survival of Hodgkin's disease tumor cells. J Clin Invest 100(12):2961–2969

Barth S, Pfuhl T, Mamiani A, et al (2008) Epstein–Barr virus-encoded microRNA miR-BART2 down-regulates the viral DNA polymerase BALF5. Nucleic acids Res 36(2):666–675

Baumforth KR, Young LS, Flavell KJ, et al (1999) The Epstein–Barr virus and its association with human cancers. Mol Pathol 52(6):307–322

Bernheim A, Rousselet G, Massaad L, et al (1993) Cytogenetic studies in three xenografted nasopharyngeal carcinomas. Cancer genet cytogenet 66(1):11–15

Bhatia K, Raj A, Guitierrez MI, et al (1996) Variation in the sequence of Epstein–Barr virus nuclear antigen 1 in normal peripheral blood lymphocytes and in Burkitt's lymphomas. Oncogene 13(1):177–181

Billaud M, Busson P, Huang D, et al (1989) Epstein–Barr virus (EBV)-containing nasopharyngeal carcinoma cells express the B-cell activation antigen blast2//CD23 and low levels of the EBV receptor CR2. J Virol 63(10):4121–4128

Borza CM, Hutt-Fletcher LM (2002) Alternate replication in B cells and epithelial cells switches tropism of Epstein–Barr virus. Nat med 8(6):594–599

Bouzid M, Sheng W, Buisson M, et al (1998) Different distribution of H1-H2 Epstein–Barr virus variant in oropharyngeal virus and in biopsies of Hodgkin's disease and in nasopharyngeal carcinoma from Algeria. Int J Cancer 77(2):205–210

Buell P (1974) The effect of migration on the risk of nasopharyngeal cancer among Chinese. Cancer res 34(5):1189–1191

Burgos JS (2005) Involvement of the Epstein–Barr virus in the nasopharyngeal carcinoma pathogenesis. Med oncol 22(2): 113–121

Cai X, Lu S, Zhang Z, et al (2005) Kaposi's sarcoma-associated herpesvirus expresses an array of viral microRNAs in latently infected cells. Proc Natl Acad Sci U S A 102(15):5570–5575

Cai X, Schafer A, Lu S, et al (2006) Epstein–Barr virus microRNAs are evolutionarily conserved and differentially expressed. PLoS pathog 2(3):e23

Chan AT, Teo PM, Johnson PJ (2002) Nasopharyngeal carcinoma. Ann Oncol 13(7):1007–1015

Chang JT, Liao CT, Jung SM, et al (2000) Telomerase activity is frequently found in metaplastic and malignant human nasopharyngeal tissues. Br J Cancer 82(12):1946–1951

Chang YS, Lin SY, Lee PF, et al (1989) Establishment and characterization of a tumor cell line from human nasopharyngeal carcinoma tissue. Cancer Res 49(23):6752–6757

Chang YS, Tyan YS, Liu ST, et al (1990) Detection of Epstein–Barr virus DNA sequences in nasopharyngeal carcinoma cells by enzymatic DNA amplification. J Clin Microbiol 28(11):2398–2402

Chan SL, Cui Y, van Hasselt A, et al (2007) The tumor suppressor Wnt inhibitory factor 1 is frequently methylated in nasopharyngeal and esophageal carcinomas. Lab invest 87(7):644–650

Chen HL, Lung MM, Sham JS, et al (1992) Transcription of BamHI-A region of the EBV genome in NPC tissues and B cells. Virology 191(1):193–201

Chen YJ, Ko JY, Chen PJ, et al (1999) Chromosomal aberrations in nasopharyngeal carcinoma analyzed by comparative genomic hybridization. Genes Chromosomes Cancer 25(2):169–175

Chien G, Yuen PW, Kwong D, et al (2001) Comparative genomic hybridization analysis of nasopharygeal carcinoma: consistent patterns of genetic aberrations and clinicopathological correlations. Cancer Genet Cytogenet 126(1):63–67

Cho EY, Hildesheim A, Chen CJ, et al (2003) Nasopharyngeal carcinoma and genetic polymorphisms of DNA repair enzymes XRCC1 and hOGG1. Cancer Epidemiol Biomarkers Prev 12(10):1100–1104

Choi PH, Suen MW, Huang DP, et al (1993) Nasopharyngeal carcinoma: genetic changes, Epstein–Barr virus infection, or both. A clinical and molecular study of 36 patients. Cancer 72(10):2873–2878
Chou J, Lin YC, Kim J, et al (2008) Nasopharyngeal carcinoma – review of the molecular mechanisms of tumorigenesis. Head Neck 30(7):946–963
Chow LS, Lo KW, Kwong J, et al (2004) RASSF1A is a target tumor suppressor from 3p21.3 in nasopharyngeal carcinoma. Int J Cancer 109(6):839–847
Choy EY, Kok KH, Tsao SW, et al (2008) Utility of Epstein–Barr virus-encoded small RNA promoters for driving the expression of fusion transcripts harboring short hairpin RNAs. Gene ther 15(3):191–202
Cleary ML, Smith SD, Sklar J (1986) Cloning and structural analysis of cDNAs for bcl-2 and a hybrid bcl-2//immunoglobulin transcript resulting from the t (14;18) translocation. Cell 47(1):19–28
Cohen JI (2000) Epstein–Barr virus infection. N Engl J Med 343(7):481–492
Costinean S, Zanesi N, Pekarsky Y, et al (2006) Pre-B cell proliferation and lymphoblastic leukemia//high-grade lymphoma in E (mu)-miR155 transgenic mice. Proc Natl Acad Sci U S A 103(18):7024–7029
Dambaugh T, Hennessy K, Chamnankit L, et al (1984) U2 region of Epstein–Barr virus DNA may encode Epstein–Barr nuclear antigen 2. Proc Natl Acad Sci U S A 81(23):7632–7636
Dawson CW, Eliopoulos AG, Dawson J, et al (1995) BHRF1, a viral homologue of the Bcl-2 oncogene, disturbs epithelial cell differentiation. Oncogene 10(1):69–77
Dawson CW, Rickinson AB, Young LS (1990) Epstein–Barr virus latent membrane protein inhibits human epithelial cell differentiation. Nature 344(6268):777–780
Deng L, Jing N, Tan G, et al (1998) A common region of allelic loss on chromosome region 3p25.3–26.3 in nasopharyngeal carcinoma. Genes Chromosomes Cancer 23(1):21–25
Dolcetti R, Masucci MG (2003) Epstein–Barr virus: induction and control of cell transformation. J Cell Physiol 196(2): 207–218
Edwards RH, Marquitz AR, Raab-Traub N (2008) Epstein–Barr virus BART microRNAs are produced from a large intron prior to splicing. J Virol 82(18):9094–9106
Edwards RH, Seillier-Moiseiwitsch F, Raab-Traub N (1999) Signature amino acid changes in latent membrane protein 1 distinguish Epstein–Barr virus strains. Virology 261(1):79–95
Eis PS, Tam W, Sun L, et al (2005) Accumulation of miR-155 and BIC RNA in human B cell lymphomas. Proc Natl Acad Sci U S A 102(10):3627–3632
Eliopoulos AG, Stack M, Dawson CW, et al (1997) Epstein–Barr virus-encoded LMP1 and CD40 mediate IL-6 production in epithelial cells via an NF-kappaB pathway involving TNF receptor-associated factors. Oncogene 14(24):2899–2916
Epstein MA, Achong BG, Barr YM (1964) Virus particles in cultured lymphoblasts from Burkitt's lymphoma. Lancet 1(7335):702–703
Epstein MA, Barr YM, Achong BG (1966) Preliminary observations on new lymphoblast strains (EB4, EB5) from Burkitt tumours in a British and a Ugandan patient. Br J Cancer 20(3):475–479
Fang Y, Guan X, Guo Y, et al (2001) Analysis of genetic alterations in primary nasopharyngeal carcinoma by comparative genomic hybridization. Genes Chromosomes Cancer 30(3):254–260
Friborg JT, Yuan JM, Wang R, et al (2007) A prospective study of tobacco and alcohol use as risk factors for pharyngeal carcinomas in Singapore Chinese. Cancer 109(6):1183–1191
Friborg J, Wohlfahrt J, Koch A, et al (2005) Cancer susceptibility in nasopharyngeal carcinoma families – a population-based cohort study. Cancer Res 65(18):8567–8572
Fulci V, Chiaretti S, Goldoni M, et al (2007) Quantitative technologies establish a novel microRNA profile of chronic lymphocytic leukemia. Blood 109(11):4944–4951
Gilligan KJ, Rajadurai P, Lin JC, et al (1991) Expression of the Epstein–Barr virus BamHI A fragment in nasopharyngeal carcinoma: evidence for a viral protein expressed in vivo. J Virol 65(11):6252–6259
Grundhoff A, Sullivan CS, Ganem DA (2006) combined computational and microarray-based approach identifies novel microRNAs encoded by human gamma-herpesviruses. RNA 12(5):733–750
Gullo C, Low WK, Teoh G (2008) Association of Epstein–Barr virus with nasopharyngeal carcinoma and current status of development of cancer-derived cell lines. Ann Acad Med Singapore 37(9):769–777
Guo W, Lasky JL, Chang CJ, et al (2008) Multi-genetic events collaboratively contribute to Pten-null leukaemia stem-cell formation. Nature 453(7194):529–533
Gutierrez MI, Raj A, Spangler G, et al (1997) Sequence variations in EBNA-1 may dictate restriction of tissue distribution of Epstein–Barr virus in normal and tumour cells. J Gen Virol 78(Pt 7):1663–1670
Hahn P, Novikova E, Scherback L, et al (2001) The LMP1 gene isolated from Russian nasopharyngeal carcinoma has no 30-bp deletion. Int J Cancer 91(6):815–821
Hepeng J (2008) Zeng Yi profile. A controversial bid to thwart the 'Cantonese cancer'. Science 321(5893):1154–1155
He Z, Xin B, Yang X, et al (2000) Nuclear factor-kappaB activation is involved in LMP1-mediated transformation and tumorigenesis of rat-1 fibroblasts. Cancer Res 60(7):1845–1848
Hildesheim A, Anderson LM, Chen CJ, et al (1997) CYP2E1 genetic polymorphisms and risk of nasopharyngeal carcinoma in Taiwan. J Natl Cancer Inst 89(16):1207–1212
Hildesheim A, Apple RJ, Chen CJ, et al (2002) Association of HLA class I and II alleles and extended haplotypes with nasopharyngeal carcinoma in Taiwan. J Natl Cancer Inst 94(23):1780–1789
Hildesheim A, Chen CJ, Caporaso NE, et al (1995) Cytochrome P4502E1 genetic polymorphisms and risk of nasopharyngeal carcinoma: results from a case-control study conducted in Taiwan. Cancer Epidemiol Biomarkers Prev 4(6):607–610
Hudson GS, Farrell PJ, Barrell BG (1985) Two related but differentially expressed potential membrane proteins encoded by the EcoRI Dhet region of Epstein–Barr virus B95-8. J Virol 53(2):528–535
Hui AB, Cheung ST, Fong Y, et al (1998) Characterization of a new EBV-associated nasopharyngeal carcinoma cell line. Cancer Genet Cytogenet 101(2):83–88
Hui AB, Lo KW, Leung SF, et al (1999) Detection of recurrent chromosomal gains and losses in primary nasopharyngeal carcinoma by comparative genomic hybridisation. Int J Cancer 82(4):498–503

Hui AB, Lo KW, Teo PM, et al (2002) Genome wide detection of oncogene amplifications in nasopharyngeal carcinoma by array based comparative genomic hybridization. Int J Oncol 20(3):467–473

Humme S, Reisbach G, Feederle R, et al (2003) The EBV nuclear antigen 1 (EBNA1) enhances B cell immortalization several thousandfold. Proc Natl Acad Sci U S A 100(19): 10989–10994

Imai S, Nishikawa J, Takada K (1998) Cell-to-cell contact as an efficient mode of Epstein–Barr virus infection of diverse human epithelial cells. J Virol 72(5):4371–4378

Itakura O, Yamada S, Narita M, et al (1996) High prevalence of a 30-base pair deletion and single-base mutations within the carboxy terminal end of the LMP-1 oncogene of Epstein–Barr virus in the Japanese population. Oncogene 13(7):1549–1553

Jeyakumar A, Brickman TM, Jeyakumar A, et al (2006) Review of nasopharyngeal carcinoma. Ear Nose Throat J 85(3):168–170, 172–163, 184

Jiang X, Yao KT (1996) The clonal progression in the neoplastic process of nasopharyngeal carcinoma. Biochem Biophys Res Commun 221(1):122–128

Jia WH, Feng BJ, Xu ZL, et al (2004) Familial risk and clustering of nasopharyngeal carcinoma in Guangdong, China. Cancer 101(2):363–369

Kilger E, Kieser A, Baumann M, et al (1998) Epstein–Barr virus-mediated B-cell proliferation is dependent upon latent membrane protein 1, which simulates an activated CD40 receptor. EMBO J 17(6):1700–1709

Kim CF, Jackson EL, Woolfenden AE, et al (2005) Identification of bronchioalveolar stem cells in normal lung and lung cancer. Cell 121(6):823–835

Kim do N, Chae HS, Oh ST, et al (2007) Expression of viral microRNAs in Epstein–Barr virus-associated gastric carcinoma. J Virol 81(2):1033–1036

Kluiver J, Poppema S, de Jong D, et al (2005) BIC and miR-155 are highly expressed in Hodgkin, primary mediastinal and diffuse large B cell lymphomas. J Pathol 207(2):243–249

Korsmeyer SJ (1992) Bcl-2: an antidote to programmed cell death. Cancer Surv 15:105–118

Kouvidou C, Stefanaki K, Dai Y, et al (1997) P21//waf1 protein expression in nasopharyngeal carcinoma. Comparative study with PCNA, p53 and MDM-2 protein expression. Anticancer Res 17(4A):2615–2619

Kwong J, Lo KW, To KF, et al (2002) Promoter hypermethylation of multiple genes in nasopharyngeal carcinoma. Clin Cancer Res 8(1):131–137

Landgraf P, Rusu M, Sheridan R, et al (2007) A mammalian microRNA expression atlas based on small RNA library sequencing. Cell 129(7):1401–1414

Laux G, Perricaudet M, Farrell PJ (1988) A spliced Epstein–Barr virus gene expressed in immortalized lymphocytes is created by circularization of the linear viral genome. EMBO J 7(3):769–774

Levine PH, Pocinki AG, Madigan P, et al (1992) Familial nasopharyngeal carcinoma in patients who are not Chinese. Cancer 70(5):1024–1029

Liebowitz D (1994) Nasopharyngeal carcinoma: the Epstein–Barr virus association. Semin Oncol 21(3):376–381

Liebowitz D, Mannick J, Takada K, et al (1992) Phenotypes of Epstein–Barr virus LMP1 deletion mutants indicate transmembrane and amino-terminal cytoplasmic domains necessary for effects in B-lymphoma cells. J Virol 66(7):4612–4616

Lin CT, Chan WY, Chen W, et al (1993) Characterization of seven newly established nasopharyngeal carcinoma cell lines. Lab invest 68(6):716–727

Lin J, Johannsen E, Robertson E, et al (2002) Epstein–Barr virus nuclear antigen 3C putative repression domain mediates coactivation of the LMP1 promoter with EBNA-2. J Virol 76(1):232–242

Li SN, Chang YS, Liu ST (1996) Effect of a 10-amino acid deletion on the oncogenic activity of latent membrane protein 1 of Epstein–Barr virus. Oncogene 12(10):2129–2135

Lo AK, Huang DP, Lo KW, et al (2004) Phenotypic alterations induced by the Hong Kong-prevalent Epstein–Barr virus-encoded LMP1 variant (2117-LMP1) in nasopharyngeal epithelial cells. Int J Cancer 109(6):919–925

Lo AK, To KF, Lo KW, et al (2007) Modulation of LMP1 protein expression by EBV-encoded microRNAs. Proc Natl Acad Sci U S A 104(41):16164–16169

Lo K, Huang PW, Lee CK (1997) Genetic changes in nasopharyngeal carcinoma. Chin Med J 110(7):548–549

Lo KW, Cheung ST, Leung SF, et al (1996) Hypermethylation of the p16 gene in nasopharyngeal carcinoma. Cancer Res 56(12):2721–2725

Lo KW, Huang DP (2002) Genetic and epigenetic changes in nasopharyngeal carcinoma. Semin Cancer Biol 12(6): 451–462

Lo KW, Teo PM, Hui AB, et al (2000) High resolution allelotype of microdissected primary nasopharyngeal carcinoma. Cancer Res 60(13):3348–3353

Lo KW, To KF, Huang DP (2004) Focus on nasopharyngeal carcinoma. Cancer cell 5(5):423–428

Longnecker R (2000) Epstein–Barr virus latency: LMP2, a regulator or means for Epstein–Barr virus persistence? Adv Cancer Res 79:175–200

Longnecker R, Miller CL, Miao XQ, et al (1992) The only domain which distinguishes Epstein–Barr virus latent membrane protein 2A (LMP2A) from LMP2B is dispensable for lymphocyte infection and growth transformation in vitro; LMP2A is therefore nonessential. J Virol 66(11): 6461–6469

Lung ML, Lam WP, Sham J, et al (1991) Detection and prevalence of the "f" variant of Epstein–Barr virus in southern China. Virology 185(1):67–71

Marks JE, Phillips JL, Menck HR (1998) The National Cancer Data Base report on the relationship of race and national origin to the histology of nasopharyngeal carcinoma. Cancer 83(3):582–588

Martin JM, Veis D, Korsmeyer SJ, et al (1993) Latent membrane protein of Epstein–Barr virus induces cellular phenotypes independently of expression of Bcl-2. J Virol 67(9): 5269–5278

Mazeron MC (1996) Value of anti-Epstein–Barr antibody detection in the diagnosis and management of undifferentiated carcinoma of the nasopharynx. Bull Cancer Radiother 83(1):3–7

Moorthy RK, Thorley-Lawson DA (1993) All three domains of the Epstein–Barr virus-encoded latent membrane protein LMP-1 are required for transformation of rat-1 fibroblasts. J Virol 67(3):1638–1646

Morrison JA, Raab-Traub N (2005) Roles of the ITAM and PY motifs of Epstein–Barr virus latent membrane protein 2A in the inhibition of epithelial cell differentiation and activation of {beta}-catenin signaling. J Virol 79(4):2375–2382

Murray PG, Young LS (2000) Themed issue: the biology and pathology of the Epstein-Barr virus. Mol Pathol 53(5):219–221
Murray RJ, Kurilla MG, Brooks JM, et al (1992) Identification of target antigens for the human cytotoxic T cell response to Epstein-Barr virus (EBV): implications for the immune control of EBV-positive malignancies. J Exp Med 176(1):157–168
Nasrin N, Taiba K, Hannan N, et al (1994) A molecular study of EBV DNA and p53 mutations in nasopharyngeal carcinoma of Saudi Arab patients. Cancer Lett 82(2):189–198
Nazar-Stewart V, Vaughan TL, Burt RD, et al (1999) Glutathione S-transferase M1 and susceptibility to nasopharyngeal carcinoma. Cancer Epidemiol Biomarkers Prev 8(6):547–551
Nemerow GR, Mold C, Schwend VK, et al (1987) Identification of gp350 as the viral glycoprotein mediating attachment of Epstein-Barr virus (EBV) to the EBV//C3d receptor of B cells: sequence homology of gp350 and C3 complement fragment C3d. J Virol 61(5):1416–1420
Niedobitek G (2000) Epstein-Barr virus infection in the pathogenesis of nasopharyngeal carcinoma. Mol Pathol 53(5): 248–254
Niedobitek G, Agathanggelou A, Barber P, et al (1993) P53 overexpression and Epstein-Barr virus infection in undifferentiated and squamous cell nasopharyngeal carcinomas. J Pathol 170(4):457–461
Niedobitek G, Agathanggelou A, Nicholls JM (1996) Epstein-Barr virus infection and the pathogenesis of nasopharyngeal carcinoma: viral gene expression, tumour cell phenotype, and the role of the lymphoid stroma. Semin Cancer Biol 7(4):165–174
Niedobitek G, Agathanggelou A, Steven N, Young LS (2000) Epstein-Barr virus (EBV) in infectious mononucleosis: detection of the virus in tonsillar B lymphocytes but not in desquamated oropharyngeal epithelial cells. Mol Pathol 53(1):37–42
Niedobitek G, Hansmann ML, Herbst H, et al (1991) Epstein-Barr virus and carcinomas: undifferentiated carcinomas but not squamous cell carcinomas of the nasopharynx are regularly associated with the virus. J Pathol 165(1):17–24
Niedobitek G, Young LS (1994) Epstein-Barr virus persistence and virus-associated tumours. Lancet 343(8893):333–335
Niemhom S, Kitazawa S, Murao S, et al (2000) Co-expression of p53 and bcl-2 may correlate to the presence of Epstein-Barr virus genome and the expression of proliferating cell nuclear antigen in nasopharyngeal carcinoma. Cancer Lett 160(2):199–208
Ning JP, Yu MC, Wang QS, et al (1990) Consumption of salted fish and other risk factors for nasopharyngeal carcinoma (NPC) in Tianjin, a low-risk region for NPC in the People's Republic of China. J Natl Cancer Inst 82(4):291–296
Old LJ, Boyse EA, Oettgen HF, et al (1966) Precipitating antibody in human serum to an antigen present in cultured Burkitt's lymphoma cells. Proc Natl Acad Sci U S A 56(6):1699–1704
Parkin DM, Muir CS (1992) Cancer incidence in five continents. Comparability and quality of data. IARC sci publ (120):45–173
Pathmanathan R, Prasad U, Sadler R, et al (1995) Clonal proliferations of cells infected with Epstein-Barr virus in preinvasive lesions related to nasopharyngeal carcinoma. N Engl J Med 333(11):693–698
Pfeffer S, Zavolan M, Grasser FA, et al (2004) Identification of virus-encoded microRNAs. Science 304(5671):734–736
Pratt ZL, Kuzembayeva M, Sengupta S, et al (2009) The microRNAs of Epstein-Barr virus are expressed at dramatically differing levels among cell lines. Virology
Raab-Traub N (2002) Epstein-Barr virus in the pathogenesis of NPC. Semin Cancer Biol 12(6):431–441
Raab-Traub N, Flynn K (1986) The structure of the termini of the Epstein-Barr virus as a marker of çlonal cellular proliferation. Cell 47(6):883–889
Rickinson A (2002) Epstein-Barr virus. Virus Res 82(1–2):109–113
Rowe M (2001) Cell transformation induced by Epstein-Barr virus – living dangerously. Semin Cancer Biology 11(6): 403–405
Roy NS, Nakano T, Keyoung HM, et al (2004) Telomerase immortalization of neuronally restricted progenitor cells derived from the human fetal spinal cord. Nat Biotechnol 22(3):297–305
Sakai E, Tsuchida N (1992) Most human squamous cell carcinomas in the oral cavity contain mutated p53 tumor-suppressor genes. Oncogene 7(5):927–933
Sample J, Young L, Martin B, et al (1990) Epstein-Barr virus types 1 and 2 differ in their EBNA-3A, EBNA-3B, and EBNA-3C genes. J Virol 64(9):4084–4092
Sandvej K, Gratama JW, Munch M, et al (1997) Sequence analysis of the Epstein-Barr virus (EBV) latent membrane protein-1 gene and promoter region: identification of four variants among wild-type EBV isolates. Blood 90(1): 323–330
Scholle F, Longnecker R, Raab-Traub N (1999) Epithelial cell adhesion to extracellular matrix proteins induces tyrosine phosphorylation of the Epstein-Barr virus latent membrane protein 2: a role for C-terminal Src kinase. J Virol 73(6):4767–4775
Sham JS, Wei WI, Zong YS, et al (1990) Detection of subclinical nasopharyngeal carcinoma by fibreoptic endoscopy and multiple biopsy. Lancet 335(8686):371–374
Shanmugaratnam K (1978) Histological typing of nasopharyngeal carcinoma. IARC Sci Publ (20):3–12
Shannon-Lowe C, Baldwin G, Feederle R, et al (2005) Epstein-Barr virus-induced B-cell transformation: quantitating events from virus binding to cell outgrowth. J Gen Virol 86(Pt 11):3009–3019
Shao YM, Poirier S, Ohshima H, et al (1988) Epstein-Barr virus activation in Raji cells by extracts of preserved food from high risk areas for nasopharyngeal carcinoma. Carcinogenesis 9(8):1455–1457
Sheu LF, Chen A, Meng CL, et al (1997) Analysis of bcl-2 expression in normal, inflamed, dysplastic nasopharyngeal epithelia, and nasopharyngeal carcinoma: association with p53 expression. Hum Pathol 28(5):556–562
Shih-Hsin Wu L (2006) Construction of evolutionary tree models for nasopharyngeal carcinoma using comparative genomic hybridization data. Cancer Genet Cytogenet 168(2):105–108
Sixbey JW, Yao QY (1992) Immunoglobulin A-induced shift of Epstein-Barr virus tissue tropism. Science 255(5051): 1578–1580
Smith P (2001) Epstein-Barr virus complementary strand transcripts (CSTs//BARTs) and cancer. Semin Cancer Biol 11(6):469–476
Smith PR, de Jesus O, Turner D, et al (2000) Structure and coding content of CST (BART) family RNAs of Epstein-Barr virus. J Virol 74(7):3082–3092

Snudden DK, Smith PR, Lai D, et al (1995) Alterations in the structure of the EBV nuclear antigen, EBNA1, in epithelial cell tumours. Oncogene 10(8):1545–1552
Song LB, Zeng MS, Liao WT, et al (2006) *Bmi-1* is a novel molecular marker of nasopharyngeal carcinoma progression and immortalizes primary human nasopharyngeal epithelial cells. Cancer Res 66(12):6225–6232
Spruck CH III, Tsai YC, Huang DP, et al (1992) Absence of p53 gene mutations in primary nasopharyngeal carcinomas. Cancer Res 52(17):4787–4790
Sriamporn S, Vatanasapt V, Pisani P, et al (1992) Environmental risk factors for nasopharyngeal carcinoma: a case-control study in northeastern Thailand. Cancer Epidemiol Biomarkers Prev 1(5):345–348
Strowig T, Brilot F, Arrey F, et al (2008) Tonsilar NK cells restrict B cell transformation by the Epstein–Barr virus via IFN-gamma. PLoS pathog 4(2):e27
Suarez C, Rodrigo JP, Ferlito A, et al (2006) Tumours of familial origin in the head and neck. Oral Oncol 42(10):965–978
Sung NS, Edwards RH, Seillier-Moiseiwitsch F, et al (1998) Epstein–Barr virus strain variation in nasopharyngeal carcinoma from the endemic and non-endemic regions of China. Int J Cancer 76(2):207–215
Sun Y, Hegamyer G, Cheng YJ, et al (1992) An infrequent point mutation of the p53 gene in human nasopharyngeal carcinoma. Proc Natl Acad Sci U S A 89(14):6516–6520
Swaminathan S (2008) Noncoding RNAs produced by oncogenic human herpesviruses. J Cell Physiol 216(2):321–326
Swaminathan S, Tomkinson B, Kieff E (1991) Recombinant Epstein–Barr virus with small RNA (EBER) genes deleted transforms lymphocytes and replicates in vitro. Proc Natl Acad Sci U S A 88(4):1546–1550
Tao Q, Srivastava G, Chan AC, et al (1995) Evidence for lytic infection by Epstein–Barr virus in mucosal lymphocytes instead of nasopharyngeal epithelial cells in normal individuals. J Med Virol 45(1):71–77
Tiwawech D, Srivatanakul P, Karalak A, et al (2006) Cytochrome P450 2A6 polymorphism in nasopharyngeal carcinoma. Cancer Lett 241(1):135–141
Tjia WM, Sham JS, Hu L, et al (2005) Characterization of 3p, 5p, and 3q in two nasopharyngeal carcinoma cell lines, using region-specific multiplex fluorescence in situ hybridization probes. Cancer Genet Cytogenet 158(1):61–66
Tong JH, Lo KW, Au FW, et al (2003) Re: discrete alterations in the BZLF1 promoter in tumor and non-tumor-associated Epstein–Barr virus. J Natl Cancer Inst 95(13):1008–1009; author reply 1009
Trivedi P, Hu LF, Chen F, et al (1994) Epstein–Barr virus (EBV)-encoded membrane protein LMP1 from a nasopharyngeal carcinoma is non-immunogenic in a murine model system, in contrast to a B cell-derived homologue. Eur J Cancer 30A(1):84–88
Tumbar T, Guasch G, Greco V, et al (2004) Defining the epithelial stem cell niche in skin. Science 303(5656):359–363
Uchida J, Yasui T, Takaoka-Shichijo Y, et al (1999) Mimicry of CD40 signals by Epstein–Barr virus LMP1 in B lymphocyte responses. Science 286(5438):300–303
Vasef MA, Ferlito A, Weiss LM (1997) Nasopharyngeal carcinoma, with emphasis on its relationship to Epstein–Barr virus. Ann Otol Rhinol Laryngol 106(4):348–356
Walling DM, Ray AJ, Nichols JE, et al (2007) Epstein–Barr virus infection of Langerhans cell precursors as a mechanism of oral epithelial entry, persistence, and reactivation. J Virol 81(13):7249–7268
Wang D, Liebowitz D, Kieff E (1985) An EBV membrane protein expressed in immortalized lymphocytes transforms established rodent cells. Cell 43(3 Pt 2):831–840
Wang GL, Lo KW, Tsang KS, et al (1999) Inhibiting tumorigenic potential by restoration of p16 in nasopharyngeal carcinoma. Br J Cancer 81(7):1122–1126
Wan J, Sun L, Mendoza JW, et al (2004) Elucidation of the c-Jun N-terminal kinase pathway mediated by Estein-Barr virus-encoded latent membrane protein 1. Mol Cell Biol 24(1): 192–199
Wei MX, de Turenne-Tessier M, Decaussin G, et al (1997) Establishment of a monkey kidney epithelial cell line with the BARF1 open reading frame from Epstein–Barr virus. Oncogene 14(25):3073–3081
Weiss LM, Movahed LA, Butler AE, et al (1989) Analysis of lymphoepithelioma and lymphoepithelioma-like carcinomas for Epstein–Barr viral genomes by in situ hybridization. Am J Surg Pathol 13(8):625–631
Wei WI, Sham JS (2005) Nasopharyngeal carcinoma. Lancet 365(9476):2041–2054
Wong N, Hui AB, Fan B, et al (2003) Molecular cytogenetic characterization of nasopharyngeal carcinoma cell lines and xenografts by comparative genomic hybridization and spectral karyotyping. Cancer Genet Cytogenet 140(2):124–132
Wu HC, Lin YJ, Lee JJ, et al (2003) Functional analysis of EBV in nasopharyngeal carcinoma cells. Lab Invest 83(6):797–812
Wu YT, Luo HL, Johnson DR (1986) Effect of nickel sulfate on cellular proliferation and Epstein–Barr virus antigen expression in lymphoblastoid cell lines. Cancer Lett 32(2):171–179
Xiong W, Zeng ZY, Xia JH, et al (2004) A susceptibility locus at chromosome 3p21 linked to familial nasopharyngeal carcinoma. Cancer Res 64(6):1972–1974
Young LS, Dawson CW, Eliopoulos AG (2000) The expression and function of Epstein–Barr virus encoded latent genes. Mol Pathol 53(5):238–247
Young LS, Rickinson AB (2004) Epstein–Barr virus: 40 years on. Nat Rev 4(10):757–768
Young LS, Yao QY, Rooney CM, et al (1987) New type B isolates of Epstein–Barr virus from Burkitt's lymphoma and from normal individuals in endemic areas. J Gen Virol 68 (Pt 11):2853–2862
Yuan JM, Wang XL, Xiang YB, et al (2000) Preserved foods in relation to risk of nasopharyngeal carcinoma in Shanghai, China. Int J Cancer 85(3):358–363
Yu MC, Ho JH, Ross RK, et al (1981) Nasopharyngeal carcinoma in Chinese – salted fish or inhaled smoke? Prev Med 10(1):15–24
Yu MC, Mo CC, Chong WX, et al (1988) Preserved foods and nasopharyngeal carcinoma: a case-control study in Guangxi, China. Cancer Res 48(7):1954–1959
Yu MC, Yuan JM (2002) Epidemiology of nasopharyngeal carcinoma. Semin Cancer Biol 12(6):421–429
Zeng MS, Li DJ, Liu QL, et al (2005) Genomic sequence analysis of Epstein–Barr virus strain GD1 from a nasopharyngeal carcinoma patient. J Virol 79(24):15323–15330
Zeng YX, Jia WH (2002) Familial nasopharyngeal carcinoma. Semin Cancer Biol 12(6):443–450
Zeng Y, Zhong JM, Ye SQ, et al (1994) Screening of Epstein–Barr virus early antigen expression inducers from Chinese medicinal herbs and plants. Biomed Environ Sci 7(1):50–55

Zeng ZY, Zhou YH, Zhang WL, et al (2007) Gene expression profiling of nasopharyngeal carcinoma reveals the abnormally regulated Wnt signaling pathway. Hum Pathol 38(1): 120–133

Zhang S, Wu Y, Zeng Y, et al (1982) Cytogenetic studies on an epithelioid cell line derived from nasopharyngeal carcinoma. Hereditas 97(1):23–28

Zhang XS, Wang HH, Hu LF, et al (2004) V-val subtype of Epstein–Barr virus nuclear antigen 1 preferentially exists in biopsies of nasopharyngeal carcinoma. Cancer Lett 211(1):11–18

Zheng X, Yan L, Nilsson B, et al (1994) Epstein–Barr virus infection, salted fish and nasopharyngeal carcinoma. A case-control study in southern China. Acta oncol 33(8):867–872

Zimber U, Adldinger HK, Lenoir GM, et al (1986) Geographical prevalence of two types of Epstein–Barr virus. Virology 154(1):56–66

Molecular Signaling Pathways in Nasopharyngeal Cancer

Quynh-Thu Le and Jiade J. Lu

3

CONTENTS

Quynh T. Le, MD
Department of Radiation Therapy, 875 Blake Wilbur Dr, MC 5847, Stanford, CA 94350-5847, USA
Jiade J. Lu, MD, MBA
Department of Radiation Oncology, National University Cancer Institute, National University Health System, National University of Singapore, 5 Lower Kent Ridge Road, Singapore 119074, Republic of Singapore

3.1 Introduction

Nasopharyngeal carcinoma (NPC) is a unique type of head and neck malignancy that shows a clear regional and racial prevalence. It occurs most commonly in Asians who inhabit in the Southern Chinese provinces and Southeast Asia (Ma and Cao 2009). The biological behavior of NPC differs significantly from other types of squamous cell carcinoma of the head and neck, which are abbreviated here as SCCHN: NPC has the highest propensity of regional and distant metastases when compared with SCCHN. At the same time, NPC is more sensitive to ionizing radiation and chemotherapy.

The underlying reason for the differences in the biologic and clinical behaviors between NPC and other head and neck malignancies is of particular interest. One underlying factor mediating the biological behavior of a malignancy is the mechanisms transmitting the extracellular signals to the intracellular compartments. Such signaling pathways are critical for cell survival, growth, and metastasis. Better understanding of the molecular signaling pathways in SCCHN has provided a substantial opportunity for novel and individualized treatment in patients with these cancers. For example, the epidermal growth factor receptor (EGFR), which mediates multiple cellular processes including proliferation, survival, and angiogenesis, has been found to be highly expressed in SCCHN and is associated with worse prognosis in these tumors (Ang et al. 2002). Therefore, studies were conducted to target this pathway in combination with either radiation or chemotherapy in patients with locally advanced or metastatic SCCHN (Bonner et al. 2006; Vermorken et al. 2008). These studies have shown that EGFR targeting could enhance the effect of traditional therapies and resulted in improved survival in these patients. In addition to the EGFR pathway, several molecular pathways have also been evaluated in SCCHN and other solid cancers. These include pathways mediating angiogenesis, metabolism, survival, migration, and invasion (Le and Raben 2009; Bozec et al. 2009). Although the clinical data for targeting these other pathways are less mature than that for the EGFR molecule in SCCHN, preliminary studies have indicated that these approaches, especially those targeting angiogenesis, are feasible and promising (Seiwert et al. 2008; Cohen et al. 2009).

However, research on molecular signaling pathways and their clinical implications in NPC is in its infancy, when compared with other solid tumors such as lung cancer, breast cancer, colorectal cancer, and SCCHN. Similarly, clinical data supporting the significance of these molecular markers in NPC is scarce. In this framework, this chapter intends to summarize what is known in the literature regarding the molecular signaling pathways in NPC to clinicians, with a focus on the two pathways with readily available targeted therapy: the EGFR pathway and the angiogenesis pathway. We will also discuss briefly certain molecular signaling pathways that are more NPC-specific, such as the Wnt pathways and microRNA, which can serve as potential target for future emerging therapies.

3.2 Epidermal Growth Factor Receptor and Nasopharyngeal Carcinoma

3.2.1 Epidermal Growth Factor Receptor

The epidermal growth factor receptor (EGFR) is part of a receptor tyrosine kinase (RTK) family, which consists of four transmembrane tyrosine kinases including HER-1/EGFR (erbB-1), HER-2 (erbB-2), HER-3 (erbB-3), and HER-4 (erbB-4). All four receptors of the EGFR family have similar physical structures. HER-1/EGFR is a 170 kDa protein that has a ligand-binding extracellular domain, a hydrophobic transmembrane domain, and a tyrosine kinase intracellular cytoplasmic domain (Herbst 2004). It is the most pertinent member of the erbB RTK family in head and neck malignancies. EGFR exists on normal cells and its signaling is crucial for the survival, development, and homeostasis of these cells (Miettinen et al. 1995). However, EGFR also plays an important role in the development, progression, and metastasis of several neoplasms. Approximately 70%–100% of the SCCHN overexpress EGFR; a similar percentage of overexpression was also reported for NPC (Sheen et al. 1999; Chua et al. 2004; Pan et al. 2008). The number of receptors on the cancer cell surface can be as high as millions and elevated expression of EGFR has been associated with poor prognosis in SCCHN.

The mechanisms involved in the overexpression of EGFR in cancer cells are not fully understood, but may involve gene amplification, tumor microenvironmental stressors, and viral oncogenes (Normanno et al. 2006; Nishi et al. 2002; Yarden 2001a). Although gene amplification had been proposed to be the main reason for increased EGFR expression, high expression of EGFR has been observed without gene amplification (Normanno et al. 2006). Hypoxia, which is the condition of low oxygen, is a common phenomenon during solid tumor progression. It has been demonstrated to induce the early growth response factor 1 (Egr-1) that directly enhances the synthesis of EGFR, thus conferring hypoxic cancer cells a growth advantage (Nishi et al. 2002). As the Epstein–Barr virus (EBV) has long been recognized as a causative agent of NPC, viral oncogene is of particular interest to NPC. It has been suggested that the expression of the EBV latent membrane protein 1 (LMP1), which plays an important role in carcinoma genesis of the disease, is associated with increased expression of EGFR (Zheng et al. 1994; Miller et al. 1998). LMP1 also causes endocytosis and nuclear accumulation of EGFR, which can act as transcriptional factor to increase cell proliferation (Mainou et al. 2005). Therefore, it appears that EGFR can act as both a transcriptional factor as well as a signal tranducer in NPC.

In addition to being overexpressed, activity of EGFR and its downstream targets can be enhanced by activating mutations in the receptors themselves, resulting in the receptors being "on" all the time. These included activating mutation on the ligand-binding domain (EGFR-vIII), that has been shown to be common in glioblastoma multiforme (Pedersen et al. 2001), and activating mutations in the ATP-binding pocket, which are commonly found in nonsmall cell lung cancers arising from female gender, Asians, and nonsmokers (Eberhard et al. 2008). Such mutations, although have been reported in SCCHN, are rare, and unlikely to contribute to the effect of targeting this pathway

(Schwentner et al. 2008; Sok et al. 2006). However, the prevalence of these mutations in NPC has not been evaluated.

3.2.2 EGFR Ligands and the Effector Pathways

Members of the epidermal growth factor (EGF) family have similar structural and functional characteristics. Besides EGF, other family members include heparin-binding EGF-like growth factor (HB-EGF), transforming growth factor-α (TGF-α), amphiregulin, epiregulin, epigen, betacellulin, and neuregulin-1–4 (NRG1–4) (Dreux et al. 2006). EGF is synthesized in membrane-bound precursor forms prior to being released by proteolytic cleavage on activation (Herbst 2004). EGF is a potent mitogen with ability to stimulate cell growth and proliferation and is important for many developmental processes including promoting mitogenesis and differentiation of mesenchymal and epithelial cells (Normanno et al. 2006).

All EGF family members contain one or more common structural motif, the EGF domain, which consists of six conserved cysteine residues forming three intramolecular disulfide bonds (Herbst 2004). The binding of a ligand such as EGF to the extracellular domain initiates the homo- and hetero-dimerization of the receptor and induces the juxtaposition of cytoplasmic and catalytic domains, enabling activation of the kinase activity. The kinase domain of the receptors is subsequently activated, initiating signaling cascades of phosphorylation of downstream cytoplasmic molecule, such as in the Ras and mitogen-activated protein kinase (MAPK) pathways, leading to a cascade of processes that affect cell growth and proliferation, and the phosphatidylinositol-3 kinase (PI3K) and Akt pathway that drives cell cycle progression and cell survival (Yarden and Sliwkowski 2001b) (Fig. 3.1). The cognate ligands of EGFR can be produced exogenously from normal cells as well as from the cancer cell themselves, creating self-activating loops (Singh and Harris 2005).

The activity of EGF family members is mediated by the EGFR/ErbB RTKs. EGF and TGF-α are often overexpressed in many types of cancers including 90% of SCCHN (Ford and Grandis 2003). The co-overexpression of EGFR and its cognate ligands may be associated with poor prognosis and the development of resistance to treatment in cancers (Hsieh et al. 2000; Volante et al. 2007; DiGiovanna et al. 2005). However, such association has not been thoroughly investigated in NPC.

3.2.3 Interactions Between EGFR Signaling Pathways and Radiotherapy

Results from preclinical studies have indicated an inverse relationship between EGFR expression and the radiocurability of tumors (Akimoto et al. 1999; Milas et al. 2004). For SCCHN other than NPC, the association between poor prognoses after definitive radiation therapy and EGFR overexpression has been repeatedly demonstrated in clinical studies (Bentzen et al. 2005; Eriksen et al. 2005a, b; Chen et al. 2003, Ang et al. 2002). Similar associations between EGFR overexpression and poor prognoses such as lower overall survival and time to progression have been suggested in late-stage NPC (Ma et al. 2003, Chua et al. 2004).

Furthermore, it has been demonstrated that radiation therapy can induce the activation of EGFR signaling without ligand binding (Bowers et al. 2001). Such activity may result in activation of the PI3K/Akt and Ras/MAPK pathways and enhance radiation resistance of cancer cells, a proposed mechanism for tumor accelerated repopulation during radiation therapy (Yarden and Sliwkowski 2001b). However, whether radiation therapy is able to activate EGFR signaling in NPC specifically has not been demonstrated clinically.

The results from a large randomized trial by Bonner et al. (2006) confirmed the synergistic effect between radiation therapy and anti-EGFR monoclonal antibody cetuximab on SCCHN. Patients with locoregionally advanced SCCHN (excluding NPC) were randomized and received definitive dose of radiation therapy with or without cetuximab (C-225). At a 54 months of median follow-up, the median overall survival and duration of locoregional control was superior for the cetuximab arm (median survival of 49 vs. 29.3 months, $p = 0.03$, and median duration of locoregrional control 24.4 vs. 14.9 months, $p = 0.005$, both favoring the radiation plus cetuximab arm). Another study compared platinum-based chemotherapy alone to the same chemotherapy with cetuximab in patients with recurrent or metastatic SCCHN. The addition of cetuximab to chemotherapy significantly prolonged the median survival from 7.4 to 10.4 months ($p = 0.04$) and median progression-free survival from 3.3 to 5.6 months ($p < 0.001$)

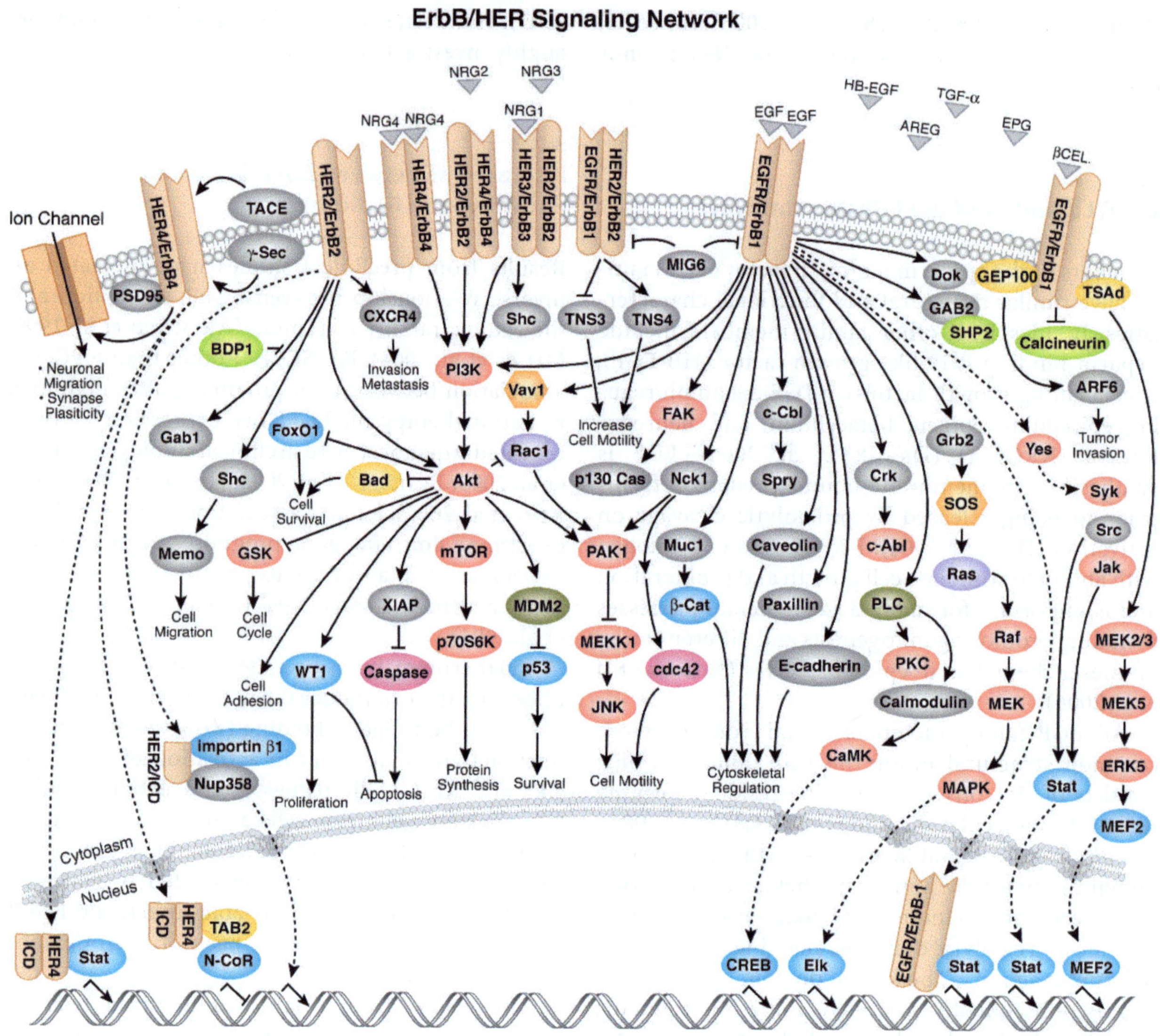

Fig. 3.1. ErbB/HER Signaling Network (Pathway diagram reproduced courtesy of Cell Signaling Technology, Inc. [www.cellsignal.com])

(Vermorken et al. 2008). Since the pathogenesis and biological behavior of NPC are substantially different from other head and neck malignancies, it is not surprising that NPC was not included in the abovementioned trials and the results of these studies therefore cannot be directly extrapolated to NPC.

3.2.4
EGFR in Nasopharyngeal Carcinoma

Similar to SCCHN, overexpression of EGFR in NPC is quite frequent and has been reported to be as high as 80% in primary tumor biopsies (Sheen et al. 1999; Chua et al. 2004; Soo et al. 2005; Pan et al. 2008). Similarly, clinical studies have shown that EGFR overexpression is a negative prognostic factor for NPC as for other SCCHN: The expression of EGFR (as well as that of cytoplasmic VEGF and COX-2) has been shown to correlate with tumor AJCC staging in patients with stage II to IV NPC, with higher expression found in more advanced stage tumors (Zheng et al. 1994; Pan et al. 2008). Overexpression of EGFR was also shown to be an independent prognostic factor for treatment outcome in patients with locoregionally advanced NPC. In a prospective study from the Prince of Wales Hospital in Hong Kong, strong pretreatment EGFR expression in the primary tumor by immunohistochemical (IHC) staining was significantly linked to shorter overall survival and time to

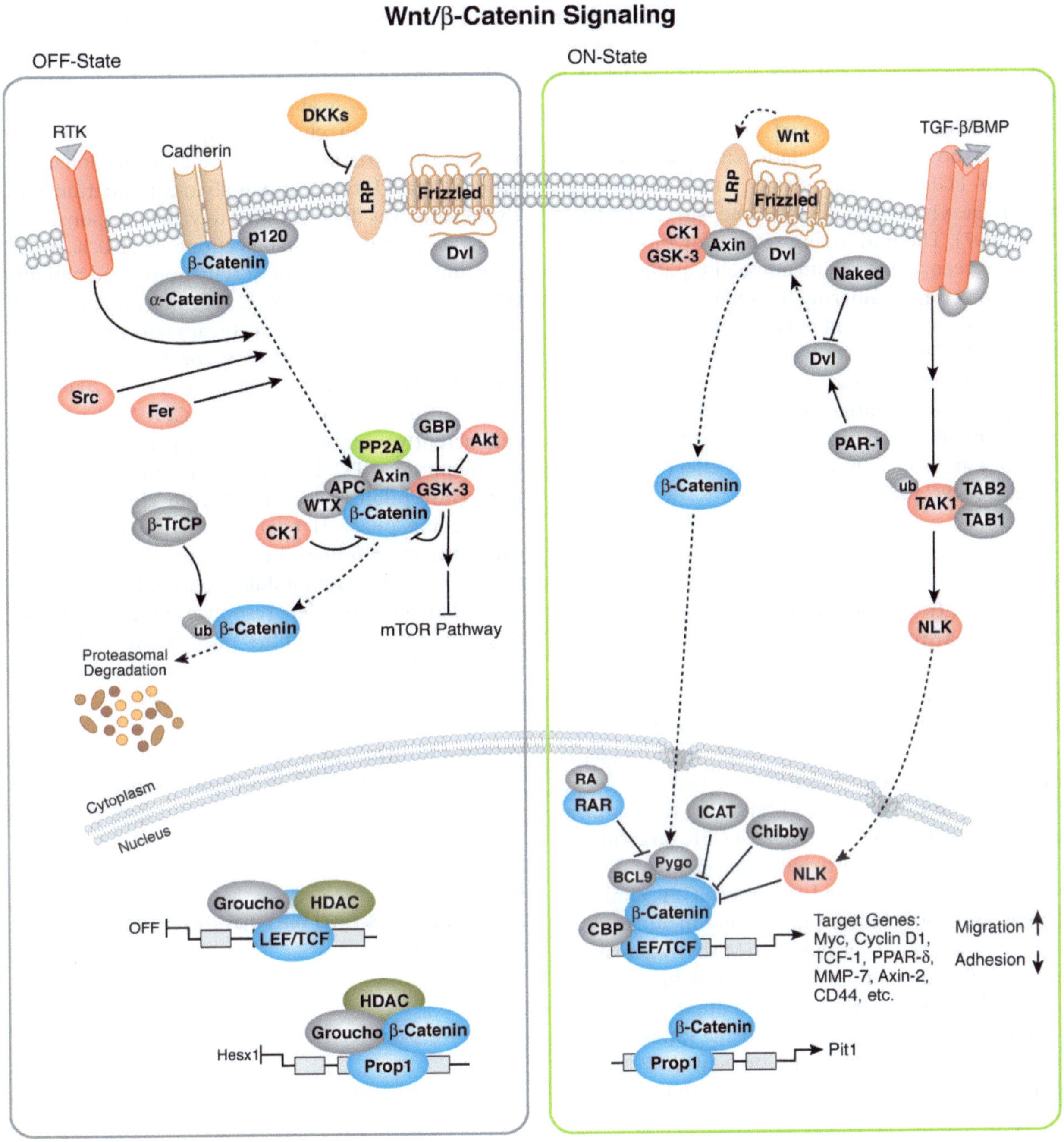

Fig. 3.2. The Wnt/β-Catenin Signaling Pathways. (Diagram reproduced courtesy of Cell Signaling Technology, Inc. [www.cellsignal.com])

progression in 78 NPC patients treated with definitive radiation therapy on multivariate analysis (Ma et al. 2003). These findings were similarly confirmed in a more recently published series. Chua et al. (2004) reported on the association between EGFR expression and disease-specific survival, relapse-free survival, locoregional relapse-free, and distant metastasis-free rates in 54 patients with stage III–IV NPC treated with induction chemotherapy and radiation therapy: Those rates for patients with EGFR extent of > 25% were 48%, 36%, 60%, and 55%, respectively, when compared with 86%, 80%, 93%, and 86%, respectively, for EGFR extent <25%. In multivariate analysis, EGFR extent was the only independent factor that predicted for disease relapse, locoregional failure, and cancer death in this series.

Interestingly, the above-illustrated relationship between EGFR and prognoses of NPC was not demonstrated in pediatric patients. In a small series of 20 juvenile NPC patients of < 20 years old, overexpression of EGFR was observed in 65% of the cases. However, no significant relationship was identified between EGFR overexpression and disease stage, overall survival, and disease-free survival (Fang et al. 2007). The underlying reason for this discrepancy between pediatric and adult NPC patients is not clear. However, considering the small sample size, the variability in treatment strategy for the different patients (~50% received radiation alone whereas the remainder received combined chemoradiation therapy), and potential intrinsic differences in the biology of adult and pediatric tumors, further investigations are needed to address the effect of EGFR in pediatric NPC patients.

3.2.5 Targeting EGFR for Nasopharyngeal Cancer Treatment

The association between overexpression of EGFR and poor prognoses after definitive radiation therapy, the potential activation of EGFR signaling pathway by radiation, the availability of EGFR targeting drugs, and prior successes in targeting this pathway in other SCCHN together make EGFR targeting an ideal treatment strategy in NPC management. Several strategies have been used to target EGFR clinically. The two relatively mature approaches include (1) the use of monoclonal antibodies (MAbs) against the extracellular domain to block ligand binding and signal transduction such as cetuximab and panatunumab and (2) the use of tyrosine kinase inhibitors (TKI) to compete and prevent ATP-binding intracellularly, thereby inhibiting tyrosine autophosphorylation an downstream intracellular signaling.

Although the effect of anti-EGFR MAbs and TKI on tumor cell cytotoxicity, angiogenesis, invasion, and metastasis are well studied in several solid tumors including nonsmall cell lung cancer, colorectal cancer, and SCCHN (Vokes and Chu 2006), little is known about the effect of these drugs in NPC preclinically or clinically. Only one study showed that Cetuximab has single agent activity in certain NPC cell lines and has additive cytotoxic effect with cisplatin and paclitaxel in vitro (Sung et al. 2005). No study has evaluated the effect of this drug in combination with radiation in NPC and there is no published report on the effect of TKIs on NPC cells either in vitro or in vivo setting.

Nevertheless, clinical trials have started to employ these drugs, specifically cetuximab and gefitinib, in combination with chemotherapy in patients with recurrent/metastatic NPC. In a multi institutional single arm phase II trial, cetuximab in combination with carboplatin was demonstrated to yield a response rate of 11.7% and a disease stabilization rate of 48%, which is promising in a group of heavily pretreated patients (Chan et al. 2005). However, gefitinib, an anti-EGFR TKI, provided no significant efficacy with no observed response in a similar setting according to two other phase II trials (Ma et al. 2008a, Chua et al. 2008).

The utilization of either anti-EGFR MAbs or TKI concurrently with radiation therapy in the definitive treatment of NPC has not been fully addressed. A recently published abstract from Hong Kong on an ongoing phase II trial indicated that neoadjuvant cetuximab followed by concurrent cetuximab–cisplatin and intensity-modulated radiotherapy (IMRT) yielded an 83% complete response and a 17% partial response rate at 3 months post-radiation therapy (Ma et al. 2008b). However, long-term outcomes from this treatment strategy are not available.

A thorough discussion of the clinical utilization of anti-EGFR agents as well as their associated treatment outcome in NPC is out of the scope of this chapter, and is detailed in Chap. 11.

3.3 Angiogenesis and Nasopharyngeal Carcinoma

3.3.1 Angiogenesis

Angiogenesis is the process of the development and formation of new blood vessels from an existing vascular network to support tissue growth. It is an important physiological phenomenon in the embryonic phase of human development. However, it is normally suppressed in adulthood and is a rare physiological event (Folkman 1995a; Risau 1997).

The process of angiogenesis involves degradation of basement membranes, migration and proliferation of endothelial cells, lumen formation, and stabilization of neovasculatures, which are crucial for the development, invasion, and metastasis of tumor. It has been demonstrated that without neovasculatures, transportation of oxygen and nutrients are largely via diffusion and solid tumor growth is limited to 2–3 mm in diameter (FOLKMAN 1990, 1995a, 1995b, 2002).

Angiogenesis is controlled by pro- and antiangiogenic factors for endothelial cells. However, the tight suppression of angiogenesis that is present in physiologic state is absent in tumor tissues (FERRARA 2002). Any one step from the expression of ligands and receptors, ligand–receptor engagement, or efferent signal transduction cascade can be upregulated in tumors. As such, not only the process of angiogenesis is active, the characteristics of tumoral endothelial cells and perivascular structures are substantially different from their normal counterparts.

3.3.2 Vascular Endothelial Growth Factors and Receptors

Vascular endothelial growth factor (VEGF) is a specific growth factor group for endothelial cells, and is considered to be the most cardinal vascular growth factor prompting tumor angiogenesis. The VEGF family consists of seven ligands derived from distinct genes: VEGF A–E, as well as placenta growth factor (PGF) 1 and PGF 2 (FERRARA et al. 2003). Among all family members of VEGF, VEGF-A is the most potent and specific growth factor for endothelial cells (FERRARA 2004). VEGF-A has been shown to stimulate endothelial cell mitogenesis and migration. It is also a vasodilator and increases microvascular permeability; it was originally referred to as vascular permeability factor and eventually renamed VEGF (FERRARA 2009; VERHEUL and PINEDO 2007). Figure 3.3 illustrated the biological functions of VEGF (Fig. 3.3).

VEGF is associated with most steps in angiogenesis. In addition to the functions described above, it can also induce proteinases leading to remodeling of the extracellular matrix and suppress dendritic cell maturation. (PEPPER et al. 1991; GERBER et al. 1998; MANDRIOTA et al. 1995). The production of VEGF and subsequent angiogenesis can be triggered by a number of cellular and microenvironmental factors, including hypoxia, balance between oncogenes and tumor suppressor genes, expression of certain cellular receptors, and circulating levels of other growth factors and cytokines (HICKLIN and ELLIS 2005). Among the known promoting factors, hypoxia is of particular importance in tumor growth. Hypoxia remains an important trigger of VEGF expression even after formation of neovascularization in tumor tissues (LEVY et al. 1997; MAXWELL et al. 1999; FERRARA et al. 2003).

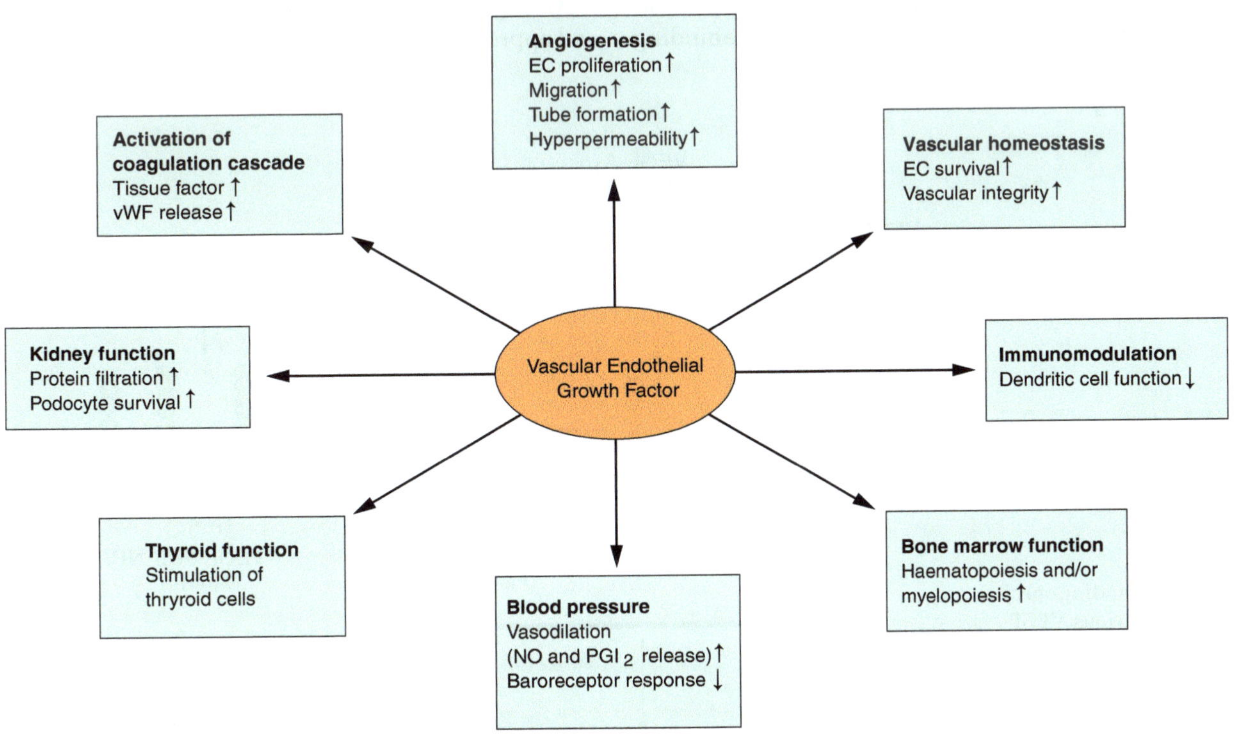

Fig. 3.3. The various biological functions of VEGF EC endothelial cell; NO nitric oxide; PGI2 prostacyclin; VEGF vascular endothelial growth factor; vWF von Willebrand factor

The growth of tumors usually outgrows its existing blood supply, thus leaving a center of necrotic and hypoxic tissue. The tumor responds by upregulating VEGF gene expression via the hypoxia-inducible factor (HIF), which is a major transcriptional factor regulating gene expression under hypoxic stress (GIACCIA et al. 2003). Such positive feedback loop keeps the angiogenesis cascade perpetually active (BERGERS and BENJAMIN 2003). Interestingly, a recent study suggested that in NPC, the EBV oncoprotein LMP1 can induce VEGF expression via HIF, independent of hypoxia. Under normoxia, the HIF protein is marked for degradation by certain proteins known as prolyl HIF hydroxylases (PHDs). These PHDs are themselves degraded by interacting with certain proteins known as Siah proteins. LMP1 has been shown to stabilize one of the Siah protein family member, specifically Siah-1, resulting in increased degradation of PHDs, therefore, leaving HIF protein present and active at high level even under normal oxygen condition (KONDO et al. 2006). Such aberrant HIF function resulted in overexpression of VEGF and enhanced angiogenesis even in the absence of hypoxia.

Action of VEGF is primarily mediated through binding to the RTKs, VEGF receptors (VEGFR). VEGFR have an extracellular portion consisting of seven immunoglobulin-like domains, a single transmembrane spanning region, and an intracellular portion containing a split tyrosine-kinase domain. The binding of VEGF ligands to their corresponding tyrosine kinase receptor (VEGFR) causes dimerization of the receptors and activation through transphosphorylation. VEGF-A binds to VEGFR-1 (Flt-1) and VEGFR-2 (KDR/Flk-1). VEGFR-2 appears to mediate most known cellular responses to VEGF (DVORAK 2002).

The function of VEGFR-1 is less well defined, although it is thought to modulate VEGFR-2 signaling (AUTIERO et al. 2003), and is critical for physiologic and developmental angiogenesis (FONG et al. 1995). VEGF-C and VEGF-D, but not VEGF-A, are ligands for a third receptor (VEGFR-3), which mediates lymphangiogenesis (MANDRIOTA et al. 2001; STACKER et al. 2001) (Fig. 3.4).

The extent of angiogenesis can be evaluated by measuring the microvessel density (MVD) in the tumor tissue. VEGF levels in the primary tumor tissue or in serum have been suggested to be a useful marker for predicting prognosis of cancer patients including NPC.

3.3.3 Angiogenesis in Nasopharyngeal Cancer

Angiogenesis plays a major role in the development, progression, as well as metastasis in SCCHN including NPC. VEGF and its receptor VEGFR2 and VEGFR2 are expressed in close to 90% of SCCHN, and approximately two-third of all NPC have positive

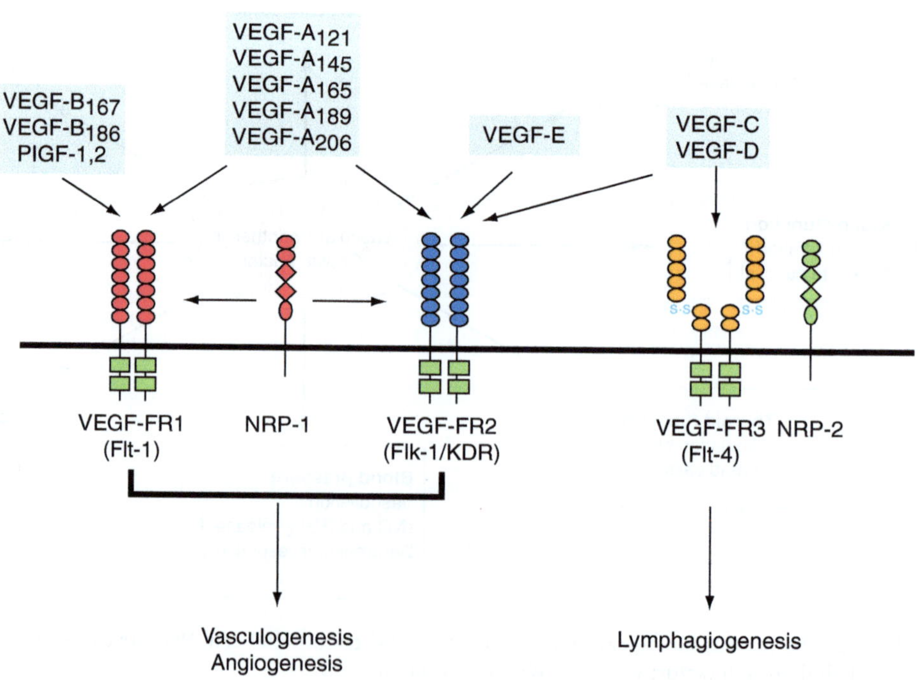

Fig. 3.4. Binding specificity of various VEGF family members and their receptors. Adapted from Hicklin and Ellis (2005). (Used with permission from Journal of Clinical Oncology)

expression of VEGF in the primary tumor (Krishna et al. 2006; Pan et al. 2008). Overexpression of VEGF-A is associated with poor prognosis in head and neck cancers. A meta-analysis of 12 studies and 1002 SCCHN patients (7% of cases were NPC) revealed that positive VEGF-A staining by IHC was associated with a doubled death rate at 2 years after treatment (Kyzas et al. 2005). However, the meta-analysis did not demonstrate an association between VEGF staining and cervical nodal metastasis in SCCHN, possibly due to the heterogeneity of the included patient population and the lack of direct assessment of VEGF-C expression, which plays a larger role on lymphangiogesis and possibly nodal spread. In an NPC-specific study, Wakisaka et al. (1999) found that the VEGF intensity by IHC staining correlated with the microvessel count in the tumor tissue and regional nodal spread in 29 NPC patients, indicating that VEGF-induced angiogenesis may be related to nodal metastasis in this disease (Wakisaka et al. 1999). A different study of 73 NPC patients (49 with locoregional disease and 24 with metastatic disease) demonstrated a significant increase of MVD and VEGF expression in tumor tissue when compared with normal nasopharyngeal mucosa. Similarly, both MVD and VEGF expression were significantly elevated in metastatic NPC when compare with non-metastatic disease (Guang-Wu et al. 2000). In the previously mentioned study by Krishna et al. (2006), higher expression of VEGF in EBV positive tumors was associated with a higher rate of tumor recurrence, regional nodal involvement, and poorer survival. Similar results were reported in the study by Pan et al. (2008). The intensity of VEGF expression correlated tumor extent by the TNM staging.

Interestingly, in an attempt to validate prior small institutional reports, the RTOG (Radiation Therapy Oncology Group) evaluate MVD in 123 NPC patients treated with definitive radiation therapy and found no significant association between the two parameters (Foote et al. 2005). Measurements of tumor angiogenesis are dependent on tumor size, the size of the sampled specimens, location of measurement (tumor edge “hot spots” vs. average), immunostaining technique, the scoring system, and method of measurement. The difference in any of the measurement parameters, treatment techniques, and patient cohort sample size can account for the different results noted from this and the above-mentioned studies. A large prospective study using samples from a homogenously treated group of patients is warranted to address this important question.

The serum VEGF level as an indicator of angiogenesis has also been studied in SCCHN including NPC. In a study of 65 male patients with NPC, serum VEGF was found to be significantly associated with metastatic disease when compared with healthy individuals and patients with nonmetastatic NPC, although no significant differences in the levels of VEGF were detected among various T classifications, N classifications, and clinical stages of nonmetastatic disease (Qian et al. 2000). However, the significance of the serum level of VEGF in predicting the outcome including overall survival, disease- or progression-free survival, and local/regional control rates have not been thoroughly investigated in clinical studies.

3.3.4 Targeting VEGF and VEGFR in Nasopharyngeal Cancer Treatment

Potential treatment strategies for targeting tumor angiogenesis include VEGF ligand-targeted therapy, VEGFR-2 receptor inhibitor, endothelial cytotoxic medication, inhibitors of enzymes that degrade the extracellular matrix, and integrin antagonists. Anti-angiogenic therapies have been extensively studied, and their efficacy has been confirmed in the treatment of several malignancies including colorectal cancer, lung cancer, renal cell carcinoma, and liver cancer. However, their use in head and neck cancers is relatively limited, especially when used with definitive radiotherapy (Mauceri et al. 1998).

The feasibility of combining antiangiogenic treatment and chemoradiation therapy to the head and neck cancers has been reported in a phase I trial, which combined bevacizumab, a recombinant humanized monoclonal antibody to VEGFs, dosed at 10 mg/kg IV q2 weeks and fluorouracil- and hydroxyurea-based (FXH) chemoradiotherapy. The results demonstrated no major additive toxicities and the feasibility of such combination (Seiwert et al. 2008).

A number of phase II clinical trials are currently ongoing to test the efficacy of other anti-angiogenic therapies such as small molecule TKIs in the treatment of SCCHN.

With the technological advances in the diagnosis and treatment of NPC, local and regional control rates exceed 90% after IMRT or combined chemotherapy and IMRT. Distant metastasis has become the most commonly observed mode of treatment failure. As higher level of VEGF is noted in tumor tissue and serum of patients with metastatic disease, it is reasonable to postulate that the addition of anti-angiogenic treatment to chemoradiation therapy may result in less distant failure rates and improved survival in NPC patients. A prospective phase II trial from the RTOG, Protocol 0615, evaluating the toxicity and efficacy of adding bevacizumab to concurrent chemoradiation (IMRT based) and adjuvant chemotherapy, has just completed accrual (Lee et al. 2006). Analysis of the results of this study is ongoing. These results, if positive, will pave the way for a future multi-institution randomized phase III study to address the role of anti-angionesis therapy in NPC (Nancy Lee and Kian Ang, Personal communication).

Since antiangiogenic treatment has been shown to normalize the tumor vasculature (Jain 2008), we also theorize that bevacizumab treatment will decrease tumor hypoxia and improve chemotherapy delivery. A phase II study evaluating bevacizumab delivered with three cycles of TPF induction chemotherapy (taxotere, 5-fluorouracil, cisplatin), followed by bevacizumab and concurrent cisplatin-based chemoradiation, has recently been activated for NPC patients treated at Stanford University. Patients will undergo serial hypoxia PET imaging with F-misonidazole and the changes in imaging hypoxia will be correlated to treatment response and EBV DNA level in the blood. This study will also address the theoretical concern that antiangiogenesis could induce hypoxia within the tumor and may counteract the effect of radiation therapy.

Aside from bevacizumab, other antiangiogenesis strategies such as the use of VEGFR TKIs, drugs that inhibit endothelial cell function, drugs that block breakdown of extracellular matrix, and vascular disrupting therapies have not yet been investigated in nasopharyngeal cancer. Since different targeting strategies may have different toxicity and efficacy profiles, clinical studies to evaluate the role of these drugs in NPC are sorely needed.

3.4 Wnt Pathway in NPC

The Wnt signaling pathway is critical for normal development; however, it is often aberrantly activated in cancer. Secreted signaling proteins of the Wnt family bind to cell surface receptors of the Frizzled (Fzd) family. In the absence of a Wnt signal, the transcriptional activator β-catenin is actively degraded by the actions of a protein complex known as the "destruction box," whose scaffold consists of Axin and the adenomatous polyposis coli (APC) protein. These proteins facilitate phosphorylation of β-catenin by casein-kinase 1α (CK1α) and glycogen synthase kinase 3β (GSK3β). Phosphorylated β-catenin is then ubiquitinylated and targeted for proteosomal degradation. Levels of free β-catenin consequently remain low under normal condition (Fig. 3.2.). Binding of Wnt to Fzd receptor complexes at the membrane results in the dissolution of the "destruction box" due to relocation of Axin to the cell membrane. This allows β-catenin to accumulate and enter the nucleus, where it interacts with various other transcriptional factors to activate Wnt target genes including C-myc (Barker and Clevers 2006). Cytoplasmic β-catenin also binds to E-cadherin in normal cells to maintain cellular adhesion; therefore, removal of such β-catenin can result in loss of cell–cell anchoring process (Jou et al. 1995).

Abnormal Wnt signaling has been implicated in the development and progression in several solid tumors including SCCHN, liver tumors, lung cancers, and colorectal cancers (Barker and Clevers 2006). Similary, there exist several strong pieces of evidence to suggest that the Wnt pathway also plays an important role in NPC development. Over 90% of NPC tumors showed increased Wnt protein expression and approximately 75% exhibited decreased expression of Wnt inhibitory factor (WIF), an endogenous Wnt antagonist (Shi et al. 2006; Zeng et al. 2007). WIF expression has also been found to be silent by promoter hypermethylation in several NPC cell lines (Lin et al. 2006). A gene expression study confirmed upregulation of Fzd7 receptor and downregulation of Axin2 in NPC tumors (Sriuranpong et al. 2004). Nuclear β-catenin level is increased in over 90% of NPC tumors and NPC cells show increased phosphorylation of GSK3β (Morrison et al. 2004). Downstream targets of β-catenin have also been found to be upregulated in NPC. These include IL8, a highly pro-angiogenic factor and C-myc, a well-known oncogene (Ren et al. 2004; Chou et al. 2008). Taken together, these dates suggest that Wnt signaling pathway is a likely contributor to NPC development and a new potential therapeutic target for this cancer.

3.5 MicroRNA in NPC

Recently, microRNAs (miRNA) have emerged as a new class of noncoding genes involved in regulating cell proliferation, differentiation, and viability (Bartel 2004; Stefani and Slack, 2008). MiRNA are 22–24 nucleotide noncoding RNAs that are processed from a primary transcript, or pri-miRNA, usually found in introns or other noncoding regions. Pri-RNA are cleaved in the nucleus by an enzyme called Drosha to yield hairpin pre-miRNA, which are transported to the cytoplasm where it is cleaved further by Dicer to yield the final miRNA. These RNA fragments perform their regulatory role as a component of the RISC complex, which either inhibits protein translation or promote mRNA degradation (Ambros, 2004; Bartel, 2004). Close to 40 miRNA have been found to be expressed in the different regions of the EBV genome (Cosmopoulos et al. 2009) and the expression pattern of these miRNA is dependent on cell type and the overall pattern of EBV gene expression. For example, while one cluster of miRNA from BamHI-A regions (BART miRNAs) is robustly expressed in NPC, a second cluster encoded in the HamHI-H region known as BHRFI miRNA is not detected in these cells at all. The reverse, on the other hand, is true for EBV-related lymphoma (Swaminathan 2008). One of the major targets of EBV-encoded BART miRNA is LMP1, which is a major EBV-derived oncogene (Lo et al. 2007). Although LMP1 has transforming properties, overexpression of this protein may inhibit cell proliferation and increased susceptibility to apoptotic stress (Kaykas and Sugden 2000). Therefore, suppression of excessive LMP1 production on NPC by BART miRNA appeared to protect LMP1 expressing NPC cells from apoptotic stimuli and enhance cisplatin resistance (Lo et al. 2007). BART miRNA regulation of LMP1 protein synthesis also explains for the observed discrepancies between LMP1 transcripts and protein expression that are often noted in NPC tumor tissues (Lo et al. 2007).

In addition to EBV-derived miRNA, several cellular miRNAs, which are encoded in the host cells, are also found to be aberrantly expressed in NPC and such aberrant expression can promote aggressive tumor phenotype through changes in the expression of their downstream targets. For examples, miR-29c is consistently downregulated in primary NPC tumors when compared with normal nasopharyngeal mucosa. On further investigation, most of miR-29c's target genes encodes for extracellular matrix proteins such as laminin-γ1, which are associated with tumor cell invasiveness and metastatic protential (Sengupta et al. 2008,). Another large-scale miRNA profiling study of 13 NPC tumor samples and 9 adjacent normal tissues yielded 35 cellular miRNA with altered expression in the tumor. Changes included upregulation of oncogenic miRNA such as miR-155 and downregulation of tumor suppressive miRNA such as miR-34 and miR-143. Computational analysis of the 22 downregulated miRNAs showed that these potentially target several signaling pathways that are known to play an important role in NPC development and progression. These include the previously discussed Wnt and VEGF pathways, cell cycle regulators, and survival pathways (Chen et al. 2009).

These data together indicate that the miRNA from both the virus and the host cells play a critical role in mediating NPC development and spread. However, our understanding of the function of these miRNAs and their dowstream targets is still at the infancy level. A better knowledge of the complex network involving miRNAs and their targets leading to a coordinated pattern of gene expression in NPC will undoubtedly provide important tools to develop novel therapeutic strategies for these tumors. In addition, selective regulation of particular miRNAs targeting tumor cell survival, invasion, and angiogenesis is a promising prospect for future antitumor therapy.

3.6 Summary

The highly integrated and complex circuitry of cellular molecular signaling in NPC remains only partially understood. However, it is certain that molecular signaling pathways such as EGFR, VEGF, the Wnt pathway, and miRNA regulation are vitally important in the understanding of the biological behavior of the disease and its treatment. Expression of EGFR and VEGF appear to be predictive for the prognosis of NPC. Although still in early phases of investigation, therapeutic strategies directed against EGFR and angiogenesis signaling pathways, using existing drugs, represent promising advances in the management of NPC. Preclinical and clinical data indicate that both the Wnt signaling pathways and miRNA play a major role in NPC development and progression. Active research is ongoing in several laboratories to identify the best approaches to mediate the function of these molecules. Better understanding of the Wnt signaling network, their protein structural function, miRNA regulation, and the function of their respective targets will offer new therapeutic strategies in the management of nasopharyngeal cancer.

References

Akimoto T, Hunter NR, Buchmiller L, et al (1999) Inverse relationship between epidermal growth factor receptor expression and radiocurability of murine carcinomas. Clin Cancer Res 5:2884–2890

Ambros V (2004) The functions of animal microRNAs. Nature 431:350–355

Ang KK, Berkey BA, Tu X, et al (2002) Impact of epidermal growth factor receptor expression on survival and pattern of relapse in patients with advanced head and neck carcinoma. Cancer Res 62:7350–7356

Autiero M, Waltenberger J, Communi D, et al (2003) Role of PlGF in the intra- and intermolecular cross talk between the VEGF receptors Flt1 and Flk1. Nat Med 9:936–943

Barker N, Clevers H (2006) Mining the Wnt pathway for cancer therapeutics. Nat Rev Drug Discov 5:997–1014

Bartel DP (2004) MicroRNAs: genomics, biogenesis, mechanism, and function. Cell 116:281–297

Bentzen SM, Atasoy BM, Daley FM, et al (2005) Epidermal growth factor receptor expression in pretreatment biopsies from head and neck squamous cell carcinoma as a predictive factor for a benefit from accelerated radiation therapy in a randomized controlled trial. J Clin Oncol 23: 5560–5567

Bergers G, Benjamin LE (2003) Tumorigenesis and the angiogenic switch. Nat Rev Cancer 3:401–410

Bonner JA, Harari PM, Giralt J, et al (2006) Radiotherapy plus cetuximab for squamous-cell carcinoma of the head and neck. N Engl J Med 354:567–578

Bowers G, Reardon D, Hewitt T, et al (2001) The relative role of ErbB1-4 receptor tyrosine kinases in radiation signal transduction responses of human carcinoma cells. Oncogene 20:1388–1397

Bozec A, Peyrade F, Fischel JL, et al (2009) Emerging molecular targeted therapies in the treatment of head and neck cancer. Expert Opin Emerg Drugs 14:299–310

Chan AT, Hsu MM, Goh BC, et al (2005) Multicenter, phase II study of cetuximab in combination with carboplatin in patients with recurrent or metastatic nasopharyngeal carcinoma. J Clin Oncol 23:3568–3576

Chen HC, Chen GH, Chen YH, et al (2009) MicroRNA deregulation and pathway alterations in nasopharyngeal carcinoma. Br J Cancer 100:1002–1011

Chen IH, Chang JT, Liao CT, et al (2003) Prognostic significance of EGFR and Her-2 in oral cavity cancer in betel quid prevalent area cancer prognosis. Br J Cancer 89:681–686

Chou J, Lin YC, Kim J, et al (2008) Nasopharyngeal carcinoma – review of the molecular mechanisms of tumorigenesis. Head Neck 30:946–963

Chua DT, Nicholls JM, Sham JS (2004) Prognostic value of epidermal growth factor receptor expression in patients with advanced stage nasopharyngeal carcinoma treated with induction chemotherapy and radiotherapy. Int J Radiat Oncol Biol Phys 59:11–20

Chua DT, Wei WI, Wong MP, et al (2008) Phase II study of gefitinib for the treatment of recurrent and metastatic nasopharyngeal carcinoma. Head Neck 30:863–867

Cohen EE, Davis DW, Karrison TG, et al (2009) Erlotinib and bevacizumab in patients with recurrent or metastatic squamous-cell carcinoma of the head and neck: a phase I/II study. Lancet Oncol 10:247–257

Cosmopoulos K, Pegtel M, Hawkins J, et al (2009) Comprehensive profiling of Epstein–Barr virus microRNAs in nasopharyngeal carcinoma. J Virol 83:2357–2367

DiGiovanna MP, Stern DF, Edgerton SM, et al (2005) Relationship of epidermal growth factor receptor expression to ErbB-2 signaling activity and prognosis in breast cancer patients. J Clin Oncol 23:1152–1160

Dreux AC, Lamb DJ, Modjtahedi H, et al (2006) The epidermal growth factor receptors and their family of ligands: their putative role in atherogenesis. Atherosclerosis 186(1):38–53

Dvorak HF (2002) Vascular permeability factor/vascular endothelial growth factor: a critical cytokine in tumor angiogenesis and a potential target for diagnosis and therapy. J Clin Oncol 20:4368–4380

Eberhard DA, Giaccone G, Johnson BE (2008) Biomarkers of response to epidermal growth factor receptor inhibitors in Non-Small-Cell Lung Cancer Working Group: standardization for use in the clinical trial setting. J Clin Oncol 26: 983–994

Eriksen JG, Steiniche T, Overgaard J; Danish Head and Neck Cancer study group (DAHANCA) (2005a) The influence of epidermal growth factor receptor and tumor differentiation on the response to accelerated radiotherapy of squamous cell carcinomas of the head and neck in the randomized DAHANCA 6 and 7 study. Radiother Oncol 74:93–100

Eriksen JG, Steiniche T, Overgaard J; Danish Head and Neck Cancer study group (DAHANCA) (2005b) The role of epidermal growth factor receptor and E-cadherin for the outcome of reduction in the overall treatment time of radiotherapy of supraglottic larynx squamous cell carcinoma. Acta Oncol 44:50–58

Fang FM, Li CF, Chien CY, et al (2007) Immunohistochemical expression of epidermal growth factor receptor and cyclooxygenase-2 in pediatric nasopharyngeal carcinomas: no significant correlations with clinicopathological variables and treatment outcomes. Int J Pediatr Otorhinolaryngol 71:447–455

Ferrara N (2002) Role of vascular endothelial growth factor in physiologic and pathologic angiogenesis: therapeutic implications. Semin Oncol 29:10–14

Ferrara N (2004) Vascular endothelial growth factor: Basic science and clinical progress. Endocr Rev 25:581–611

Ferrara N (2009) Vascular endothelial growth factor. Arterioscler Thromb Vasc Biol 29:789–791

Ferrara N, Gerber HP, LeCouter J (2003) The biology of VEGF and its receptors. Nat Med 9:669–676

Folkman J (1990) What is the evidence that tumors are angiogenesis dependent? J Natl Cancer Inst 82:4–6

Folkman J (1995a) Angiogenesis in cancer, vascular, rheumatoid and other disease. Nat Med 1:27–31

Folkman J (1995b) Seminars in medicine of the Beth Israel hospital, Boston. Clinical applications of research on angiogenesis. N Engl J Med 333:1757–1763

Folkman J (2002) Role of angiogenesis in tumor growth and metastasis. Semin Oncol 29:15–18

Fong GH, Rossant J, Gertsenstein M, et al (1995) Role of the Flt-1 receptor tyrosine kinase in regulating the assembly of vascular endothelium. Nature 376:66–70

Foote RL, Weidner N, Harris J, et al (2005) Evaluation of tumor angiogenesis measured with microvessel density (MVD) as a prognostic indicator in nasopharyngeal carcinoma: results of RTOG 9505. Int J Radiat Oncol Biol Phys 61: 745–753

Ford AC, Grandis JR (2003) Targeting epidermal growth factor receptor in head and neck cancer. Head Neck 25:67–73

Gerber HP, McMurtrey A, Kowalski J, et al (1998) Vascular endothelial growth factor regulates endothelial cell survival through the phosphatidylinositol 3′-kinase/Akt signal transduction pathway. Requirement for Flk-1/KDR activation. J Biol Chem 273:30336–30343

Giaccia A, Siim BG, Johnson RS (2003) HIF-1 as a target for drug development. Nat Rev Drug Discov 2:803–811

Guang-Wu H, Sunagawa M, Jie-En L, et al (2000) The relationship between microvessel density, the expression of vascular endothelial growth factor (VEGF), and the extension of nasopharyngeal carcinoma. Laryngoscope. 110: 2066–9

Herbst RS (2004) Review of epidermal growth factor receptor biology. Int J Radiat Oncol Biol Phys 59:21–26

Hicklin DJ, Ellis LM (2005) Role of the vascular endothelial growth factor pathway in tumor growth and angiogenesis. J Clin Oncol 23:1011–1027

Hsieh ET, Shepherd FA, Tsao MS (2000) Co-expression of epidermal growth factor receptor and transforming growth factor-alpha is independent of ras mutations in lung adenocarcinoma. Lung Cancer 29:151–157

Jain RK (2008) Lessons from multidisciplinary translational trials on anti-angiogenic therapy of cancer. Nat Rev Cancer 8:309–316

Jou TS, Stewart DB, Stappert J, et al (1995) Genetic and biochemical dissection of protein linkages in the cadherin-catenin complex. Proc Natl Acad Sci USA 92:5067–5071

Kaykas A, Sugden B (2000) The amino-terminus and membrane-spanning domains of LMP1 inhibit cell proliferation. Oncogene 19:1400–1410

Kondo S, Seo SY, Yoshizaki T, et al (2006) EBV latent membrane protein 1 up-regulates hypoxia-inducible factor 1alpha through Siah1-mediated down-regulation of prolyl hydroxylases 1 and 3 in nasopharyngeal epithelial cells. Cancer Res 66:9870–9877

Krishna SM, James S, Balaram P (2006) Expression of VEGF as prognosticator in primary nasopharyngeal cancer and its relation to EBV status. Virus Res 115:85–90

Kyzas PA, Cunha IW, Ionnidis JPA (2005) Prognostic significance of vascular endothelial growth factor immunohistochemical expression in head and neck squamous cell carcinoma: A meta-analysis. Clin Cancer Res 11: 1434–1440

Lee N, Pfister DG, Garden A, et al RTOG 0615, A phase II study of concurrent chemoradiotherapy using three-dimentional conformal radiotherapy (3D-CRT) or intensity-modulated radiation therapy (IMRT) + bevacizumab (BV) for locally or regionally advanced nasopharyngeal cancer. http://www.rtog.org/members/protocols/0615/0615.pdf. Accessed 19 Jun 2009

Le QT, Raben D (2009) Integrating biologically targeted therapy in head and neck squamous cell carcinomas. Semin Radiat Oncol 19:53–62

Levy AP, Levy NS, Iliopoulos O, et al (1997) Regulation of vascular endothelial growth factor by hypoxia and its modulation by the von Hippel–Lindau tumor suppressor gene. Kidney Int 51:575–578

Lin YC, et al (2006) Wnt signaling activation and WIF-1 silencing in nasopharyngeal cancer cell lines. Biochem Biophys Res Commun 341:635–40

Lo AK, To KF, Lo KW, et al (2007) Modulation of LMP1 protein expression by EBV-encoded microRNAs. Proc Natl Acad Sci U S A 104:16164–16169

Ma BB, Hui EP, King A, et al (2008a) A phase II study of patients with metastatic or locoregionally recurrent nasopharyngeal carcinoma and evaluation of plasma Epstein–Barr virus DNA as a biomarker of efficacy. Cancer Chemother Pharmacol 62:59–64

Ma BB, Leung SF, Kam MK, et al (2008b) Phase II study of concurrent cetuximab-cisplatin and intensity-modulated radiotherapy (IMRT) in locoregionally advanced nasopharyngeal carcinoma (NPC) with correlation using dynamic contrast-enhanced magnetic resonance imaging (DCE-MRI). J Clin Oncol 26:abstract 6055

Ma BB, Poon TC, To KF, et al (2003) Prognostic significance of tumor angiogenesis, Ki 67, p53 oncoprotein, epidermal growth factor receptor and HER2 receptor protein expression in undifferentiated nasopharyngeal carcinoma – a prospective study. Head Neck 25:864–872

Mainou BA, Everly DN Jr, Raab-Traub N (2005) Epstein–Barr virus latent membrane protein 1 CTAR1 mediates rodent and human fibroblast transformation through activation of PI3K. Oncogene 24:6917–6924

Ma J, Cao S (2009) Epidemiology and etiology. In: Lu JJ, Cooper JS, Lee AW (eds) Nasopharyngeal carcinoma: multidisciplinary management. Springer, New York

Mandriota SJ, Jussila L, Jeltsch M, et al (2001) Vascular endothelial growth factor-C-mediated lymphangiogenesis promotes tumour metastasis. EMBO J 20:672–682

Mandriota SJ, Seghezzi G, Vassalli JD, et al (1995) Vascular endothelial growth factor increases urokinase receptor expression in vascular endothelial cells. J Biol Chem 270: 9709–9716

Mauceri HJ, Hanna NN, Beckett MA, et al (1998) Combined effects of angiostatin and ionizing radiation in antitumour therapy. Nature 394:287–291

Maxwell PH, Wiesener MS, Chang GW, et al (1999) The tumour suppressor protein VHL targets hypoxia-inducible factors for oxygen-dependent proteolysis. Nature 399:271–275

Miettinen PJ, Berger JE, Meneses J, et al (1995) Epithelial immaturity and multiorgan failure in mice lacking epidermal growth factor receptor. Nature 376:337–341

Milas L, Fan Z, Andratschke NH, et al (2004) Epidermal growth factor receptor and tumor response to radiation: in vivo preclinical studies. Int J Radiat Oncol Biol Phys 58: 966–971

Miller WE, Cheshire JL, Baldwin AS Jr, et al (1998) The NPC derived C15 LMP1 protein confers enhanced activation of NF-kappa B and induction of the EGFR in epithelial cells. Oncogene 16:1869–1877

Morrison JA, Gulley ML, Pathmanathan R, et al (2004) Differential signaling pathways are activated in the Epstein–Barr virus-associated malignancies nasopharyngeal carcinoma and Hodgkin lymphoma. Cancer Res 64: 5251–5260

Nishi H, Nishi KH, Johnson AC (2002) Early growth response-1 gene mediates up-regulation of epidermal growth factor receptor expression during hypoxia. Cancer Res 62: 827–834

Normanno N, De Luca A, Bianco C, et al (2006) Epidermal growth factor receptor (EGFR) signaling in cancer. Gene 366:2–16

Pan J, Kong L, Lin S, et al (2008) The clinical significance of coexpression of cyclooxygenases-2, vascular endothelial growth factors, and epidermal growth factor receptor in nasopharyngeal carcinoma. Laryngoscope 118:1970–1975
Pedersen MW, Meltorn M, Damstrup L, et al (2001) The type III epidermal growth factor receptor mutation. Biological significance and potential target for anti-cancer therapy. Ann Oncol 12:745–760
Pepper MS, Ferrara N, Orci L, et al (1991) Vascular endothelial growth factor (VEGF) induces plasminogen activators and plasminogen activator inhibitor-1 in microvascular endothelial cells. Biochem Biophys Res Commun 181: 902–906
Qian CN, Zhang CQ, Guo X, et al (2000) Elevation of serum vascular endothelial growth factor in male patients with metastatic nasopharyngeal carcinoma. Cancer 88:255–61
Ren Q, Sato H, Murono S, et al (2004) Epstein–Barr virus (EBV) latent membrane protein 1 induces interleukin-8 through the nuclear factor-kappa B signaling pathway in EBV-infected nasopharyngeal carcinoma cell line. Laryngoscope 114:855–859
Risau W (1997) Mechanisms of angiogenesis. Nature 386(6626): 671–674
Schwentner I, Witsch-Baumgartner M, Sprinzl GM, et al (2008) Identification of the rare EGFR mutation p.G796S as somatic and germline mutation in white patients with squamous cell carcinoma of the head and neck. Head Neck 30:1040–1044
Seiwert TY, Haraf DJ, Cohen EE, et al (2008) Phase I study of bevacizumab added to fluorouracil- and hydroxyurea-based concomitant chemoradiotherapy for poor-prognosis head and neck cancer. J Clin Oncol 26:1732–1741
Sengupta S, den Boon JA, Chen IH, et al (2008) MicroRNA 29c is down-regulated in nasopharyngeal carcinomas, up-regulating mRNAs encoding extracellular matrix proteins. Proc Natl Acad Sci U S A 105:5874–5878
Sheen TS, Huang YT, Chang YL, et al (1999) Epstein–Barr virus-encoded latent membrane protein 1 co-expresses with epidermal growth factor receptor in nasopharyngeal carcinoma. Jpn J Cancer Res 90:1285–1292
Shi W, Bastianutto C, Li A, Perez-Ordonez B, et al (2006) Multiple dysregulated pathways in nasopharyngeal carcinoma revealed by gene expression profiling. Int J Cancer 119:2467–2475
Singh AB, Harris RC (2005) Autocrine, paracrine and juxtacrine signaling by EGFR ligands. Cell Signal 17: 1183–1193
Sok JC, Coppelli FM, Thomas SM, et al (2006) Mutant epidermal growth factor receptor (EGFRvIII) contributes to head and neck cancer growth and resistance to EGFR targeting. Clin Cancer Res 12:5064–5073
Soo R, Putti T, Tao Q, et al (2005) Overexpression of cyclooxygenase-2 in nasopharyngeal carcinoma and association with epidermal growth factor receptor expression. Arch Otolaryngol Head Neck Surg 131:147–152
Sriuranpong V, Mutirangura A, Gillespie JW, et al (2004) Global gene expression profile of nasopharyngeal carcinoma by laser capture microdissection and complementary DNA microarrays. Clin Cancer Res 10:4944–4958
Stacker SA, Caesar C, Baldwin ME, et al (2001) VEGF-D promotes the metastatic spread of tumor cells via the lymphatics. Nat Med 7:186–191
Stefani G, Slack FJ (2008) Small non-coding RNAs in animal development. Nat Rev Mol Cell Biol 9:219–230
Sung FL, Poon TC, Hui EP, et al (2005) Antitumor effect and enhancement of cytotoxic drug activity by cetuximab in nasopharyngeal carcinoma cells. In Vivo 19: 237–245
Swaminathan S (2008) Noncoding RNAs produced by oncogenic human herpesviruses. J cell physiol 216:321–6
Verheul HM, Pinedo HM (2007) Possible molecular mechanisms involved in the toxicity of angiogenesis inhibition. Nat Rev Cancer 475–485
Vermorken JB, Mesia R, Rivera F, et al (2008) Platinum-based chemotherapy plus cetuximab in head and neck cancer. N Engl J Med 359:1116–1127
Vokes EE, Chu E (2006) Anti-EGFR therapies: clinical experience in colorectal, lung, and head and neck cancers. Oncology (Williston Park) 20:15–25
Volante M, Saviozzi S, Rapa I, et al (2007) Epidermal growth factor ligand/receptor loop and downstream signaling activation pattern in completely resected nonsmall cell lung cancer. Cancer 110:1321–1328
Wakisaka N, Wen QH, Yoshizaki T, et al (1999) Association of vascular endothelial growth factor expression with angiogenesis and lymph node metastasis in nasopharyngeal carcinoma. Laryngoscope 109:810–814
Yarden Y (2001a) The EGFR family and its ligands in human cancer. signalling mechanisms and therapeutic opportunities. Eur J Cancer 37:S3–8
Yarden Y, Sliwkowski MX (2001b) Untangling the ErbB signalling network. at Rev Mol Cell Biol 2:127–137
Zeng ZY, Zhou YH, Zhang WL, et al (2007) Gene expression profiling of nasopharyngeal carcinoma reveals the abnormally regulated Wnt signaling pathway. Hum Pathol 38: 120–133
Zheng X, Hu L, Chen F, et al (1994) Expression of Ki67 antigen, epidermal growth factor receptor and Epstein–Barr virus-encoded latent membrane protein (LMP1) in nasopharyngeal carcinoma. Eur J Cancer B Oral Oncol 30B:290–295

Natural History, Presenting Symptoms, and Diagnosis of Nasopharyngeal Carcinoma

4

Simon S. Lo and Jiade J. Lu

CONTENTS

Simon S. Lo, MD
Department of Radiation Medicine, Arthur G. James Cancer Hospital, Ohio State University Medical Center, 300 West 10th Avenue, Columbus, OH 43210, USA
Jiade J. Lu, MD, MBA
Department of Radiation Oncology, National University Cancer Institute, National University Health System, National University of Singapore, 5 Lower Kent Ridge Road, Singapore 119074, Republic of Singapore

4.1 Introduction

Early diagnosis has been demonstrated to correlate with favorable treatment outcomes in patients with nasopharyngeal carcinoma (NPC). Unfortunately, the clinical manifestation can often be very deceptive and confusing until the disease progresses into a relatively advanced stage. Coupled with the difficulty associated with thorough examination of the nasopharynx, this disease presents a diagnostic challenge to physicians. Only about 10% of all new patients present with early disease despite recent advances in diagnostic techniques such as fiberoptic examination, diagnostic imaging, and tumor serology. The presenting symptoms are closely related to the location of the tumor in nasopharynx, the extent of local tumor invasion, and the degree of regional nodal metastasis. Because early symptoms are frequently minimal in nature, they are easily ignored by the physician and the patient. A high index of suspicion is crucial in a timely diagnosis of nasopharyngeal carcinoma, especially in endemic areas like Southeast Asia and areas with a large number of Chinese immigrants. As mentioned earlier, the treatment outcomes of NPC depend on the stage of the disease, and delaying the diagnosis of NPC can potentially be detrimental.

Apart from a correct diagnosis, detailed interpretation of the presenting symptoms can facilitate accurate delineation of the extent of disease. Certain symptoms and signs will direct further detailed review of areas of suspected involvement, especially in the base of skull area, on diagnostic imaging studies such as computerized tomography (CT) and magnetic resonance imaging (MRI). A geographic miss can potentially occur if the target volume is underestimated, especially in the modern era where highly conformal radiation therapy techniques such as intensity-modulated radiation therapy are used to minimize toxicities. This chapter reviews the natural history, presenting symptoms, and diagnosis of NPC.

4.2 Natural History

As originally described by Ho from Hong Kong, there are three clinical types of NPC (Ho 1970). The types include: (1) the mainly invasive type, (2) the mainly metastatic type, and (3) mixed type. In the mainly invasive type, the main pattern of disease progression is local invasion. Metastasis to cervical lymph nodes is either absent or insignificant. However, hematogenous spread to distant sites such as the spine, the lungs, and the liver can occur when the tumor invades the basal venous sinus. In the mainly metastatic type, there is early metastasis to the cervical lymph nodes. Hematogenous spread usually occurs after cervical lymph node metastasis. The most common sites of metastases are bone, lung, liver, and superior mediastinal and hilar lymph nodes. In the mixed type, invasion of adjacent structures by the NPC and metastases may occur concurrently or sequentially.

4.3 Presenting Symptoms and Signs

The presenting symptoms and signs of NPC can be classified according to the involved anatomic regions and they include cervical mass, nasal symptoms, ear symptoms, neurologic symptoms, eye symptoms, headache, paraneoplastic syndrome, and miscellaneous symptoms.

4.3.1 Cervical Mass

This is the most common presenting symptom prompting the patient to seek medical evaluation and 43% of patients present with unilateral or bilateral cervical mass on physical examination (Skinner et al. 1991). In nearly all cases, the upper cervical nodes enlarge before the middle and lower cervical nodes (Sham et al. 1990). The upper cervical nodes are usually more bulky than the lower cervical nodes, indicative of an orderly spread in the craniocaudal direction. In most cases, the cervical node enlargement is unilateral, but it is not uncommon to see bilateral cervical adenopathy. The cervical node enlargement is usually painless unless it is accompanied by concurrent inflammatory or infectious process.

4.3.2 Nasal Symptoms

The most common nasal symptoms include blood-stained nasal discharge, unilateral or bilateral nasal obstruction, and posterior nasal discharge, which is blood-stained, and approximately 30% of patients present with these symptoms (Skinner et al. 1991). Some patients may experience epistaxis or hawking and coughing up of blood-stained sputum in the morning secondary to postnasal dripping of blood-stained discharge down the airway at night. Because of the nasal blockage, patients frequently speak with a nasal twang. Many of these symptoms can be confused with those caused by sinusitis or rhinitis. When such symptoms are present, it is crucial to examine the nasopharynx thoroughly.

4.3.3 Ear Symptoms

The most common ear symptom is conductive hearing loss as a result of middle ear effusion caused by the blockage of the Eustachian tube. The hearing loss is usually unilateral (Skinner et al. 1991). Since serious otitis media is relatively rare in adults when compared with that in children, the new onset of unilateral conductive hearing loss can be a warning sign for nasopharyngeal carcinoma. Therefore, a thorough examination of the nasopharynx is necessary if serious otitis media does not clear out in 2–3 weeks in an adult patient. Other common symptoms include tinnitus, which can occur in approximately 1/3 of patients with NPC. Again, tinnitus in the setting of NPC is usually unilateral. In cases where there is infiltration of the glossopharyngeal nerve by NPC, severe unilateral otalgia can occur.

4.3.4 Neurological Symptoms

Neurological symptoms are usually indicative of locally advanced disease. Depending on the extent of involvement by the primary tumor, any of the cranial nerves, the upper cervical sympathetic nerves, the lesser occipital nerve, and the greater auricular nerve

Table 4.1. Incidence of cranial nerve deficit from selected series

Series	Country	*N*	Percentage of patients with cranial nerve deficit
Turgut et al. (1998)	Turkey	124	39
Sham et al. (1991)	Hong Kong	262	13
Leung et al. (1990)	Hong Kong	564	12
Lee et al. (1992)	Hong Kong	5037	18
Chang et al. (2005)	Taiwan	3871	10
Heng et al. (1999)	Singapore	677	12
Sanguineti et al. (1997)	USA (Houston, TX)	378	8
Perez et al. (1992)	USA (St. Louis, MO)	143	23

can be involved. The reported rates of cranial nerve palsy vary among studies (Chang et al. 2005; Heng et al. 1999; Lee et al. 1992; Leung et al. 1990; Perez et al. 1992; Sanguineti et al. 1997; Sham et al. 1991; Turgut et al. 1998). Cranial nerve deficits can occur as isolated or multiple cranial nerve palsies. Table 4.1 summarizes the incidence of cranial nerve deficit from selected series.

The most commonly involved cranial nerves are the V and the VI cranial nerves (Li et al. 2006; Stanley and Fong 1997). Impairment of the function of these nerves will result in paresthesia or numbness of the face and diplopia, respectively. Their involvement is a result of tumor invasion of the skull base into the cavernous sinus (the V and the VI nerves are located inferiorly in the cavernous sinus and are of the closest proximity to the roof of the nasopharynx). Other cranial nerves in the cavernous sinus such as the III nerve may be involved in more advanced cases but an isolated III nerve palsy will never occur alone without associated involvement of the V and the VI nerves (Leung et al. 1990).

The involvement of cranial nerves IX, X, XI, and XII can occur in locally advanced disease. Horner's syndrome may be present in conjunction with deficits of one or more of the last four cranial nerves, but rarely occurs alone. In rare circumstances where the sympathetic nerve fibers surrounding the internal carotid artery inside the carotid canal are involved, an isolated Horner's syndrome can occur.

4.3.5 Eye Symptoms

Diplopia on lateral gaze is a manifestation of VI nerve palsy as a result of tumor infiltration of the cavernous sinus. In very rare circumstances, proptosis can occur as a result of tumor infiltration of the orbit through the orbital fissures.

4.3.6 Headache

Headache can occur in patients of NPC and usually indicates the presence of skull base involvement. The headache is usually unilateral and temporoparietal in location. The headache associated with NPC is usually neuralgic in nature and is due to the irritation of the meningeal branch of the second division of the V nerve. The patient may experience pain caused by lifting of head as a result of posterior infiltration of the prevertebral muscles or retropharyngeal lymphadenopathy.

4.3.7 Paraneoplastic Syndrome

In rare circumstances, the patients with NPC may present with a condition called dermatomyositis as the initial manifestation. In one of the large series from Hong Kong, 1% of the 1,154 patients with NPC had associated dermatomyositis (Teo et al. 1989). Three of the ten patients with dermatomyositis had the presentation of paraneoplastic syndrome prior to the clinical detection of their NPC.

The skin lesions consist of distinctive hyperkeratotic, follicular, erythematous papules (Teo et al. 1989). The first lesions usually appear on the face and eyelids and eventually, the neck, shoulders, and upper extremities are involved. Muscular weakness always follows the skin manifestation. Figure 4.1 shows the typical skin rash associated with dermatomyositis.

4.3.8 Miscellaneous Symptoms

Trismus can occur when there is involvement of the pterygoid muscles. The patient will usually be able to locate the site of the tightness approximately 3–4 cm anterior to the temporal mandibular joint. It is very

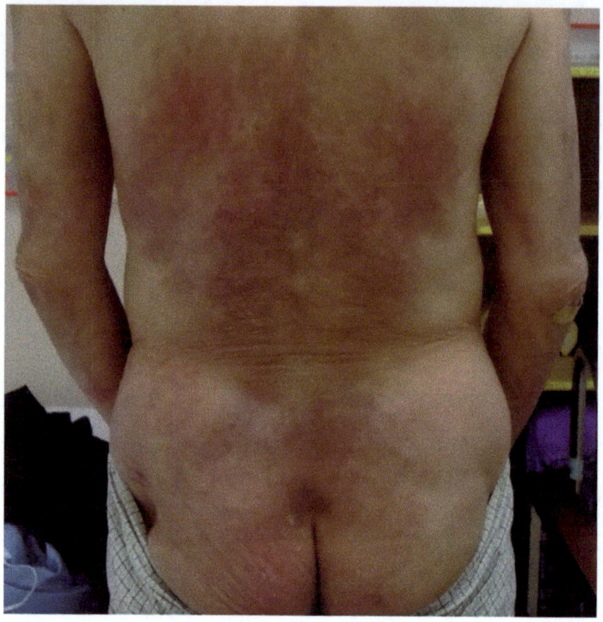

Fig. 4.1. This was a patient diagnosed with NPC who presented with dermatomyositis; his rash improved after treatment with steroid. (Courtesy of Department of Clinical Oncology, Queen Elizabeth Hospital, Hong Kong)

uncommon to see patients with NPC presenting with symptoms related to distant metastases. In most studies, approximately 1–5% of the patients have distant metastasis at the time of first presentation (Lee et al. 1992; Lee and Fu 2004; Skinner et al. 1991; Stanley and Fong 1997). Bone, specifically the thoracolumbar spine, is the most common site of metastasis (Stanley and Fong 1997). Other sites include lung and liver. The presenting symptoms depend on the site and extent of the metastatic lesions.

4.4 Neurological Syndromes

A few syndromes associated with neurologic deficits caused by NPC have been described (Lee and Fu 2004):

1. Petrosphenoidal syndrome of Jacod – This is a result of direct intracranial extension of the NPC with involvement of the II to the VI nerves. This will cause unilateral trigeminal type neuralgia, unilateral ptosis (caused by III nerve involvement), complete ophthalmoplegia (caused by involvement of the III, IV, and VI nerves), and amaurosis (caused by involvement of the optic nerve).
2. The syndrome of the retroparotid space of Villaret – This is a result of the involvement of the last four cranial nerves and cervical sympathetic nerve caused by lateral retropharyngeal lymph node metastasis in the retroparotid space. Patients presenting with this syndrome will have difficulty in swallowing (as a result of the involvement of the IX and X nerves), perversion of taste in the posterior 1/3 of the tongue (caused by involvement of the IX nerve), hyperesthesia, hypoesthesia, or anesthesia of the mucous membranes of the soft palate, pharynx, and larynx, and problems with respiration and salivation (caused by the involvement of the X nerve), paralysis and atrophy of the trapezius and sternocleidomastoid muscles and unilateral weakness of the soft palate (caused by the involvement of the XI nerve), and unilateral paralysis and atrophy of the tongue (caused by the involvement of the XII nerve). When the cervical sympathetic nerves are also involved, the patient may present with Horner's syndrome.
3. Trotter's syndrome – This is a clinical trait of unilateral deafness, neuralgia affecting the branches of the trigeminal nerve, and defective mobility of the soft palate as a result of the NPC involving the fossa of Rosenmüller. It can masquerade as dental masticatory pain. Trismus may also occur as a result of involvement of the medial pterygoid muscle.

4.5 Routes of Tumor Spread

As radiation therapy is the mainstay of treatment for NPC, accurate target delineation is of utmost importance. To facilitate proper target delineation, the knowledge of the anatomy of the nasopharynx and the patterns of spread of NPC is crucial.

4.5.1 Clinical Anatomy and Lymphatic Drainage

The nasopharynx is a space without many natural barriers to spread of tumor growth, but with many critical structures in the immediate vicinity. It is located below the base of skull and behind the nasal cavity. The nasopharynx is in continuity with the nasal cavity near the posterior choanae. The first two cervical vertebral bodies constitute the posterior wall. The basisphenoid, basiocciput, and the anterior arch of the atlas constitute the roof of the nasopharynx. The roof houses abundant lymphoid tissue (adenoids) and if it persists in adulthood, it may be confused with tumor during examination of the nasopharynx. The Eustachian tube opening is located in each of the lateral walls of the nasopharynx and is surrounded by the torus tubarius. The fossa of Rosenmüller, which is the most common site of occurrence of NPC, is a recess located behind the torus tubarius. It is bounded superiorly by the base of the skull with the foramen lacerum medially, the petrous apex and carotid canal posteriorly, and the foramina ovale and spinosum anterolaterally; anterolaterally by the levator veli palatini muscle, posteriorly by the retropharyngeal space, inferiorly by the upper edge of the superior constrictor muscle, and laterally by the tensor veli palatini muscle and pharyngeal space. The proximity of the nasopharynx to foramen lacerum and foramen ovale provide easy access of NPC to the cranium including the cavernous sinus. The hypoglossal canal is located posterior to the posterior nasopharyngeal wall. The upper surface of the soft palate forms the floor of the nasopharynx. The nasopharynx is separated from the oropharynx by the pharyngeal isthmus.

The posterior wall of the nasopharynx consists of four anatomical layers including the mucous membrane, the pharyngeal aponeurosis, the superior constrictor muscle of the pharynx, and the buccopharyngeal fascia. The sinus of Morgagni is an area of muscular deficiency in the upper nasopharynx where the cartilaginous part of the Eustachian tube and levator veli palatine muscle enter the pharyngeal wall. This area of potential weakness allows easy invasion of the NPC into the parapharyngeal area.

There is abundant lymphoid tissue in the nasopharynx and this accounts for the high rate of nodal metastases found at diagnosis. There are three main groups of submucosal collecting lymphatic channels draining the pharynx, the superior, middle, and inferior pathways. The superior pathway provides the primary drainage of the nasopharynx along with a small contribution by the middle pathway and is divided into medial and lateral groups. The medial group provides lymphatic drainage of the roof and posterior border of the nasopharynx into the lateral retropharyngeal node of Röuviere. However, the lymphatic drainage may bypass this node and goes directly to the upper deep cervical lymph node chain (jugulodigastric nodes or level II nodes) located near the internal jugular vein. The lateral group provides lymphatic drainage of the lateral nasopharynx, including the fossa of Rosenmüller directly into the deep nodes of the posterior triangle (the spinal accessory nodes or upper level V nodes), which are located beneath the sternocleidomastoid muscle at the tip of the mastoid process, or into the lateral retropharyngeal node of Röuviere. Further drainage of these primary groups of nodes proceed down the jugular and spinal chains in the cranio-caudal direction. Lymphatic channels can cross the midline and this accounts for contralateral or bilateral nodal involvement. In rare circumstances, lymphatics can drain to the submandibular, submental, and parotid nodes.

4.5.2 Local Spread

Because of the lack of natural barriers to tumor spread, the structures surrounding the nasopharynx are at risk of invasion by NPC. The spread of NPC typically follows several well-established routes. The direction of spread is determined by the site of origin of the NPC. The modes of local spread by NPC can be classified according to the relationships to the nasopharynx:

1. Anterior spread – It is common to see tumor invasion into the nasal cavity through the choanae. Invasion of the paranasal sinuses including the posterior ethmoid and maxillary sinuses can occur although it is less common. In very advanced cases, one or both orbits can be involved.
2. Lateral spread – As mentioned before, the sinus of Morgagni represents an area of weakness in the upper pharyngeal wall and NPC can invade the parapharyngeal space through it. Lateral spread into the parapharyngeal space leading to invasion of the levator and tensor veli palatini muscles can occur early in the disease process. Compression or invasion of the last four cranial nerves and cervical sympathetic nerves can occur as a result of direct tumor extension or lateral retropharyngeal lymph node of Röuviere metastasis. Invasion of the internal carotid artery, pterygoid muscles, and the middle ear (through the Eustachian tube) can occur in more advanced cases.
3. Superior and posterior spread – The superior and posterior aspects of the nasopharynx are bounded by the base of skull and the first two cervical vertebral bodies. Superior extension of NPC can result in erosion of the base of skull, the sphenoid sinus,

and the clivus. There are multiple foramina in the base of skull that can serve as the portals of entry into the cranium. The tumor can gain access to the cavernous sinus and the middle cranial fossa, invading cranial nerves II–VI through the foramen lacerum, which is located immediately above the fossa of Rosenmüller. The tumor can gain access to the middle cranial fossa, the petrous temporal bone, and the cavernous sinus through the foramen ovale. Posterior extension of NPC can result in direct invasion of the prevertebral muscles.

4. Inferior spread – Inferior extension of NPC into the oropharynx can occur. However, direct involvement of the soft palate is relatively uncommon.

4.5.3 Regional Nodal Spread

Lymphatic spread to the ipsilateral neck occurs in 85–90% of cases and to bilateral neck in 50% of the cases (Lee and Fu 2004; Lindberg 1972; Mao et al. 2008; Ng et al. 2004). It is uncommon to see contralateral cervical nodal metastasis alone. The lateral and medial retropharyngeal lymph nodes are regarded as the first echelon nodal stations for NPC. Because of their deep location, retropharyngeal nodal metastases are not palpable. Metastatic involvement of jugulodigastric (Level II) and superior/posterior cervical nodes (upper Level V) is also very common. Some oncologists also consider level II as first echelon nodes. Further nodal metastasis proceeds in the craniocaudal direction. In patients with very extensive cervical nodal metastases, spread to unusual lymph node locations like the submental and occipital regions can occur due to lymphatic channel obstruction. Mediastinal lymph node metastasis can occur in patients with supraclavicular nodal metastasis. Because of the high incidence of cervical nodal metastasis, the entire neck including the retropharyngeal nodes and Level I–V lymph nodes are considered at risk for involvement. For this reason, all these nodal regions are to be included in the clinical target volume for radiation therapy. However, results from a number of recently reported series questioned the necessity of encompassing the lower neck in patients with no cervical adenopathy, as nodal spread usually occurs in an orderly fashion (Gao et al. 2009; Tang et al. 2009). Table 4.2 summarizes the distribution of metastatic nodes based on MRI ± 18-fluorodeoxyglucose positron-emission tomography (^{18}FDG PET).

Table 4.2. Distribution of metastatic nodes in NPC

Nodal sites	Percentage (Ng et al. 2004)[a]	Percentage (Mao et al. 2008)[b]
Retropharyngeal nodes	82	86.4
Level I nodes	a:– b:2.2[c]	a:0 b:3.1
Level II nodes	95.5	a:42.7 b:65
Level III nodes	60.7	28.8
Level IV nodes	34.8	7.1
Level V nodes	27	11.1
Supraclavicular nodes	22.5	3.9
Level VI nodes	2.2	–
Level VII nodes	1.1	–
Parotid nodes	3.4	–
Mediastinal nodes	4.5	–
Abdominal nodes	3.4	–
Retrostyloid nodes	–	0

[a]Study was done based on the findings on MRI and ^{18}FDG PET of 101 patients
[b]Study was done based on the findings on MRI of 924 patients
[c]Designated as submandibular nodes in the study

4.5.4 Distant Spread

Distant metastasis occurs in 3% of the cases at presentation and may occur in a much higher percentage (ranging from 18% to above 50%) of the cases in the disease course (Ahmad and Stefani 1986; Bedwinek et al. 1980; Chu et al. 1984; Hoppe et al. 1976; Lee and Fu 2004; Moench and Phillips 1972). The incidence of distant metastases correlate with the presence of advanced nodal metastasis, especially in the supraclavicular region (Lee et al. 1996a, b; Teo et al. 1991a,b, 1992). The skeleton is the most common site of distant metastasis. Other common sites of metastases include the lungs and the liver.

4.6 Diagnosis

Since the stage of disease is the most important determinant of prognosis in NPC, a delay in diagnosis can be detrimental to the patient in terms of local regional tumor control and survival. The early presenting symptoms of NPC can be confused with benign conditions such as upper respiratory tract infection, sinusitis, and allergies. As stated above, the most common presenting symptoms is a neck mass as a result of cervical nodal metastasis. A good understanding of the epidemiology of NPC and its presenting symptoms and signs and a high index of suspicion in individuals with high risk of developing NPC are necessary for a prompt diagnosis. In all patients with symptoms and signs suspicious for NPC, a very thorough examination of nasopharynx is necessary. If indicated, a biopsy is necessary to provide pathologic diagnosis. This should be supplemented with further diagnostic tests including diagnostic imaging studies and serology test.

4.6.1 History and Physical Examination

The symptoms of NPC can mimic other benign conditions and can vary tremendously among patients. It is important to inquire about a family history of NPC. Patients with early stage disease typically present with nasal and/or ear symptoms including nasal blockage (speech with nasal twang), blood-stained nasal discharge, postnasal drip, hearing loss, and tinnitus, and they are of greater concern to the physician if the presentation is unilateral. In more advanced disease, the above symptoms will become more obvious and there may be presence of cervical nodal metastasis, cranial nerve involvement, and distant metastasis. Patients with dermatomyositis should be screened for NPC in endemic areas. The clinical presentation of NPC has been described in detail in the previous sections of this chapter.

In all patients suspected to have NPC, a full head and neck examination including a nasopharyngoscopy should be performed. On the general head and neck examination, the neck is carefully palpated to detect any cervical nodal involvement. The levels involved should be carefully documented. It is also important to document whether the cervical lymphadenopathy is mobile, partially fixed, or fixed. The oral cavity and oral pharynx should be inspected to look out for tumor invasion of the oral pharynx and trismus. The nasal cavity is inspected with a nasal speculum to detect any tumor extension to the nasal cavity. The cranial nerves and cervical sympathetic nerves should be examined systematically and any deficit present should be carefully documented.

In the clinic, the nasopharynx is best examined using a flexible fiberoptic endoscope under local anesthesia. Alternatively, a rigid Hopkins rod endoscope can be used to visualize the nasopharynx. An indirect mirror examination may be used if an endoscope is not available. The most important aspect in the detection of NPC during an endoscopic examination is the familiarity with its appearance and usual subsites of involvement. Figure 4.2 shows a normal nasopharynx under the endoscope. Most NPC arise from the fossa of Rosenmüller. However, owing to the variation of its anatomy, some early tumors may be obscured. As the tumor progresses, it will encroach on the torus tubaris. Occasionally, NPC may arise from the superior posterior wall, appearing as a well-circumscribed or an ulcerated mass (Woo 1999). Figure 4.3 shows an NPC under endoscopic view. In more advanced tumors, as a result of more extensive involvement of the nasophar-

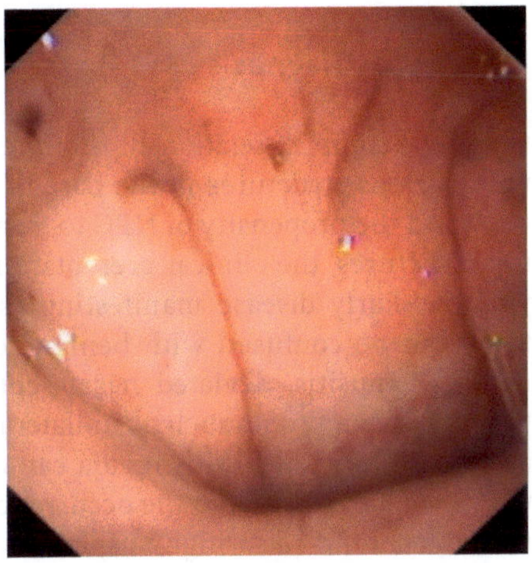

Fig. 4.2. This is an endoscopic view of a normal nasopharynx

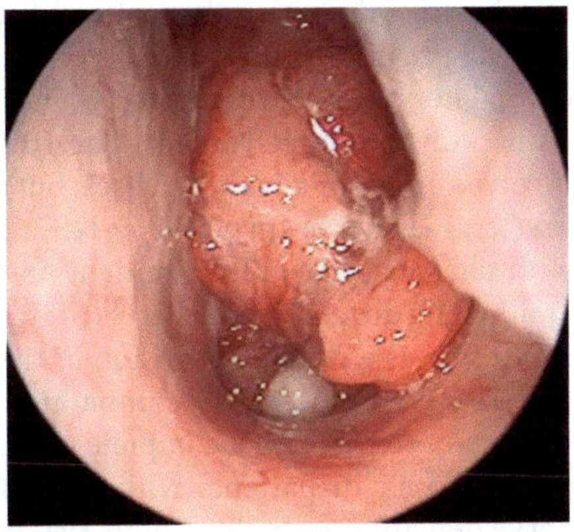

Fig. 4.3. This is an endoscopic view of a nasopharyngeal carcinoma

ynx, it may not be possible to determine where the tumor arises from locally. Most tumors are pale-looking and have moderate vascularity. It is not uncommon to see contact bleeding when the tip of the scope touches the tumor. The mucosal surface of the nasopharynx may appear to be normal despite involvement by NPC (submucosally) and the only sign of involvement may just be some asymmetry in the nasopharynx. Random biopsies should be considered in such cases.

Apart from the head and neck examination, a general physical examination is essential to screen for distant metastasis. This should include percussion and ausculatation of the chest, palpation of the abdomen for an enlarged liver, which may be indicative of liver metastasis, and percussion of bones including the spine to detect any bony tenderness that may indicate bony metastasis.

4.6.2 Differential Diagnosis

Given the complex relationships of the nasopharynx with various structures in the base of skull and the neck and the propensity of NPC to invade surrounding structures, the clinical presentation can be very variable. Early disease manifesting as nasal symptoms can be confused with benign conditions like rhinitis, sinusitis, deviated nasal septum, or nasal polyp. Ear symptoms such as unilateral hearing loss as a result of serous otitis media can occur without the existence of NPC, but the occurrence in any adult patients should raise high suspicion of NPC, especially in individuals from endemic areas.

NPC associated with cranial nerve palsies without accompanying nasal or ear symptoms may be confused with other neurological conditions. As mentioned previously, the most commonly involved cranial nerves are V and VI nerves in NPC associated with skull base involvement. The III nerve may be involved in more advanced cases, but it is rarely the first cranial nerve involved by NPC. Some patients with parapharyngeal involvement may present with swallowing difficulty, hoarseness of voice, or Horner's syndrome as a result of invasion of the last four cranial nerves and cervical sympathetic plexus. It is important to perform a complete examination of the nasopharynx in patients with unexplained cranial nerve deficits, especially in high-risk individuals.

During the endoscopic examination, if a mass is detected in the nasopharynx, the location and the appearance of the lesion should be carefully noted because in some circumstances, a diagnosis can be made with confidence just based on the examination findings (Woo 1999). For instance, a large adenoid, which may be present in some adults, usually has a smooth surface with some longitudinal furrows and is usually located centrally in the nasopharynx. The diagnosis of juvenile angiofibroma, which occurs in adolescent male, is usually made based on the appearance on endoscopic examination and this is confirmed by diagnostic imaging such as MRI. A biopsy of the angifibroma should be avoided because of the risk of massive hemorrhage from this vascular tumor. A pulsatile smooth cystic lesion in nasopharynx should only be biopsied after MRI excludes the possibility of a meningiocele or meningio-encephalocele. Other tumors that can arise from the nasopharynx include lymphoma, sinonasal undifferentiated carcinoma, chordoma, salivary gland tumor, rhabdomyosarcoma, melanoma, teratoma, fibrous tumor, and giant cell tumors (Woo 1999).

In a patient presenting with a cervical neck mass, a biopsy of the node should be deferred until a thorough examination of the upper aerodigestive tract is completed. Conditions that can manifest as a cervical mass include inflammatory or infectious condition, lymphoma, and malignant tumors of the head and neck region and other parts of the body.

4.6.3 Biopsy

A biopsy of the nasopharyngeal tumor is necessary in the definitive diagnosis of NPC. With direct visualization of the nasopharynx under the endoscope, it is possible to obtain representative biopsies from suspicious areas. Biopsies are usually performed under local anesthesia. The endoscopy should enter through the nostril opposite to the site of the suspected tumor to allow clear passage for the biopsy forceps. It is important to obtain adequate tissue for microscopic examination. The specimens obtained should be sent fresh for microscopic examination. The biopsy is usually painless if it is directed at the tumor, which is friable and without sensation. However, if the biopsy is taken from the normal mucosa, the patient may experience some discomfort. Although some degree of bleeding may occur from the biopsy sites, massive hemorrhage is seldom seen.

In patients where there is a clinical suspicion of NPC but with no tumor visible or in patients with a negative biopsy under local anesthesia, a repeat biopsy of the nasopharynx under general anesthesia is recommended. The fossa of Rosenmüller, which is the only region of the nasopharynx that in some circumstances cannot be adequately visualized on endoscopic examination, should be examined in detail under general anesthesia. Multiple deep biopsies and/or curettage should be obtained from bilateral fossae of Rosenmüller and from the superior/posterior wall of nasopharynx.

4.6.4 Diagnostic Imaging Studies Required

In the past when CT and MRI were less available, plain radiographs of the nasopharynx were used for the evaluation of the nasopharynx and skull base. In the modern era, CT and MRI of the nasopharynx and bilateral neck are recommended for accurate delineation of the disease extent. Bony erosion of the skull base can readily be detected with CT scan using the bone window. However, MRI is more sensitive than CT in detecting marrow replacement by the tumor in the skull base. It can also detect perineural and intracranial tumor extension. In patients who present with cranial nerve deficits, attention should be directed to the relevant areas of the skull base to evaluate disease extent. ^{18}FDG PET/CT is increasingly used in the diagnosis of NPC. Some studies show that ^{18}FDG–PET/CT is superior to other conventional studies in terms of detection of cervical nodal and distant metastases, though other studies do not show any benefit. In general, MRI is superior to PET/CT in the delineation of the primary tumor, especially in the skull base and intracranial regions. Diagnostic imaging for NPC is covered in details in a separate chapter.

4.6.5 Serology

Epstein–Barr virus specific serology is useful in the diagnosis of NPC. The IgA antibody to the viral capsid antigen (VCA) of EBV is a highly sensitive diagnostic test for NPC although it has a much lower specificity. Data in the literature showed that approximately 75%–100% of the patients with NPC had elevated IgA VCA levels (Tam 1999). On the other hand, the IgA antibody to the early antigen (EA) has a high specificity and a raised titer almost certainly indicated the presence of NPC. However, it is a much less sensitive test when compared with IgA VCA. In some circumstances, the IgA EA titer may return to a normal level during the later phase of the disease process. These tests are particularly useful to physicians managing NPC in endemic area because raised titers of the antibodies will raise the suspicion of the presence of NPC. In patients with an apparently normal clinical examination but with raised titers of IgA antibodies to VCA and EA, further detailed examination of nasopharynx is warranted to avoid a missed diagnosis of NPC.

4.7 Algorithm of a Standardized Diagnostic Procedure

In patients suspected to have NPC, a thorough examination of the posterior nasal space, along with a complete physical examination including a neck examination, should be the initial step. In patients with an obvious NPC, endoscopically guided biopsy under local anesthesia should be performed to obtain tissue for definitive diagnosis. If the biopsy does not yield a pathologic diagnosis, a repeat biopsy under local anesthesia or deep biopsies/curettage under general anesthesia would be necessary. In patients with suspicious clinical features such as unilateral serous otitis media, persistently elevated IgA to EBV, impairment of V and VI nerve function, or suspicious skull base lesion on diagnostic imaging, but with a normal looking nasopharynx, endoscopically guided biopsies of the nasopharynx including bilateral fossae of Rosenmüller and the superior/posterior wall under local anesthesia should be performed. If the first biopsy does not yield the diagnosis, a repeat biopsy under local anesthesia or deep biopsies/curettage under general anesthesia is recommended. In patients who have suspected NPC with cervical adenopathy but with a normal nasopharynx, pathologic diagnosis can be obtained from one of the enlarged cervical nodes using fine needle aspiration. If squamous cell carcinoma or undifferentiated carcinoma is confirmed, endoscopically guided biopsies of the nasopharynx under local anesthesia or deep biopsies/curettage of the nasopharynx under general anesthesia should be performed. Figure 4.4 summarizes the diagnostic algorithm.

4.8 Summary

Nasopharyngeal carcinoma (NPC) is uncommon in most parts of the world and often presents a diagnostic challenge to physicians who have limited

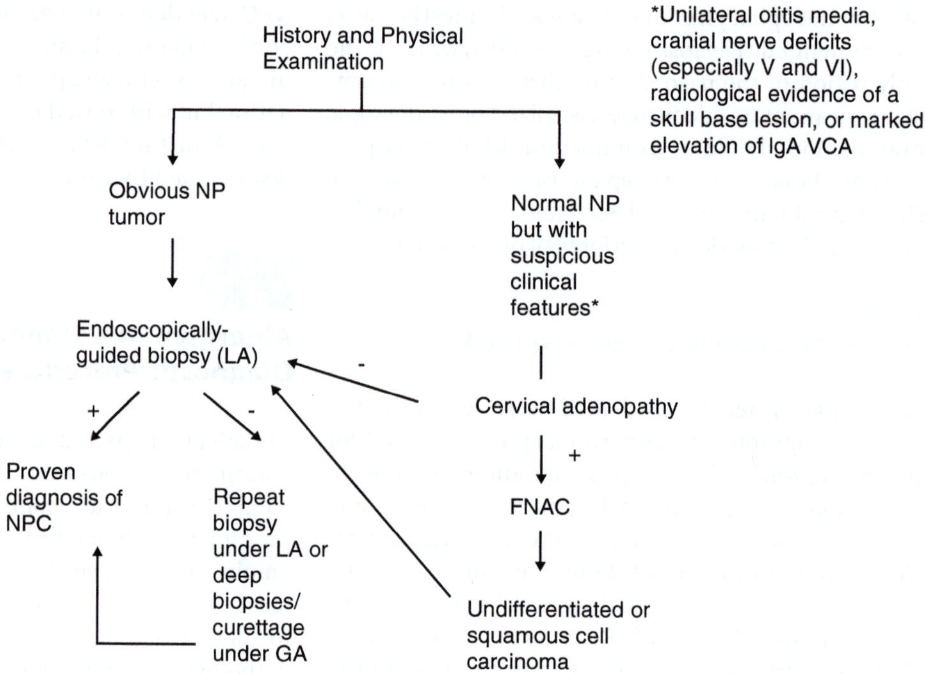

Fig. 4.4. Diagnostic algorithm for NPC

experience with this disease. As the prognosis of NPC is dependent on the stage of the disease, a timely diagnosis leading to appropriate treatment is crucial. An awareness of the presenting symptoms and signs of NPC and a high index of suspicion in individuals with high risk of developing NPC are necessary for a prompt diagnosis. Secondary to its lack of natural barriers to tumor invasion and its proximity to various critical structures, NPC can exhibit multiple routes of spread leading to different combinations of clinical manifestation. A good understanding of the routes of spread of NPC is crucial in the management of this disease because radiotherapy is the mainstay of treatment and an accurate target delineation is important to avoid a geographic miss, especially in the modern radiotherapy era, where highly conformal techniques are often used.

References

Ahmad A, Stefani S (1986) Distant metastases of nasopharyngeal carcinoma: a study of 256 male patients. J Surg Oncol 33: 194–197

Bedwinek JM, Perez CA, Keys DJ (1980) Analysis of failures after definitive irradiation for epidermoid carcinoma of the nasopharynx. Cancer 45: 2725–2729

Chang JT, Lin CY, Chen TM, et al (2005) Nasopharyngeal carcinoma with cranial nerve palsy: the importance of MRI for radiotherapy. Int J Radiat Oncol Biol Phys 63: 1354–1360

Chu AM, Flynn MB, Achino E, et al (1984) Irradiation of nasopharyngeal carcinoma: correlations with treatment factors and stage. Int J Radiat Oncol Biol Phys 10: 2241–2249

Gao Y, Zhu G, Lu JJ, et al (2009) Is prophylactic irradiation to the lower neck necessary for nasopharyngeal cancer patients with N0 disease? Int J Radiat Oncol Biol Phys

Heng DM, Wee J, Fong KW, et al (1999) Prognostic factors in 677 patients in Singapore with nondisseminated nasopharyngeal carcinoma. Cancer 86: 1912–1920

Ho JH (1970) The natural history and treatment of nasopharyngeal carcinoma (NPC). In: Lee-Clark R (ed) Oncology, yearbook (Proceedings of the tenth International Cancer Congress, Chicago), pp 1–14

Hoppe RT, Goffinet DR, Bagshaw MA (1976) Carcinoma of the nasopharynx. Eighteen years' experience with megavoltage radiation therapy. Cancer 37: 2605–2612

Lee AW, Foo W, Law CK, et al (1996a) N-staging of nasopharyngeal carcinoma: discrepancy between UICC/AJCC and Ho systems. Union Internationale Contre le Cancer. American Joint Committee for Cancer. Clin Oncol (R Coll Radiol) 8: 155–159

Lee AW, Foo W, Poon YF, et al (1996b) Staging of nasopharyngeal carcinoma: evaluation of N-staging by Ho and UICC/AJCC systems. Union Internationale Contre le Cancer. American Joint Committee for Cancer. Clin Oncol (R Coll Radiol) 8: 146–154

Lee AW, Poon YF, Foo W, et al (1992) Retrospective analysis of 5037 patients with nasopharyngeal carcinoma treated during 1976–1985: overall survival and patterns of failure. Int J Radiat Oncol Biol Phys 23: 261–270

Lee N, Fu KK (2004) Cancer of the nasopharynx. In: Leibel SA, Phillips TL (eds) Textbook of radiation oncology. Saunders, Philadelphia, pp 579–600

Leung SF, Tsao SY, Teo P, et al (1990) Cranial nerve involvement by nasopharyngeal carcinoma: response to treatment and clinical significance. Clin Oncol (R Coll Radiol) 2: 138–141

Li JC, Mayr NA, Yuh WT, et al (2006) Cranial nerve involvement in nasopharyngeal carcinoma: response to radiotherapy and its clinical impact. Ann Otol Rhinol Laryngol 115: 340–345

Lindberg R (1972) Distribution of cervical lymph node metastases from squamous cell carcinoma of the upper respiratory and digestive tracts. Cancer 29: 1446–1449

Mao YP, Liang SB, Liu LZ, et al (2008) The N staging system in nasopharyngeal carcinoma with radiation therapy oncology group guidelines for lymph node levels based on magnetic resonance imaging. Clin Cancer Res 14: 7497–7503

Moench HC, Phillips TL (1972) Carcinoma of the nasopharynx. Review of 146 patients with emphasis on radiation dose and time factors. Am J Surg 124: 515–518

Ng SH, Chang JT, Chan SC, et al (2004) Nodal metastases of nasopharyngeal carcinoma: patterns of disease on MRI and FDG PET. Eur J Nucl Med Mol Imaging 31: 1073–1080

Perez CA, Devineni VR, Marcial-Vega V, et al (1992) Carcinoma of the nasopharynx: factors affecting prognosis. Int J Radiat Oncol Biol Phys 23: 271–280

Sanguineti G, Geara FB, Garden AS, et al (1997) Carcinoma of the nasopharynx treated by radiotherapy alone: determinants of local and regional control. Int J Radiat Oncol Biol Phys 37: 985–996

Sham JS, Cheung YK, Choy D, et al (1991) Cranial nerve involvement and base of the skull erosion in nasopharyngeal carcinoma. Cancer 68: 422–426

Sham JS, Choy D, Wei WI (1990) Nasopharyngeal carcinoma: orderly neck node spread. Int J Radiat Oncol Biol Phys 19: 929–933

Skinner DW, Van Hasselt CA, Tsao SY (1991) Nasopharyngeal carcinoma: modes of presentation. Ann Otol Rhinol Laryngol 100: 544–551

Stanley RE, Fong KW (1997) Clinical presentation and diagnosis. In: Chong VF (ed) Nasopharyngeal carcinoma. Armour, Singapore, pp 29–41

Tam JS (1999) Epstein–Barr virus serological markers. In: van Hasselt CA, Gibb AG (eds) Nasophryngeal carcinoma. The Chinese University of Hong Kong Press && Greenwich Medical Media, Hong Kong, pp 161–176

Tang L, Mao Y, Liu L, et al (2009) The volume to be irradiated during selective neck irradiation in nasopharyngeal carcinoma: analysis of the spread patterns in lymph nodes by magnetic resonance imaging. Cancer 115: 680–688

Teo P, Shiu W, Leung SF, et al (1992) Prognostic factors in nasopharyngeal carcinoma investigated by computer tomography – an analysis of 659 patients. Radiother Oncol 23: 79–93

Teo P, Tai TH, Choy D (1989) Nasopharyngeal carcinoma with dermatomyositis. Int J Radiat Oncol Biol Phys 16: 471–474

Teo PM, Leung SF, Yu P, et al (1991a) A comparison of Ho's, International Union Against Cancer, and American Joint Committee stage classifications for nasopharyngeal carcinoma. Cancer 67: 434–439

Teo PM, Tsao SY, Ho JH, et al (1991b) A proposed modification of the Ho stage-classification for nasopharyngeal carcinoma. Radiother Oncol 21: 11–23

Turgut M, Erturk O, Saygi S, et al (1998) Importance of cranial nerve involvement in nasopharyngeal carcinoma. A clinical study comprising 124 cases with special reference to clinical presentation and prognosis. Neurosurg Rev 21: 243–248

Woo JK (1999) Clinical Diagnosis. In: van Hasselt CA, Gibb AG (eds) Nasophryngeal carcinoma. The Chinese University of Hong Kong Press & Greenwich Medical Media, Hong Kong, pp 111–125

Screening and Early Diagnosis of Nasopharyngeal Carcinoma

5

Pei-Jen Lou, Wan-Lun Hsu, Yin-Chu Chien, and Chien-Jen Chen

CONTENTS

Pei-Jen Lou, MD, PhD
Department of Otolaryngology, College of Medicine, National Taiwan University, Taipei 100, Taiwan, ROC
Wan-Lun Hsu, PhD
Yin-Chu Chien, PhD
Chien-Jen Chen, ScD
Genomics Research Center, Academia Sinica, Academia Road Section 2, Nankang, Taipei 115, Taiwan, ROC

5.1 Introduction

Nasopharyngeal carcinoma (NPC) is a relatively rare disease in most parts of the world, but is the most commonly diagnosed head and neck cancer in certain regions of Southeast Asia. The age-standardized incidence rate is less than 1 per 100,000 persons per year for either gender worldwide, while the annual incidence in southern China and Southeast Asia approaches 20 per 100,000 persons. In most populations, the age-standardized annual incidence rate of NPC is higher in males than in females. The male-to-female ratio is around 2–3:1 in high- and moderate-risk areas. Although it has been reported in NPC patients ranging from 4 to 91 years of age in various countries, it is uncommon under the age of 20 years (<1%). More than 80% of patients were diagnosed between 30 and 59 years of age. In high-risk areas such as Hong Kong, the NPC incidence in both genders rises sharply after the age of 20, reaching a plateau between 40 and 60 years of age. Otherwise, the age distribution curves rise late in moderate- and low-risk areas.

According to the World Health Organization International Histological Classification of Tumors, NPC are classified into three classes: keratinizing carcinoma, differentiated nonkeratinizing carcinoma, and undifferentiated carcinoma. Most NPC diagnosed in the high-risk areas belong to the second and third groups. As NPC is highly sensitive to radiation therapy and chemoradiotherapy, it has a relatively good prognosis compared to other types of malignancies, especially when the disease is diagnosed at an earlier stage.

Epstein–Barr virus (EBV) was classified by the International Agency for Cancer Research (IARC) as a Class I carcinogen for NPC in 1997; however, EBV alone is not sufficient to cause NPC. NPC has a multifactorial etiology involving viral, genetic, and environmental factors, and other genetic and environmental cofactors also play contributory roles in the development of NPC. Results from published literatures indicated that dietary intake of nitrite and nitrosamine, especially in Cantonese salted fish and preserved foods, occupational exposures to wood dust and formaldehyde, familial tendency, and host genetic susceptibilities are significantly associated with an increased risk of NPC (Chien and Chen, 2003). Therefore, certain subgroups of population might be at higher risk for NPC, and screening of NPC in those patients may be of value to improve patients' prognoses by early detection. The aim of this chapter is to discuss the tumor markers that are clinically relevant to NPC and their potential use in screening and early diagnosis.

5.2 Potential Advantage of Early Diagnosis

The relative survival rate for NPC at 1 year in endemic regions such as Taiwan after conventional radiation therapy was 89% for males and 91% for females in 2002; the rate at 5 years was 63% for males and 68% for females (http://crs.cph.ntu.edu.tw). With the utilization of intensity-modulated radiation therapy, the long-term survival rate of 90% for early-stage NPC has been reported (Lee et al. 2002; Lin et al. 2009). In addition to gender, age is also an important predictor of NPC prognosis. The older the age at the diagnosis of NPC, the lower was the relative survival rate. Patients affected with keratinizing squamous cell carcinoma have poorer prognosis than those affected with differentiated nonkeratinizing carcinoma, and undifferentiated carcinoma.

NPC relatively has an overall good prognosis compared to other types of human cancer. Radiation is the standard therapeutic modality for NPC, and radiation alone is usually sufficient for patients in early-stage NPC. Stage is one of the most important prognostic predictor of NPC (Fleming et al. 1997). Although combined chemoradiation therapy can substantially improve the treatment outcome of locoregionally advanced NPC, the overall prognosis of patients, especially disease-free survival, metastasis-free survival, and overall survival are usually better in patients diagnosed and treated in earlier stages.

There is a striking difference in prognosis between NPC at early and late stages; therefore, early diagnosis is considered a key factor to assure the good prognosis of NPC.

5.3 Screening of NPC by Epstein–Barr Virus Seromarkers

The association of EBV and NPC has been demonstrated for decades. Through salivary infection, resting memory B-cells are thought to be the site of persistence of EBV within the body. EBV-associated diseases generally show viral gene expression limited to three patterns of latency. Latency II was first recognized in a proportion of NPC, and is also common in most EBV-carrying non-B-cell tumors and Hodgkin's disease. In this latent type, expression of EBV-encoded RNA (*EBER*), *LMP1*, *LMP 2*, and *EBNA1* was detected (IARC 1997; Baumforth et al. 1999; Niedobitek 2000; Raab-Traub 2002). *EBNA1* and *EBER* genes were found to be expressed in all EBV-positive NPCs, and *LMP1* was present in up to 65% of NPCs (Young et al. 1988; Niedobitek et al. 1992). Associations with NPC development for *EBNA1, LMP1, and LMP2* were also observed in other studies. (Brooks et al. 1992; Busson et al. 1992; Lennette et al. 1995; Lin et al. 2001).

5.3.1 Anti-EBV Antibodies for the Early Detection and Prognostic Prediction of NPC

After wide application of molecular biological approaches, it has been demonstrated that EBV is harbored in almost every NPC tumor, irrespective of histological differentiation or geographical distribution (Chang et al. 1990, Chen et al. 1993, Wu et al. 1991, Lung and Chang, 1992). A variety of methods have been used to detect various antibodies against EBV antigens (anti-EBV) in patients with the disease (Gratama and Ernberg 1995, Cohen 2000). Numerous studies have documented the utility of anti-EBV antibodies for the early detection and prognostic prediction of NPC. The anti-EBV antibodies frequently studied include IgA antibodies against EBV capsid antigen (anti-EBV VCA IgA), antibodies against EBV DNase (anti-EBV DNase), antibodies against nuclear antigen-1 (anti-EBNA1), and antibodies against early antigen (anti-EBV EA) (de-The et al. 1975; Wara et al. 1975; Henle and Henle 1976; Lynn et al. 1976; Lin et al. 1977; Lanier et al. 1981; Zeng et al. 1982; Chen et al. 1987, 1989; De-Vathaire et al. 1988). Based on the findings of several case-control studies in which a significantly increased seropositive prevalence of anti-EBV seromarkers was consistently observed in NPC cases than unaffected controls, EBV was classified by the IARC as a Class I carcinogen for NPC in 1997. There have been several case-control and cohort studies on the association between EBV and NPC since then.

5.3.2 Discovery of Circulating EBV DNA and mRNA in NPC Patients

Since EBV DNA is identified in the tumor cells of tissue samples, it is reasonable to speculate that these DNA could be detected in the circulation of NPC patients. Mutirangura et al. (1998) showed that circulating extracellular EBV DNA could be detected in the sera of 31% (13/42) of NPC patients by PCR amplification of the *EBNA-2*. All the 82 controls were seronegative for EBV DNA. The detection rate was further improved by the same group using a modified nested PCR approach. The EBV DNA (*EBNA-2*) was detected in plasma/serum of 98 of 167 (59%) NPC patients and 10 of 77 (13%) samples derived from healthy blood donors (Shotelersuk et al. 2000). Hsiao et al. (2002) used similar PCR approach to detect EBV DNA (*EBNA-1*) from sera of NPC patients, and the seropositive rate increased from 39% to 75% through increasing the number of PCR cycles from 35 to 50. The major drawback of these studies that use PCR and gel electrophoresis assays is that the test *per se* is only qualitative and provides no quantitative information. Thus, the detection rates were highly variable in both NPC patients and healthy controls among these studies.

Lo et al. (1999b) developed a real-time quantitative PCR assay for the detection of EBV DNA in the plasma of NPC patients. Cell-free EBV DNA (*Bam* HI-W and *EBNA-1*) was detectable in the plasma of 96% (55 of 57) of NPC patients and 7% (3 of 43) of controls. The EBV DNA concentrations were positively correlated with the clinical staging of the NPC patients. Advanced-stage NPC patients had higher plasma EBV DNA levels than those with early-stage disease. At 1 month after completion of radiotherapy, plasma EBV DNA was undetectable in 7 of 15 subjects (47%). These findings suggest that the concentration of circulating EBV DNA may reflect the tumor load in NPC patients, and that quantitative analysis of plasma EBV DNA may be a useful tool in the screening and monitoring of NPC patients. Compared to the gel electrophoresis assay, real-time quantification using fluorescence detection appears to be a more sensitive method in the detection of circulating EBV DNA. This quantitative assay also has the advantage of greater flexibility because the threshold of EBV DNA can be adjusted to optimize the sensitivity and specificity required for a particular diagnosis or monitoring purpose (Chan and Lo 2002).

Following the discovery of EBV DNA in the circulation of NPC patients, Lo et al. (1999a) demonstrated that EBV RNA could also be detected in the plasma of NPC patients. *EBER-1* mRNA was detectable in the plasma of 88% of NPC patients and 21% of healthy controls. Given that the RNase is identified in the blood of both healthy individuals and cancer patients (Reddi and Holland 1976), the presence of EBV RNA in the plasma of NPC patients is an interesting finding and the mechanism by which EBV RNA escapes from RNase digestion still awaits elucidation.

5.3.3 Case-Control Studies on NPC and Anti-EBV Seromarkers

The association between EBV seromarkers and NPC has been reported in several case-control studies since 1997. In a cross-sectional case-control study of 139 NPC patients and 178 healthy controls in Hong Kong (Leung et al. 2004), the seroprevalence of anti-EBV VCA IgA was 81% for NPC patients and 4% for healthy controls, showing a relative risk as high as 400. Patients affected with Stage III and IV NPC had higher seroprevalence than those with Stage I and II NPC. In another cross-sectional case-control study of 124 NPC patients (93 pretreatment, 13 relapsed, and 18 in remission) and 40 controls in Hong Kong (Fan et al. 2004), the seroprevalence of anti-EBV EA IgA was 73% for untreated NPC patients, 88% for relapsed NPC patients, 44% for remission patients, and 0% for health controls. The seroprevalence of anti-EBV EA IgG was 93% for untreated NPC patients, 88% for relapsed NPC patients, 94% for remission patients, and 40% for health controls.

In the other cross-sectional case-control study of 314 NPC patients, 244 hospital controls and 263 community controls in Taiwan (Chen et al. 2001), the seroprevalence of anti-EBNA-1 was 78.7%, 11.5%, and 3.8%, respectively, for these three groups. The anti-EBV VCA IgA seroprevalence was 77.1% for NPC cases and 5.1% for community controls, while the anti-EBV DNase seroprevalence was 84.5% for NPC cases and 11.7% for community controls. The crude relative risk comparing NPC cases and community controls was 176, 63, and 41, respectively, for anti-EBNA-1, anti-EBV VCA IgA, and anti-EBV DNase.

5.3.4 Case-Control Studies on NPC and EBV DNA in Serum

Several recent studies have compared EBV DNA in serum/plasma samples of NPC patients and their controls. In a cross-sectional case-control study of 42 NPC patients and 82 normal controls in Thailand (Mutirangura et al. 1998), the seroprevalence of EBV DNA (*EBNA*-2) was 31% for NPC patients and 0% for healthy controls. In another cross-sectional case-control study of 57 NPC patients and 43 family controls in Hong Kong (Lo et al. 1999b), seroprevalence of EBV DNA (*Bam* HI-W and *EBNA*-1) was 96% for cases and 7% (3/43) for controls. In the other cross-sectional case-control study of 139 NPC patients and 178 healthy controls in Hong Kong (Leung et al. 2004), the seroprevalence of EBV DNA was 95% for NPC patients and 2% for healthy controls showing a crude relative risk of 180.

In a cross-sectional case-control study of 99 patients with advanced NPC, 20 cured NPC patients and 40 healthy controls in Taiwan (Lin et al. 2004), the seroprevalence of EBV DNA (*Bam* HI-W) was 94% for advanced NPC patients and 0% for cured NPC patients and healthy controls. The more advanced the NPC stage, the higher the plasma levels of EBV DNA. In another cross-sectional case-control study of 124 NPC patients (93 pretreatment, 13 relapsed, and 18 in remission) and 40 controls in Hong Kong (Fan et al. 2004), the seroprevalence of EBV DNA was 69% for untreated NPC patients, 85% for relapsed NPC patients, 0% for remission patients, and 2.5% for healthy controls. The more advanced the NPC stage, the higher the positive prevalence and the mean level of EBV DNA.

5.3.5 Cohort Studies on NPC and Anti-EBV Seromarkers

In a 13-year follow-up study of 9,699 men in Taiwan (Chien et al. 2001), both anti-EBV VCA IgA and anti-EBV DNase tested at study entry were significantly associated with the risk of NPC developed during the follow-up. After adjustment for age and family NPC history, the relative risk (95% CI) of developing NPC was 22.0 (7.3–66.9) for anti-EBV VCA IgA-seropositivity and 3.5 (1.4–8.7) for anti-EBV DNase-seropositivity. Compared with those who were seronegative for both anti-EBV markers as the reference group, the adjusted relative risk (95% CI) was 32.8 (7.3–147.2) for those who were seropositive for both anti-EBV markers. In another cohort study of 3,093 anti-EBV VCA IgA-seropositive and 38,955 seronegative participants in southern China (Ji et al. 2007), seropositivity of anti-EBV VCA IgA was associated with an increased risk of NPC during follow-up, showing a crude relative risk of 9.4. However, the schedule and method for follow-up and NPC ascertainment were different between anti-EBV- seropositives and seronegatives.

5.3.6 Sensitivity and Specificity of EBV Seromarkers for NPC Screening

Anti-EBV VCA IgA was reported to be a sensitive and specific seromarker for the screening of NPC in endemic areas like Taiwan (Zeng et al. 1982, 1983, 1985). The sensitivity and specificity of EBV seromarkers for the screening of NPC in studies published after 1997 are shown in Table 5.1. Both the sensitivity and specificity vary by seromarker type, laboratory method, cutoff point, geographical area, NPC stage, and control group. The sensitivity of anti-EBV VCA IgA (FA test) and anti-EBV DNase (ELISA test) for the screening of NPC in Taiwan was 74 and 72%, respectively (Liu et al. 1997). The combination of these two seromarkers increased the sensitivity to 88%. In another study in Taiwan (Hsu et al. 2001), the combination of IgA antibodies against EBV EA and EBNA1 (ELISA test) had the sensitivity and specificity of 98%, and 82%, respectively.

In a study comparing the sensitivity and specificity for NPC screening among anti-EBV Rta, anti-EBV VCA IgA, and anti-EBV EA IgA in Singapore (Feng et al. 2001), the sensitivity was highest for anti-EBV EA IgA (96%) and the specificity was highest for anti-EBV VCA IgA (98%). However, another study comparing the sensitivity and specificity for NPC screening among anti-EBV TK, anti-EBV VCA IgA, and anti-EBV EA IgA in China (Connolly et al. 2001), anti-EBV TK had the highest sensitivity (96%) and both anti-EBV VCA IgA and anti-EBV EA IgA had higher specificity (98%). In another study in China (Cheng et al. 2002), the combination of anti-EBNA1 IgA, anti-EBNA1 IgG, and anti-EBV Zta IgA using ELISA method had a sensitivity of 92% and a specificity of 93% when any two seropositivity was used as the cutoff point.

The sensitivity of anti-EBV VCA IgA and anti-EBV EA IgA was found to vary more than the respective specificity when different cutoff points were used (Tsang et al. 2004). The sensitivity and specificity of anti-EBV VCA IgA and anti-EBV EA IgA were found to vary by laboratory methods. The specificity of anti-EBV VCA IgA was higher by using the ELISA test than the FA test, while the sensitivity of anti-EBV EA IgA was lower by using the ELISA test than the FA test for NPC screening. Recently, Chang et al. (2008) reported the anti-EBV EA/EBNA1 (ELISA) had the best sensitivity of 94% and EBV DNA in serum had the best specificity of 97% among three EBV seromarkers including anti-EBV VCA IgA (FA), anti-EBV EA/EBNA1m, and EBV DNA. The area under ROC curve (AUC) was best for anti-EBV EA/EBNA1.

The sensitivity and specificity of DNA-based and antibody-based assays in the diagnosis of NPC have been compared in several studies. Chan et al. (2003) reported the highest sensitivity of 93% for anti-EBV VCA IgA and the highest specificity of 97% for anti-EBV EA IgA for the screening of NPC in Hong Kong among four anti-EBV seromarkers against VCA (IgA), EA (IgA), EBNA1 (IgA), and Zta (IgG). The sensitivity and specificity of EBV DNA in serum were 75 and 98%, respectively, in this study. On the other hand, another study in Hong Kong (Leung et al. 2004) showed the EBV DNA had a better sensitivity (95%) and a similar specificity (96%) for the NPC screening than anti-EBV VCA IgA (sensitivity 81 and specificity 98%). However, in a study in China, the sensitivity for NPC screening was not different between anti-EBV VCA IgA and EBV DNA in serum (both around 96%), but with a better specificity for EBV DNA in serum (89%) than anti-EBV VCA IgA (85%) (Shao et al. 2004).

5.4 Screening for Family Members of Patients with NPC

It has been observed that individuals with a family history of NPC are at a higher risk of developing the disease (Williams and de The 1974). Screening for family members of patients with NPC may provide an opportunity for early detection and thus improve the outcome of the subjects who are at high risk of developing NPC. Ng et al. (2005) screened 929 family members of NPC with EBV seromarkers (anti-EBV VCA IgA and anti-EBNA-1 IgA), physical examination (to exclude cervical lymphadenopathy and cranial nerve palsy), and endoscopic examination of the nasopharyngeal region. Twelve cases of NPC were identified, of whom 5 (41%) had Stage I disease (note that only 2% of patients referred for primary treatment presented with such early disease), during a median follow-up of 29 months. Based on the initial serology results, the sensitivity and specificity of EBV serology was 75% and 92%, respectively. There is a supplementary role for the use of routine endoscopy: one additional case of NPC with negative EBV serology was diagnosed among the 12 diseased patients. On the other hand, the DNA-based assays have not been tested in this setting.

Taken together, results from earlier studies suggest that both EBV DNA and anti-EBV antibodies are sensitive markers in the screening and diagnosis of NPC. However, the validity for prediction of NPC using multiple seromarkers has not been extensively investigated partly due to the lack of longitudinal follow-up data, and also because only one or two seromarkers have been examined in most of the earlier studies. Further evaluation of this topic is warranted in larger studies or those with longer follow-up to better define the specific performance characteristics of using repeated screening for specific EBV markers for NPC prediction. Feasibility and cost-effectiveness of using these seromarkers in EBV screening programs aimed at the prevention of NPC in endemic areas also require evaluation.

5.5 Clinical Methods for Screening and Early Diagnosis of NPC

The majority of NPCs arise in the lateral walls, especially from the fossa of Rosenmüller and Eustachian cushions. Few initial symptoms are directly referable to NPC. Neck mass, blood tinged sputum and/or rhinorrhea are common clinical presentations. Sometimes the tumor can present a variety of local, regional, and distant signs and symptoms, such as nasal symptoms (nasal obstruction, and increasing nasal discharge), aural symptoms (tinnitus, stuffiness, and hearing loss), headache, facial pain or paresthesia, diplopia, and weight loss. The nasopharynx

Table 5.1. Sensitivity and specificity of various Epstein–Barr virus seromarkers for the screening of nasopharyngeal carcinoma

Author and year	Area	Case and controls	Method	Result
Chang et al. (2008)	Taiwan	156 NPC patients 264 healthy volunteers 97 patients of head and neck squamous cell carcinomas (HNSCC)	VCA IgA (FA) EA/EBNA1 (ELISA) EBV DNA (PCR)	VCA IgA (1:40) Sen: 86% Spe: 86% (controls) 84% (HNSCC) AUC: 0.89 (controls) 0.88 (HNSCC) EA/EBNA1 (≥3.0 (EU/ml)) Sen: 94% Spe: 83% (controls) 89% (HNSCC) AUC: 0.95 (controls) 0.96 (HNSCC) DNA (>0/ml) Sen: 81% Spe: 97% (controls) AUC: 0.90 (controls)
Tang et al. (2007)	Hong Kong	163 NPC patients 98 medical students	VCA IgA (ELISA, commercial FA, IN-house FA) EA IgA (ELISA, commercial FA, IN-house FA)	VCA IgA (ELISA) Sen: 93% Spe: 95% AUC: 0.98 VCA IgA (commercial FA) Sen: 97% Spe: 42% AUC: 0.95 VCA IgA (in-house FA) Sen: 98% Spe: 72% AUC: 0.97 EA IgA (ELISA) Sen: 47% Spe: 100% AUC: 0.85 EA IgA (commercial FA) Sen: 77% Spe: 100% AUC: 0.89 EA IgA (in-house FA) Sen: 78% Spe: 99% AUC: 0.89
Tsang et al. (2004)	Hong-Kong	215 NPC patients 448 nonNPC patients	VCA IgA (FA) EA IgA (FA)	VCA IgA Sen Spe 1:5 89% 80% 1:10 83% 89% 1:20 82% 91% EA IgA Sen Spe 1:5 63% 97% 1:10 61% 98% 1:20 56% 99%
Shao et al. (2004)	China	120 primary NPC cases 8 locally recurrent NPC cases 21 metastatic NPC cases 47 healthy controls 38 nonNPC tumor patients	VCA IgA (ELISA) EBV DNA (PCR)	VCA IgA DNA Primary NPC 96% 96% Recurrent NPC 100% 100% Metastatic NPC 100% 100% Normal controls 15% 11% NonNPC tumor 21% 13%

Table 5.1. (cont.) Sensitivity and specificity of various antibodies against Epstein–Barr virus for screening of nasopharyngeal carcinoma

Author and year	Area	Case and controls	Method	Result
LEUNG et al. (2004)	Hong-Kong	139 NPC cases 178 healthy controls	VCA IgA (FA) EBV DNA (PCR)	VCA IgA Sen: 81% Spe: 98% DNA (≥60 copies/ml) Sen: 95% Spe: 96% Combined marker panel: Sen: 99%
CHAN et al. (2003)	Hong-Kong	218 samples 51 NPC + 4 LELC of the lung 23 other cancer + 140 did not have tumor	VCA IgA (FA) EA IgA (FA) EBNA1 IgA (ELISA) Zta IgG (ELISA) EBV DNA (PCR)	VCA IgA (1:40) Sen: 93% Spe: 60% EA IgA (1:10) Sen: 73% Spe: 97% EBNA1 IgA Sen: 84% Spe: 87% Zta IgG Sen: 75% Spe: 83% DNA Sen: 76% Spe: 98%
CHENG et al. (2002)	Hong-Kong and Zhongshan	121 NPC cases 332 healthy controls	EBNA1 IgG (ELISA) EBNA1 IgA (ELISA) Zta IgG (ELISA) VCA IgA (FA)	EBNA IgG Sen: 83% Spe: 86% EBNA IgA Sen: 85% Spe: 86% Zta IgG Sen: 79% Spe: 80% VCA IgA (1:10) Sen: 93% Spe: 87% 3 ELISA combined (any two seropositivity) Sen: 92% Spe: 93%
CONNOLLY et al. (2001)	China	52 NPC cases 52 nonNPC patients matched by age and gender	TK(ELISA) VCA IgA (FA) EA IgA (FA)	TK Sen: 96% Spe: 96% VCA IgA Sen: 85% Spe: 98% EA IgA Sen: 72% Spe: 98%
FENG et al. (2001)	Singapore	51 NPC cases 115 nonNPC ENT controls	Rta (ELISA) VCA IgA (FA) EA IgA (FA)	Rta Sen: 82% Spe: 85% VCA IgA Sen: 84% Spe:98% EA IgA Sen: 96% Spe: 69%
HSU et al. (2001)	Taiwan	123 NPC cases 149 nonNPC ENT contorls	VCA IgA (FA) VCA IgG (FA) EA IgA (FA) EA IgG (FA) EA + EBNA1 IgA (ELISA)	VCA IgA Sen: 87% Spe: 81% VCA IgG Sen: 85% Spe: 54% EA IgA Sen: 58% Spe: 94% EA IgG Sen: 70% Spe: 78% EA + EBNA1 Sen: 98% Spe: 82%
LIU et al. (1997)	Taiwan	100 NPC outpatients 7 pre-NPC patients	VCA IgA (FA) DNAse (NT and ELISA) MDBP (ELISA) DP (NT)	NPC pre-NPC VCA 74% 71% DNase (NT) 72% 86% DNase (ELISA) 82% 86% MDBP 82% 57% DP 71% 86%

Sen Sensitivity; *Spe* specificity; *AUC* area under ROC curve; *FA* Fluorescence assay; *ELISA* enzyme-linked immunosorbant assay; *NT* neutralization test; *PCR* polymerase chain reaction has abundant supply of regional lymphatic vessels, so metastasis is frequently found in NPC rather than in other head-and-neck cancers. Any type of NPC most commonly metastasizes to regional lymph nodes. Cervical lymphadenopathy is often the only clinical manifestation of NPC patients. The usual sites of distant metastasis are bone, lung, and liver. Metastasis to the brain, breast, or other parts of the body is occasionally found.

5.5.1 Early Symptoms

For early diagnosis of NPC, it is important to recognize the early symptoms of this disease. Discussion on symptoms from NPC and their implication to the diagnosis has been presented in the previous chapter. Therefore, only symptoms related to early diagnosis and screening is detailed here.

The nasopharynx is situated at the skull base with close proximity to the surrounding head and neck spaces. It is a clinical blind spot in many aspects. Tumors arising here may masquerade their symptoms to regions other than the primary site. The marked invasive and metastatic powers of the NPC are responsible for the symptomatology. Most patients have multiple symptoms which are insidious at the onset, and are sometimes disregarded by the patients and doctors. This has often led to delayed diagnosis and treatment. However, in endemic areas, patients with the following symptoms should be presumed to have NPC, until proven otherwise.

Blood-stained rhinorrhea or saliva. Blood-stained nasal mucus and/or saliva on hawking are frequently encountered as an early symptom of NPC. Epistaxis, on the other hand, is more commonly seen in advanced NPC.

Tinnitus and aural symptoms. Unilateral tinnitus, aural stuffiness, and mild hearing loss that are caused by serous otitis media are not an uncommon presentation of NPC. These symptoms are related to the dysfunctional Eustachian tube due to peritubal tumor infiltration.

Painless neck lumps. NPC has a tendency for early lymphatic spread. Statistically, cervical lymphadenopathy is the most frequent presenting symptom of NPC by many centers. The lateral retropharyngeal lymph node (of Röuviere) is the first lymphatic filter, but is not palpable. The first common palpable node is the jugulodigastric node under the sternocleidomastoideus muscle.

Headache, neurological symptoms such as diplopia and facial numbness are also clinical symptoms of NPC, but are considered as late symptoms of the disease.

5.5.2 Nasopharyngeal Examination

Mirror examination is the quickest and most commonly used method to assess the nasopharynx. However, it is restricted by the pharyngeal reflex, patient cooperation, and inability to open the mouth. With the introduction of transnasal fiberoptic nasopharyngoscopes, close-up, end-on viewing of the nasopharynx becomes possible. Any tiny growth which escapes detection with routine mirror examination can be identified. Biopsy can also be performed under direct visual guidance. Care must be taken that the tumors in the early stage may be indistinguishable from the surrounding nasopharyngeal lymphoid tissues. This is especially true in young subjects whose adenoid tissues have not completely degenerated (Fig. 5.1). In some cases, tumors in early stage are so insignificant that they cannot even be identified by the nasopharyngoscope. In such cases, the vascular pattern in the nasopharynx becomes an important clue in assisting the diagnosis of NPC (Fig. 5.2). A gentle touch with a cotton stick may be

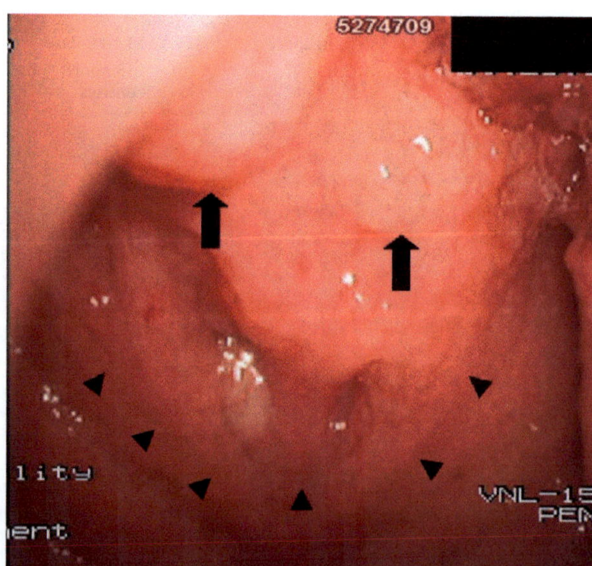

Fig. 5.1. Endoscopic view of a T1 tumor in the nasopharynx. *Arrowheads* indicate the normal adenoid tissue in the nasopharynx. *Arrows* indicate the tumor

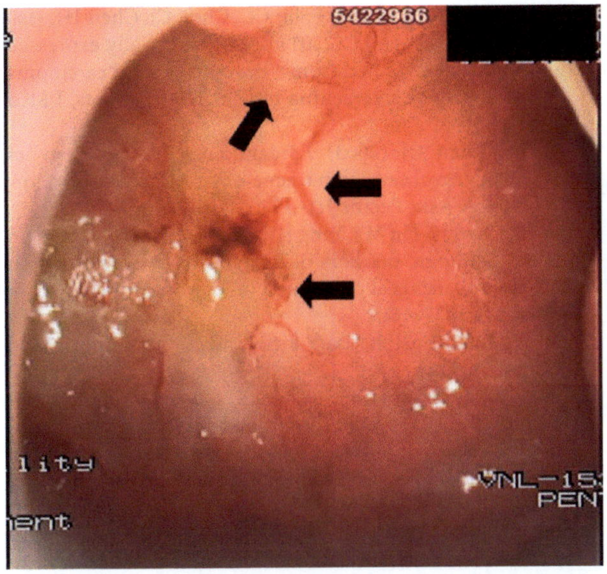

Fig. 5.2. Endoscopic view of an insignificant tumor in the nasopharynx. *Arrows* indicate the areas of hypervascularity with mild touch bleeding. Biopsy from the hypervascular areas confirmed the diagnosis of NPC

applied to the hypervascular areas. If there is any touch bleeding of these lesions, biopsies should be taken to rule out the possibility of NPC.

The diagnosis of NPC depends on the histological examination of tissue biopsies. Although endoscopic examination enables the clinicians to have direct visualization of the nasopharynx, and allows tissue biopsy for pathological diagnosis, this invasive procedure is not ideal for mass screening. In patients with relevant symptoms but without significant tumors in the nasopharynx, it is also difficult for the clinicians to decide which patient should receive biopsy. Efforts have been taken in the past decades to develop cheap, fast, and reliable methods to assist clinical decision making, and to facilitate mass screening in the community. Implementation of EBV DNA in nasal swab as a tumor marker for NPC is an important example.

5.5.3 Nasopharyngeal Swab for EBV DNA in the Screening of NPC

The EBV DNA can be identified in the nasopharyngeal swabs of NPC patients. Sheen et al. (1998) investigated the presence of EBV DNA (*Bam* HI-W) by PCR and gel electrophoresis in 133 different tissues from nasopharynx, nose, and sinus and found that EBV DNA was present in 91% (85/93) of NPC tissues and in 25% (10/40) of nonNPC tissues. Nasopharyngeal swabs were subsequently performed in 55 cases to check the presence of EBV DNA and to investigate the feasibility of using such approach in the screening of NPC patients. Anti-EBV VCA IgA and IgG serostatus were tested for comparison. EBV DNA was present in 87% (26/30) of NPC patients and 42% (8/19) of nonNPC controls. Its sensitivity (87%) and specificity (58%) were similar to those of anti-EBV seromarkers (88% and 44%). Lin et al. (2001) used a modified nasopharyngeal swab method to check the presence of EBV DNA (*LMP1*) in NPC patients by PCR and gel electrophoresis. There were 95% (36/38) of the NPC swab samples and none of 28 control samples positive for EBV DNA, showing a sensitivity of 95% and a specificity of 100%. Using nasopharyngeal swabs, NPC was diagnosed with a sensitivity of 87% and a specificity of 98% by detection of *LMP1* (Hao et al. 2003). The combination of EBV *LMP1* and *EBNA* could detect NPC with a sensitivity of 91% and a specificity of 98% (Hao et al. 2004). The combination of *VCA-BALF4* and *EBNA1* was found to have a sensitivity of 90% and a specificity of 93% (Hu et al. 2007).

The EBV DNA seems to be a good tumor marker for the diagnosis of NPC. For the benefit of further development in this field, the standardization of specimen collection, sample preparation protocol, target DNA region (*EBNA-1* or *Bam* HI-W or *LMP-1*), and assay methodology (PCR and gel electrophoresis or real-time quantitative PCR) is necessary. Furthermore, a well-designed large-scale epidemiologic study is needed to confirm the reliability and feasibility of EBV DNA in the screening and diagnosis of NPC.

5.6 Summary

Nasopharyngeal carcinoma (NPC) is a commonly diagnosed head and neck malignancy in Southeast Asia, and is associated with a number of potential causative factors. The EBV seromarkers and EBV DNA have been demonstrated to be associated with the presence of the malignancy.

NPC in its early stages are highly curable with radiation therapy, thus early diagnosis of the disease is critical for the malignancy. As individuals with a family history of NPC are at higher risk for the disease, screening for early diagnosis of the disease in high-risk group population may improve overall outcome after treatment. The EBV DNA seems to be a good tumor marker for early diagnosis of NPC, supplemented with physical (include endoscopic) examination. However, further investigation is needed to validate the findings in currently available research results and optimize the testing technique before clinical screening can be advocated for NPC in the endemic area.

References

Baumforth KR, Young LS, Flavell KJ, Constandinou C, Murray PG (1999) The Epstein-Barr virus and its association with human cancers. Mol Pathol 52:307–322

Brooks L, Yao QY, Rickinson AB, Young LS (1992) Epstein–Barr virus latent gene transcription in nasopharyngeal carcinoma cells: coexpression of EBNA1, LMP1, and LMP2 transcripts. J Virol 66:2689–2697

Busson P, McCoy R, Sadler R, Gilligan K, Tursz T, Raab-Traub N (1992) Consistent transcription of the Epstein–Barr virus LMP-2 gene in nasopharyngeal carcinoma. J Virol 66: 3257–3262

Chang KP, Hsu CL, Chang YL, Tsang NM, Chen CK, Lee TJ, Tsao KC, Huang CG, Chang YS, Yu JS, Hao SP (2008) Complementary serum test of antibodies to Epstein–Barr virus nuclear antigen-1 and early antigen: a possible alternative for primary screening of nasopharyngeal carcinoma. Oral Oncol 44:784–792

Chang YS, Tyan YS, Liu ST, Tsai MS, Pao CC (*1990*) Detection of Epstein–Barr virus DNA sequences in nasopharyngeal carcinoma cells by enzymatic DNA amplification. *J Clin Microbiol* 28:2398–2402

Chan KCA, Lo YMD (2002) Circulating EBV DNA as a tumor marker for nasopharyngeal carcinoma. Semin Cancer Biol 12:489–496

Chan KH, Gu YL, Ng F, Ng PS, Seto WH, Sham JS, Chua D, Wei W, Chen YL, Luk W, Zong YS, Ng MH (2003) EBV specific antibody-based and DNA-based assays in serologic diagnosis of nasopharyngeal carcinoma. Int J Cancer 105:706–709

Chen CL, Wen WN, Chen JY, Hsu MM, Hsu HC (*1993*) Detection of Epstein–Barr virus genome in nasopharyngeal carcinoma by in situ DNA hybridization. *Intervirology* 36:91–98

Cheng WM, Chan KH, Chen HL, Luo RX, Ng SP, Luk W, Zheng BJ, Ji MF, Liang JS, Sham JS, Wang DK, Zong YS, Ng MH (2002) Assessing the risk of nasopharyngeal carcinoma on the basis of EBV antibody spectrum. Int J Cancer 97:489–492

Chen JY, Chen CJ, Liu MY, Cho SM, Hsu MM, Lynn TC, Shieh T, Tu SM, Lee HH, Kuo SL (1987) Antibodies to Epstein–Barr virus-specific DNase in patients with nasopharyngeal carcinoma and control groups. J Med Virol 23:11–21

Chen JY, Chen CJ, Liu MY, Cho SM, Hsu MM, Lynn TC, Shieh T, Tu SM, Beasley RP, Hwang LY (1989) Antibody to Epstein–Barr virus specific DNase as a marker for field survey of patients with nasopharyngeal carcinoma in Taiwan. J Med Virol 27:269–273

Chen MR, Liu MY, Hsu SM, Fong CC, Chen CJ, Chen IH, Hsu MM, Yang CS, Chen JY (2001) Use of bacterially expressed EBNA-a protein cloned from a nasopharyngeal carcinoma (NPC) biopsy as a screening test for NPC patients. J Med Virol 64:51–57

Chien YC, Chen CJ (2003) Epidemiology and etiology of nasopharyngeal carcinoma: gene-environment interaction. Cancer Rev Asia-Pacific 1:1–19

Chien YC, Chen JY, Liu MY, Yang HI, Hsu MM, Chen CJ, Yang CS (2001) Serologic markers of Epstein–Barr virus infection and nasopharyngeal carcinoma in Taiwanese men. N Engl J Med 345:1877–1882

Cohen JI (2000) Epstein–Barr virus infection. N Engl J Med 343:481–492

Connolly Y, Littler E, Sun N, Chen X, Huang PC, Stacey SN, Arrand JR (2001) Antibodies to Epstein–Barr virus thymidine kinase: a characteristic marker for the serological detection of nasopharyngeal carcinoma. Int J Cancer 91:692–697

de-The G, Ho JHC, Ablashi DV, Day NE, Macario AJ, Martin-Berthelon MC, Pearson G, Sohier R (1975) Nasopharyngeal carcinoma. IX. Antibodies to EBNA and correlation with response to other EBV antigens in Chinese patients. Int J Cancer 16:713–721

De-Vathaire F, Sancho-Garner H, De-The H, Pieddeloup C, Schwaab G, Ho JH, Ellouz R, Micheau C, Cammoun M, Cachin Y (1988) Prognostic value of EBV markers in the clinical management of nasopharyngeal carcinoma (NPC): a multicenter follow-up study. Int J Cancer 42:176–181

Fan H, Nicholls J, Chua D, Chan KH, Sham J, Lee S, Gulley ML (2004) Laboratory markers of tumor burden in nasopharyngeal carcinoma: a comparison of viral load and serologic tests for Epstein–Barr virus. Int J Cancer 112: 1036–1041

Feng P, Chan SH, Soo MY, Liu D, Guan M, Ren EC, Hu H (2001) Antibody response to Epstein–Barr virus Rta protein in patients with nasopharyngeal carcinoma: a new serologic parameter for diagnosis. Cancer 92:1872–1880

Fleming ID, Cooper JS, Henson DE, et al. (1997) AJCC cancer staging manual, 5th edn. Lippincott-Raven, Philadelphia

Gratama JW, Ernberg I (1995) Molecular epidemiology of Epstein–Barr virus infection. Adv Cancer Res 67:197–255

Hao SP, Tsang NM, Chang KP (2003) Screening nasopharyngeal carcinoma by detection of the latent membrane protein 1 (LMP-1) gene with nasopharyngeal swabs. Cancer 97:1909–1913

Hao SP, Tsang NM, Chang KP, Ueng SH (2004) Molecular diagnosis of nasopharyngeal carcinoma: detecting LMP-1 and EBNA by nasopharyngeal swab. Otolaryngol Head Neck Surg 131:651–654

Henle G, Henle W (1976) Epstein–Barr virus-specific IgA serum antibodies as an outstanding feature of nasopharyngeal carcinoma. Int J Cancer 17:1–7

Hsiao JR, Jin YT, Tsai ST (2002) Detection of cell free Epstein–Barr virus DNA in sera from patients with nasopharyngeal carcinoma. Cancer 94:723–729

Hsu MM, Hsu WC, Sheen TS, Kao CL (2001) Specific IgA antibodies to recombinant early and nuclear antigens of Epstein–Barr virus in nasopharyngeal carcinoma. Clin Otolaryngol 26:334–338

Hu B, Hong G, Li Z, Xu J, Zhu Z, Li L (2007) Expression of VCA (viral capsid antigen) and EBNA1 (Epstein-Barr-virus-encoded nuclear antigen 1) genes of Epstein-Barr virus in *Pichia pastoris* and application of the products in a screening test for patients with nasopharyngeal carcinoma. Biotechnol Appl Biochem 47:59–69

IARC monographs on the evaluation of carcinogenic risks to humans (1997) Epstein–Barr virus and Kaposi's sarcoma herpesvirus/human herpesvirus 8, Vol. 70. IARC Press, Lyon, France, pp 47–373

Ji MF, Wang DK, Yu YL, Guo YQ, Liang JS, Cheng WM, Zong YS, Chan KH, Ng SP, Wei WI, Chua DT, Sham JS, et al. (2007) Sustained elevation of Epstein-Barr virus antibody levels preceding clinical onset of nasopharyngeal carcinoma. Br J Cancer 96:623–630

Lanier AP, Bornkamm GW, Henle W, Henle G, Bender TR, Talbot ML, Dohan PH (1981) Association of EBV with NPC in Alaskan native patients: serum antibodies and tissue EBNA and DNA. Int J Cancer 28:301–305

Lee N, Xia P, Quivey JM, et al. (2002) Intensity-modulated radiotherapy in the treatment of nasopharyngeal carcinoma: an update of the UCSF experience. Int J Radiat Oncol Biol Phys 53(1):12–22

Lennette ET, Winberg G, Yadav M, Enbald G, Klein G (1995) Antibodies to LMP2A/2B in EBV-carrying malignancies. Eur J Cancer 31:1875–1878

Leung SF, Tam JS, Chan AT, Zee B, Chan LY, Huang DP, Van Hasselt A, Johnson PJ, Lo YM (2004) Improved accuracy of detection of nasopharyngeak carcinoma by combined application of circulation Epstein-Barr virus DNA and anti-Epstein Barr virus casid antigen IgA antibody. Clin Chem 50:339–345

Lin S, Pan J, Lu H, et al. (2009) Nasopharyngeal carcinoma treated with reduced-volume intensity-modulated radiation therapy: report on the 3-year outcome of a prospective series. Int J Radiat Oncol Biol Phys 2009 Apr 11 [Epub ahead of print]

Lin SY, Tsang NM, Kao SC, Hsieh YL, Chen YP, Tsai CS, Kuo TT, Hao SP, Chen IH, Hong JH (2001) Presence of Epstein–Barr virus latent membrane protein 1 gene in the nasopharyngeal swabs from patients with nasopharyngeal carcinoma. Head Neck 23:194–200

Lin JC, Wang WY, Chen KY, Wei YH, Liang WM, Jan JS, Jiang RS (2004) Quantification of plasma Epstein-Barr virus DNA in patients with advanced nasopharyngeal carcinoma. N engl J Med 350:2461-70

Lin TM, Yang CS, Chiou JF, Tu SM, Chen TY, Tu YC, Lin PJ, Kawamura A Jr, Hirayama T (1977) Antibodies to Epstein–Barr virus capsid antigen and early antigen in nasopharyngeal carcinoma and comparison groups. Am J Epidemiol 106:336–339

Liu MY, Chang YL, Ma J, Yang HL, Hsu MM, Chen CJ, Chen JY, Yang CS (1997) Evaluation of multiple antibodies to Epstein–Barr virus as markers for detecting patients with nasopharyngeal carcinoma. J Med Virol 52:262–269

Lo KW, Lo YMD, Leung SF, Tsang YS, Chan LY, Johnson PJ, Hjelm NM, Lee JC, Huang DP (1999a) Analysis of cell-free Epstein–Barr virus associatedRNAin the plasma of patients with nasopharyngeal carcinoma. Clin Chem 45: 1292–1294

Lo YMD, Chan LY, Lo KW, Leung SF, Zhang J, Chan AT, Lee JC, Hjelm NM, Johnson PJ, Huang DP (1999b) Quantitative analysis of cell-free Epstein–Barr virus DNA in plasma of patients with nasopharyngeal carcinoma. Cancer Res 9:1188–1191

Lo YMD, Chan LY, Chan AT, Leung SF, Lo KW, Zhang J, Lee JC, Hjelm NM, Johnson PJ, Huang DP (1999c) Quantitative and temporal correlation between circulating cell-free Epstein–Barr virus DNA and tumour recurrence in nasopharyngeal carcinoma. Cancer Res 59:5452–5455

Lung ML, Chang GC (1992) Detection of distinct Epstein–Barr virus genotypes in NPC biopsies from southern Chinese and Caucasians. Int J Cancer 52:34–37

Lynn TC, Hsu MM, Hsieh T, Tu SM, Hamajima K (1976) Nasopharyngeal carcinoma and Epstein–Barr virus. III. The detection of anti-nuclear antibodies. Jpn J Exp Med 46:289–295

Mutirangura A, Pornthanakasem W, Theamboonlers A, Sriuranpong V, Lertsanguansinchi P, Yenrudi S, Voravud N, Supiyaphun P, Poovorawan Y (1998) Epstein–Barr viral DNA in serum of patients with nasopharyngeal carcinoma. Clin Cancer Res 4:665–669

Ng WT, Yau TK, Yung RWH, Sze WM, Tsang AHL, Law ALY, Lee AWM (2005) Screening for family members of patients with nasopharyngeal carcinoma. Int J Cancer 113: 998–1001

Niedobitek G (2000) Epstein–Barr virus infection in the pathogenesis of nasopharyngeal carcinoma. Mol Pathol 53: 248–254

Niedobitek G, Young LS, Sam CK, Brooks L, Prasad U, Rickinson AB (1992) Expression of Epstein–Barr virus genes and of lymphocyte activation molecules in undifferentiated nasopharyngeal carcinomas. Am J Pathol 140:879–887

Raab-Traub N (2002) Epstein–Barr virus in the pathogenesis of NPC. Semin Cancer Biol 12:431–441

Reddi KK, Holland JF (1976) Elevated serum ribonuclease in patients with pancreatic cancer. Proc Natl Acad Sci USA 73:2308–2310

Shao JY, Li YH, Gao HY, Wu QL, Cui NJ, Zhang L, Cheng G, Hu LF, Ernberg I, Zeng YX (2004) Comparison of plasma Epstein–Barr virus (EBV) DNA levels and serum EBV immunoglobulin A/virus capsid antigen antibody titers in patients with nasopharyngeal carcinoma. Cancer 100:1162–1170

Sheen TS, Ko JY, Chang YL, et al. (1998) Nasopharyngeal swab and PCR for the screening of nasopharyngeal carcinoma in the endemic area: a good supplement to the serologic screening. Head Neck 20:732–738

Shotelersuk K, Khorprasert C, Sakdikul S, Pornthanakasem W, Voravud N, Mutirangura A (2000) Epstein–Barr virus DNA in serum/plasma as a tumour marker for nasopharyngeal cancer. Clin Cancer Res 6:1046–1051

Tang JW, Rohwäder E, Chu IM, Tsang RK, Steinhagen K, Yeung AC, To KF, Chan PKJ (2007) Evaluation of Epstein–Barr virus antigen-based immunoassays for serological diagnosis of nasopharyngeal carcinoma. J Clin Virol 40: 284–288

Tsang RK, Vlantis AC, Ho RW, Tam JS, To KF, van Hasselt CA (2004) Sensitivity and specificity of Epstein–Barr virus IGA titer in the diagnosis of nasopharyngeal carcinoma: a three-year institutional review. Head Neck 26: 598–602

Wara WM, Wara DW, Phillips TL, Ammann AJ (1975) Elevated IgA in carcinoma of the nasopharynx. Cancer 35: 1313–1315

Williams EH, de The G (1974) Letter: familial aggregation in nasopharyngeal carcinoma. Lancet 2:295–296

Wu TC, Mann RB, Epstein JI, et al. (*1991*) Abundant expression of EBER1 small nuclear RNA in nasopharyngeal carcinoma. *Am J Pathol* 138:1461–1469

Young LS, Dawson CW, Clark D, et al. (1988) Epstein–Barr virus gene expression in nasopharyngeal carcinoma. J Gen Virol 69:1051–1065

Zeng Y, Zhang LG, Li HY, Jan MG, Zhang Q, Wu YC, Wang YS, Su GR (1982) Serological mass survey for early detection of nasopharyngeal carcinoma in Wuzhou city, China. Int J Cancer 29:139–141

Zeng Y, Zhong JM, Li LY, Wang PZ, Tang H, Ma YR, Zhu JS, Pan WJ, Lin YX, Wei ZN (1983) Follow-up studies on Epstein–Barr virus IgA/VCA antibody-positive persons in Zangwu county, China. Intervirology 20:190–194

Zeng Y, Zhang LG, Wu YC, Huang YS, Huang NQ, Li JY, Wang YB, Jiang MK, Fang Z, Meng NN (1985) Prospective studies on nasopharyngeal carcinoma in Epstein–Barr virus IgA/VCA antibody-positive persons in Wuzhou city, China Int J Cancer. 36:545–547

Familial Nasopharyngeal Carcinoma

6

Kwok Seng Loh

CONTENTS

Familial nasopharyngeal carcinoma (NPC) is defined as NPC occurring in two or more first-degree relatives. The rate of familial NPC is likely to be about 8% in any cohort of NPC patients in a high-risk region. The risk of a first-degree relative of an NPC patient being diagnosed with NPC is 2–15 times that of the general population in the endemic regions. Genetic factors are most likely the major causal associations for familial NPC, though environmental factors cannot be excluded. The current evidence shows that familial NPC is not a clinical syndrome. Treatment outcomes of familial NPC patients are not established and hence the protocols used for managing these patients should not be different from the sporadic NPC patients. Screening the first-degree relatives of NPC patients may increase the proportion of early NPC in a high-risk population.

6.1 Introduction

Nasopharyngeal carcinoma (NPC) is the most commonly diagnosed head and neck cancer in South East Asia. The vast majority of the newly diagnosed cases are sporadic without family history of NPC. However, it is well recognized that NPC does occur in families in the endemic regions (Loh et al. 2006; Jia et al. 2004; Ng et al. 2009; Zeng 2002). In addition, familial NPC is a well-reported entity in the nonendemic regions such as United States, though most of these are case reports of small number of familial clusters (Nevo et al. 1971; Williams and De-The 1974; Brown et al. 1976; Lanier et al. 1979; Gajwani et al. 1980; Fischer et al. 1984; Coffin et al. 1991; Levine et al. 1992; Albeck et al. 1993). Although information on NPC that exists in multiple members of the same family began to emerge in the past two decades, knowledge on familial NPC remains limited. One will

Kwok Seng Loh, MD, FRCS
Department of Otolaryngology Head & Neck Surgery, National University Health System, 5 Lower Kent Ridge Road, Singapore 119074, Republic of Singapore

obviously surmise that with multiple members in a family diagnosed with NPC, genetic factors must play a leading role. However, epidemiological and clinical evidences have demonstrated that genetic factors alone might be just one of the several causative factors for familial NPC (Jia et al. 2005). It is generally accepted that the carcinogenesis of NPC is the interplay between genetic and environmental factors and the Epstein–Barr virus. Thus, shared environmental factors may also be responsible for NPC occurring in families.

NPC observed in multiple members of a single family is not uncommon. Comparing with other commonly diagnosed malignancies such as colorectal cancer, the probability of NPC diagnosed in siblings is higher. Clearly, familial NPC is not likely to be a random entity. Understanding of the pathogenesis as well as clinical manifestation may lead to early detection and the development of an effective and efficient screening program in high-risk populations.

6.2 Definition

The National Cancer Institute (NCI) of the United States defined familial cancers as cancers occurring in families more often than would be expected by chance. Classic examples of cancers fulfilling this definition include retinoblastoma, familial medullary carcinoma, and certain forms of breast, ovarian, and colon cancers. The connotation of familial cancer is that inheritable factors are responsible for its occurrence. However, even in the stated list of examples of familial cancers, not all are absolutely familial but may occur in a sporadic manner. Furthermore, there is no internationally accepted definition for familial NPC.

Familial cancers are best described as cancers that occur within a family related by shared genetic components. For simplicity, familial NPC may be defined as NPC occurring in two or more first-degree relatives of a family. First-degree relatives within a family include parents, children (offspring of the parents), and siblings from the same parents. First-degree relatives are not only genetically related but also more likely to share common environmental factors. Most cases reported in the literature define familial NPC as a disease entity if two or more first-degree relatives within a family are affected by NPC (Loh et al. 2006; Jia et al. 2004; Zeng et al. 2002; Chen et al. 1990; Ung et al. 1999).

6.3 Causal Associations in Familial NPC

6.3.1 Risks of NPC in First-Degree Relatives

It is tempting to attribute familial NPC to genetic factors alone; however, such an assumption could only be true if most first- or second-degree relatives in the same family are also diagnosed with NPC. In other commonly diagnosed malignancies with a predilection for familial aggregation such as colorectal and breast cancers, the incidence of the same pathology diagnosed in the same family is relatively high (Hemminki et al. 2004). The rate of familial NPC in any cohort is very likely to fall between 2 and 15%, and most reports suggest a rate varying from 6 to 8% (Table 6.1) (Loh et al. 2006; Chen and Huang 1997; Yu et al. 1990; Yuan et al. 2000). Although such rate is higher than many other types of familial cancers, the incidence of 2–15% is not sufficient to suggest that genetic factors play the only role. It is suggested that shared environmental factors such as diet can also explain the rate of familial aggregation in NPC (Yu et al. 1986).

The discrepancies between the incidences reported in the above-mentioned studies need further discussion. The incidence of familial NPC reported in certain endemic regions such as Singapore was substantially higher than other countries or regions. The underlying reason for this high incidence is not clear. However, a study reported from China for patients with intermediate-risk for NPC, i.e., patients of nonendemic areas of China origin demonstrated a low incidence of familial NPC (Yuan et al. 2000). If only the series of patients from high-risk regions were reviewed, more than 8.3% of NPC are familial (Table 6.1). Therefore, the risk of familial NPC probably is associated with

Table 6.1. Familial NPC rates in different studies

Study	Region	Cohort	Rate
Loh et al. (2006)	Singapore	200	31/200, 15.5%
Yuan et al. (2000)	Shanghai	918	17/918, 1.9%
Ung et al. (1999)	Taiwan	375	25/375, 6.7%
Chen et al. (1997)	Hong Kong	104	8/104, 7.7%
Yu et al. (1990)	Guangzhou	306	18/306, 5.9%

the underlying risk of NPC in the general population in the endemic area.

The reported standardized incidence ratio (SIR) was 2.09 in a high-risk cohort of 13,833 first-degree relatives (Jia et al. 2004). The SIRs for brothers, sisters, father, and mother were 2.17, 2.91, 1.46, and 2.76, respectively. These data demonstrated a higher risk amongst siblings of an NPC patient compared with other direct relatives. A similar study reported by Yu et al. (2009) analyzed 358 high-risk families with two or more NPC cases. Over a 10-year period, the reported SIR of NPC was 15 (95% CI 10, 23). Guo et al. (2009) reported that the attributable risk of having a first-, second-, or third-degree relative with NPC is 6% (OR = 3.1 [95% C.I. 2.0, 4.9]). The latter two studies provide clear evidence for the risk of NPC in first-degree relatives of NPC patients.

6.3.2 Genetic Associations in Familial NPC

Genetic changes associated with familial NPC have been well documented. In 2002, Feng et al. (2002) had reported that genome wide scans of 20 high-risk families with multiple members having NPC identified linkage to chromosome 4. On average, there were more than three family members with NPC in these families, although the number of the first- or second-degree relatives affected was not clearly reported. However, no further reports are available in the literature to confirm similar findings of linkage to chromosome 4 in familial NPC. A study reported in 2004 by Xiong et al. (2004) indicated that familial NPC was linked to a susceptibility locus on chromosome 3p21. This study involved 18 families with two or more members involved with NPC, and did not demonstrate linkage to any other chromosomes. Fine mapping located the locus to a region on 3p21.31–21.2 where a cluster of tumor suppressor genes resided.

In a study of 15 families with two or more members diagnosed with NPC, Hu et al. (2008) reported linkage of chromosome 5 to familial NPC. A possible linkage was suggested and mapped to chromosome 5p13.1. However, the study did not confirm any linkage to chromosomes 3 or 4.

The association of HLA haplotypes with NPC had been established for more than 30 years (Simons et al. 1975, 1976). The HLA loci are located on chromosome 6. It was because of this strong association between HLA haplotypes and NPC that the HLA region was thought of being a possible region where tumor susceptibility genes were present (Lu et al. 1990). Ooi et al. (1997) had reported that in an analysis of a large pool of sib-pairs, a susceptibility region was localized to the major histocompatibility complex (MHC) region of chromosome 6. Subsequent studies have also corroborated this finding (Lu et al. 2003) and it is clear that there is an association in the region of HLA-A with NPC. Despite the reported association between chromosome 6 and the development of NPC, no study has supported a significant linkage to the familial type of NPC.

6.3.3 Non-Genetic Associations in Familial NPC

Since a consistent association between a genetic factor with familial NPC has not been identified, shared environment factors may play a role in the development of NPC including its familial type. A number of nongenetic factors including dietary and nondietary factors have been postulated. The dietary factors associated with NPC have mainly been the use of salted fish, especially during a young age (Yu et al. 1986, 1989; Ning et al. 1990). Other preserved foods have also been reported to be associated with NPC (Yu et al. 1988). Like in other types of squamous cell carcinoma of the head and neck areas (SCCHN), cigarette smoking is associated with the development of NPC, although the magnitude of the risk is not as substantial as in other SCCHN (Yu et al. 1990; Yuan et al. 2000). Lending further weight to the role that environmental and lifestyle factors play in the carcinogenesis of NPC, Luo et al. (2007) had studied the trends of NPC in Singapore, Hong Kong, and Los Angeles. There was a clear reduction in incidence of NPC over the period from 1973 to 1997. In addition, cohorts born in the 1940s in Hong Kong and 1958 in Singapore showed significant reduction in NPC. The authors concluded that the reductions in the incidence of NPC over time in the endemic regions suggest a strong role for environmental factors. However, all the above-mentioned risk factors of NPC were largely associated with the sporadic form, and their link with familial NPC has not been reported. Nevertheless, it is reasonable to postulate that the occurrences of familial NPC, at least in part, were due to environmental exposures by the first-degree family members to both dietary and/or nondietary factors.

Well-designed case control studies are needed to determine the nongenetic risk factors in the development of familial NPC. However, sufficient power

Table 6.2. Causal associations in familial NPC

Study	Region	Cohort (families)	Linkage
Feng et al. (2002)	Guangdong	20	4p15.1-q12
Xiong et al. (2004)	Hunan	18	3p21.31-21.2
Hu et al. (2008)	Guangdong	15	5p13.1

needed to detect small but significant risk factors in such setting may require a vast number of cases of patients fulfilling the criteria of familial NPC. In addition, a good proportion of affected family members may not be alive, the parents of the proband may be deceased, or the affected first-degree members could have succumbed owing to the progression of their disease. Furthermore, reliability of data recall of specific dietary habits and/or occupational exposures may not be accurate. Controlling for the multiple variables is a mammoth task in case control studies like these. Determining causal relationship of nongenetic factors for familial NPC seems to be an insurmountable task.

Current evidence suggests that genetic factors play a more significant role in the development of NPC in multiple first-degree relatives of a family than environmental factors. The genetic associations in familial NPC are summarized Table 6.2. It is important to remember that no consistent linkage between familial NPC and a single chromosome has been confirmed in the reported literature. The fact that chromosomes 3, 4, 5, and 6 have been reported as possible associations in familial NPC suggests that substantial heterogeneity may exist among familial clusters with NPC. Based on these findings, a number of tumor susceptibility genes may be responsible for NPC. Furthermore, it is also possible that NPC patients from different geographical regions may possess different susceptibility genes. And even different families from the same region may have differing susceptibility locus. However, prediction for the likelihood of NPC among first-degree relatives of a patient is not currently possible using genetic markers due to such heterogeneity.

6.4 Clinical Manifestation of Familial NPC

The available data in the current literature confirms that the clinical characteristics of familial NPC does not present any differently from sporadic NPC (Loh et al. 2006). Hence, it is expected that patients who fit the definition of familial NPC will most likely present with typical NPC presenting symptoms like nodal metastasis, blood stained saliva, and/or otitis media with effusion. In addition, no specific features are present on imaging studies of the primary tumor and nodal disease. There is also no significant difference in the levels of IgA viral capsid antigen (VCA) and IgA early antigen (Ea) titers between familial and sporadic NPC patients. The rate of distant metastasis is not higher than in patients with sporadic NPC, and the stage of disease is expected to be similar in both groups of patients, with patients predominantly diagnosed with stage III or stage IV NPC. Interestingly, some authors believe that patients with familial NPC tend to be diagnosed at an earlier age (Ng et al. 2009; Zeng et al. 2002). The pattern of earlier onset of disease, if it is confirmed, will lend weight to the belief that familial NPC is strongly associated with genetic predisposition. However, other authors do not report any differences in the age at diagnosis of familial NPC patients (Loh et al. 2006; Chen et al. 1990). It is also thought that first-degree relatives have a higher risk if the proband was diagnosed at age 40 years or less (Zeng et al. 2002). None of the reported series conclude any gender difference between familial NPC and the sporadic form, and the majority of NPC patients are male, like in its sporadic form.

Clinically, familial NPC does not seem to be a distinct disease entity, as clinical behavior does not differ from the more commonly diagnosed sporadic NPC. The significance of this lack of a clear clinical pattern of familial NPC is that one is unable to use objective clinical criteria to define familial NPC. In fact, it suggests that the factors that cause both sporadic and familial forms of NPC produce the same phenotypic results. The more obvious features of familial NPC are in Table 6.3.

Although all first-degree family members are at risk of NPC once a new diagnosis is made, the available data suggest a clear predominance of the disease in siblings over other first-degree relatives of the family. It is estimated that 30% of the affected first-degree family members are parents and 70% are siblings in the affected families. The period from an affected parent to a child being diagnosed with NPC is reported to be about 25 years; however, the period between affected siblings is about 5 years (Loh et al. 2006). These findings provided significant implications for screening protocols for first-degree relatives, which suggested that siblings might need to be

Table 6.3. Salient characteristics of familial NPC

Rate of familial NPC in high-risk populations	Likely 8%, ranging from 6 to 15%
Risk of first-degree relative of NPC patients being diagnosed with NPC	2–15 times of general population
Genetic associations	Chromosomes 3, 4, 5 reported. Possible chromosome 6
Environmental factors associated with familial NPC	None reported
Gender difference	No gender difference
Age at diagnosis	Familial NPC patients may be diagnosed younger than sporadic patients
TNM stage	No difference from sporadic NPC
Specific radiological features	None reported
Specific EBV antibody levels	None reported
Outcomes of familial NPC after definitive treatment	No evidence outcomes different from sporadic NPC

screened once an NPC patient is diagnosed. Such a suggestion is relatively practical as the life expectancy of most siblings of the newly diagnosed patients could be well over 5 years.

6.5 Clinical Significance of Familial NPC

The relatively high incidence indicated that screening for early diagnosis in the first-degree relative of NPC patients might be beneficial. Available data reported by Ng et al. and Friborg et al. supported screening first-degree relatives, especially in high-risk populations, mostly due to the higher incidence of the condition when compared with other commonly diagnosed malignancies (Ng et al. 2005; Friborg et al. 2005). Both authors suggested that screening should be performed in the siblings and children of NPC patients. And when a case of NPC is diagnosed, screening should be offered to the siblings as soon as possible. The children of NPC patients can be screened from 25 to 30 years old. However, whether screening among first-degree family members of NPC patients would result in early diagnosis of the disease and the long-term effect of such screening programs remain to be confirmed. Furthermore, specifics such as the test utilized and the frequency of an optimal screening protocol are open to debate. A detailed discussion of such protocols is out of the scope of this chapter; however, no evidence supports one protocol over another currently.

The outcomes after definitive treatment of familial NPC have not been reported; however, as the biological behavior of NPC in familial NPC is similar to the sporadic form, significant differences in treatment outcome are not likely to be identified. Presently, standard management strategy using radiotherapy or chemoradiation is suggested for patients with familial NPC as in the sporadic cases.

6.6 Summary

Approximately 2%–15% of all nasopharyngeal cancer cases are familial with two or more first-degree members of the same family diagnosed with the malignancy. Clinical evidence suggests that first-degree relatives especially siblings are at a higher risk of developing NPC than the general population. Although genetic factors are very likely to be responsible for the majority of the familial NPC cases, no clear-cut chromosomal changes have been confirmed. Clinically, familial NPC does not represent a distinct entity regarding its presentation and treatment strategy. Cancer syndromes associated with familial NPC have yet to be reported. It is suggested that first-degree relatives of newly diagnosed NPC patients in the endemic population be targeted for screening.

References

Albeck H, Bentzen J, Ockelmann HH, et al (1993) Familial clusters of nasopharyngeal carcinoma and salivary gland carcinomas in Greenland natives. Cancer 72:196–200

Brown TM, Heath Jr CW, Lang RM, et al (1976) Nasopharyngeal cancer in Bermuda. Cancer 37:1464–1468

Chen CJ, Liang KY, Chang YS, et al (1990) Multiple risk factors of nasopharyngeal carcinoma: Epstein–Barr virus, malarial infection, cigarette smoking and familial tendency. Anticancer Res 10:547–554

Chen DL, Huang TB (1997) A case-control study of risk factors of nasopharyngeal carcinoma. Cancer Lett 117:17–22

Coffin CM, Rich SS, Dehner LP (1991) Familial aggregation of nasopharyngeal carcinoma and other malignancies: a clinicopathologic description. Cancer 68:1323–1328

Feng BJ, Huang W, Shugart YY, et al (2002) Genome wide scan for familial nasopharyngeal carcinoma reveals evidence for linkage to chromosome 4. Nat Genet 31:395–399
Fischer A, Fischer GO, Cooper E (1984) Familial nasopharyngeal carcinoma. Pathology 16:23–24
Friborg J, Wohlfart J, Koch A, et al (2005) Cancer susceptibility in nasopharyngeal familes – a population based cohort study. Cancer Res 65:8567–8572
Gajwani BW, Devereaux JM, Beg JA (1980) Familial clustering of nasopharyngeal carcinoma. Cancer 46:2325–2327
Guo X, Johnson RC, Deng H, et al (2009) Evaluation of nonviral risk factors for nasopharyngeal carcinoma in a high-risk population of Southern China. Int J Cancer 124(12): 2942–2947.
Hemminki K, Li X, Czene K (2004) Familial risk of cancer: data for clinical counseling and cancer genetics. Int J Cancer 108:109–114
Hu LF, Qiu QH, Fu SM, et al (2008) A genome wide scan suggests a susceptibility locus on 5p13 for nasopharyngeal carcinoma. Eur J Hum Genet 16:343–349
Jia WH, Collins A, Zeng YX, et al (2005) Complex segregation analysis of nasopharyngeal carcinoma in Guangdong, China. Evidence for a multifactorial mode of inheritance (complex segregation analysis of NPC in China). Eur J Hum Genet 13:248–252
Jia WH, Feng BJ, Xu ZL, et al (2004) Familial risk and clustering of nasopharyngeal carcinoma in Guangdong, China. Cancer 101:363–369
Lanier AP, Bender TR, Tschopp CF, et al (1979) Nasopharyngeal carcinoma in an Alaskan Eskimo family: report of three cases. JNCI 62:1121–1124
Levine PH, Pocinki AG, Madigan P, et al (1992) Familial nasopharyngeal carcinoma in patients who are not Chinese. Cancer 70:1024–1029
Loh KS, Goh BC, Lu J, et al (2006) Familial nasopharyngeal carcinoma in a cohort of 200 patients. Arch Otolaryngol Head Neck Surg 132:82–85
Lu CC, Chen JC, Jin YT, et al (2003) Genetic susceptibility to nasopharyngeal carcinoma within the HLA-A locus in Taiwanese. Int J Cancer 103:745–751
Luo J, Chia KS, Chia SE, et al (2007) Secular trends of nasopharyngeal carcinoma incidence in Singapore, Hong Kong and Los Angeles Chinese populations, 1973–1997. Eur J Epidemiol 22:513–521
Lu SJ, Day NE, Degos L, et al (1990) Linkage of a nasopharyngeal carcinoma susceptibility locus to the HLA region. Nature 346:470–471
Nevo S, Meyer W, Altman M (1971) Carcinoma of nasopharynx in twins. Cancer 28:807–809
Ng WT, Cheuk WC, Lee MCH, et al (2009) Familial nasopharyngeal carcinoma in Hong Kong: epidemiology and implication in screening. Fam Cancer 8(2):103–108
Ng WT, Yau TK, Yung RW, et al (2005) Screening for family members of patients with nasopharyngeal carcinoma. Int J Cancer 113:998–1001
Ning JP, Yu MC, Wang QS, et al (1990) Consumption of salted fish and other risk factors for nasopharyngeal carcinoma (NPC) in Tianjin, a low-risk region for NPC in the People's Republic of China. J Natl Cancer Inst 82:291–296
Ooi EE, Ren EC, Chan SH (1997) Association between microsatellites within the human MHC and nasopharyngeal carcinoma. Int J Cancer 74:229–232
Simons MJ, Wee GB, Chan SH, et al (1975) Probable identification of an HL-A second-locus antigen associated with a high risk of nasopharyngeal carcinoma. Lancet 1:142–143
Simons MJ, Wee GB, Goh EH, et al (1976) Immunogenetic aspects of nasopharyngeal carcinoma. IV. Increased risk in Chinese of nasopharyngeal carcinoma associated with a Chinese-related HLA profile (A2, Singapore 2). J Natl Cancer Inst 57:977–980
Ung A, Chen CJ, Levine PH, et al (1999) Familial and sporadic cases of nasopharyngeal carcinoma in Taiwan. Anticancer Res 19:661–665
Williams EH, De-The G (1974) Familial aggregation in nasopharyngeal carcinoma. Lancet 2:295–296
Xiong W, Zeng ZY, Xia JH, et al (2004) A susceptibility locus at chromosome 3p21 linked to familial nasopharyngeal carcinoma. Cancer Res 64:1972–1974.
Yuan JM, Wang XL, Xiang YB, et al (2000) Non-dietary risk factors for nasopharyngeal carcinoma in Shanghai, China. Int J Cancer 85:364–369
Yu KJ, Hsu WL, Chiang CJ, et al (2009) Cancer patterns in nasopharyngeal carcinoma multiplex families in Taiwan. Int J Cancer 124:1622–1625
Yu MC, Garabrant DH, Huang TB, et al (1990) Occupational and other non-dietary risk factors for nasopharyngeal carcinoma in Guangzhou, China. Int J Cancer 45:1033–1039
Yu MC, Ho JH, Lai SH, et al (1986) Cantonese style salted fishes as a cause of nasopharyngeal carcinoma: report of a case-control study in Hong Kong. Cancer Res 46:956–961
Yu MC, Huang TB, Henderson BE (1989) Diet and nasopharyngeal carcinoma: a case-control study in Guangzhou, China. Int J Cancer 43:1077–1082
Yu MC, Mo CC, Chong WX, et al (1988) Preserved foods and nasopharyngeal carcinoma:a case-control study in Guangxi, China. Cancer Res 48:1954–1959
Zeng YX, Jia WH (2002) Familial nasopharyngeal carcinoma. Semin Cancer Biol 12:443–450

Pathology of Nasopharyngeal Carcinoma

7

Thomas Choudary Putti and Kong-Bing Tan

CONTENTS

Thomas Choudary Putti, MD
Kong-Bing Tan, MD
Department of Pathology, National University Health System, National University of Singapore, 5 Lower Kent Ridge Road, Singapore 119074, Republic of Singapore

7.1 Introduction

Nasopharyngeal carcinoma (NPC) features prominently in the field of head and neck cancers (Chan et al. 2005). In centers with an active otolaryngology service, in particular those servicing NPC-endemic populations, nasopharyngeal biopsies form a significant part of a histopathologist's workload. In the vast majority of such biopsies, the diagnosis is straightforward – either benign (reactive lymphoid hyperplasia) or malignant (NPC). In a minority of cases, diagnostic challenges may arise: either a reactive process that mimics malignancy or the unusual occurrence of other forms of malignancy that histologically resemble NPC. A correct diagnosis is required for the institution of the appropriate follow-up or therapy.

The archetypical histological type of NPC, the undifferentiated carcinoma, has a histologically distinctive appearance featuring cohesively arranged syncytial tumor cells occurring in association with admixed lymphocytes. Such a tumor has been termed "*lymphoepithelial carcinoma*." Although such a histological phenotype has been reported in tumors arising in other body sites as diverse as the salivary glands, skin, lung, and the gastrointestinal tract, the nasopharynx is by far the major origin of this type of tumor. This site is thus the priority for evaluation as a source of a *lymphoepithelial carcinoma* when such a tumor presents in the context of a metastatic carcinoma of uncertain origin. The aim of this chapter is to discuss the histological varieties of NPC, the use of ancillary techniques in the diagnostic evaluation of the tumor, the salient histological differential diagnoses, the posttreatment histological alterations, and potential diagnostic pitfalls.

7.2 Histopathological Types of Nasopharyngeal Carcinoma NPC

Most cases of NPC can broadly be classified as nonkeratinizing and keratinizing. The nonkeratinizing group can further be separated into undifferentiated carcinoma and differentiated carcinoma group.

7.2.1 Undifferentiated Carcinoma

Undifferentiated carcinoma is the major histopathological type of NPC, although the exact percentage in different populations varies. In endemic populations, undifferentiated carcinoma takes up between 47% and 92% of all cases of NPC (Shanmugaratnam et al. 1979; Tan and Putti 2005). In a major series on a western (non-endemic) population, this subtype of NPC constituted only 44% of all NPCs (Al-Sarraf et al. 1998). Undifferentiated carcinoma is characterized microscopically by tumor cells with spindle-to-oval vesicular or hyperchromatic nuclei bearing prominent nucleoli and which also feature scattered mitotic activity (Figs. 7.1–7.3). Variable numbers of intermixed lymphocytes and plasma cells are seen. There are two classically described patterns of growth: the "*Regaud*" pattern denotes a solid sheet-like tumor cell growth pattern, while the "*Schmincke*" pattern is typified by the presence of apparently separated or loosely attached tumor cells (sometimes described as a reticulated pattern) with prominent intermixed lymphocytes (Glanzmann et al. 1976). This latter pattern exemplifies the previous terms for NPC: "*lymphoepithelial carcinoma or lymphoepithelioma*" (*vide supra*). These histological patterns have no prognostic significance.

7.2.2 Differentiated Nonkeratinizing Carcinoma

Differentiated nonkeratinizing NPC is very similar histopathologically to undifferentiated carcinoma, except that the tumor cells have a stratified or pavemented arrangement with cell borders being readily discernable (Chan et al. 2005) (Fig. 7.4). The tumor cells may have a plexiform arrangement, a growth pattern akin to that of transitional cell carcinoma of the urinary tract. In series from Singapore, this tumor subtype constitutes between 7% and 49% of cases of NPC (Shanmugaratnam et al. 1979; Tan and Putti 2005). Nonkeratinizing NPC can rarely have a papillary architecture with tumor epithelium covering fibrovascular tissue cores (Fig. 7.5). Apart from histological similarities, differentiated nonkeratinizing NPC and undifferentiated NPC have comparable prognosis and their distinction is not thought to have clinical significance (Chan et al. 2005).

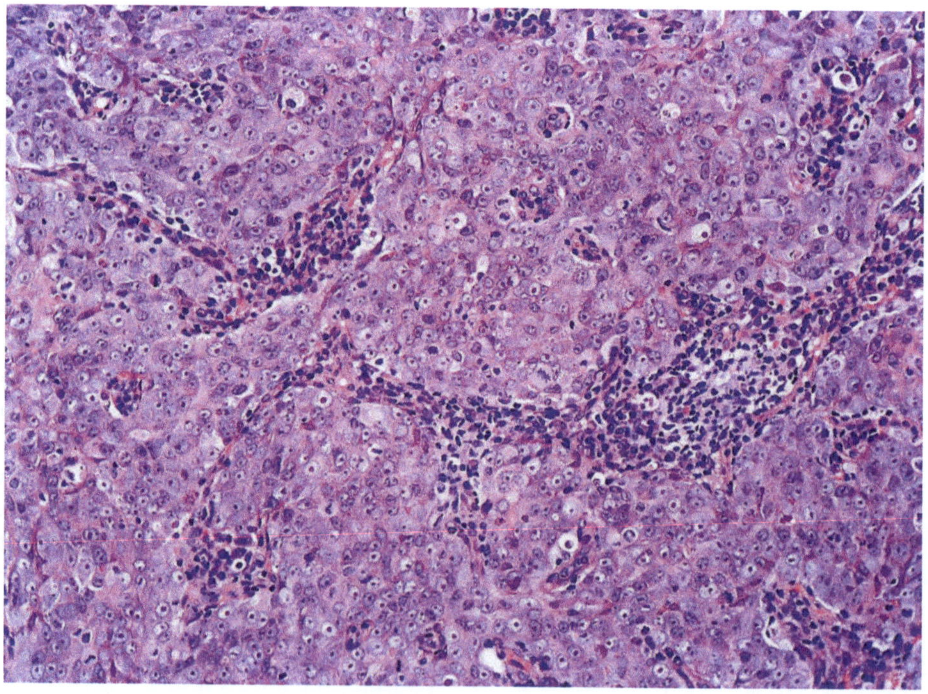

Fig. 7.1. Undifferentiated carcinoma featuring cohesive sheet of tumor cells with few intermixed lymphocytes (Hematoxylin and Eosin, original magnification ×200)

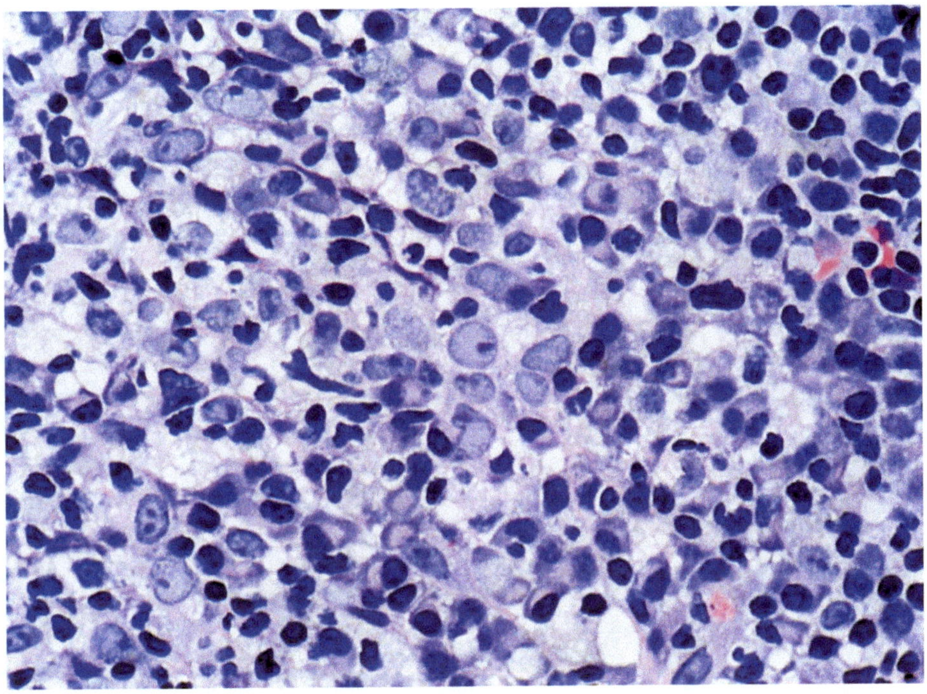

Fig. 7.2. Undifferentiated carcinoma featuring scattered loosely attached tumor cells with plentiful intermixed lymphocytes. (Hematoxylin and Eosin, original magnification ×600)

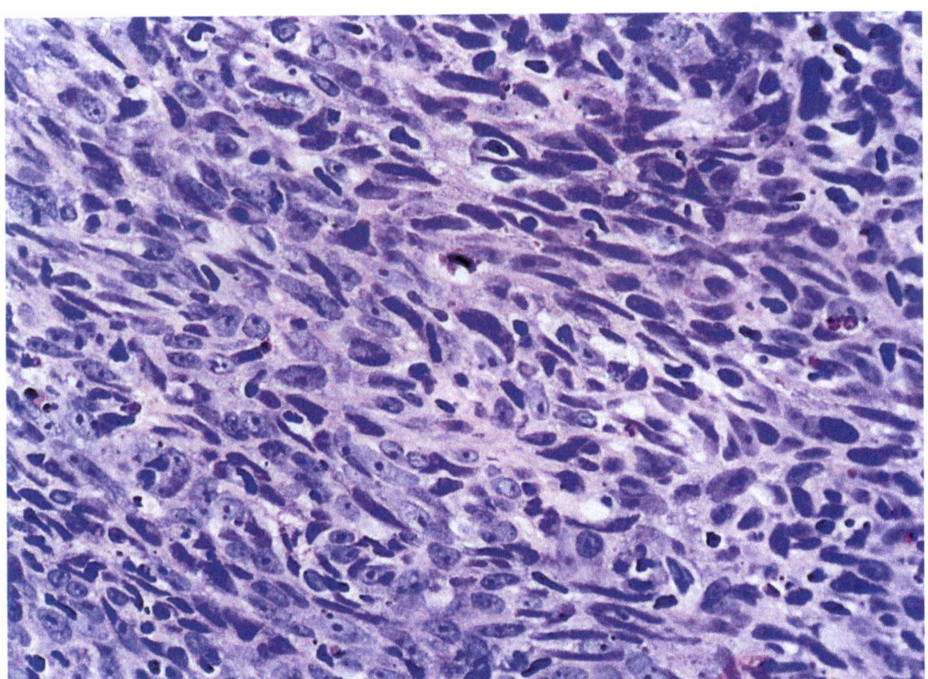

Fig. 7.3. Not uncommonly, undifferentiated carcinoma is composed of spindle-shaped tumor cells (hematoxylin and eosin, original magnification ×400)

7.2.3 Keratinizing Squamous Cell Carcinoma

Keratinizing squamous cell carcinoma (SCC) is uncommon in NPC-endemic regions. In endemic areas such as Singapore, it constituted between 1% and 20% of all cases of NPC (Shanmugaratnam et al. 1979; Tan and Putti 2005). In contrast, the proportion of this subtype in non-endemic western populations has been reported in up to 67% of cases

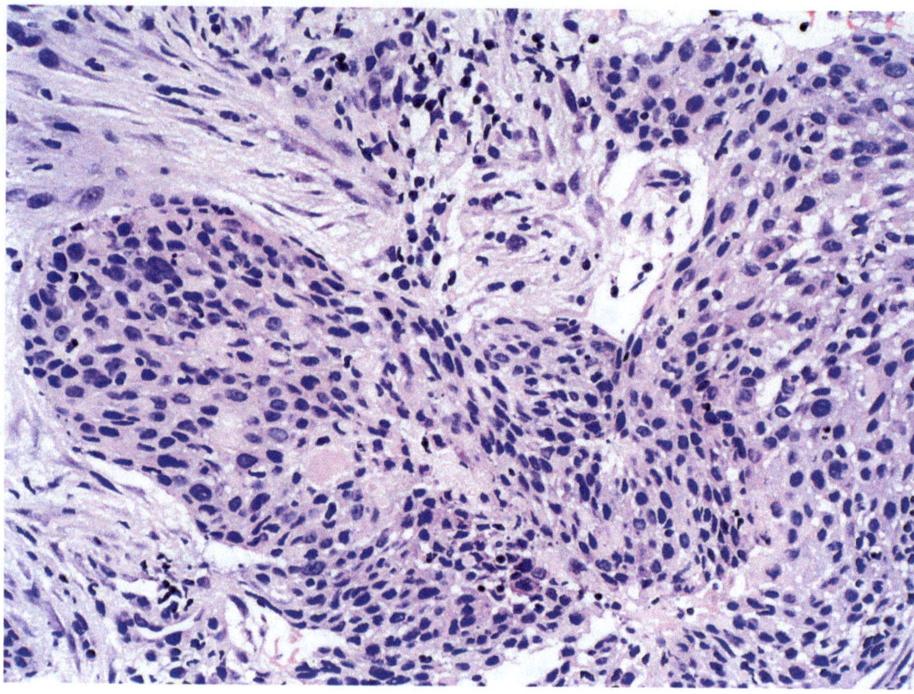

Fig. 7.4. Differentiated nonkeratinizing carcinoma showing cohesive tumor cells with well-defined cell borders (hematoxylin and eosin, original magnification ×400)

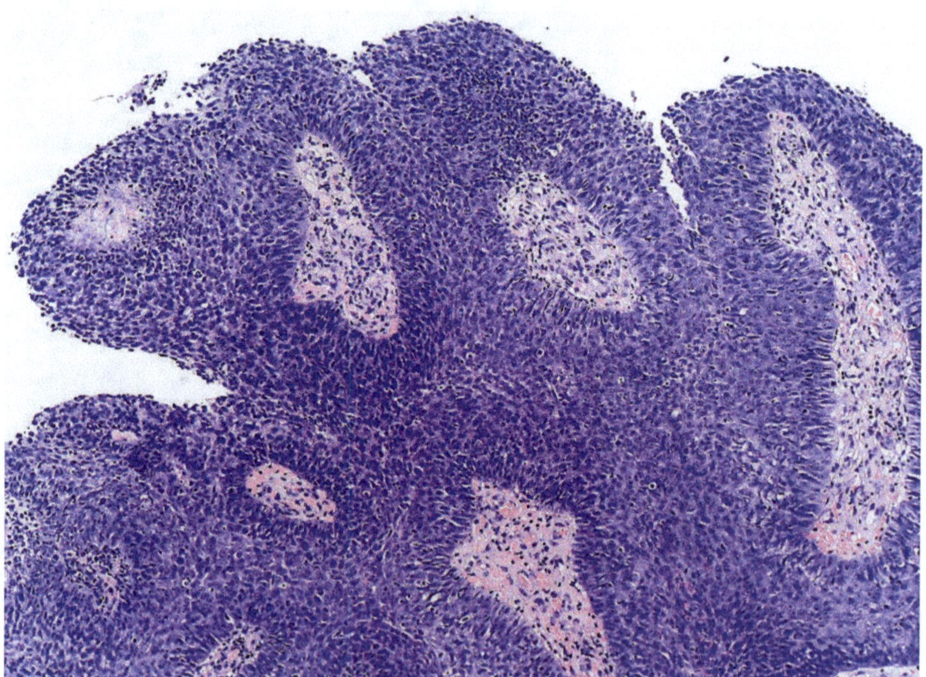

Fig. 7.5. Nonkeratinizing NPC, papillary type (hematoxylin and eosin, original magnification ×200)

of NPC (Shedd et al. 1967). Histologically, the tumor shows prominent features of keratinization, including presence of squamous pearl formation and evident intercellular bridges (Fig. 7.6). The tumor islands infiltrate within a desmoplastic stroma and the tumor can be graded as well, moderately and poorly differentiated, as in SCCs of other body sites. This subtype of NPC has been described to have the most guarded prognosis of all NPC subtypes, probably contributed by its relative radioresistance

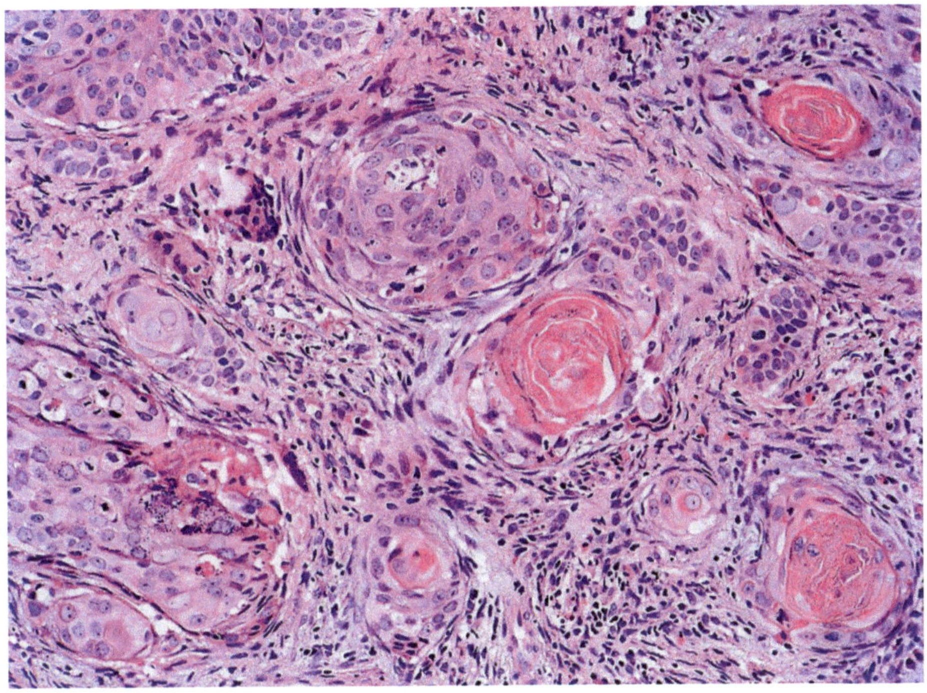

Fig. 7.6. Keratinizing squamous cell carcinoma showing clusters of malignant squamous cells infiltrating within desmoplastic stroma (hematoxylin and eosin, original magnification ×200)

(Weiland 1985; Wenig 2007). The 5-year survival is reportedly 20%–40% as compared with about 65% for nonkeratinizing NPC subtypes (Wenig 2007).

Basaloid SCC is the most unusual variant of NPC with only a handful of cases reported in the literature (Wan et al. 1995; Müller et al. 2000). It is histologically very similar to other basaloid SCCs that occur in the rest of the upper aerodigestive tract and displays tumor cells with hyperchromatic nuclei, increased nuclear–cytoplasmic ratio with peripheral palisading of tumor nuclei.

7.2.4 In Situ Nasopharyngeal Cancer

In keeping with precursor lesions seen in other carcinomas, in situ NPC as a precursor to invasive NPC is conceptually sound, although it is not easily recognizable in diagnostic practice. Several synonyms have been used: atypia, dysplasia, carcinoma in situ, and nasopharyngeal intraepithelial neoplasia (Chan et al. 1992; Pathmanathan et al. 1995; Lee 1991). Various series of NPC have reported the incidence of these lesions present in nasopharyngeal biopsies to be between 3% and 73% (Pathmanathan et al. 1995; Lee 1991), a variability that may be partially attributed to the previous lack of widely acceptable criteria in this tumor. Current consensus is that this lesion is typified by cytological and architectural atypia that affects the whole thickness of the nasopharyngeal epithelium. The cytological atypia incorporates nuclear enlargement and irregularity, with prominence of nucleoli (Chan et al. 2005) (Fig. 7.7). Intraepithelial lymphocytes are often present, although the usefulness of this is questionable as non-neoplastic nasopharyngeal epithelium also commonly shows this feature.

In common with invasive NPC, in situ lesions are characteristically positive for the presence of Epstein–Barr virus (EBV), while non-neoplastic nasopharyngeal epithelium is negative (Pak et al. 2002). Other studies of protein marker expression in NPC have shown an intermediate level of expression of antiapoptotic proteins, Bcl-2 and Cyclooxygenase-2, in in situ NPC when compared with non-neoplastic epithelium and invasive tumors (Sheu et al. 1997; Tan and Putti 2005). Such biomarker findings tend to support the relationship of in situ NPC to its invasive counterpart. While most cases of in situ NPC are identified as being coexistent with an invasive NPC, a few cases of progression of pure in situ NPC to invasive NPC have been recorded (Pak et al. 2002).

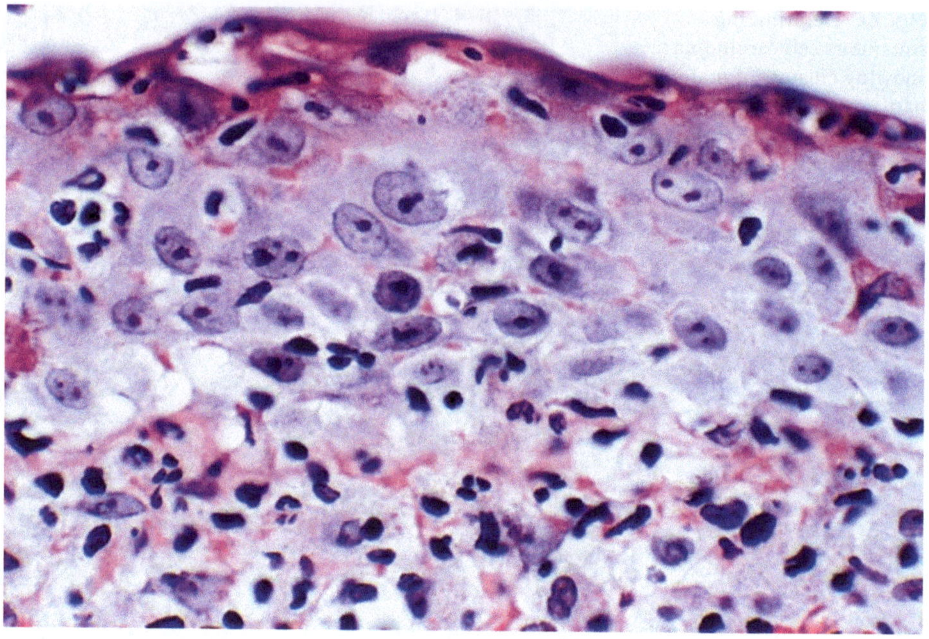

Fig. 7.7. In situ NPC featuring loss of polarity of the nasopharyngeal epithelium with nuclear atypia and prominent nucleoli (hematoxylin and eosin, original magnification ×600)

7.3 Adjunctive Pathological Procedures in the Diagnosis of Nasopharyngeal Carcinoma

7.3.1 Immunohistochemistry

Although the evaluation of routine Hematoxylin and Eosin-stained tissue sections is the mainstay of the histological diagnosis of NPC, cytokeratin immunohistochemistry has become a very useful ancillary technique to help elucidate the diagnosis in challenging cases. Immunoperoxidase reaction using antibodies to broad spectrum cytokeratins (e.g., AE1/3, MNF-116) is commonly used with good effect. In non-neoplastic nasopharyngeal biopsies, the regular and predictable surface or crypt epithelium is highlighted with such immunohistochemistry. In biopsies bearing a small quantity of NPC, the irregular clusters of tumor cells may be better seen with cytokeratin immunohistochemistry (Fig. 7.8). Nonkeratinizing undifferentiated carcinoma shows cytokeratin-positive cells in cohesive groups or in a reticulated pattern intermingled with lymphocytes while the nonkeratinizing differentiated NPC demonstrates cellular sheets composed of tightly associated polygonal tumor cells. The use of an immunohistochemical panel for reacting against cytokeratins and with other relevant protein markers is especially useful to help distinguish NPC from other differential diagnoses, both neoplastic and non-neoplastic (*vide infra*).

7.3.2 Detection of EBV

The etiological association of latent EBV infection with NPC carcinogenesis has provided the opportunity for EBV detection to be used as a diagnostic adjunct for this tumor. Epstein–Barr virus encoded early RNA (EBER) in situ hybridization (ISH) or EBER-ISH has emerged as another useful histological ancillary technique that allows for the elucidation of diagnostically challenging cases using the convenience of conventional light microscopy. EBER-ISH is almost invariably positive (Fig. 7.9) in nonkeratinizing NPC, while it is less often positive in keratinizing SCC (Hwang et al. 1998; Inoue et al. 2002; Ertan et al. 2008). Hence, in a nasopharyngeal biopsy, the greatest diagnostic utility of EBER-ISH is to help distinguish reactive or inflammatory atypia of the nasopharynx (negative) from NPC (invasive or in situ) (positive) in diagnostically difficult cases. Furthermore, in metastatic undifferentiated carcinoma in which the primary is not apparent, EBER-ISH positivity lends support to the likelihood of a nasopharyngeal origin of the tumor (Chan et al. 2005).

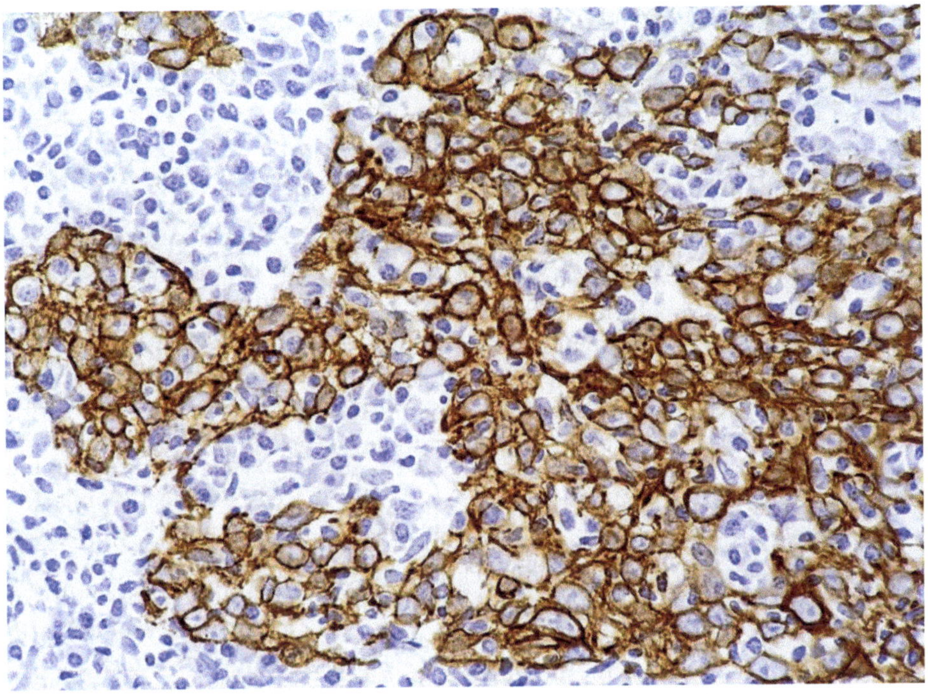

Fig. 7.8. Undifferentiated carcinoma showing positivity for cytokeratin (AE1/3) (immunoperoxidase, original magnification ×200)

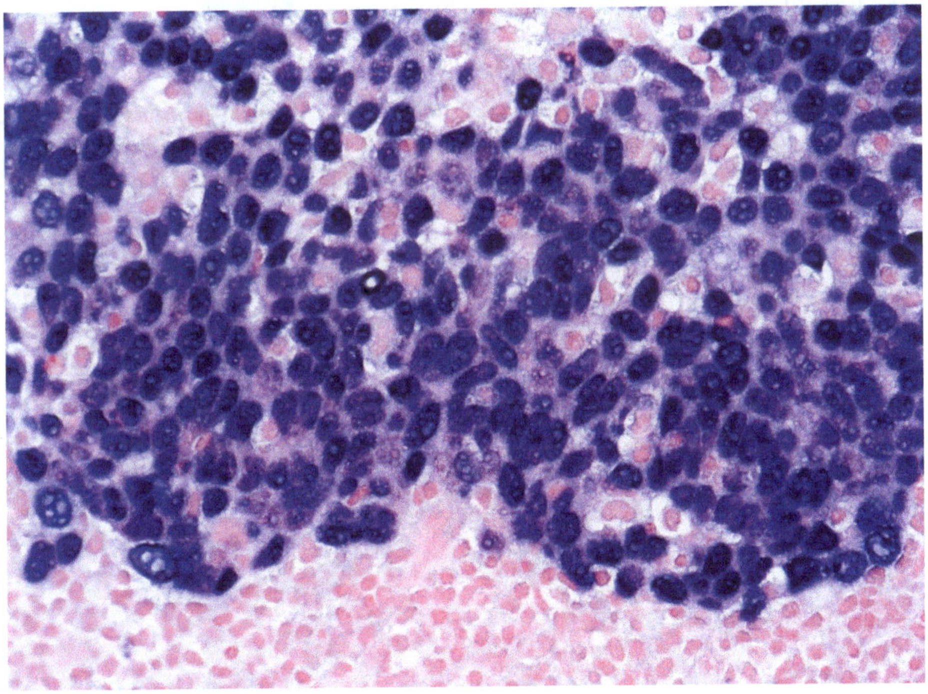

Fig. 7.9. Undifferentiated carcinoma showing EBER positivity by in situ hybridization (original magnification ×400)

7.3.3 Role of Fine Needle Aspiration Cytology

Fine needle aspiration cytology (FNAC) is a convenient, minimally invasive, low-cost, and fairly accurate method to assess for the presence of NPC tumor cells (Viguer et al. 2005). The technique helps sample cells for diagnostic evaluation from sites of suspected tumor involvement, most often the cervical lymph nodes. Hence, its functions are threefold: for the diagnosis of NPC, as an aid to initial tumor staging, and for the confirmation of tumor recurrence or metastasis.

Cytological smears are prepared and conventionally stained with Papanicolaou (alcohol-fixed) and Giemsa (air-dried). The former helps highlight nuclear features of the cells, while the latter better delineates the cytoplasmic detail; hence the two are complementary. Nonkeratinizing NPC features cohesive groups of tumor cells, although some dispersed single tumor cells are often present as well. The almost obligatory presence of associated lymphocytes is also noted. The hyperchromatic nuclei of NPC tumor cells are elongated-to-oval in configuration, are frequently overlapping, and often bear prominent nucleoli (Fig. 7.10). The cytoplasm is scanty in amount. The keratinizing SCC subtype of NPC discloses tumor cells with keratinized (dense) cytoplasm with hyperchromatic nuclei; nucleoli are usually not prominent.

In assessing a suspected case of nonkeratinizing NPC, the cytological features may occasionally be very challenging and may mimic those seen in other tumors, notably small cell neuroendocrine carcinoma and large cell lymphoma. In such instances, a cell block prepared at the time of FNAC can be very useful as it provides a source of cellular material on which ancillary studies can be performed. NPC tumor cells are positive for cytokeratin immunhistochemistry as well as EBER-ISH (*vide supra*). Large cell lymphoma is negative for cytokeratins and positive for leukocyte common antigen (LCA), while small cell carcinoma is negative for EBER-ISH and positive for neuroendocrine markers such as Synaptophysin and CD56.

7.3.4 Diagnosis of Metastases

The cervical lymph nodes are generally the first site of tumor metastases. Extranodal distant metastases can occur in bone, lung, and liver. For confirmation of metastases in the cervical lymph nodes, FNAC is preferred (*vide supra*). In those cases with inadequate material, an open biopsy can be performed. The tumor cells generally form cohesive islands intermixed with variable number of lymphocytes, plasma cells, and eosinophils. In a small percentage of metastatic tumors, epithelioid granulomas can be noted, some even with caseous necrosis. A diligent search to exclude the possibility of mycobacterial infection is imperative, especially following radiation therapy (Chan et al. 2004).

7.4 Pathological Differential Diagnosis

Crush artifacts: Sometimes, severe crush artifacts of small nasopharyngeal biopsies may give rise to a mistaken diagnosis of NPC, especially in the presence

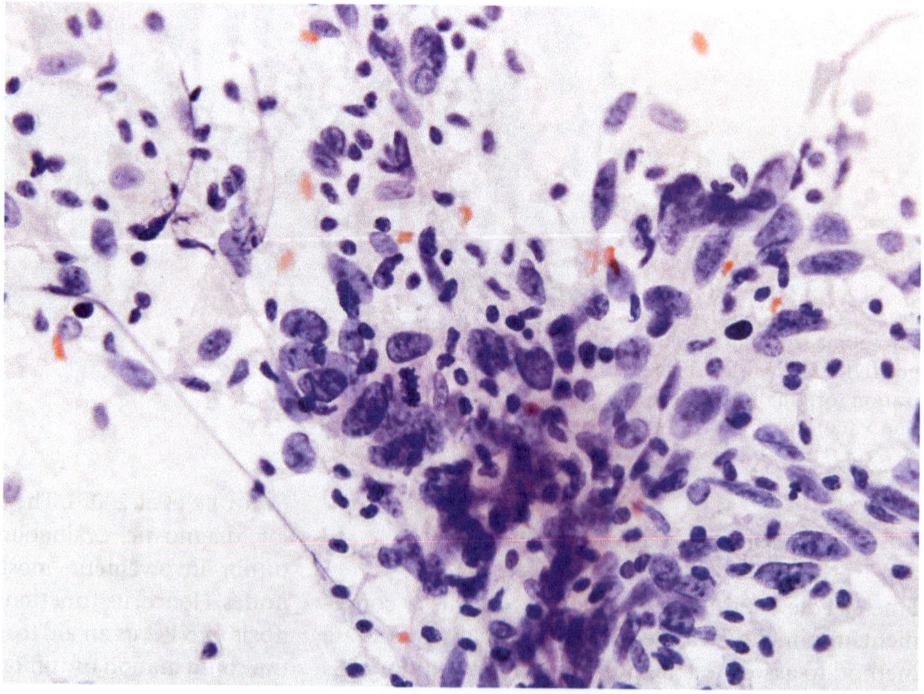

Fig. 7.10. Cytological smear showing cohesive spindle-shaped undifferentiated carcinoma cells (papanicolaou, original magnification ×600)

of clinical symptoms and a mass. It is prudent not to make a firm diagnosis of carcinoma in such cases. Depending on the morphological features, immunohistochemical staining for cytokeratin may or may not be helpful. A crushed crypt with irregular borders and cytokeratin positivity may mimic carcinoma. A repeat biopsy is a better alternative over a false-positive diagnosis.

Reactive germinal centers: Nasopharyngeal mucosa is rich in lymphoid tissue and may contain several reactive lymphoid follicles. Germinal center cells can easily mimic malignant cells, as they contain large cells with vesicular nuclei and prominent nucleoli. This is a problem when the mantle zone is indistinct and the biopsy sample is small, compounded by crush artifacts. A useful clue is identification of tingible body macrophages. Immunohistochemistry for LCA (positive) and cytokeratins (negative) can be used for confirmation of follicular center cells in difficult cases.

Lymphoma: Occasionally, a large cell lymphoma of nasopharyngeal tissue can be difficult to differentiate from carcinoma on morphological features alone. Generally, carcinomatous cells form cohesive groups and have ill-defined cell borders. Again, an immunohistochemistry panel (LCA and cytokeratin) would be of great value.

Sinonasal carcinoma: Sinonasal undifferentiated carcinoma is a rare aggressive neoplasm arising in the nasal cavity and rarely nasopharyngeal region. These tumors may resemble undifferentiated NPC but are consistently negative for EBER-ISH (Jeng et al. 2002).

Rhabdomyosarcoma: These tumors can resemble undifferentiated NPC but are most commonly seen in younger individuals while NPC occurs mostly in adults and the elderly population. They present with aural symptoms, nasal obstruction, and pain. Immunohistochemical stains are strongly positive for desmin and myoglobin. Embryonal and spindle cell variants are the common subtypes (Nascimento et al. 2005).

Melanoma: Melanoma can uncommonly be encountered in the nasopharyngeal location. The presence of melanin pigment, multinucleate tumor giant cells, or positivity for S-100, HMB-45, and melan-A excludes NPC. Histologically, these tumors can be epithelioid, spindled, or undifferentiated (Thompson et al. 2003).

Olfactory neuroblastoma: Olfactory neuroblastoma (Esthesioneuroblastoma) is a malignant neuroendocrine tumor originating in the olfactory mucosa. It is a *small blue cell neoplasm* with a characteristic lobular architecture, neuroendocrine immunophenotype, and a sustentacular S-100-positive staining pattern (Ingeholm et al. 2002).

7.5 Pathological Aspects of Post-treatment Changes

Postradiation changes – Radiation therapy is the mainstay treatment modality for nonmetastatic NPC. Generally, a reasonable tumor response occurs in 10–12 weeks following radiation therapy. Residual tumor cells may display vacuolated cytoplasm and bizarre nuclei. Normal epithelium, either surface or cryptal, may sometimes show changes resembling carcinoma. A negative EBER-ISH would in most cases rule out malignancy. The stromal cells also exhibit atypical changes in the form of enlarged abnormal nuclei with prominent nucleoli, but these are negative for cytokeratin.

Secondary malignancies – Second malignancies after definitive treatment of NPC is a rare but devastating complication. The two most commonly diagnosed malignancies following treatment for NPC include SCC and sarcomas of varying types including osteosarcoma, malignant fibrous histiocytoma, malignant schwannoma, extraskeletal chondrosarcoma, and angiosarcoma. Of about 3,000 patients treated with radiotherapy for NPC over a 10-year period in Singapore, only one patient developed postradiation sarcoma of the sphenoid bone (Teo et al. 2006). The latency period can be anytime from 2 to 40 years.

7.6 Summary

Nasopharyngeal carcinoma (NPC) has important and unique clinicopathological features in the field of head and neck pathology. NPC is histopathologically classified as nonkeratinizing or keratinizing. The former is further subdivided into undifferentiated carcinoma and differentiated carcinoma subgroups and is the predominant form of NPC encountered worldwide, particularly in NPC-endemic regions. Microscopically, nonkeratinizing NPC is characterized by tumor cells growing in either a cohesive or reticulated pattern with a typical admixture of lymphocytes, while keratinizing NPC shows the features of a well-differentiated SCC. While light microscopy of H and E-stained sections remains the cornerstone of NPC diagnosis, EBV encoded early RNA in situ hybridization (EBER-ISH) and cytokeratin immunohistochemistry are useful adjuncts in diagnostically challenging cases. EBER-ISH is almost always positive in nonkeratinizing NPC, while it is negative in benign nasopharyngeal epithelium and most other malignant differential diagnoses of NPC. Cytokeratin immunohistochemistry helps highlight the irregular infiltrative nature of NPC, contrasting with the regular surface and cryptal epithelium of normal biopsies. Malignant differential diagnoses that need to be distinguished from NPC include lymphoma, sinonasal carcinoma, and melanoma, while benign mimics include reactive lymphoid germinal centers, crush artifacts, and postradiation changes. For the assessment of suspected metastatic sites, FNAC has been shown to be a convenient and fairly accurate technique.

References

Al-Sarraf M, LeBlanc M, Giri PG, et al (1998) Chemotherapy versus radiotherapy in patients with advanced nasopharyngeal cancer: phase III randomized intergroup study 0099. J Clin Oncol 16:1310–1317

Chan AB, Ma TK, Yu BK, et al (2004) Nasopharyngeal granulomatous inflammation and tuberculosis complicating undifferentiated carcinoma. Otolaryngol Head Neck Surg 130:125–130

Chan CW, Nicholls JM, Sham JST, et al (1992) Nasopharyngeal carcinoma in situ in nasopharyngeal carcinoma. J Clin Pathol 45:898–901

Chan JKC, Pilch BZ, Kuo TT, et al (2005) Nasopharyngeal carcinoma. In: Barnes L, Eveson JW, Reichart P, Sidransky D (eds) World Health Organization classification of tumors. Pathology and genetics. Head and neck tumors. IARC Press, Lyon, pp 83–97

Ertan Y, Hekimgil M, Karaarslan S, et al (2008) Expression of Epstein–Barr-virus-encoded small nuclear RNA in nasopharyngeal carcinomas of Aegean Turkish patients. Virchows Arch 452:411–414

Glanzmann C, Aberle HG, Horst W (1976). Radiotherapy results of nasopharyngeal carcinomas (41 patients)]. Strahlentherapie 152:310–315

Hwang TZ, Jin YT, Tsai ST (1998) EBER in situ hybridization differentiates carcinomas originating from the sinonasal region and the nasopharynx. Anticancer Res 18:4581–4584

Ingeholm P, Theilgaard SA, Buchwald C, et al (2002) Esthesioneuroblastoma: a Danish clinicopathological study of 40 consecutive cases. APMIS 110:639–645

Inoue H, Sato Y, Tsuchiya B, et al (2002) Expression of Epstein–Barr virus-encoded small nuclear RNA 1 in Japanese nasopharyngeal carcinomas. Acta Otolaryngol Suppl 547: 113–117

Jeng YM, Sung MT, Fang CL, et al (2002) Sinonasal undifferentiated carcinoma and nasopharyngeal-type undifferentiated carcinoma: two clinically, biologically, and histopathologically distinct entities. Am J Surg Pathol 26: 371–376

Lee JCK (1991) Precancerous changes. In: van Hasselt CA (ed) Nasopharyngeal carcinoma. Chinese University Press, Hong Kong, pp 37–45

Müller E, Beleites E (2000) The basaloid squamous cell carcinoma of the nasopharynx. Rhinology 38:208–211

Nascimento AF, Fletcher CD (2005) Spindle cell rhabdomyosarcoma in adults. Am J Surg Pathol 29:1106–1113

Pak MW, To KF, Lo YM, et al (2002) Nasopharyngeal carcinoma in situ (NPCIS)-pathologic and clinical perspectives. Head Neck 24:989–995

Pathmanathan R, Prasad U, Sadler R, et al (1995) Clonal proliferations of cells infected with Epstein–Barr virus in preinvasive lesions related to nasopharyngeal carcinoma. N Engl J Med 333:693–698

Shanmugaratnam K, Chan SH, de-Thé G, et al (1979) Histopathology of nasopharyngeal carcinoma: correlations with epidemiology, survival rates and other biological characteristics. Cancer 44:1029–1044

Shedd DP, von Essen CF, Eisenberg H (1967) Cancer of the nasopharynx in Connecticut, 1935 through 1959. Cancer 20:508–511

Sheu LF, Chen A, Meng CL, et al (1997) Analysis of bcl-2 expression in normal, inflamed, dysplastic nasopharyngeal epithelia, and nasopharyngeal carcinoma: association with p53 expression. Hum Pathol 28:556–562

Tan KB, Putti TC (2005) Cyclooxygenase 2 expression in nasopharyngeal carcinoma: immunohistochemical findings and potential implications. J Clin Pathol 58:535–538

Teo WY, Tan HK, Goh BC, et al (2006) Postirradiation sarcoma of the sphenoid bone – a case report. Ann Acad Med Singapore 35:104–107

Thompson LD, Wieneke JA, Miettinen M (2003) Sinonasal tract and nasopharyngeal melanomas: a clinicopathologic study of 115 cases with a proposed staging system. Am J Surg Pathol 27:594–611

Viguer JM, Jiménez-Heffernan JA, López-Ferrer P, et al (2005) Fine-needle aspiration cytology of metastatic nasopharyngeal carcinoma. Diagn Cytopathol 32:233–237

Wan SK, Chan JK, Lau WH, et al (1995) Basaloid-squamous carcinoma of the nasopharynx. An Epstein–Barr virus-associated neoplasm compared with morphologically identical tumors occurring in other sites. Cancer 76:1689–1693

Weiland LH (1985) Nasopharyngeal carcinoma. In: Barnes L (ed) Surgical pathology of the head and neck. Marcel Dekker, New York, pp 453–466

Wenig BM (2007) Tumors of the upper respiratory tract: part A: nasal cavity, paranasal sinuses and nasopharynx. In: Fletcher CDM (ed) Diagnostic Histopathology of Tumors, 3rd edn. Elsevier, London, pp 83–149

Imaging in the Diagnosis and Staging of Carcinoma of Nasopharynx

8

Cheng Kang Ong and Vincent Fook Hin Chong

CONTENTS

Dr. Cheng Kang Ong, MBBS (Hons), MRCS (Eng), FRCR
Vincent Fook Hin Chong, MBBS, MBA, FRCR
Department of Diagnostic Radiology, National University Health System, National University of Singapore, 5 Lower Kent Ridge Road, Singapore 119074, Republic of Singapore

8.1 Introduction

Endoscopy often allows direct visualization of a nasopharyngeal carcinoma (NPC) that involves the pharyngeal mucosal surface, with a definitive histopathologic diagnosis achieved through biopsy of the lesion. However, staging of the disease is primarily dependent on imaging, which delineates the full extent of the submucosal, osseous, or intracranial tumor infiltration, as well as the nodal and visceral metastases. Accurate tumor mappings on imaging enable precise radiotherapy treatment planning and administration, which in turn effectively improve the outcomes of patients (Cellai et al. 1990; Emami et al. 2003).

This chapter first presents the imaging anatomy of the nasopharynx, followed by the specific imaging features of nasopharyngeal carcinoma including tumor spread, tumor volume, nodal and systemic metastasis. The differential diagnosis of nasopharyngeal carcinoma is also briefly discussed.

8.2 Imaging Anatomy of the Nasopharynx

The nasopharynx is essentially an inverted J-shaped muscular-aponeurotic sling suspended from the central skull base (Teresi et al. 1987). Anteriorly, it merges with the nasal cavity. Inferiorly, the mobile soft palate separates the nasopharynx from the oropharynx. On imaging studies, the C1/C2 junction is also generally accepted as the level of demarcation between nasopharynx and oropharynx (Dubrulle et al. 2007).

The roof of the nasopharynx abuts the basisphenoid (sphenoid sinus floor), and slopes postero-inferiorly along the clivus/basiocciput to the upper

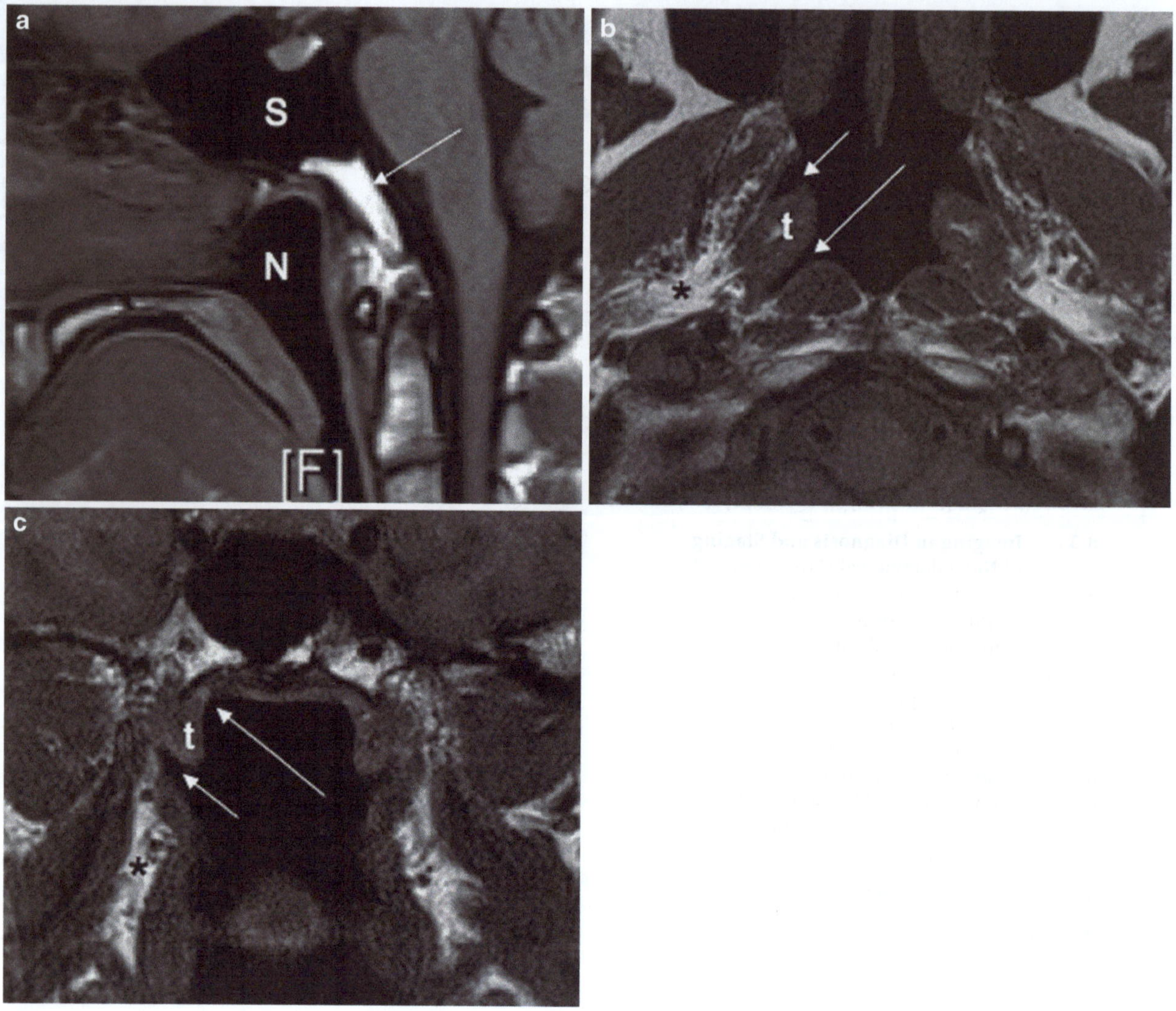

Fig. 8.1. Normal anatomy of the nasopharynx. (**a**) Sagittal T1-weighted MR image shows the nasopharynx (*N*) with its roof abutting the sphenoid sinus (*S*) and more posteriorly, the clivus (*arrow*). (**b**) Axial T1-weighted MR image shows the right lateral pharyngeal recess (*long arrow*), torus tubarius (*t*), and eustachian tube opening (*short arrow*). The hyperintense fat of the parapharyngeal space (*asterisk*) lies laterally. Note asymmetry of the lateral pharyngeal recesses, a common finding. (**c**) Coronal T1-weighted MR image shows the right lateral pharyngeal recess (*long arrow*), torus tubarius (*t*), and eustachian tube opening (*short arrow*). The hyperintense parapharyngeal fat (*asterisk*) is again seen laterally

cervical vertebrae (Fig. 8.1). The adenoids occupy the roof of the nasopharynx. These lymphoid tissues involute with age but may persist as tags of tissue into adulthood.

The pharyngobasilar fascia, a tough aponeurosis that connects the superior constrictor muscle to the skull base, provides the principal framework for maintaining the configuration of the nasopharynx (Dillon et al. 1984). This fascia attaches to the medial plate of the pterygoid process anteriorly and extends posteriorly to the occipital pharyngeal tuber, before reflecting medially over the prevertebral muscles. The foramen lacerum (the fibrocartilagous floor in the anterior aspect of the horizontal carotid canal) is within the confines of the pharyngobasilar fascia and is thus part of the nasopharyngeal roof. This foramen presents a route for nasopharyngeal tumors to access the cavernous sinus and intracranial cavity.

The eustachian tube and levator veli palatini muscle enter the nasopharynx through a posterolateral defect in the pharyngobasilar fascia, known as the sinus of Morgagni. The eustachian tube opens anterior (on axial images) and inferior (on coronal images) to the torus tubarius (distal cartilaginous end of the eustachian tube). The lateral pharyngeal recess (fossa of Rosenmuller) is seen posterior (on axial images) and superior (on coronal images) to the torus tubarius, partly due to the inverted J-configuration of the torus tubarius (Fig. 8.1). The lateral pharyngeal recess is the most common site of origin of NPC. However, these recesses can be notoriously asymmetric in normal individuals, which should not be mistaken as tumors.

The parapharyngeal space is located lateral to the nasopharynx, separating it from the masticator space (Fig. 8.1). Displacement or obliteration of the parapharyngeal fat serves as an important marker of tumor infiltration. The carotid space is located posterior to the parapharyngeal space and forms the posterolateral border of the nasopharynx. Between the nasopharyngeal mucosal space and the prevertebral muscles is the retropharyngeal space, within which are the medial and lateral retropharyngeal nodes. The lateral retropharyngeal nodes (nodes of Röuviere) constitute the first echelon nodes in the lymphatic drainage of the nasopharynx. The medial retropharyngeal nodes are less often visible on imaging.

Table 8.1 Nasopharyngeal carcinoma: sixth edition TNM classification (2002)

T - primary tumor	
T1	Tumor confined to nasopharynx
T2	Tumor extends to soft tissue of oropharynx and/or nasal fossa
T2a	Without parapharyngeal extension
T2b	With parapharyngeal extension
T3	Tumor invades bony structures and/or paranasal sinuses
T4	Tumor with intracranial extension and/or involvement of cranial nerves, infratemporal fossa, hypopharynx or orbit
N - regional lymph nodes	
Nx	Regional lymph nodes cannot be assessed
N0	No regional lymph node metastasis
N1	Unilateral lymph node(s) metastasis, 6 cm or less in greatest dimension, above supraclavicular fossa
N2	Bilateral lymph nodes metastasis, 6 cm or less in greatest dimension, above supraclavicular fossa
N3	
N3a	Lymph node(s) metastasis greater than 6 cm in dimension
N3b	Lymph node(s) metastasis in the supraclavicular fossa

Table 8.2 Nasopharyngeal carcinoma: stage grouping

Stage 0	Tis	N0	M0
Stage I	T1	N0	M0
Stage IIA	T2a	N0	M0
Stage IIB	T1	N1	M0
	T2a	N1	M0
	T2b	N0, N1	M0
Stage III	T1	N2	M0
	T2a, T2b	N2	M0
	T3	N0, N1, N2	M0
Stage IVA	T4	N0, N1, N2	M0
Stage IVB	Any T	N3	M0
Stage IVC	Any T	Any N	M1

8.3 Imaging in Diagnosis and Staging of Nasopharyngeal Carcinoma

8.3.1 Imaging Issues and Features

Multi-planar magnetic resonance imaging (MRI), using a dedicated head and neck coil, is the modality of choice for evaluation of NPC. Axial and coronal contrast-enhanced T1-weighted images with fat saturation allow precise mapping of the tumor (notably perineural and intracranial spreads), and thus accurate staging of the disease (Tables 8.1 and 8.2) (Chong et al. 1999; Lau et al. 2004). Bone-algorithm computed tomography (CT) is valuable in depicting early skull base cortical bone erosions.

NPC is generally isodense to muscle on nonenhanced CT. It is usually hypo- to isointense and relatively hyperintense to muscle on T1-weighted and T2-weighted MR images, respectively. Mild to moderate tumor enhancement is evident following intravenous contrast on both CT and MRI.

8.3.2
Staging: Tumor Spread

Most NPC originate in the lateral pharyngeal recess. The tumors tend to spread submucosally with early infiltration of the deeper neck spaces. Serous otitis media secondary to eustachian tube dysfunction is frequently encountered, owing to tumor involvement of the adjacent levator veli palatini or eustachian tube orifice (Fig. 8.2) (Hsu et al. 1995). Parapharyngeal tumor extension may also affect eustachian tubal function (Sham et al. 1992).

When NPC extends beyond the nasopharynx, it spreads along well-defined routes and the following patterns of spread may be seen in various combinations (Sham et al. 1991a; Chong and Fan 1998).

8.3.2.1
Anterior Spread

NPC often extends anteriorly into the nasal cavity, and subsequently through the sphenopalatine foramen into the pterygopalatine fossa (Chong and Fan 1997). The

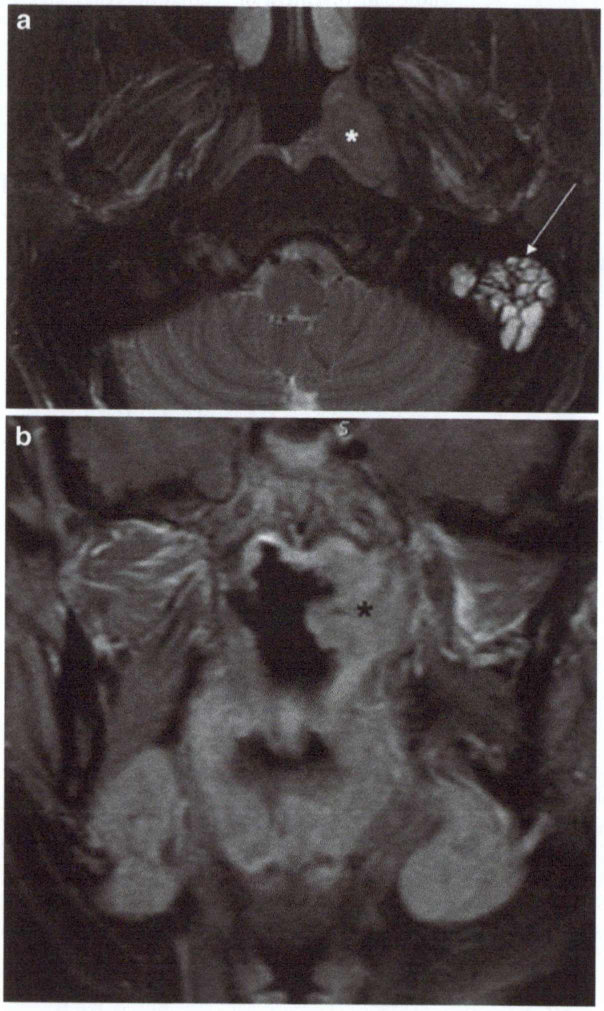

Fig. 8.2. 49-year-old man with left-sided conductive hearing loss. (**a**) Axial fat-saturated T2-weighted MR image reveals an early nasopharyngeal carcinoma arising from the left lateral pharyngeal recess (*asterisk*). Hyperintense fluid is noted in the left mastoid air-cells (*arrow*) owing to underlying eustachian tube dysfunction. (**b**) Coronal contrast-enhanced fat-saturated T1-weighted MR image shows moderate enhancement of the left nasopharyngeal tumor (*asterisk*)

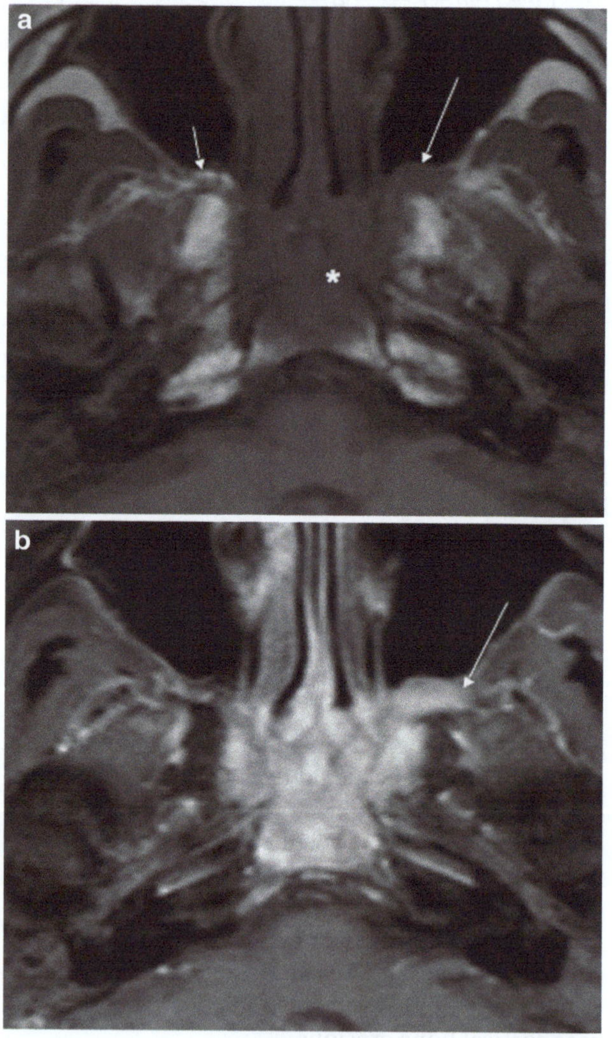

Fig. 8.3. (**a**) Axial T1-weighted MR image shows a nasopharyngeal carcinoma (*asterisk*) extending into the left pterygopalatine fossa (*long arrow*). Note the contralateral pterygopalatine fossa with its normal hyperintense fat (*short arrow*). (**b**) Axial contrast-enhanced fat-saturated T1-weighted MR image shows the tumor encroaching on the left masticator space through the pterygomaxillary fissure (*arrow*)

earliest imaging sign of pterygopalatine fossa involvement is obliteration of its normal fat content (Fig. 8.3). The pterygopalatine fossa is a major crossroad within the deep face, from where tumors may infiltrate:

- The maxillary nerve and extend perineurally through the foramen rotundum into the intracranial cavity (Chong and Fan 1996a).
- Along the vidian canal posteriorly through the foramen lacerum into the petrous carotid canal.
- Laterally through the pterygomaxillary fissure into the masticator space (Fig. 8.3).
- Superiorly through the inferior orbital fissure into the orbital apex, with subsequent intracranial extension via the superior orbital fissure (Fig. 8.4).

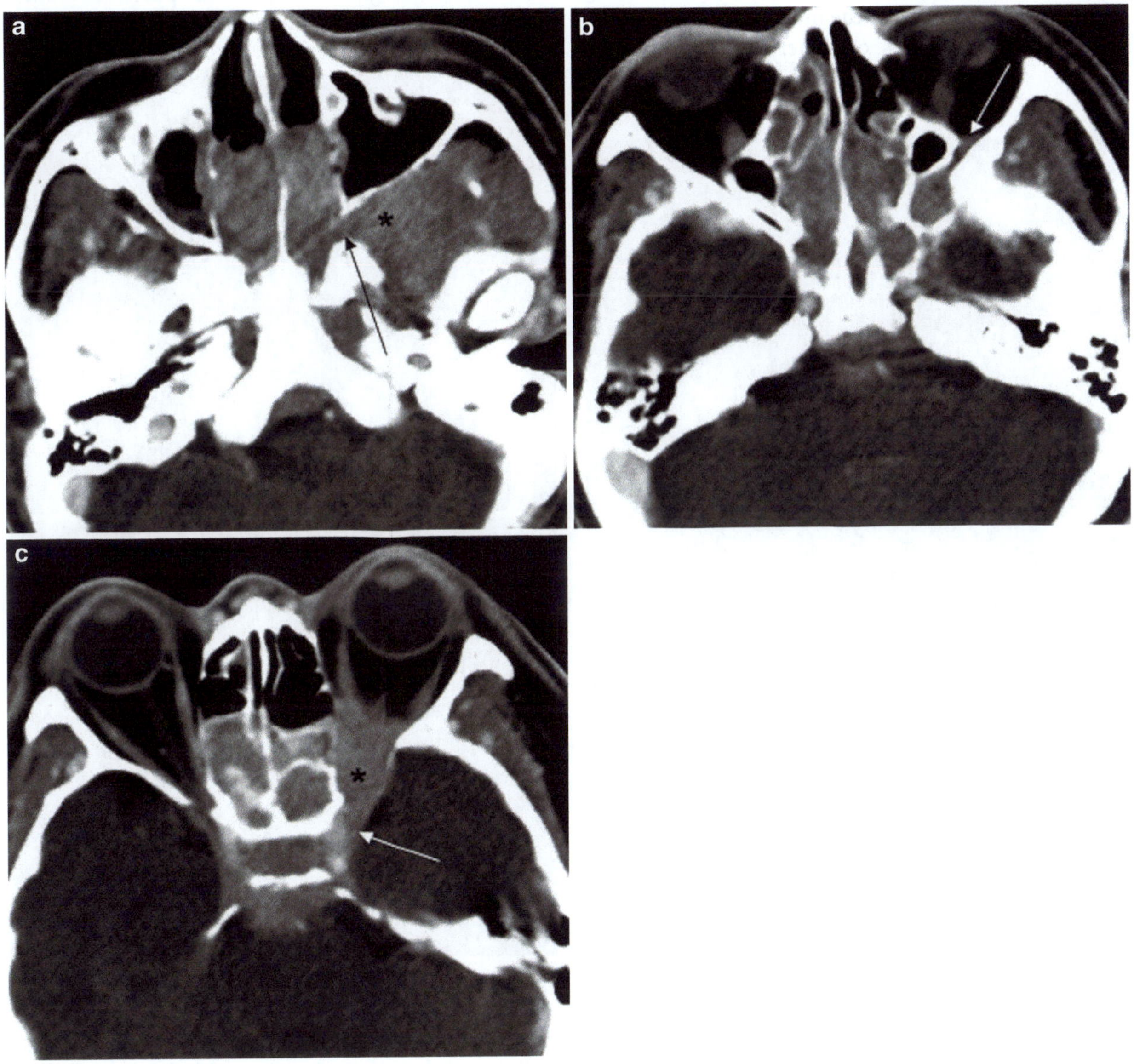

Fig. 8.4. A series of three axial contrast-enhanced CT images from inferior to superior. Image (**a**) shows a nasopharyngeal carcinoma invading the left pterygopalatine fossa and masticator space (*asterisk*) through an enlarged sphenopalatine foramen (*arrow*). Image (**b**) shows that the tumor infiltrates superiorly through the inferior orbital fissure into the left orbital apex (*arrow*). Image (**c**) shows that the tumor (*asterisk*) extends via the superior orbital fissure into the intracranial cavity and involves the left cavernous sinus (*arrow*)

8.3.2.2 Lateral Spread

NPC readily gain access into the parapharyngeal space through the sinus of Morgagni, essentially a gap in the barrier that is the pharyngobasilar fascia. Further laterally, the tumor may spread into the masticator space (Fig. 8.5). When the muscles of mastication (notably the medial and lateral pterygoid muscles) are involved, the patient often complains of trismus (Chong 1997). The mandibular nerve within the masticator space may also be infiltrated, resulting in denervation atrophy of the muscles of mastication. However, MRI features of denervation atrophy of these muscles (T2 hyperintensity and postcontrast enhancement) are more commonly seen during tumor recurrence rather than at primary staging (Chong and Ong 2008). Perineural extension along the mandibular nerve through the foramen ovale is a common route of intracranial tumor spread (Fig. 8.6) (Chong et al. 1996; Su and Lui 1996).

Posterolateral extension of tumor often involves the nasopharyngeal carotid space and compromises and IX, X, XI, and XII cranial nerves. Superior perineural or perivascular spread may then invade the jugular foramen and gain access into the posterior cranial fossa (Fig. 8.7) (Chong and Fan 1996b, c).

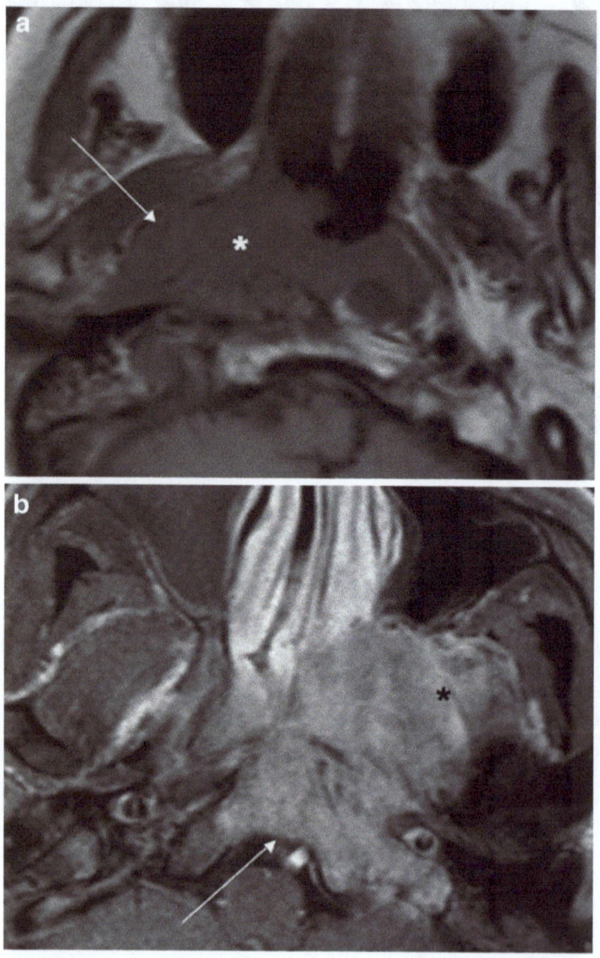

Fig. 8.5. (**a**) Axial T1-weighted MR image shows a right-sided nasopharyngeal carcinoma (*asterisk*) spreading laterally, effacing the parapharyngeal fat (*arrow*). (**b**) Axial contrast-enhanced fat-saturated T1-weighted MR image in another patient shows a more advanced tumor invading the left masticator space (*asterisk*). Tumor infiltration of the clivus is also demonstrated (*arrow*)

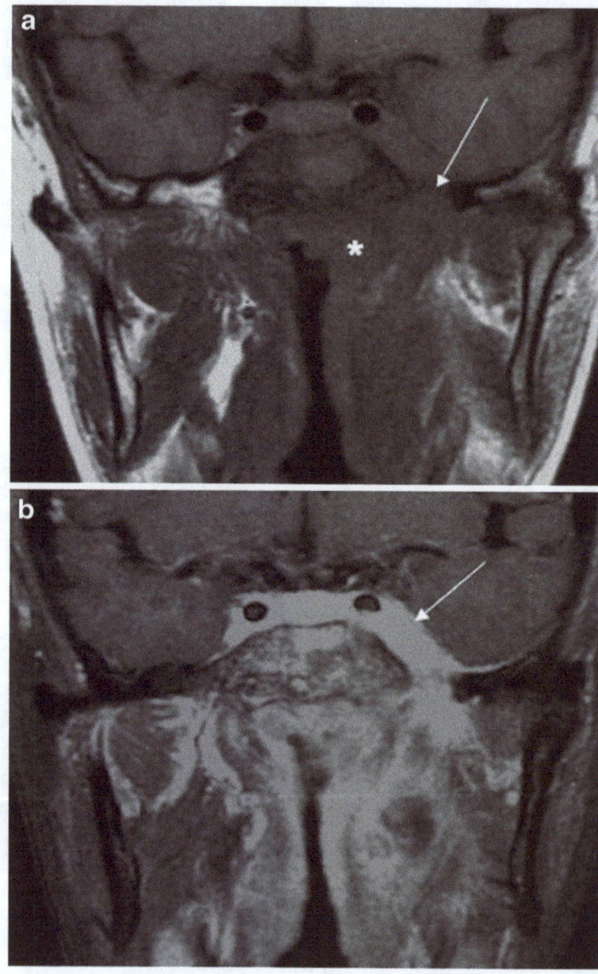

Fig. 8.6. Nasopharyngeal carcinoma with perineural spread. (**a**) Coronal T1-weighted MR image shows a left-sided nasopharyngeal carcinoma (*asterisk*). Obliteration of the normally hyperintense fat in the region of the left foramen ovale (*arrow*) is indicative of underlying perineural tumor spread along the mandibular nerve. (**b**) Coronal contrast-enhanced fat-saturated T1-weighted MR image reveals intracranial tumor spread via the left foramen ovale, infiltrating the left cavernous sinus (*arrow*)

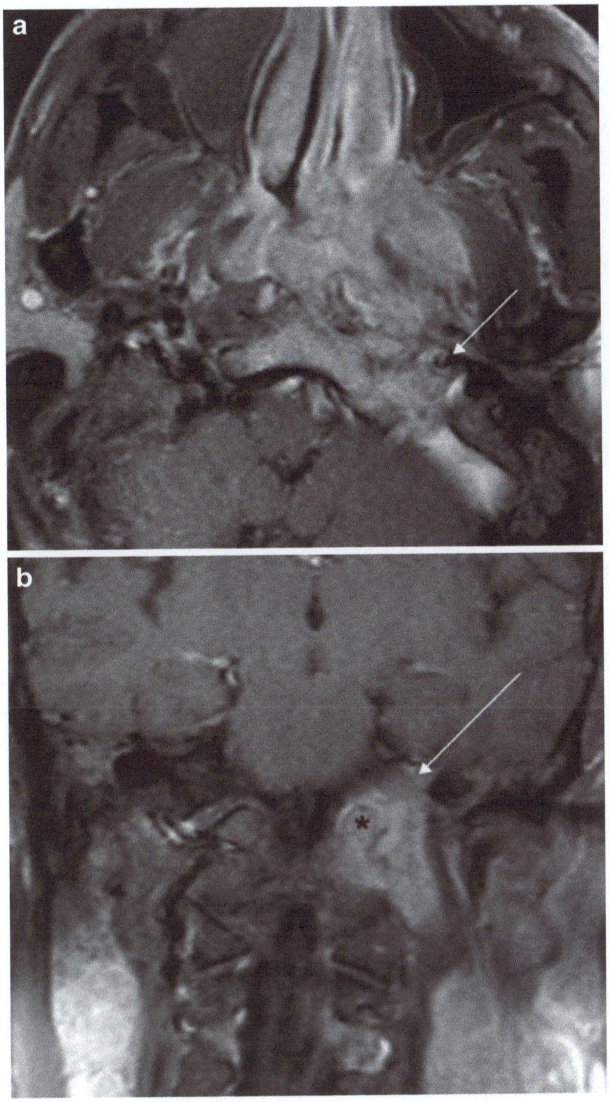

Fig. 8.7. Nasopharyngeal carcinoma with lower cranial neuropathies. (**a**) Axial contrast-enhanced MR image shows an advanced nasopharyngeal carcinoma involving the left carotid space, encircling the internal carotid artery (*arrow*). (**b**) Coronal contrast-enhanced T1-weighted image reveals further superior spread of the tumor into the left jugular foramen (*arrow*). Note tumor infiltration of the left occipital condyle (*asterisk*)

8.3.2.3
Posterior Spread

Posteriorly, NPC may infiltrate the retropharyngeal space and the prevertebral muscles of the perivertebral space (Fig. 8.8a). In advanced diseases, the vertebrae are destructed with tumor extension into the spinal canal.

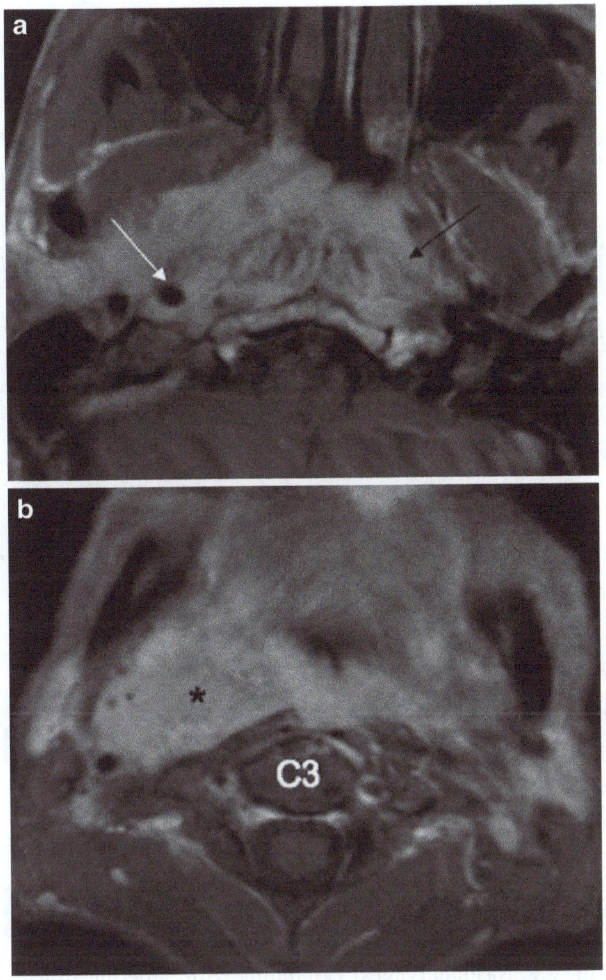

Fig. 8.8. (**a**) Axial contrast-enhanced T1-weighted MR image shows posterior spread of a nasopharyngeal carcinoma, with infiltration of the prevertebral muscles (*black arrow*). The tumor has also invaded the right carotid space, surrounding the internal carotid artery (*white arrow*). (**b**) Axial contrast-enhanced T1-weighted MR image more inferiorly at the level of C3 shows tumor extension into the oropharynx (*asterisk*)

8.3.2.4
Inferior Spread

Many NPC show preferential spread inferiorly along the submucosal plane, which may not be apparent on clinical inspection or endoscopic examination. Inferior tumor extension into the oropharynx is readily appreciated on coronal or sagittal MR images. On axial sections, the oropharynx is deemed involved when the tumor is seen inferior to the C1/C2 junction (Fig. 8.8b).

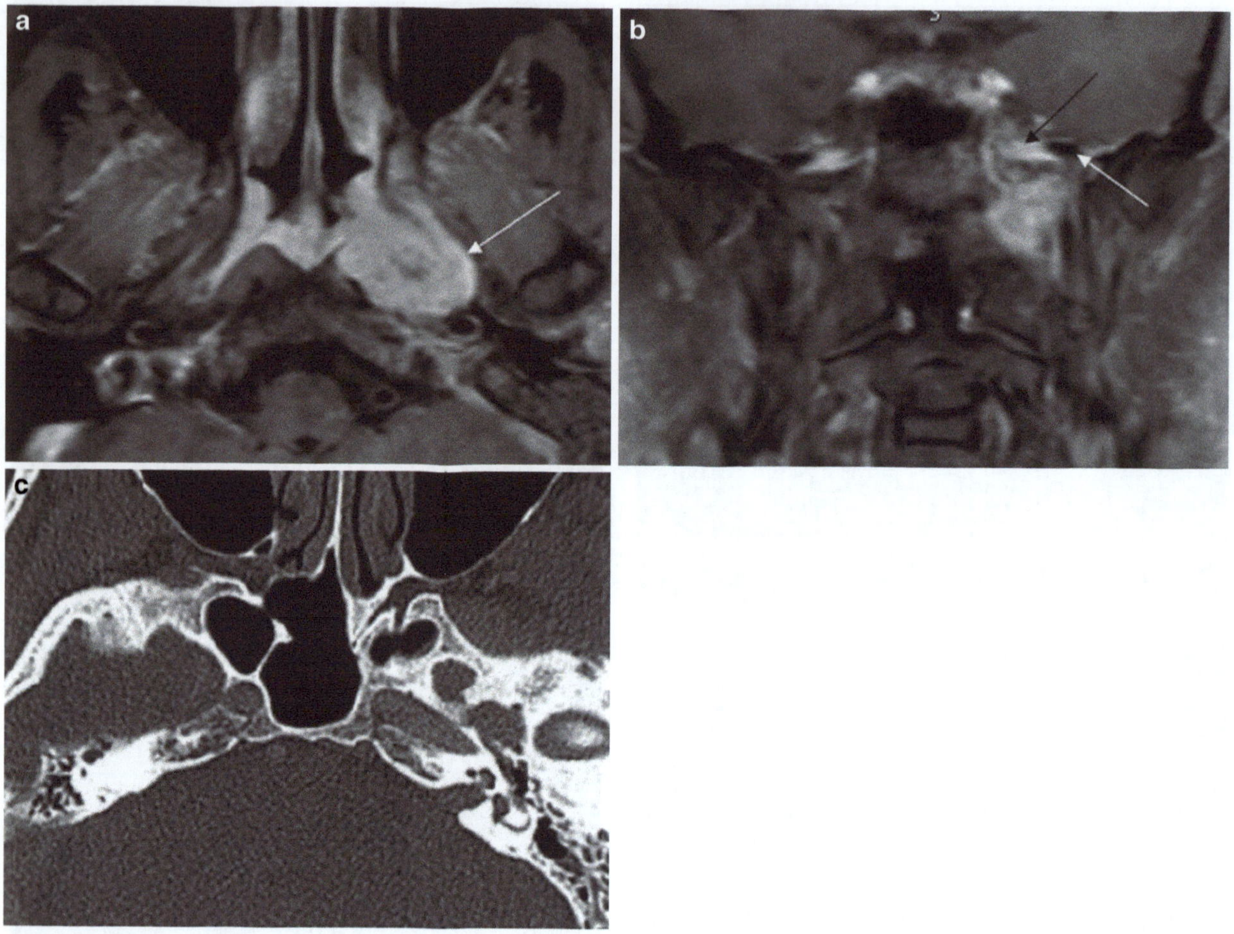

Fig. 8.9. Nasopharyngeal carcinoma with superior spread through the foramen lacerum. (**a**) Axial contrast-enhanced fat-saturated T1-weighted MR image shows a left-sided nasopharyngeal carcinoma with predominantly posterolateral spread (*arrow*). (**b**) Coronal contrast-enhanced fat-saturated T1-weighted MR image reveals further superior extension through the left foramen lacerum (*black arrow*). Note the adjacent petrous internal carotid artery (*white arrow*). (**c**) High-resolution bone algorithm CT image shows no evidence of skull base erosion

8.3.2.5 Superior Spread

As noted earlier, foramen lacerum is within the confines of the pharyngobasilar fascia and for a long time, it was believed to provide an unimpeded route of tumor infiltration into the intracranial cavity (Fig. 8.9). However, many studies have since showed that more NPC spread intracranially via direct erosion of the skull base (Fig. 8.10) (Sham et al. 1991b). Skull base invasion is seen in up to one-third of the patients, 12% on CT, and 31% on MRI (Chong et al. 1996; Roh et al. 2004). MRI is able to detect early marrow signal changes secondary to osseous infiltration without cortical bone erosion.

8.3.3 Staging: Tumor Volume

Primary tumor volume represents a significant independent prognostic factor in the treatment of malignant tumors, including NPC (Wei and Sham 2005). Larger tumors are related to increased number of tumor clonogens, as well as other adverse radiobiologic factors including tumor hypoxia and thus their relative radioresistance (Johnson et al. 1995; Lartigau et al. 1993; Bentzen et al. 1991). There is an estimated 1% increase in risk of local control failure with every 1 cm^3 increase in primary tumor volume (Sze et al. 2004). Such observations have prompted suggestions to incorporate tumor volume into the TNM staging

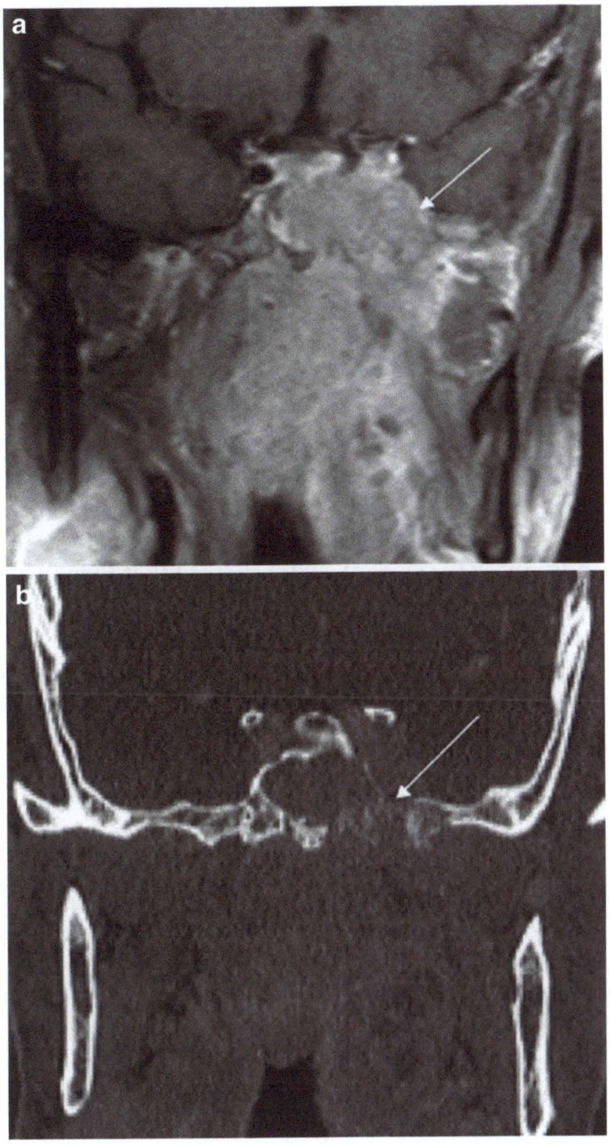

Fig. 8.10. (**a**) Coronal contrast-enhanced fat-saturated T1-weighted MR image shows a large nasopharyngeal carcinoma with superior extension into the intracranial cavity (*arrow*). (**b**) Coronal bone-algorithm CT image reveals underlying skull base erosion (*arrow*)

system. In the current system, a small tumor involving a critical area is often assigned a higher T-classification when compared with a larger tumor confined within a defined anatomic site (Willner et al. 1999; Chen et al. 2004; Chua et al. 1997). Early studies have indeed showed a positive relationship between NPC tumor volume and the TNM classification system (Chong et al. 2006).

However, technical difficulty in standardizing accurate tumor volume measurement has prevented it from being used routinely in daily practice. The measurement of tumor volume is tedious and involves operator-dependent tracing of the tumor outline. Several semi-automated systems of tumor volume measurement have been developed and are now available for NPC, reducing inter-operator as well as intra-operator variability (Clarke et al. 1995; Rasch et al. 1997; Chong et al. 2004).

8.3.4 Staging: Nodal Metastasis

Cervical lymphadenopathy is very common in NPC, and is usually the initial presenting complaint (Fig. 8.11). Enlarged cervical nodes are evident in up to 75% of patients at presentation, 80% of who have bilateral lymphadenopathy (Chong and Ong 2008). Although retropharyngeal nodes are generally considered as the first echelon nodes of NPC, they are only seen in 65% of patients with nodal involvement (Chong et al. 1995). In the other 35% of patients, the metastases bypass the retropharyngeal nodes and spread directly to the internal jugular nodes.

On imaging, the diagnosis of metastatic cervical lymphadenopathy in NPC (as well as other head and neck cancers) relies on the size and morphology of the lymph node. Generally, nodes along the jugular chain are considered malignant if their shortest axes are greater than 10 mm. A group of three or more lymph nodes that are borderline in size may also be deemed malignant (Van Der Brekel et al. 1990). In addition, a lymph node is considered involved where there is imaging evidence of central necrosis or extracapsular extension (Van Der Brekel et al. 1990; Som et al. 1992).

On MRI, the short axes of normal lateral retropharyngeal nodes are usually less than 4.5 mm. Any lateral retropharyngeal node with short axis of 5 mm or more should be regarded as malignant (Lam et al. 1997; King et al. 2000). As medial retropharyngeal nodes are usually not visible, any medial retropharyngeal nodes detected on MRI are highly suspicious of metastatic involvement (Wang et al. 2009). Note that retropharyngeal lymphadenopathy is not included in the current TNM classification, as its prognostic significance remains inconclusive and controversial (Ma et al. 2007; Tang et al. 2008; Wang et al. 2009).

Cervical nodal metastases in NPC, as a rule, show an orderly inferior spread and the affected nodes in the upper neck are generally larger than those more inferiorly. This reflects the route of spread of the

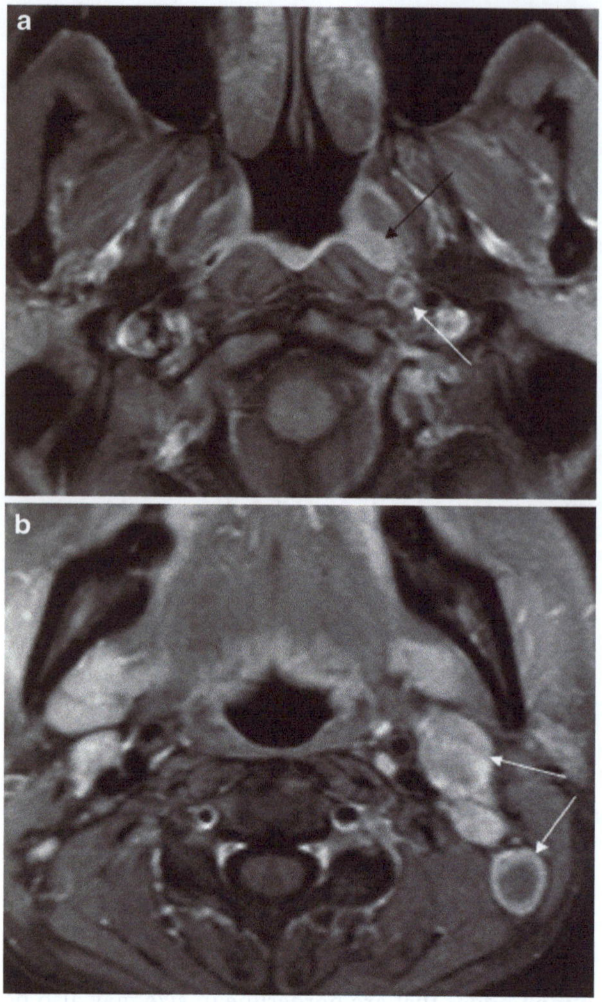

Fig. 8.11. 39-year-old female presented with left cervical lymphadenopathy. (**a**) Axial contrast-enhanced fat-saturated T1-weighted MR image shows a small nasopharyngeal carcinoma arising from the left lateral pharyngeal recess (*black arrow*). An adjacent necrotic retropharyngeal node is evident (*white arrow*). (**b**) Axial contrast-enhanced fat-saturated T1-weighted MR image more inferiorly shows multiple enlarged cervical nodes (*arrows*), despite the small and seemingly localized primary tumor. One of the nodes is necrotic

tumor cells along the lymphatic system and has prognostic significance. The internal jugular nodes may be viewed as successive defensive barriers, with the supraclavicular nodes being the last line of defense. Failure of supraclavicular nodes to contain the malignant cells results in them spilling into the thoracic duct and eventually the systemic circulation. Supraclavicular lymphadenopathy (N3 disease) is therefore associated with a high risk of systemic metastasis.

8.3.5 Staging: Systemic Metastasis

NPC has a relatively high incidence of systemic metastasis (up to 41%) when compared with the other head and neck tumors (5%–24%). The most common sites of metastases are bone (20%), lung (13%), and liver (9%) (Sham et al. 1990).

The risk of systemic metastasis increases in individuals with more advanced primary tumors and/or extensive lymph node involvement. Advanced tumors infiltrating the parapharyngeal space are related to higher incidence of systemic metastasis (Xiao et al. 2002). Tumor invasion of the parapharyngeal veins (which drain via the retropharyngeal and facial veins into the internal jugular vein) results in dissemination of disease through the systemic circulation. In addition, (Kumar et al. 2004) showed that there was a direct correlation between the prevalence of distant metastasis and the N-classification as well as the overall stage of NPC. The positive yield of their metastatic work-up (chest X-ray, liver ultrasound, and whole body bone scan) was 0, 1.8%, 4.8%, and 14.3% for N0, N1, N2, and N3 disease, respectively.

Imaging surveillance (which may include chest X-ray or CT of the thorax, ultrasound or CT of the abdomen, and whole body bone scan) is indicated in patients with advanced disease who are more susceptible to metastasis. On the other hand, as the probability of systemic metastasis is relatively low in patients with early NPC (stage I and II) diseases, the validity of metastatic work-up in every single patient diagnosed with NPC is debatable.

There is some evidence that fludeoxyglucose positron emission tomography (FDG-PET) or PET/CT has a higher sensitivity and specificity in detecting visceral and skeletal metastases when compared with CT thorax and abdomen and whole body radioisotope bone scan, respectively (Liu et al. 2007; Chua et al. 2009; Ng et al. 2009). Nevertheless, the role of PET or PET/CT in the detection of systemic metastasis and staging of NPC is yet to be fully established.

8.3.6 Differential Diagnosis

Several other tumors, albeit much less common, may arise from the nasopharynx. At times, it may be impossible to differentiate these tumors from NPC on imaging along, and histologic confirmation is necessary.

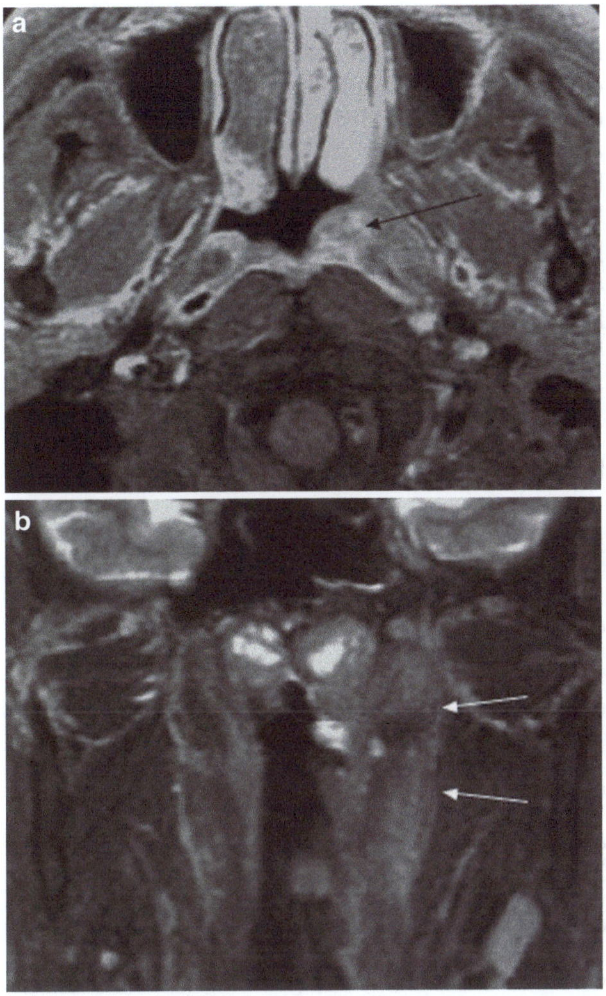

Fig. 8.12. Nasopharyngeal lymphoma. (**a**) Axial contrast-enhanced T1-weighted MR image shows a left nasopharyngeal tumor (*arrow*). (**b**) Coronal fat-saturated T2-weighted image demonstrates inferior spread of the tumor along the left pharyngeal mucosal space (*arrows*). No infiltration of the deep neck spaces is evident

The principal differential diagnoses of NPC include nasopharyngeal non-Hodgkin's lymphoma (NHL) and minor salivary gland carcinoma. Nasopharyngeal NHL, in contrast to NPC, usually shows no or minimal infiltration of the deep neck spaces (Fig. 8.12) (King et al. 2003). Skull base erosion is also rare. The lymph nodes in NHL are usually non-necrotic, except in immunocompromised patients. Nodal metastasis is rare in nasopharyngeal minor salivary gland malignancy, which is otherwise often indistinguishable from NPC on imaging (Jones et al. 1998; Sigal et al. 1992). Nasopharyngeal plasmacytoma, hemangiopericytoma, melanoma, and rhabdomyosarcoma have also been reported (King et al. 2003; Palacios et al. 2005; Mortele et al. 2001; Nikolidakis et al. 2000) (Figs. 8.13 and 8.14).

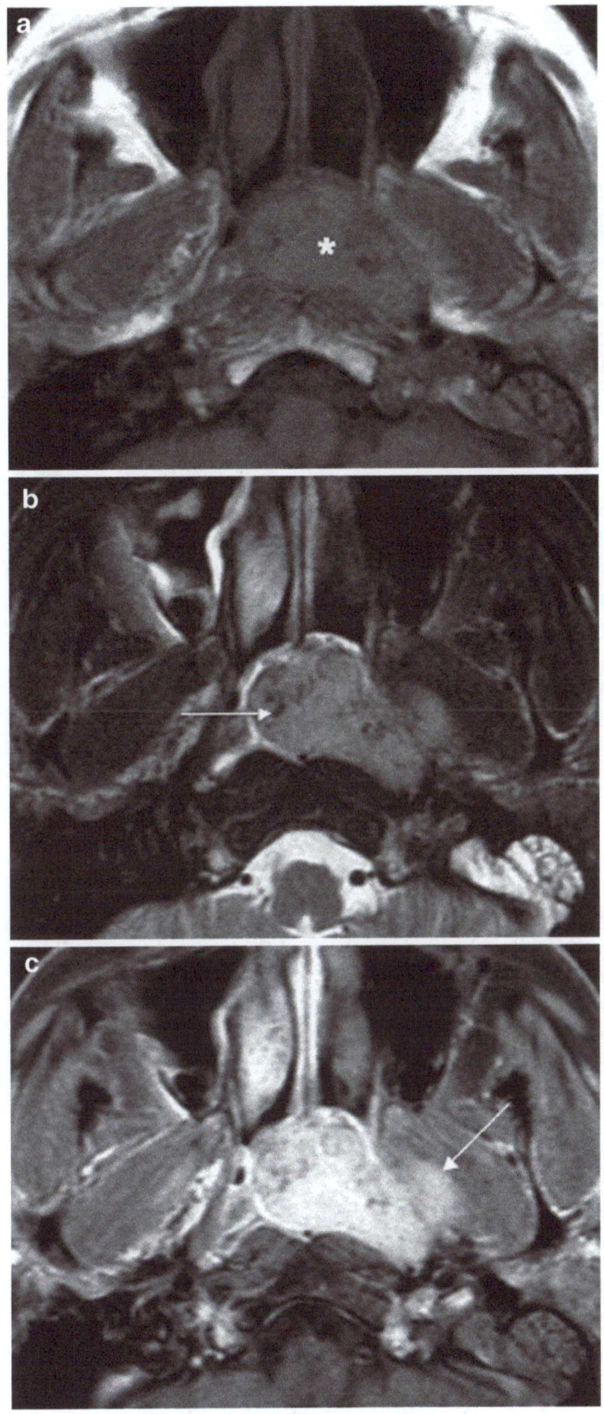

Fig. 8.13. Nasopharyngeal hemangiopericytoma. (**a**) Axial T1-weighted MR image shows a fairly well-delineated, isointense tumor (*asterisk*) arising from the left pharyngeal recess protruding into the nasopharyngeal airway. (**b**) Axial fat-saturated T2-weighted MR image reveals serpentine flow-voids (*arrow*) within the hyperintense tumor, owing to prominent intratumoral vessels. (**c**) Axial contrast-enhanced T1-weighted MR image shows intense tumor enhancement. Infiltration of the adjacent left lateral pterygoid muscle is noted (*arrow*)

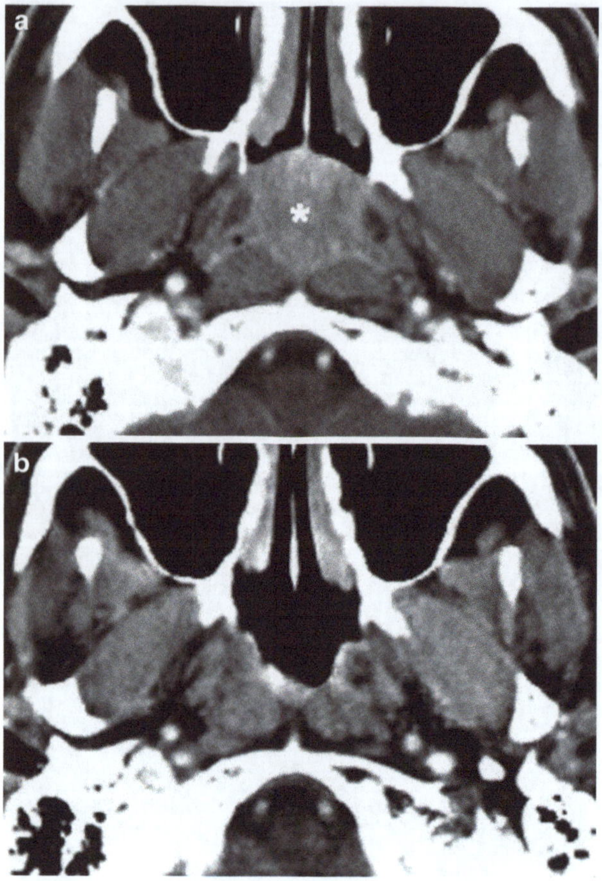

Fig. 8.14. Extramedullary plasmacytoma of the nasopharynx. (**a**) Axial contrast-enhanced CT image shows a mild to moderately enhancing tumor (*asterisk*) arising from the nasopharyngeal mucosal wall, occluding the nasopharyngeal airway. (**b**) Axial contrast-enhanced CT image following radiotherapy shows significant disease resolution

8.4 Summary

NPC commonly arises from the lateral pharyngeal recess and spreads widely into the surroundings along well-defined routes. Primary tumor volume is a significant independent prognostic factor of the disease, but technical complexity often limits its use in daily practice. Cervical lymphadenopathy is very common in NPC and is usually the initial presenting complaint. NPC has a relatively high incidence of systemic metastasis, and the risk increases in individuals with parapharyngeal tumor extension and supraclavicular lymphadenopathy.

Diagnosis of NPC is often achievable through endoscopic examination and biopsy, but imaging is essential for accurate staging of the tumor, delineating the full scale of submucosal, osseous, or intracranial tumor spread, the detection of which eludes clinical and endoscopic examinations. Multi-planar contrast-enhanced MRI is the best tool for full evaluation of the disease extent, while high-resolution bone algorithm CT is of value in assessing cortical bone erosion. A thorough understanding of the complex anatomy of the nasopharynx and the natural history of the disease facilitates accurate tumor mapping and treatment planning, which are crucial for favorable therapeutic outcome.

References

Bentzen SM, Johansen LV, Overgaard J, et al (1991) Clinical radiobiology of squamous cell carcinoma of the oropharynx. Int J Radiat Oncol Biol Phys 206:1197–1206

Cellai E, Olmi P, Chiavacci A, et al (1990) Computed tomography in nasopharyngeal carcinoma – part II: impact on survival. Int J Radiat Oncol Biol Phys 19:1177–1182

Chen MK, Chen TH, Liu JP, et al (2004) Better prediction of prognosis for patients with nasopharyngeal carcinoma using primary tumor volume. Cancer 100:2160–2166

Chong VFH (1997) Masticator space in nasopharyngeal carcinoma. Ann Otol Rhinol Laryngol 106:979–982

Chong VFH, Fan YF (1996a) Pictorial essay: maxillary nerve involvement in nasopharyngeal carcinoma. AJR 167: 1309–1312

Chong VFH, Fan YF (1996b) Radiology of the carotid space. Clin Radiol 51:762–768

Chong VFH, Fan YF (1996c) Jugular foramen involvement in nasopharyngeal carcinoma. J Laryngol Otol 110:897–900

Chong VFH, Fan YF (1997) Pterygopalatine fossa and maxillary nerve infiltration in nasopharyngeal carcinoma. Head Neck 19:121–125

Chong VFH, Fan YF (1998) Nasopharyngeal carcinoma. Semin Ultrasound CT MR 19:449–462

Chong VFH, Fan YF, Khoo JBK (1995) Retropharyngeal lymphadenopathy in nasopharyngeal carcinoma. Eur J Radiol 21:100–105

Chong VFH, Fan YF, Khoo JBK (1996) Nasopharyngeal carcinoma with intracranial spread: CT and MRI characteristics. J Comput Assist Tomogr 20:563–639

Chong VFH, Ong CK (2008) Nasopharyngeal carcinoma. Eur J Radiol 66:437–447

Chong VFH, Zhou JY, Khoo JBK, et al (2004) Tumor volume measurement in nasopharyngeal carcinoma. Radiology 231:914–921

Chong VFH, Zhou JY, Khoo JBK, et al (2006) Correlation between MR imaging-derived nasopharyngeal carcinoma tumor-volume and TNM system. Int J Radiat Oncol Biol Phys 64:72–76

Chong VF, Mukherji SK, Ng SH, et al (1999) Nasopharyngeal carcinoma: review of how imaging affects staging. J Comput Assist Tomogr 23:984–993

Chua DT, Sham JS, Kwong DL, et al (1997) Volumetric analysis of tumor extent in nasopharyngeal carcinoma and correlation with treatment outcome. Int J Radiat Oncol Biol Phys 39:711–719

Chua ML, Ong SC, Wee JT, et al (2009) Comparison of 4 modalities for distant metastasis staging in endemic nasopharyngeal carcinoma. Head Neck 31:346–354

Clarke LP, Velthuizen RP, Camacho MA, et al (1995) MRI segmentation: methods and applications. Magn Reson Imaging 13:343–368

Dillon WP, Mills CM, Kjos B, et al (1984) Magnetic resonance imaging of the nasopharynx. Radiology 152:731–738

Dubrulle F, Souillard R, Hermans R (2007) Extension patterns of nasopharyngeal carcinoma. Eur Radiol 17:2622–2630

Emami B, Sethi A, Petruzzelli GJ (2003) Influence of MRI on target volume delineation and IMRT planning in nasopharyngeal carcinoma. Int J Radiat Oncol Biol Phys 57: 481–488

Hsu MM, Young YH, Lin KL (1995) Eustachian tube function of patients with nasopharyngeal carcinoma. Ann Otol Rhinol Laryngol 104:453–455

Johnson CR, Thames HD, Huang DT, et al (1995) The tumor volume and clonogens number relationship: tumor control predictions based upon tumor volume estimates derived from computed tomography. Int J Radiat Oncol Biol Phys 332:281–337

Jones AS, Beasley NJ, Houghton DJ, et al (1998) Tumors of the minor salivary glands. Clin Otolaryngol Allied Sci 23: 27–33

King AD, Ahuja AT, Leung SF, et al (2000) Neck node metastases from nasopharyngeal carcinoma: MR imaging of patterns of disease. Head Neck 22:275–281

King AD, Lei KI, Richards PS, et al (2003) Non-Hodgkin's lymphoma of the nasopharynx: CT and MRI imaging. Clin Radiol 58:621–625

Kumar MB, Lu JJ, Loh KS, et al (2004) Tailoring distant metastatic imaging for patients with clinically localized undifferentiated nasopharyngeal carcinoma. Int J Radiat Oncol Biol Phys 58:688–693

Lam WW, Chan YL, Leung SF, et al (1997) Retropharyngeal lymphadenopathy in nasopharyngeal carcinoma. Head Neck 19:176–181

Lartigau E, Le Ridant AM, Lambin P, et al (1993) Oxygenation of head and neck tumors. Cancer 717:2319–2325

Lau KY, Kan WK, Sze WM, et al (2004) Magnetic resonance for T-staging of nasopharyngeal carcinoma, the most informative pair of sequences. Jpn J Clin Oncol 34:171–175

Liu FY, Lin CY, Chang JT, et al (2007) 18F-FDG PET can replace conventional work-up in primary M staging of nonkeratinizing nasopharyngeal carcinoma. J Nucl Med 48: 1614–9161

Ma J, Liu L, Tang L, et al (2007) Retropharyngeal lymphadenopathy in nasopharyngeal carcinoma: prognostic value and staging categories. Clin Cancer Res 13:1445–1452

Mortele B, Lemmerling M, Seynaeve P, et al (2001) Hemangiopericytoma of the parotid gland: CT and MR features. Eur Radiol 11:1073–1075

Ng SH, Chan SC, Yen TC, et al (2009) Staging of untreated nasopharyngeal carcinoma with PET/CT: comparison with conventional imaging work-up. Eur J Nucl Med Mol Imaging 36:12–22

Nikolidakis A, Skoulakis C, Papadakis C, et al (2000) Solitary extramedullary plasmacytomas of the nasopharynx. J Otolaryngol 29:254–257

Palacios E, Restrepo S, Mastrogiovanni L, et al (2005) Sinonasal hemangiopericytomas: clinicopathologic and imaging findings. Ear Nose Throat J 84:99–102

Rasch C, Keus R, Pameijer FA, et al (1997) The potential impact of CT-MRI matching on tumor volume delineation in advanced head and neck cancer. Int J Radiat Oncol Biol Phys 394:841–848

Roh JL, Sung MW, Kim KH, et al (2004) Nasopharyngeal carcinoma with skull base invasion: a necessity of staging subdivision. Am J Otolaryngol 25:26–32

Sham JST, Cheung YK, Chan FL, et al (1990) Nasopharyngeal carcinoma: pattern of skeletal metastases. Br J Radiol 63: 202–205

Sham JST, Cheung YK, Choy D, et al (1991a) Nasopharyngeal carcinoma: CT evaluation of patterns of tumor spread. AJNR 12:265–270

Sham JST, Cheung YK, Choy D, et al (1991b) Cranial nerve involvement and base of skull erosion in nasopharyngeal carcinoma. Cancer 68:422–426

Sham JST, Wei WI, Lau SK, et al (1992) Serous otitis media and paranasopharyngeal extension of nasopharyngeal carcinoma. Head Neck 14:19–23

Sigal R, Monnet O, de Baere T, et al (1992) Adenoid cystic carcinoma of the head and neck: evaluation with MR imaging and clinical-pathologic correlation in 27 patients. Radiology 184:95–101

Som PM (1992) Detection of metastasis in cervical lymph nodes: CT and MR criteria and differential diagnosis. AJR Am J Roentgenol 158:961–969

Su CY, Lui CC (1996) Perineural invasion of the trigeminal nerve in patients with nasopharyngeal carcinoma. Cancer 78:2063–2069

Sze WM, Lee AW, Yau TK, et al (2004) Primary tumor volume of nasopharyngeal carcinoma: prognostic significance for local control. Int J Radiat Oncol Biol Phys 59:21–27

Tang L, Li L, Mao Y, et al (2008) Retropharyngeal lymph node metastasis in nasopharyngeal carcinoma detected by magnetic resonance imaging – prognostic value and staging categories. Cancer 113:347–354

Teresi LM, Lufkin RB, Vinuela F, et al (1987) MR imaging of the nasopharynx and floor of the middle cranial fossa – part I: Normal anatomy. Radiology 164:811–816

van der Brekel MW, Stel HV, Castelijns JA, et al (1990) Cervical lymph node metastasis: assessment of radiologic criteria. Radiology 177:379–384

Wang XS, Hu CS, Ying HM, et al (2009) Patterns of retropharyngeal node metastasis in nasopharyngeal carcinoma. Int J Radiat Oncol Biol Phys 73:194–201

Wei WI, Sham JST (2005) Nasopharyngeal carcinoma. Lancet 365:2041–2054

Willner J, Baier K, Pfreunder L, et al (1999) Tumor volume and local control in primary radiotherapy of nasopharyngeal carcinoma using primary tumor volume. Acta Oncol 38: 1025–1030

Xiao GL, Gao L, Xu GZ (2002) Prognostic influence of parapharyngeal space involvement in nasopharyngeal carcinoma. Int J Radiat Oncol Biol Phys 52:957–963

Prognostic Factors in Nasopharyngeal Cancer

9

Jin-Ching Lin

CONTENTS

Jin-Ching Lin, MD, PhD
Department of Radiation Oncology, Taichung Veterans General Hospital, Taiwan, No. 160, Sec. 3, Taichung-Kang Rd., Taichung 407, Taiwan, ROC

9.1 Introduction

The prognosis of a cancer depends on the biological aggressiveness of the tumor, the characteristic of the host, and the therapeutic interventions. Prognostic factors of nasopharyngeal carcinoma (NPC) have been one of the most important research foci, and a large number of investigations in this area have been performed and published. The extent of local invasion, regional lymphatic spread, and distant metastasis, as reflected by the TNM staging, are the most important prognostic factors in NPC. Generally, advanced T-classification is associated with worse local control and overall survival; advanced N-classification predicts increased risk of both distant failure and suboptimal survival; and patients with distant metastasis, that is, M1 disease usually are not curable and have limited life expectancy. In addition, advances in imaging modalities, such as computerized tomography (CT) scan, magnetic resonance imaging (MRI), and positron emission tomography (PET) scan, make it possible to measure tumor volume and extension more precisely. A number of radiological criteria other than those required by the TNM staging have been reported to affect treatment outcome significantly. Furthermore, NPC has been proven as an EBV-associated disease. Recently, cell-free circulating EBV DNA has been detected in plasma and serum of NPC patients, and has been shown as a reliable prognosticator.

Because of the anatomic constraints of NPC and its high radiosensitivity, NPC is traditionally treated by radiation therapy. Advances in radiation technology and fractionation schedule have significantly improved the treatment results. NPC is a chemosensitive malignancy as well, and chemotherapy has been incorporated into the management of advanced disease. Various strategies of combined chemoradiation therapy have demonstrated a different impact on the outcome. The aim of this chapter is to present a systemic discussion of the above-mentioned disease- and treatment-related prognosticators, as well as other factors, such as pathological type, age, gender, race, performance status, and potential biomarkers in prediction of the clinical outcome.

9.2 Presenting Stage as a Prognostic Factor

The extent of a malignancy after a confirmed diagnosis is usually measured by clinical or pathological staging. However, as NPC is usually treated in a nonsurgical fashion, it is usually staged clinically based on results of physical and radiological examinations. Although staging for NPC is out of the scope of this chapter and is detailed in Chapter 24, it is important to recognize that clinical staging is not only important in the reporting of the extent of the disease and predicting outcome of patients, but also crucial in determining the proper management strategy.

A number of clinical staging systems, including the American Joint Committee on Cancer (AJCC) staging, the International Union Against Cancer (UICC) staging, the Ho's staging from Hong Kong, the Fuzhou 1992 staging from Mainland China, Huang's or Hsu's staging from Taiwan had been developed for NPC. Each system had different criteria for T and N classification. The staging for NPC remained relatively confused until 1987 when two large staging systems – the AJCC and UICC – merged. The fourth edition of the AJCC/UICC cancer staging system in 1992 offered no changes to the guidelines for staging NPC. In 1997, the AJCC/UICC revised the fifth edition of the NPC staging classification by incorporating data from both Western and Eastern studies, particularly those from high incidence areas in Southern Asia. An ideal staging system should correctly distinguish patients with different prognoses, assign them to stage groups of relatively uniform size, and guide appropriate treatment. Several studies confirm the superiority of the 1997 staging system over the 1992 system in terms of more even distribution of cases across stage and accurate prediction of patients' survival (Cooper et al. 1998; Heng et al. 1999; Ozyar et al. 1999; Lee et al. 1999, 2004; Hong et al. 2000; Chua et al. 2001; Ma et al. 2001a). The sixth edition of the AJCC/UICC cancer staging system in 2002 used the same criteria as in the 1997 version for NPC staging. The significance of TNM staging in the prediction of prognosis was demonstrated in a large retrospective series from Hong Kong. In this report which studied 2687 patients, more than 2000 cases were treated with conventional radiation alone, and demonstrated that the presenting stage was the most important prognostic factor for both overall survival and distant failure-free survival with locoregional control (Lee et al. 2005b).

In general, T-classification predominantly affects local control, whereas N-classification significantly predicts neck and distant control. Thus, the overall stage derived from both the T- and N-classifications can affect local, regional, and distant control rates. Table 9.1 presents major series published recently regarding staging on patient's prognoses. All studies included used the 1997 AJCC/UICC staging criteria. The local control rate decreases as the T-classification increases (Ma et al. 2001a; Au et al. 2003; Lee et al. 2005b; Leung et al. 2005); and the regional control rate decreases as the N-classification increases (Au et al. 2003; Lee et al. 2005b; Leung et al. 2005). T-classification also affects locoregional failure-free survival (Ozyar et al. 1999; Cheng et al. 2006a, b), overall survival (Heng et al. 1999; Yeh et al. 2005), disease-free survival (Yeh et al. 2005; Lu et al. 2006), distant metastasis-free survival (Au et al. 2003), and disease-specific survival (Hong et al. 2000). The N-classification also affects distant metastasis-free survival (Ozyar et al. 1999; Ma et al. 2001a; Au et al. 2003), overall survival (Heng et al. 1999; Yeh et al. 2005), disease-free survival (Yeh et al. 2005; Lu et al. 2006), and disease-specific survival (Hong et al. 2000). Among different endpoints of outcome analysis, overall survival is always the most important one. The overall stage has been shown as the most significant prognostic factor for overall survival and also affects other survival endpoints. Several studies using multivariate analysis also confirmed the results of aforementioned univariate analysis (Lee et al. 2004; Tang et al. 2008; Liu et al. 2008; Mao et al. 2009).

Despite the proven accuracy of the 1997 version of the TNM-staging system, one must note that it is derived based on patients treated prior to the mid 1990s, when conventional radiation therapy was the gold standard treatment modality. Significant changes in the management of nonmetastatic NPC have occurred in the past decade. However, updated staging classification accommodating the advances in the management of NPC has not been developed. Among all the improvement in NPC treatment, the use of combined chemoradiotherapy and intensity-modulated radiation therapy (IMRT) can be considered revolutionary, and has significantly changed the paradigm of the management of NPC. Recently, several studies have proposed some modifications for T-classification, N-classification, and overall stage grouping (Au et al. 2003; Lu et al. 2006; Ma et al. 2007; Ng et al. 2007; Liu et al. 2008; Mao et al. 2008, 2009; Tang et al. 2008). Each modification was based on their survival data and showed better prognostic discrimination between patients with different subgroup. Future revision of the staging system should incorporate these suggestions.

It is reasonable to question the magnitude of the predictive value of the 1997 version of staging system (or its 2002 updates) in the new era of combined chemoradiotherapy and IMRT for NPC. Nevertheless, the follow-up periods of literatures on IMRT for NPC were limited. The long-term effect of these new treatment technology or strategy on the patients' outcome awaits further investigation. We expect that the effect of presenting staging on prognosis will change more or less under different treatment modality in the future. Since the locoregional control has been greater than 90% using modern radiation technique, distant failure rate will continue to be the critical point affecting patient's prognosis. Future staging modification should focus on risk grouping according to the distant failure rate. For patients with high risk of distant failure, more intensive systemic treatment strategy deserves to be investigated.

9.3 Predictive Value of the Volumes of the Primary Disease and Cervical Lymph Adenopathy on Prognosis

Tumor volume or size has been well recognized as one of the major prognostic factors in the management of most malignancies. The main purpose of staging systems in cancer is to segregate patients into subgroups with different prognosis, and to guide appropriate treatment. Thus, tumor bulk has been adopted in the staging systems of several malignancies, which often employed a crude measurement of tumor diameter as well as assessment of tumor extension. For resectable tumors, tumor size may be of less importance to predict local control. However, for diseases treated with radiation therapy or chemotherapy, tumor bulk will have a great impact in local control because bulky tumor usually have increasing numbers of tumor clonogens to be sterilized. In addition, larger tumor volume is also likely to contain hypoxic regions thus more resistant to radiation therapy. A number of publications have suggested a positive correlation between tumor volume and treatment outcome (Hamilton et al. 2004; Plataniotis et al. 2004; Cheng SW et al. 2006).

NPC is a highly infiltrative tumor, with propensity to spread along adjacent soft tissues as well as the skull base and foramina (Sham and Choy 1991). Tumor volume of NPC cannot be easily assessed clinically without CT scan and MRI. However, accurate assessment of tumor volume in NPC requires delineation of the tumor extent from series imaging slides and calculation of tumor volume from a 3D perspective. With the prevailing utilization of computerized treatment-planning system in radiation therapy, the calculation of tumor volume becomes easier. As the T-classification of NPC is based on the anatomical location and cranial nerve involvement, a large variation in tumor extension or tumor volume exists within the same T-classification, especially in advanced primary diseases. Although advanced T-disease is usually associated with poorer local control and survival, patients with different tumor volume within the same T-category may possess different prognosis. Several studies have addressed the prognostic impact of tumor volume in NPC (Chua et al. 1997b, 2004b; Chang et al. 2002; Chen et al. 2004, 2009; Sze et al. 2004; Kim and Lee 2005; Lee et al. 2008; Shen et al. 2008). Overall, the results of these studies showed a large variation in primary tumor volume in the same T-category, irrespective of the staging systems or imaging modalities used. Although the median and range of primary tumor volume differs largely in different studies, most studies reported a positive correlation between primary tumor volume and various survivals (Table 9.2).

In a study reported by Chua et al. (1997b) from the Queen Mary Hospital of Hong Kong, the primary and nodal tumor of 290 NPC patients were contoured followed by summation of areas in sequential CT scan slides. All patients received radiation therapy and 67 patients also received neoadjuvant chemotherapy before radiotherapy. On univariate analyses, large primary disease (>60 ml) was associated with a significantly poorer local control ($p < 0.001$) and disease-specific survival ($p < 0.001$). In patients with a small primary disease (≤20 ml), there were no significant differences in local control among different T-classification. Large nodal volume was significantly associated with poor distant failure rate ($p = 0.002$), nodal control rate ($p = 0.001$), and disease-specific survival ($p < 0.001$). In multivariate analyses, primary

Table 9.1. Summary of prognostic impact of presenting stage in nasopharyngeal carcinoma

Series	No. of cases	Treatment	T-stage				
			Category	T1	T2	T3	T4
Ma et al. (2001a)	621	RT	5-year LFFS	93%	84%	71%	58%
Au et al. (2003)	1294	RT	5-year LFFS	82%	82%–77%[a]	70%	66%
			5-year MFS	85%	82%–72%	72%	63%
Lee et al. (2005b)	2687	RT ± Ch	5-year LFFS	91%	87%	80%	77%
Leung et al. (2005)	1070	RT ± Ch	5-year LFFS	88%	87%–82%	69%	69%
Ozyar et al. (1999)	90	RT ± Ch	3-year LRFFS	92%	82%	100%	86%
Cheng et al. (2006a, b)	630	RT ± Ch	5-year LRFFS	95%	91%	87%	81%
Lee et al. (1999)	4515	RT ± Ch					
Hong et al. (2000)	411	RT	5-year DSS	83%	82%–65%	48%	22%
Chua et al. (2001)	324	RT ± Ch					
Heng et al. (1999)	677	RT	5-year OS	76%	56%–66%	63%	31%
Yeh et al. (2005)	849	RT	5-year OS	74%	64%	47%	41%
			5-year DFS	69%	57%	39%	30%
Lu et al. (2006)	159	RT	5-year DFS	91%	77%	65%	61%
Liu et al. (2008)	749	RT ± Ch	OS (HR)	0.48*	1 (T2b)	1.30	2.43*
			LFFS (HR)	0.27	1 (T2b)	1.83*	3.22*
Mao et al. (2009)	924	RT ± Ch	DFS (HR)	0.45*	1 (T2b)	0.98	2.52*
			LFFS (HR)	0.95	1 (T2b)	1.96	3.92[a]

RT radiotherapy; *y* year; *LFFS* local failure-free survival; MFS distant metastasis failure-free survival; OS overall survival; *RFS* relapse-free survival; *Ch* chemotherapy; *NFFS* neck failure-free survival; *DSS* disease-specific survival; *PFS* progression-failure survival; *CSS* cancer-specific survival; *LRFFS* locoregional failure-free survival; *DFS* disease-free survival; *HR* hazard ratio

[a]When two numbers appear in one field, it represents data of T2a and T2b for T-classification, N3a and N3b for N-stage, IIA and IIB for overall stage II, IVA and IVB for overall stage IV

*Indicates statistically significant difference

N-stage					Overall stage				
Category	N0	N1	N2	N3	Category	I (%)	II (%)	III (%)	IV (%)
5-year MFS	90%	81%	62%	51%	5-year OS	89	70	53	37
					5-year RFS	84	69	51	36
5-year NFFS	96%	84%	86%	59%–70%[a]	5-year DSS	82	80–72[a]	69	39
5-year MFS	87%	76%	70%	73%–54%					
5-year NFFS	98%	95%	92%	83%	5-year OS	90	84	75	58
					5-year DSS	92	87	79	65
					5-year PFS	85	73	62	44
					5-year MFS	93	87	80	67
5-year NFFS	97%	96%	90%	75%–83%	5-year OS	85	92–78	62	44–43[a]
					5-year CSS	91	95–82	67	50–46
					5-year PFS	84	87–71	57	42–43
					5-year MFS	93	95–84	76	58–56
3-year MFS	93%	76%	80%	40%	3-year OS	100	72	65	55
					3-year LRFFS	88	90	89	85
					10-year DSS	77	65	54	29
5-year DSS	66%	53%	40%	26%	5-year DSS	96	74	50	24
					5-year OS	98	79	80	61
					5-year RFS	96	65	55	41
					5-year LFFS	98	83	76	69
					5-year NFFS	98	98	86	75
					5-year MFS	98	77	78	71
5-year OS	73%	60%	43%	43%–20%	5-year OS	88	75–74	60	35–28
5-year OS	68%	61%	54%	35%	5-year OS	82	72–71	55	42–39
5-year DFS	62%	54%	44%	30%	5-year DFS	76	72–65	47	31–30
5-year DFS	83%	66%	69%	53%					
OS (HR)	1	2.13*	3.70*	4.01–5.60*					
MFS (HR)	1	2.89*	5.66*	7.85–9.49*					
OS (HR)	1	1.37	2.46*	5.20–4.91*					
MFS (HR)	1	1.72	2.86[a]	6.43–6.52[a]					

Table 9.2. Summary of prognostic impact of tumor volume in nasopharyngeal carcinoma

Series	No. of cases	Stage	Treatment	Image	RPLN included	Tumor volume	Univariate analysis	
							LFFS	NFFS
Chua et al. (1997b)	290	I–IV	RT ± Ch	CT	Yes	TV-NP	$p < 0.001$	–
						≤20 (n = 142)	88%	–
						20–40 (n = 78)	80%	–
						40–60 (n = 34)	78%	–
						>60 (n = 36)	56%	–
						TV-Neck	–	$p = 0.0001$
						≤ 10 (n = 202)	–	96%
						10–20 (n = 45)	–	87%
						20–30 (n = 22)	–	81%
						>30 (n = 21)	–	81%
Chua et al. (2004b)	116	I–II	RT	CT	Yes	TV-NP	$p = 0.033$	–
						≤15	93%	–
						>15	82%	–
						TV-Neck	–	–
						≤4	–	–
						>4	–	–
Chen et al. (2004)	129	I–IV	RT ± Ch	CT	–	TV-NP	–	–
Chang et al. (2002)	76	T3–4	RT ± Ch	CT	–	TV-NP	–	–
						<30 (n = 22)	–	–
						30–60 (n = 26)	–	–
						>60 (n = 28)	–	–
Shen et al. (2008)	154	I–IV	RT	CT	Yes	TV-NP	$p = 0.002$	–
						≤20 (n = 53)	92%	–
						20–40 (n = 64)	90%	–
						40–60 (n = 22)	81%	–
						>60 (n = 15)	49%	–
						TV-NP	$p = 0.002$	–
						≤60 (n = 139)	89%	–
						>60 (n = 15)	49%	–
Kim and Lee (2005)	60	I–IV	RT ± Ch	CT	Yes	TV-NP	$p = 0.004$	–
						≤30 (n = 46)	84%	–
						>30 (n = 14)	47%	–
						TV-Neck	–	$p = 0.019$
						≤5 (n = 27)	–	100%
						>5 (n = 33)	–	64%
Lee et al. (2008)	91	I–IV	RT ± Ch	CT	Yes	TV-NP	–	–
						≤ 20	–	–
						20–40	–	–
						>40	–	–
Sze et al. (2004)	308	I–IV	RT ± Ch	MRI	Yes	TV-NP	$p < 0.01$	–
						<15 (n = 106)	97%[b]	–
						≥15 (n = 202)	82%[b]	–
Chen et al. (2009)	69	III–IV	Ch + RT	MRI	No	TV-NP	$p = 0.51$	–
						<median	87%	–
						≥median	91%	–
						TV-NP	p=0.80	–
						<mean	90%	–
						≥mean	87%	–

RPLN retropharyngeal lymph node; *LFFS* local failure-free survival; *NFFS* neck failure-free survival; *MFS* distant metastasis failure-free survival; *DSS* disease-specific survival; *OS* overall survival; *RT* radiotherapy; *Ch* chemotherapy; *CT* computerized tomography scan; *TV-NP* tumor volume of nasopharynx; *TV-Neck* tumor volume of neck nodes; *n.s.* not statistically significant difference; *MRI* magnetic resonance image

[a]Number was estimated from the survival curve

[b]Indicates 3-year rates of survival, otherwise indicates 5-year rates of survival

			Multivariate analysis				
MFS	DSS	OS	LFFS	NFFS	MFS	DSS	OS
$p = 0.01$	$p < 0.001$	–	$p < 0.001$	–	–	$p < 0.001$	–
83%	87%	–					
79%	80%	–					
64%	68%	–					
64%	53%	–					
$p = 0.002$	$p < 0.001$	–		$p = 0.003$	$p < 0.001$	–	–
81%	82%	–					
74%	90%	–					
75%	62%	–					
54%	40%	–					
–	n.s.	–	n.s.	–	n.s.	n.s.	–
–	89%	–					
–	83%	–					
$p = 0.011$	$p = 0.038$	–	–	n.s.	n.s.	n.s.	–
90%	94%	–					
72%	76%	–					
–	–	$p < 0.001$	–				$p < 0.001$
	$p < 0.0001$	–		–	–	$p < 0.001$	–
–	80%[a]	–					
	46%[a]	–					
–	10%[a]	–					
$p = 0.0001$	$p = 0.001$	–	$p = 0.035$	–	$p = 0.355$	$p = 0.325$	
78%	65%	–					
66%	57%	–					
44%	35%	–					
17%	0%	–					
$p = 0.0001$	$p = 0.001$	–					
67%	56%	–					
17%	0%	–					
–	$p = 0.27$	–	$p = 0.015$	–		n.s.	
–	65%	–					
–	44%	–					
–	$p = 0.046$	–	–	$p = 0.039$	–	$p = 0.012$	–
–	74%	–					
–	49%	–					
–	$p < 0.0001$	–		–	–	$p < 0.05$	–
–	90%[a]	–					
–	65%[a]	–					
–	20%[a]	–					
–	$p < 0.01$	$p = 0.13$	$p < 0.05$	–	–	n.s.	n.s.
–	85%[b]	93%[b]					
–	65%[b]	80%[b]					
$p = 0.37$	–	$p = 0.90$	$p = 0.75$	–	–	–	$p = 0.89$
79%	–	70%					
66%	–	74%					
$p = 0.45$	–	$p = 0.94$					
65%	–	73%					
76%	–	72%					

tumor volume was found to be the only independent factor in predicting local control and one of independent factors in predicting disease-specific survival; nodal volume was the only independent factor in predicting neck control. In a subsequent study on 116 patients with stage I–II NPC using similar method, Chua et al. (2004b) found that patients with a primary disease volume of >15 ml had significantly worse 5-year local control rates (82% vs. 93%, p = 0.033), but no statistically significant difference was noted in survival (5-year disease-specific survival rates, 83% vs. 89%, p = 0.30). Multivariate analyses, however, demonstrated that only parapharyngeal extension (T2b) and N1 stage were independent factors that predicted locoregional control and survival, and N1 stage was the only factor that predicted distant failure. The authors concluded that the pretreatment volume of the primary disease has a limited prognostic value in early-stage NPC compared with the usual T- and N-classification, with stage T2b and N1 as independent factors that predicted treatment outcome.

Willner et al. (1999) tried to estimate the correlation between CT scan-derived tumor volume and a dose-response relation. The authors demonstrated that tumor volume was an important factor influencing local control of NPC, and suggested that tumor volume larger than 64 ml are unlikely to be controlled with a total dose of 72 Gy.

Four groups from Mainland China, Taiwan, and Korea using CT scan-derived measurement consistently demonstrated results similar to the aforementioned trials (Shen et al. 2008; Chen et al. 2004; Chang et al. 2002; Lee et al. 2008; Kim and Lee 2005). Shen et al. (2008) analyzed 154 NPC patients treated by accelerated hyperfractionated radiation alone. After a median follow-up of 61 months, the 5-year local failure-free rate, disease-free survival, and distant failure-free survival rates were 89.4% vs. 48.9% (p = 0.002), 56.6% vs. 0% (p = 0.001), and 66.9% vs. 16.5% (p = 0.0001), respectively, for patients whose primary tumor volume were ≤60 cm^3 and >60 cm^3. Multivariate analysis revealed that primary tumor volume is an independent prognostic factor for local control (hazard ratio = 3.568, p = 0.035). Two studies from Taiwan included 129 NPC patients with Stage I–IV (Chen et al. 2004) or 76 patients with Stage III–IV (Chang et al. 2002) showed that tumor volume was a significant prognostic factor in both univariate and multivariate analyses. The validation results with receiver operating characteristic (ROC) curves also revealed that, in predicting patient outcome, primary tumor volume (area under the ROC = 83.33%) was superior to T-classification (area under the ROC = 66.53%), and overall stage (area under the ROC = 58.61%). Another study of 91 NPC patients treated by radiation alone or concurrent chemoradiotherapy from Taiwan demonstrated that primary tumor volume could separate disease-specific survival more clearly than overall stage or T-classification and was the only independent prognostic factor by multivariate analysis (Lee et al. 2008). In addition, Kim and Lee (2005) from Korea investigated 60 NPC patients with Stage I–IV and found that large primary disease of >30 ml in volume was associated with a significantly lower local control (46.9% vs. 84.2%, p = 0.004) and large cervical nodal disease of >5 ml was associated with a significantly lower nodal control (64% vs. 100%, p = 0.019) and lower disease-specific survival (49.0% vs. 73.6%, p = 0.046). In multivariate analysis, the primary tumor volume and neck nodal volume were found to be independent factors in predicting the local (p = 0.015) and nodal (p = 0.039) control, respectively.

MRI has good soft tissue contrast resolution and the capacity of obtaining different multiplanar imaging (Casselman 1994). It has been proven to be superior to CT scan in determining the primary tumor extent of NPC in many studies (Jian et al. 1998; Chong et al. 1999; King et al. 1999, 2000; Sakata et al. 1999; Chung et al. 2004). The studies regarding volumetric analysis for NPC patients using MRI, however, were sparse (Sze et al. 2004; Zhou et al. 2007; Chen et al. 2009). Zhou et al. (2007) demonstrated that mean primary tumor volume increased significantly with advanced T-classification; however, the authors did not analyze the impact of primary tumor volume on prognosis. Two studies addressed the prognostic impact of tumor volume measured by MRI. Sze et al. (2004) collected 308 NPC patients in Hong Kong with stage I–IV disease and retrospectively measured the primary tumor volume including retropharyngeal nodes on MRI. The 3-year rates of local failure-free survival (97% vs. 82%, $p < 0.01$), progression-free survival (85% vs. 65%, $p < 0.01$), and overall survival (93% vs. 80%, p = 0.13) were more superior for patients with a volume <15 ml compared to those with bigger volumes. On multivariate analysis, volume of the primary disease remained an independent prognostic factor for the local failure-free rate (HR = 1.01, 95% CI = 1.00–1.02; $p < 0.01$). And the risk of local failure was estimated to increase by 1% for every 1 ml increase in volume.

A recent study from Taiwan (Chen et al. 2009) collected 69 patients with Stage III/IV NPC treated with a uniform protocol of 10-weekly neoadjuvant chemotherapy followed by radiation (Lin et al. 2003a) with a minimal follow-up time of 5 years. There were 3 local recurrences, 16 distant failures, and 4 combined local and distant failures. The authors retrospectively delineated the tumor contour without retropharyngeal nodes on pretreatment T2-weighted axial MRI and calculated the primary tumor volume in radiation treatment planning system. All survival analyses showed no statistically significant difference between patients with large or small (cutoff values by either median, or mean) primary tumor volume. The comparisons between patients with primary tumor volume ≥ 25 and $<25\,cm^3$ (mean volume) also showed no statistically significant differences in 5-year local failure-free survival, metastasis-free survival, and overall survival rates. The differences between outcomes using different cutoff values other than mean or median of the primary tumor volume were all statistically insignificant. The authors explained possible reasons of their results compared with other studies: First, MRI rather than CT scan was used, and the superior contrast resolution of MRI on soft tissue provided them with the capability to discriminate primary tumor from enlarged (RPLN), which might be included in the primary tumor volume on CT scan of previous studies. Second, all patients were treated with neoadjuvant chemotherapy prior to radiation. Third, the local-failure rate is relatively low with a minimum follow-up of five years. The few local failure events and the small patient number might preclude them from detecting a small but statistical significance in prognosis analyses.

9.4 Predictive Value of Tumor Markers and Molecular Indicators on Prognosis

Tumor biomarkers can be divided into two categories: diagnostic marker that distinguishes one tumor from another or normal control and prognostic/predictive marker that is associated with the clinical behavior of a tumor and predicts the outcome after treatment. A number of prognostic biomarkers have been reported for NPC. Among these markers, quantitative analysis of plasma/serum EBV DNA have been most thoroughly investigated and shown to be clinically useful for the early detection, monitoring, and prognostication of NPC.

9.4.1 Anti-EBV Antibody

NPC has been proved as an EBV-associated cancer by several lines of evidence: the presence of DNA, RNA, and proteins of EBV in almost all cancer cells of almost all tissue samples (primary and various metastatic sites) obtained from patients with NPC (Chang et al. 1990; Chen et al. 1993; Tsai et al. 1996), tumor cells proved to be derived from a single EBV-infected cell (Raab-Traub and Flynn 1986); and high levels of EBV protein antibodies in newly found NPC patients (Henle et al. 1970; Henle and Henle 1976; Ho et al. 1976) and in healthy individuals in whom NPC later developed (Chien et al. 2001; Zeng et al. 1983). Furthermore, EBV has been detected in premalignant (preinvasive) nasopharyngeal lesions, including carcinoma in situ and dysplasia (Pathmanathan et al. 1995; Yeung et al. 1993). Thus, EBV has been investigated as a surrogate marker for NPC during the past decades.

Various anti-EBV antibodies have been studied as surrogate markers of NPC since 1970 (Henle et al. 1970; Henle and Henle 1976; Ho et al. 1976; Liu et al. 1997; Uen et al. 1988; Neel et al. 1984a, b). However, most studies focused on the diagnostic value and used the same design-collecting blood samples from NPC patients with active disease (previously untreated or relapsed cases) plus some controls (healthy volunteer or non-NPC tumors) and compared sensitivity and specificity of different assay systems targeting on various EBV antigens (Henle et al. 1970; Henle and Henle 1976; Ho et al. 1976; Neel et al. 1984a). All studies demonstrated a higher positive detection rate of various anti-EBV antibodies for patients with active disease than those of controls. However, these data do little to help in the diagnosis of newly found NPC or relapsed cases. The definite diagnosis of a newly found NPC or a relapsed case depends on suspected symptoms/signs, nasopharyngoscopy and imaging findings and confirmatory biopsy results, irrespective of the titer of various antibodies. Furthermore, the antibody titer remains persistently high in most patients in remission after treatment (Shao et al. 2004; Fan et al. 2004). There is no reliable cutoff value in the differential diagnosis of recurrence or remission.

A clinically useful tumor marker should not only have higher sensitivity and specificity in the diagnosis setting, but also have significant impact on the prognosis prediction. The latter is more important in clinical practice. A few studies have previously addressed the prognostic effects of various anti-EBV antibodies

(Neel et al. 1984a; Neel and Taylor 1990; de Vathaire et al. 1988; Yip et al. 1994; Hsu et al. 1988; Twu et al. 2007) and are summarized in Table 9.3. By the antibody-dependent cellular cytotoxicity (ADCC) assay, which measures antibodies to an EBV-induced membrane antigen component, Neel et al. (1984a) demonstrated that patients with low ADCC titers at diagnosis had significantly worse progression-free survival and overall survival for World Health Organization (WHO) Types 2 and 3 NPC patients.

Table 9.3. Summary of prognostic impact of serum anti-EBV antibody in nasopharyngeal carcinoma

Series	No. Of cases	Stage	Histology	Sampling	Assay
Neel et al. (1984a)	27	I–IV	WHO 1	Pre-Tx	ADCC
	107	I–IV	WHO 2–3	Pre-Tx	ADCC
Neel and Taylor (1990)	93	–	WHO 1–3	Pre-Tx	ADCC
	110	–	WHO 1–3	Pre-Tx	IF
				Multiple after Tx	
de Vathaire et al. (1988)	373	–	–	Pre-Tx	IF
	132	–	–	1-year after Tx	IF
Yip et al. (1994)	110	I–IV	WHO 2–3	Pre-Tx	ELISA
				10 m after Tx	ELISA
Hsu et al. (1988)	179	I–IV	WHO 2–3	Multiple	IF
Twu et al. (2007)	114	II–IV	WHO 1–3	Pre-Tx	IF
				Post-Tx	IF

PFS progression-free survival; *OS* overall survival; *Tx* treatment; *ADCC* antibody-dependent cellular cytotoxicity; *n.s.* not statistically significant difference; *ncwp* No correlation with prognosis; *IF* indirect immunofluorescence; *cwrel* correlated with relapse; *ELISA* enzyme-linked immunosorbent assay; *m* month; *cwm* correlated with distant metastasis; *cwrec* correlated with local recurrence

Conventional antibody (VCA-IgG, EA-IgA, and EA-IgG) assays before treatment could not reflect the prognosis. After long-term follow-up, they also found that the posttreatment sequential measurements did not accurately predict the outcome (Neel and Taylor 1990). A multicenter follow-up study on 319 NPC patients showed no prognostic values of initial serology, including IgG and IgA antibodies to VCA, EA, or EBNA (de Vathaire et al. 1988). However, increasing titers of EA-IgA and EA-IgG, one year after completion of

Antibody	Cutoff	PFS	OS	Comments
EBV-MA	≥vs.<7680	$p = 0.2$	n.s.	
EBV-MA	≥vs.<7680	$p = 0.0001$	$p = 0.0008$	
EBV-MA				ncwp
VCA-IgA				ncwp
VCA-IgG				ncwp
EA-IgG				ncwp
various				ncwp
VCA-IgG				ncwp
EA-IgG				ncwp
VCA-IgA				ncwp
EA-IgA				ncwp
EBNA-IgG				ncwp
VCA-IgG				cwrel ($p<0.01$)
EA-IgG				cwrel ($p<0.01$)
VCA-IgA				cwrel ($p = 0.09$)
EA-IgA				cwrel ($p<0.001$)
EBNA-IgG				ncwp
ZEBRA-IgG	≥vs.<10240	–	$p = 0.331$	
ZEBRA-IgG	≥vs.<10240	–	$p = 0.0019$	
Initial Anti-DNase				cwm ($p<0.05$)
Initial VCA-IgA				ncwp
Last Anti-DNase				cwrec ($p<0.02$) and cwm ($p<0.05$)
Last VCA-IgA				cwm ($p<0.001$)
VCA-IgA	≥vs.<1:80	$p = 0.7099$	$p = 0.8169$	
VCA-IgG	≥vs.<1:2560	$p = 0.8383$	$p = 0.7512$	
VCA-IgA	≥vs.<1:80	$p = 0.4135$	$p = 0.1460$	
VCA-IgG	≥vs.<1:2560	$p = 0.3856$	$p = 0.3610$	

radiotherapy became highly significant for prediction of relapse, regardless of the initial titers. Yip et al. (1994) investigated the prognostic role of the IgG antibody against EBV BZLF-1 replication activators and found no significant difference in patients' survival between the low and high titers for sera taken before treatment ($p = 0.331$). In contrast, for sera taken 10 months after radiation therapy, the high titer group predicted significantly worse overall survival rates ($p = 0.0019$). Hsu et al. (1988) investigated the prognostic impact of two antibodies (VCA-IgA and anti-DNase) measured at different time-points on 179 NPC patients. The results showed that the last anti-DNase titer correlated with local recurrence and distant metastasis, the last VCA-IgA and initial anti-DNase predicted distant metastasis, the initial VCA-IgA had no correlation with local recurrence or distant metastasis. A recent study compared the prognostic impact of serum IgA and IgG antibodies titer against VCA and plasma EBV DNA level in 114 advanced NPC patients (Twu et al. 2007) and showed that both pre and posttreatment VCA antibodies titer could not predict overall and relapse-free survivals. Because of lack of evidence regarding pretreatment antibody titers on the prognosis prediction, longitudinal follow-up data of clinical results and series blood tests when disease status changed for the same patient groups, the prognostic role of anti-EBV antibodies in NPC seems to be less clear, and the precise point of blood sampling has not been well established. The lack of prognostic effect of antibody assays is thought to be attributable to individual differences in the immune responses to various antigens. This may be explained by the fact that antibody is a marker which essentially is a host response to viral tumor antigens. This kind of marker inevitably lags behind with regard to kinetics upon treatment. Also, the dynamic range of antibody responses is fairly limited in general, with only weak correlations observed between the extent of exposure and the level (titer) of the response. On the other hand, unlike conventional protein markers such as CEA or PSA, released mostly from tumor cells, EBV can be found in patients with EBV-related diseases or even in normal population in high concentration, especially after an EBV infection.

9.4.2 Tumor-Associated Genes in Peripheral Blood Cells

Distant metastasis is associated with worse prognosis. Cancer cells usually enter into circulation before establishment of a metastatic lesion in distant organs. Micrometastasis refers as occult disseminated tumor cells in peripheral blood, bone marrow, or lymph nodes that cannot be detected by conventional histopathological methods. Smith et al. (1991) first developed a nested reverse transcriptase-polymerase chain reaction (rt-PCR) assay for the detection of circulating melanoma cells by the amplification of tyrosinase mRNA, which is exclusively expressed in melanocytes and melanoma cells. Since then, this method has been widely applied in the early detection of occult metastasis from different specimens. The most important issue of an rt-PCR assay is to select a target molecule with high specificity and sensitivity. Cytokeratin 19 (CK19) is an intermediate filament protein expressed by all simple epithelia, their corresponding malignancies, and a small number of other tissues (Moll et al. 1982). It has been reported earlier that CK19 is not expressed by lymphoid or hematopoietic cells (Datta et al. 1994; Schoenfeld et al. 1997) and, therefore, may be a useful marker of occult metastasis in the peripheral blood, bone marrow, and lymph nodes of patients with cancer of epithelial origin. So far, CK19 mRNA is one of the most frequently studied target genes in the early detection of micrometastasis. By meticulous design of a nested rt-PCR system to detect circulating CK19 mRNA expression cells, Lin et al. (2002) found that 33.3% (19/57) clinically nonmetastatic NPC patients had CK19 mRNA in their pretreatment blood. The positive detection rates of CK19 mRNA in the peripheral blood increase as clinical stage increase (20.0% for Stage II, 31.6% Stage III, and 43.5% Stage IV, $p = 0.1335$). After a median follow-up time of 35 months, 9 of 19 (47.4%) CK19 mRNA positive patients and 5 of 38 (13.2%) CK19 mRNA negative patients developed distant metastasis ($p = 0.00826$). The 3-year metastasis-free survival rates were 49.9% for patients with detectable CK19 mRNA, and 85.9% for those with undetectable CK19 mRNA ($p = 0.0089$). They concluded that the presence of circulating CK19 mRNA positive cells before treatment indicated occurrence of micrometastasis and was a poor prognostic sign for NPC.

The EBV DNA has been shown in tumor cells of nearly all patients with NPC. Circulating peripheral blood cells that carry EBV DNA may be a sign of disseminated tumor cells for NPC. Based on this hypothesis, Lin et al. (2001) explored whether the presence of EBV DNA in the peripheral blood cells can serve as a prognostic indicator for NPC. The DNA extracted from peripheral blood cells of 124 previously untreated NPC patients with no evidence of distant metastasis was assayed by a nested PCR using primer specific to EBV nuclear Antigen 1 (EBNA-1). The characteristics of NPC patients with EBNA-1 positive and EBNA-1 negative showed no significant difference. After a median follow-up of 38 months, 29 of 88 EBNA-1 positive patients developed distant metastasis and only one distant metastasis was observed in the patients of the EBNA-1 negative group ($p = 0.00015$). Overall survival, metastasis-free survival, and progression-free survival were all significantly lower for the patients in the EBNA-1 positive group. Multivariate Cox analysis also confirmed the same results. The authors concluded that the presence of EBNA-1 DNA in peripheral blood cells of NPC patients was a novel biomarker in predicting a significantly higher distant failure and a lower survival rate. Consistent sequence variation of EBNA-1 in primary tumors and peripheral blood cells in addition to the results of clinical observations do support that the EBV DNA that appeared in peripheral blood cells of NPC patients may have arisen from the disseminated cancer cells (Wang et al. 2002). Table 9.4 lists prognostic effects of peripheral blood cells expressing tumor-associated genes in NPC.

9.4.3 Plasma/Serum EBV DNA

With recent advances in molecular biology, the PCR-based technique makes it possible to detect a very small amount of biomolecules in a wide array of biological samples. Cell-free circulating DNA could be detected in plasma and serum. A previous report indicated that the cancer patients had significantly higher mean free DNA in serum than did healthy controls (Leon et al. 1977). Studies on the characteristics of DNA found in the plasma and serum of cancer patients highly suggested that much of the circulating DNA originated from the tumor cells and exhibited tumor-associated alterations. The mechanisms underlying the release of cell-free DNA from the tumor tissues into the circulation have not yet been completely elucidated. Some studies indicated that such cell-free DNA was largely accountable through the release of apoptotic and necrotic cancer cells (Fournie et al. 1995; Jahr et al. 2001). As a consequence, circulating cell-free DNA may serve as an attractive alternative for protein-based tumor markers.

Besides peripheral blood cells, plasma/serum samples were used for EBV DNA detection in NPC (Mutirangura et al. 1998; Shotelersuk et al. 2000; Hsiao et al. 2002). Using EBNA-2 as a target gene and 40 cycles PCR, Mutirangura et al. (1998) demonstrated that 13 of 42 NPC patients (31%) had detectable EBV DNA in their sera but not in all 82 normal controls. In a subsequent study, the detection rate of serum/plasma EBV DNA increased to 58.7% in 167 NPC patients studied by using nested PCR, but false positive was found in 10 of 77 (13%) normal blood donors (Shotelersuk et al. 2000). Using EBNA-1 as a target and conventional PCR of 35 and 50 cycles, Hsiao et al. (2002) reported that 50-cycle PCR assay enhanced detection sensitivity from 38.9% to 75% for patients with newly untreated patients, from 27.8% to 88.9% for patients with locoregional recurrence, and from 71.4% to 100% for patients with distant metasta-

Table 9.4. Prognostic effects of peripheral blood cells expressing tumor-associated genes in nasopharyngeal carcinoma

Series	No. of cases	stage	Treatment	Timing and sample	Assay	Target	Results	3-y OS	3-y MFS	3-y PFS
Lin et al. (2001)	124	I–IV	RT ± Ch	Pretreatment, PBC	nested PCR	EBNA-1	positive	65.5%	64.6%	59.2%
							negative	97.2%	97.1%	94.3%
								$p = 0.001$	$p = 0.0004$	$p = 0.0004$
Lin et al. (2002)	57	II–IV	RT ± Ch	Pretreatment, PBC	nested rt- PCR	CK19 mRNA	positive	–	49.9%	–
							negative	–	85.9%	–
									$p = 0.0089$	

3-y 3-year; *OS* overall survival; *MFS* metastasis-free survival; *PFS* progression-free survival; *RT* radiotherapy; *Ch* chemotherapy; *PBC* peripheral blood cells; *PCR* polymerase chain reaction; *EBNA-1* Epstein–Barr Virus nuclear antigen 1; *rt* reverse transcriptase; *CK19* cytokeratin 19; – not available sis. However, the false positive rates also increased from 3.5% to 10.7% for normal controls, and from 7.1% to 36.5% for patients with disease in clinical remission. Based on the aforementioned data, the qualitative PCR of EBV genes cannot serve as a useful tool in detection and monitoring of NPC patients.

The most important contributors in the field of circulating EBV DNA research are Lo et al. from Hong Kong (Lo et al. 1999a, b, 2000a, b, c; Chan et al. 2002a, 2003; Leung et al. 2003, 2006). They first used a new technique, real-time quantitative PCR, and detected cell-free EBV DNA in plasma of 96% (55/57) NPC patients and 7% (3/43) controls (Lo et al. 1999a). In a series studies, they demonstrated that circulating EBV DNA levels highly correlated with tumor staging (Lo et al. 2000c), tumor recurrence (Lo et al. 1999b), patient's survival (Lo et al. 2000a) and posttreatment residual tumor load (Chan et al. 2002) in NPC patients receiving radiotherapy. By using DNase digestion and ultracentrifugation, they illustrated that circulating EBV DNA molecules are naked DNA fragments and most (87%) of them are shorter than 181 base pairs (Chan et al. 2003). Although different segments of viral DNA might result in different sensitivities in PCR assay, similar results and the detection limit were obtained using *Bam*HI-W region or EBNA-1 gene (Lo et al. 1999a).

The levels of plasma EBV DNA before treatment has been shown to be correlated with the tumor burden in NPC patients (Ma et al. 2006). Patients with advanced-stage disease would have higher concentrations of plasma EBV DNA. Thus, it is logical to correlate high circulating EBV DNA concentration with poor prognosis. By multivariate binary logistic regression analysis in a group of 91 NPC patients, Lo et al. (2000a) illustrated that the pretreatment plasma EBV DNA level was a powerful prognosticator for early disease recurrence, independent of stage, within one year of treatment. The relative risk of every 10-fold increase in plasma EBV DNA level was 3.8. It is especially striking that once circulating EBV DNA has been taken into account, even stage was found to be of borderline prognostic significance. In a second cohort of 139 NPC patients followed-up for a median period of 2027 days, serum EBV DNA was found to be a significant variable associated with NPC-related death in both univariate ($p = 0.001$) and multivariate ($p = 0.007$) Cox's regression analyses (Lo et al. 2000a). In a prospective study of 170 NPC patients treated by a uniform radiation therapy protocol, Chan et al. (2002) found (1) levels of posttreatment plasma EBV DNA dominated the effect of levels of pretreatment EBV DNA for progression-free survival, the risk ratio of NPC recurrence was 11.9 (95% CI = 5.53–25.43) for patients with higher posttreatment EBV DNA and 2.5 (95% CI = 1.14–5.70) for patients with higher pretreatment EBV DNA; (2) higher levels of posttreatment EBV DNA were statistically significantly associated with overall survival ($p < 0.001$). They concluded that levels of posttreatment plasma EBV DNA in patients with NPC appear to strongly predict progression-free and overall survival and to accurately reflect the posttreatment residual tumor load. Leung et al. (2003) from the same hospital explored the prognostic effect of plasma EBV DNA on 90 patients with early-stage disease treated by radiation therapy alone. After a median follow-up of 45 months, the researchers observed that the rate of distant failure was significantly higher for patients with pretherapy plasma EBV DNA ≥ 4000 copies/ml compared with those of plasma EBV DNA <4000 copies/ml ($p = 0.0001$). In a subsequent study, Leung et al. (2006) collected 376 NPC patients of Stage I–IV and evaluated the effect of combining pretherapy plasma EBV DNA and TNM-staging data in prognosis. The results revealed that pretherapy plasma EBV DNA load is an independent prognostic factor for overall survival in NPC. Patients with early-stage disease were segregated by EBV-DNA levels into a poor-risk subgroup with survival similar to that of Stage III disease and a good-risk subgroup with survival similar to Stage I disease. Combined interpretation of plasma EBV DNA data with TNM staging data leads to alteration of risk definition of patients' subsets, with improved risk discrimination in early-stage disease.

Using a similar assay of real-time quantitative PCR, Lin et al. (2003a) measured a series of plasma samples from 99 NPC patients with advanced disease who were treated by a uniform protocol of 10-weekly neoadjuvant chemotherapy followed by radiation. They first demonstrated that circulating EBV DNA could be detected in 95% (94/99) NPC patients with Stage III/IV disease. Furthermore, EBV DNA was undetectable in all control samples (healthy controls and cured NPC patients). These findings indicated that the real-time quantitative PCR for NPC patients could be a both highly sensitive and specific assay. Second, plasma EBV DNA levels highly correlated with tumor burden in NPC patients. Third, patients with tumor relapse had a higher pretreatment plasma concentration of EBV DNA than did those without relapse. The overall survival ($p < 0.001$) and relapse-free survival

($p = 0.02$) were significantly lower in the patients with pretreatment plasma EBV DNA ≥ 1500 copies/ml than in those with plasma EBV DNA < 1500 copies/ml. Fourth, the plasma EBV DNA load before, during, and at the end of neoadjuvant chemotherapy declined significantly ($p < 0.001$). In addition, the plasma EBV DNA remained persistently low or undetectable in patients with clinically complete remission. Fifth, all patients with tumor relapse showed a rebound of plasma EBV DNA concentrations, which might be detected six months before clinical evidence of relapse. In addition, the presence or absence of plasma EBV DNA one week after the whole treatment showed significant correlation with subsequent tumor relapse. Survival analyses demonstrated that the pre and post-treatment plasma EBV DNA levels were the most important prognostic factors, and dominated all other clinical parameters, including age, gender, performance status, histological type, T- and N-classifications, and overall stage. These results were confirmed by extending analysis from 99 patients to 149 patients with longer follow-up.

In order to evaluate the long-term prognostic impact of plasma EBV DNA in NPC, stock plasma of 152 NPC patients who received a uniform schedule of concurrent chemoradiation with adequate follow-up time (median 78 months) were retrospectively assayed with a real-time quantitative PCR using the minor groove binder-probe (Lin et al. 2007). They confirmed the superior effects of plasma EBV DNA compared to other clinical parameters (including age, gender, performance status, pathological type, T-classification, N-classification, and overall stage) in prognosis prediction of NPC by multivariate Cox analysis. A recent study of direct comparison of serum anti-EBV antibody titer and plasma EBV DNA level on 114 previously untreated NPC patients clearly demonstrated that plasma EBV DNA is superior to serum anti-EBV antibody in prognostic predictions (Twu et al. 2007). Table 9.5 lists major studies of plasma/serum EBV DNA in NPC.

Plasma EBV DNA level can be a very useful molecular marker in the screening, monitoring, and prognostic prediction of NPC. Of note, the circulating DNA measured by PCR-based techniques as a tumor marker has some issues to be addressed. First, different segments of the same viral DNA or different viral genes might result in varying sensitivities in PCR assay. Two groups reported similar results and detection limits using *Bam*HI-W region or EBNA-1 gene by Lo et al. (1999a), or using polymerase-1, latent membrane protein-2, and *Bam*HI-W by Le et al. (2005) in detecting plasma EBV DNA in NPC. *Bam*HI-W assay yielded the highest concentrations due to multiple repeats in different EBV genomes compared to single-copy genes (EBNA-1, polymerase-1 or latent membrane protein-2) assay. Second, a great discrepancy exists in different groups using the same primer/probe sets and experimental conditions (Lo et al. 1999a,b, 2000a, b, c; Chan et al. 2002; Lin et al. 2004; Leung et al. 2006). In Lin's study (2004), the median concentration (1461 copies/ml) of 99 previously untreated NPC patients with Stage III/IV disease was much lower than the Hong Kong group (Lo et al. 1999a,b, 2000a, b, c; Chan et al. 2002). Even in the same group's reports, the medians (2,353–41,756 copies/ml) and ranges of pretreatment circulating EBV-DNA levels in newly diagnosed NPC patients varied considerably from study to study using the same assay conditions (Lo et al. 1999a,b, 2000a, b, c; Chan et al. 2002a, b; Leung et al. 2006). Third, circulating DNA levels declined substantially in two assessments at an average rate of 30% per year (Sozzi et al. 2005). Thus, degradation rate of DNA from stored blood samples at different time intervals may produce some difficulty in data correction. These issues should be appropriately resolved before the EBV DNA assay becomes a universal clinical routine in NPC management.

9.4.4 Other Serum/Plasma Biomarkers

Table 9.6 lists some other potential serum/plasma biomarkers with prognostic impact on NPC. Among these markers, serum lactate dehydrogenase (LDH) level has been reported as a prognostic indicator in malignant lymphoma and other carcinomas of epithelial origin. High level of serum LDH usually indicates larger tumor burden or close association with distant metastasis, resulting in a poor prognosis. Liaw et al. (1997) retrospectively investigated 465 NPC patients and demonstrated that higher serum LDH levels were found in patients with distant metastasis or relapse than those in remission or normal controls. For 118 Stage IV M0 patients, pretreatment serum LDH affected overall survival significantly. Hong et al. (2001) confirmed that pretreatment serum LDH level was an independent prognostic factor of overall survival in 111 Stage III–IV NPC patients by multivariate analysis. Cheng et al. (2006a) proposed a prognostic scoring system for locoregional

Table 9.5. Summary of prognostic impact of plasma/serum EBV DNA measured by quantitative polymerase chain reaction in nasopharyngeal carcinoma

Series	No. of cases	Stage	Treatment	Sampling	Target	Cutoff
Lo et al. (2000a)	91	I–IV	RT	Pre-Tx	*Bam*HI-W	Continuous variable
	139	I–IV	RT	Pre-Tx	*Bam*HI-W	≥vs.<40568
Chen et al. (2002a)	170	I–IV	RT ± Ch	Pre-Tx	*Bam*HI-W	≥vs.<4000
				6–8 wk after Tx	*Bam*HI-W	≥vs.<500
Leung et al. (2006)	376	I–IV	RT ± Ch	Pre-Tx	*Bam*HI-W	≥vs.<4000
Leung et al. (2003)	90	I–II	RT ± Ch	Pre-Tx	*Bam*HI-W	≥vs.<4000
Le et al. (2005)	58	II–IV	RT ± Ch	Pre-Tx	Pol-1	>vs.=0
				Pre-Tx	Pol-1	>vs.=0
Lin et al. (2004)	99	III–IV	NeoCh+RT	Pre-Tx	*Bam*HI-W	≥vs.<1500
				1 wk after Tx	*Bam*HI-W	>vs.=0
Lin et al. (unpublished)	149	II–IV	NeoCh+RT	Pre-Tx	*Bam*HI-W	≥vs.<1500
				1 wk after Tx	*Bam*HI-W	>vs.=0
Lin et al. (2007)	152	II–IV	CCRT	Pre-Tx and 1 wk after Tx	*Bam*HI-W	Pre-L/post-U
					*Bam*HI-W	Pre-H/post-U
					*Bam*HI-W	Pre-L or H/post-D

OS overall survival; *RFS* relapse-free survival; *PFS* progression-free survival; *DSS* disease-specific survival; *MFS* metastasis-free survival; *RT* radiotherapy; *Tx* treatment; *Ch* chemotherapy; *wk* week; *Pol-1* polymerase 1; *n.s.* not statistically significant difference; *NeoCT* neoadjuvant chemotherapy; *X* indicates uncalculated; *CCRT* concurrent chemoradiotherapy; *Pre-L* low pretreatment EBV DNA (<1500 copies/ml); *Pre-H* high pretreatment EBV DNA (≥1500 copies/ml); *Post-U* undetectable posttreatment EBV DNA (0 copies/ml); *Post-D* detectable posttreatment EBV DNA (>0 copies/ml)

control after retrospective review of 630 NPC patients. In their model construction, serum LDH is one of the important parameter affecting locoregional control of NPC by both univariate and multivariate analyses. A Phase III randomized study compared the outcome of concurrent chemoradiation versus radiation therapy alone for 348 NPC patients with advanced nodal disease from Hong Kong, Lee et al. (2005a) also found that serum LDH was a significant predictor for distant failure, any failure, disease progression, and death. Another study from Turkey consisting of 61 NPC patients with Stage III–IV disease also showed that pretreatment serum LDH level was a significant prognosticator for overall survival and disease-free survival (Turen et al. 2007). Based on these reports, we conclude that serum LDH level is a useful prognostic factor for NPC. Of note blood sampling for LDH assay should be gently to avoid hemolysis-induced false positive results.

Other potential markers related to NPC prognosis included macrophage inflammatory protein-3α (Chang et al. 2008), endothelin-1 (Mai et al. 2006), cytoplasmic protein fragment of CK19 (Ma et al. 2004), β-2-microglobulin (Ma et al. 2004; Sundram and Aw 1986), tissue polypeptide antigen (Sundram and Aw 1986), vascular endothelial growth factor (Qian et al. 2000), and osteopontin (Hui et al. 2008). These markers may be associated with distant metastasis (macrophage inflammatory protein-3α, endothelin-1, tissue polypeptide antigen, β-2-microglobulin, vascular endothelial growth factor), overall survival (macrophage inflammatory protein-3α, cytoplasmic protein fragment of CK19, β-2-microglobulin), or response to radiation (osteopontin).

Univariate analysis			Multivariate analysis		
OS	RFS/PFS/DSS	MFS	OS	RFS/PFS/DSS	MFS
–	$p < 0.0005$	–	–	$p = 0.003$	–
$p < 0.0005$	–	–	$p = 0.007$	–	–
$p < 0.001$	$p < 0.001$	–	$p < 0.001$	$p < 0.023$	–
$p < 0.001$	$p < 0.001$	–	$p < 0.001$	$p < 0.001$	–
–	–	–	$p = 0.0053$	$p < 0.05$	$p = 0.002$
–	–	$p = 0.0001$	–	–	–
$p = 0.73$	n.s.	–	–	–	–
$p = 0.002$	$p < 0.001$	–	–	$p = 0.0006$	–
$p < 0.001$	$p = 0.02$	–	X	$p = 0.07$	–
$p < 0.001$	$p < 0.001$	–	$p = 0.002$	$p < 0.001$	–
$p < 0.0001$	$p = 0.0003$	–	$p = 0.0007$	$p = 0.0074$	–
$p < 0.0001$	$p < 0.0001$	–	$p < 0.0001$	$p < 0.0001$	–
control	control	–	control	control	–
$p = 0.004$	$p = 0.16$	–	$p = 0.01$	$p = 0.21$	–
$p < 0.001$	$p < 0.001$	–	$p < 0.001$	$p < 0.001$	–

9.4.5 Tissue Prognostic Biomarkers

Table 9.7 summarizes potential tissue biomarkers relevant to the prognoses of NPC. Although many results were encouraging, the sample size of each study was usually too small. Large cooperative studies with other uniform confounding factors to verify the prognostic impact of these tissue biomarkers is needed before clinical use.

9.5 Other Implicated Prognostic Factors

9.5.1 Patient-Related Factors

Patients' factors on survival were less specifically addressed in the literature. However, epidemiological survey and most individual reports regarding treatment outcome of NPC patients usually analyzed the prognostic effect of patient related factors.

9.5.1.1 Age

The prevalent age of NPC at diagnosis is 40–59 years. The reported median age is between 45 and 50 years from endemic regions collecting more than 500 patients during the last 10 years (Heng et al. 1999; Ma et al. 2001a, 2007; Au et al. 2003; Leung et al. 2005; Lee et al. 2005b; Yeh et al. 2005; Yi et al. 2006; Liu et al. 2008; Mao et al. 2009). Two large series from the Surveillance, Epidemiology, and End Results (SEER) program of the United States reported a mean age at diagnosis of 52.7 years from 2,436 NPC patients (Ou et al. 2007) and 56.2 years from 5,069 NPC patients (Marks et al. 1998). There are no studies focusing specifically on the prognostic impact of age in NPC. In addition, many series studying the main

Table 9.6. Summary of other serum/plasma biomarkers on the prognosis of nasopharyngeal carcinoma

Series	No. of cases	Stage	Treatment	Markers	Cutoff	Univariate analysis
						OS
Liaw et al. (1997)	118	IV, M0	RT ± Ch	LDH	>vs.≤140 U/l	$p = 0.008$
Hong et al. (2001)	111	III–IV	NeoCh+RT	LDH	>vs.≤419 U/l	–
Lee et al. (2005a)	348	III–IV	RT ± Ch	LDH	continous variable	–
Cheng SH et al. (2006a)	630	II–IV	RT+Ch	LDH	≥vs.<410 U/l	–
Turen et al. (2007)	61	III–IV	NeoCh+RT	LDH	>vs.≤460 U/l	$p = 0.01$
Chang et al. (2008)	155	I–IV	RT ± Ch	MIP-3α	>vs.<65 pg/ml	$p = 0.008$
Mai et al. (2006)	62	III–IV	RT ± NeoCh	ET-1	>vs.<4.5 pg/ml	–
Ma et al. (2004)	160	I–IV	RT	CYFRA ferritin β_2M	≥vs.<1.5 U/ml ≥vs.<144 ng/ml ≥vs.<1.6 mg/ml	$p = 0.001$ n.s. $p = 0.0007$
Sundram and Aw (1986)	38	–	–	TPA		Patients with distant metastasis have higher serum TPA ($p < 0.001$) and β_2M ($p = 0.025$)
Qian et al. (2000)	87	I–IV	–	VEGF		Levels of serum VEGF were significantly elevated in patients with distant metastasis ($p < 0.001$)
Hui et al. (2008)	44	I–IV	RT ± Ch	OPN		Higher pretreatment OPN predicts poor response to RT by univariate ($p = 0.009$) and multivariate ($p = 0.019$) analysis

OS overall survival; *LRFFS* locoregional failure-free survival; *MFS* metastasis failure-free survival; *DFS* disease-free survival; *PFS* progression-free survival; *RT* radiotherapy; *Ch* chemotherapy; *LDH* lactate dehydrogenase; *NeoCh* neoadjuvant chemotherapy; *n.s.* not statistically significant difference; *MIP-3α* macrophage inflammatory protein-3α; *ET-1* Endothelin-1; *CYFRA* cytoplasmic protein fragment of cytokeratin 19; *β2M* β-2-microglobulin; *TPA* tissue polypeptide antigen; *VEGF* Vascular endothelial growth factor; *OPN* osteopontin

purpose of other prognostic factors have reported significantly better outcome for younger patients.

Burt et al. (1992) found that overall survival and age at diagnosis are inversely related for 1645 patients from the SEER database between 1973 and 1986. Multivariate analysis confirmed that age was a significant independent variable on survival ($p < 0.001$). Ou et al. (2007) demonstrated similar results for 2436 patients from the SEER database between 1992 and 2002. Patients with younger age are associated with improved overall survival by multivariate analysis ($p < 0.0001$). The EUROCARE study of 2,054 NPC patients diagnosed between 1978 and 1989 from several European countries also showed that overall survival declined with age (Jiong et al. 1998). The 5-year survival rates were 53% for patients aged 15–44 years and 31% for patients aged 65–74 years, and younger age at diagnosis favorably influenced survival in multivariate analysis.

Several single institute reports containing more than 100 patients from nonendemic regions also

			Multivariate analysis			
LRFFS	MFS	DFS/PFS	OS	LRFFS	MFS	DFS/PFS
–	–	–	–	–	–	–
–	–	–	$p = 0.01$	–	–	–
–	–	–	$p < 0.001$	n.s.	$p = 0.005$	$p = 0.005$
$p = 0.0003$	–	–	–	$p = 0.002$	–	–
–	–	$p = 0.047$	$p = 0.03$	–	–	$p = 0.08$
–	$p = 0.007$	–	$p = 0.022$	–	$p = 0.029$	–
–	$p = 0.031$	–	–	–	$p = 0.033$	–
–	–	–	$p < 0.0001$	–	–	n.s.
n.s.	n.s.	n.s.	–	–	–	–
n.s.	n.s.	$p = 0.008$	n.s.	–	–	n.s.

demonstrated better prognosis for younger patients (Johansen et al. 2001; August et al. 2001; Chow et al. 2002; Farias et al. 2003; Khademi et al. 2006; Corry et al. 2006). Chow et al. (2002) collected 172 Stage III/IV NPC patients from Canada and showed that age <50 years was a favorable variable for overall survival by multivariate analysis with a risk ratio of 1.6 (95% CI = 1.04–2.6, $p = 0.0322$). Corry et al. (2006) from Australia reported that younger age (<45 years) was a significant factor on event-free survival by both univariate ($p = 0.01$) and multivariate ($p = 0.001$) analyses for 158 NPC patients.

Most series from endemic regions, including Mainland China, Taiwan, Honk Kong, and Singapore demonstrated similar results. Table 9.8 lists ten studies of more than 500 patients with regard to the impact of age on overall survival. Eight studies showed younger age was a statistically significant favorable prognostic factor (Teo et al. 1996; Heng et al. 1999; Ma et al. 2001a; Au et al. 2003; Leung et al. 2005; Lee et al. 2005b; Yeh et al. 2005; Liu et al. 2008), one showed borderline significance (Yi et al. 2006), and one study reported no significance (Mao et al. 2009).

Based on the aforementioned data, we conclude that age is a significant prognostic factor for NPC. Patients with younger age always have better performance status and less comorbidity, which may contribute to better tolerance to radical radio(chemo)therapy, resulting in better survival. Two large meta-analyses for non-NPC head and neck cancer also consistently demonstrated

Table 9.7. Summary of tissue biomarkers on the prognosis of nasopharyngeal carcinoma

Series	No. of cases	stage	Treatment	Assay	Target
Chua et al. (2004c)	54	III–IV	NeoCh + RT	IHC	EGFR
Ma et al. (2003)	78		RT ± Ch	IHC	EGFR p53 HER-2 Ki67 MVD
Roychowdhury et al. (1996)	30	I–IV	RT	IHC	EGFR Ki67 p53 MVD c-erbB$_2$
Rubio et al. (2000)	55	I–IV	?	IHC	MVD
Genc et al. (2000)	35	I–IV	?	IHC	Ki67 p53 PCNA
Fujii et al. (2002)	53	I–IV	NeoCh + RT	IHC	EGFR
Fang et al. (2007)	20	II–IV	RT ± Ch	IHC	EGFR COX-2
Fang et al. (2009)	233	I–IV	RT	IHC	Skp2
Chan et al. (2007)	78	II–IV	RT ± Ch	IHC	COX-2 H1F-1α VEGF
Fujieda et al. (1999)	21	II–IV	RT + Ch	IHC	IL-10
Huang et al. (2000)	73	I–IV	?	IHC	VEGF MVD
Lee et al. (2005)	66	I–IV	RT ± Ch	IHC	Ku70 DNA-PKcs
Foote et al. (2005)	123	?	RT ± misonidazole	IHC	MVD
Bar-Sela et al. (2006)	46	I–IV	?	IHC	Heparanase
Krishna et al. (2006)	103	?	?	IHC	VEGF
Masuda et al. (1998)	22	II–IV	RT ± Ch	IHC	p53 bcl-2 Ki67
Ho et al. (2001)	68	I–IV	RT	IHC	p53
Hwang et al. (2002)	66	I–IV	RT	IHC	cyclin D1 p16 pRb
Makitie et al. (2003)	84	I–IV	RT ± Ch	IHC IHC ISH	P16 pRb EBER
Porter et al. (1994)	51	?	?	IHC	c-myc ras
Bar-Sela et al. (2005)	46	I–IV	?	IHC	c-kit
Liao et al. (2007)	160	I–IV	?	IHC	CENP-H
Yip et al. (1998)	51	I–IV	RT	FC	DNA ploidy SPF, PF
Hsu et al. (2000)	70	?	?	FC	DNA ploidy SPF

NeoCh neoadjuvant chemotherapy; *RT* radiotherapy; *IHC* immunohistochemical stain; *EGFR* epidermal growth factor receptor; *DSS* disease-specific survival; *RFS* relapse-free survival; *LRFFS* locoregional failure-free survival; *Ch* chemotherapy; *OS* overall survival; *DFS* disease-free survival; *TTP* time to progression; *MVD* microvessel density; *PCNA* proliferating cell nuclear antigen; *TATE* tumor-associated tissue eosinophilia; *COX-2* Cyclooxygenase-2; *Skp2* S-phase kinase-associated protein 2; *H1F-1α* hypoxia inducible factor-1α; *VEGF* vascular endothelial growth factor; *IL-10* interleukin-10; *?* not mentioned; *DNA-PKcs* DNA-dependent protein kinase catalytic subunit; *ISH* in situ hybridization; *EBER* EBV-encoded small nuclear RNA; *CENP-M* centromere protein H; *FC* flow cytometry; *SPF* S-phase fraction; *PF* proliferation fraction

Results
1. No significant impact of EGFR intensity on survival 2. EGFR extent ≥25% predicts poorer DSS, RFS, LRFFS ($p < 0.05$) 3. Multivariate analysis: EGFR extent is the only independent factor for disease relapse, locoregional failure, cancer death
1. Positive correlation of EGFR expression and poorer OS ($p = 0.0001$), DFS ($p = 0.01$), TTP ($p = 0.0001$) 2. p53 expression predicts poor DFS ($p = 0.01$), TTP ($p = 0.06$) 3. No prognostic effect of HER-2, Ki67, and MVD 4. Multivariate analysis: only EGFR expression is significantly linked to shorter OS and TTP
1. No significant impact of EGFR, Ki67, p53 on survival 2. Intense MVD correlates with higher distant failure ($p = 0.03$), shorter OS ($p = 0.02$) and DFS ($p = 0.05$) 3. Strong c-erbB$_2$ expression correlated with shorter OS ($p = 0.02$) and DFS ($p = 0.02$)
High MVD correlated with poor OS ($p = 0.01$)
Ki67 <10% predicts longer OS ($p = 0.03$)
Among EGFR-positive patients, TATE correlates with better OS ($p = 0.0139$)
No correlation of EGFR, COX-2 with OS or DFS
1. Greater Skp2 expression correlated with OS ($p = 0.02$) and MFS ($p = 0.01$) 2. Multivariate analysis revealed similar results (both $p = 0.01$)
1. Coexpression of COX-2 and H1F-1α predicts worse PFS ($p = 0.046$) and TTP 2. Multivariate analysis failed to confirm any prognostic correlation
IL-10 expression correlated with OS by univariate ($p = 0.0348$) and multivariate ($p = 0.0014$) analyses
Patients with metastasis have higher MVD ($p < 0.01$) and VEGF expression ($p = 0.023$)
1. Expression of Ku70 predicts locoreginal control ($p = 0.0042$) 2. No significant association between DNA-PKcs expression and clinical outcome
No significant impact of MVD on OS, time to distant or locoreginal failure
Heparanase expression predicts poorer OS ($p = 0.03$)
Higher expression of VEGF in EBV (+) tumor correlated with higher rate of recurrence and lower survival, but $p > 0.05$
Expression of p53 had poor OS ($p = 0.05$)
No significant correlation between p53 expression and radiotherapy response
1. Loss of cyclin D1 ($p = 0.015$) and p16 ($p = 0.047$) correlated with poor local control 2. No correlation of pRb with local control
1. Complete absence of p16 expression predicts poor OS by multivariate analysis ($p = 0.022$) 2. No correlation of pRb with survival 3. Patients with EBER-positive have better OS by multivariate analysis ($p = 0.005$)
1. Overexpression of c-myc correlated with a poor survival ($p < 0.05$) 2. No correlation of ras with survival
Patients with positive c-kit predict better survival ($p = 0.029$)
Higher CENP-H expression correlated with shorter OS by univariate ($p = 0.021$) and multivariate ($p = 0.04$) analysis
1. Patients with aneuploidy tumors have significantly poor OS ($p < 0.01$) 2. Patients with high SPF and PF correlated with poor OS ($p < 0.004$ and $p < 0.0009$)
1. Aneuploidy tumors predict poor OS by univariate ($p = 0.042$) and multivariate ($p = 0.052$) analysis 2. Tumors with high SPF have poor OS ($p = 0.057$)

Table 9.8. Summary of prognostic impact of age in nasopharyngeal carcinoma

Series	No. of cases	cutoff	Univariate analysis		Multivariate analysis	
			5-y OS	5-y DSS	OS	DSS
Teo et al. (1996)	903	<vs.≥40	74% vs. 61%	63% vs. 54%	$p = 0.0002$	$p = 0.0050$
Heng et al. (1999)	677	–	–	–	$p < 0.0001$	–
Ma et al. (2001a)	621	<vs.≥40	–	–	$p = 0.0042$	–
Au et al. (2003)	1294	≥vs.>50	–	–	–	$p < 0.001$
Leung et al. (2005)	1070	continuous variable	–	–	$p < 0.05$	n.s.
Lee et al. (2005b)	2687	continuous variable	–	–	$p < 0.001$	$p < 0.001$
Yeh et al. (2005)	849	≤vs.>50	$p < 0.0001$	$p < 0.0001$	$p = 0.000$	$p < 0.001$
Yi et al. (2006)	905	≤vs.>48	$p = 0.00$	$p = 0.00$	$p = 0.062$	$p = 0.003$
Liu et al. (2008)	749	≤vs.>50	–	–	$p < 0.001$	–
Mao et al. (2009)	924	≤vs.>50	–	–	–	n.s.

5-y 5-year; *OS* overall survival; *DSS* disease-specific survival; *n.s.* not statistically significant difference

that the treatment benefit of concomitant chemotherapy and altered fractionated radiation decreases with increasing age (Pignon et al. 2007). The proportion of deaths not due to head-and-neck cancer increased with age, from 18% at age 50 years to 41% at age ≥ 71 years in the meta-analyses of chemotherapy in head-and-neck cancer, and from 15% to 39% in the meta-analysis of radiation therapy in carcinoma of head and neck.

9.5.1.2 Gender

The incidence rates in male populations are commonly two to threefold that of female population in NPC. There are no studies focusing specifically on the prognostic impact of gender in NPC. In addition, many reports with studying the main purpose of other prognostic factors have shown controversial results with regard to the prognostic impact of gender. Larger series from the SEER database or EUROCARE database revealed that there was no (Jiong et al. 1998; Ou et al. 2007) or a borderline (Burt et al. 1992; Sun et al. 2007) statistically significant difference between gender in overall survival by multivariate analysis. Studies containing several hundred Chinese NPC patients reported no significant difference of overall survival between gender (Lee et al. 2005b; Leung et al. 2005; Yi et al. 2006). Female gender was reported as a favorable factor on overall survival in some Chinese series (Ma et al. 2001a, 2007; Au et al. 2003; Yeh et al. 2005; Liu et al. 2008). Some studies show that gender may affect other endpoints of prognostic analyses significantly, such as local failure-free survival (Mao et al. 2009), regional failure-free survival (Au et al. 2003), metastasis failure-free survival (Ma et al. 2001a; Au et al. 2003; Lee et al. 2005b; Yeh et al. 2005; Liu et al. 2008), and disease failure (Tang et al. 2008).

9.5.1.3 Ethnic Background

NPC is a rare disease in the Western world; however, it is particularly common in Southern China, especially in Guangtong, Guangxi, Fujian, Hong Kong, and Taiwan. Results from survival studies of NPC are inconsistent, as some studies have and others have not found differences by race. Different races have different genetic susceptibility, and may also have different prognosis. Most of the population-based studies in NPC are from endemic countries where the ethnic makeup of the population was fairly homogeneous and the undifferentiated/nonkeratinizing carcinoma is the predominant histology. Thus, it remains unknown whether ethnicity is truly an independent prognostic factor for survival in NPC.

In the United States, every WHO histological type is diagnosed in each of the major racial groups. Thus, epidemiological data from the SEER of the United

States provide the best source to investigate whether race is a prognostic factor in NPC. Several study groups examined potential survival differences among NPC patients from various ethnicities in the United States by extraction different case numbers during different time periods from the database of the SEER (Levine et al. 1980; Burt et al. 1992; Bhattacharyya 2004; Lee and Ko 2005; Sun et al. 2007; Ou et al. 2007). These studies consistently found that Chinese patients had the best overall survival than other ethnic groups. In the most recent study reported by Ou et al. (2007), 2436 newly diagnosed NPC patients were analyzed and it was found that Chinese had the best 5-year overall survival rate (63.8%) followed by Caucasian (48.2%), African-American (45.4%), Hispanic (44.0%), and others (41%) ($p < 0.0001$). Multivariate analysis using Cox proportional hazards model confirmed that Chinese race was a significant independent factor affecting overall survival (vs. Caucasian; HR = 0.784, 95% CI = 0.678–0.907, $p = 0.0010$). In order to avoid the effect of some unadjusted confounders, Bhattacharyya (2004) used a matched analysis to investigate the impact of race on survival in NPC from the SEER database from 1988 to 2000. Each Chinese patient was matched to a Caucasian patient according to age at diagnosis, gender, histological type, stage, and treatment modality. In total, 171 patients were successfully matched. The author found that overall survival was substantially better for Chinese patients (mean survival, 94 months; median survival, 95 months) compared with Caucasian patients (81 and 64 months, $p = 0.037$), but that there was no difference in cause-specific survival (mean survival for Chinese vs. White patients = 116 vs. 117 months, $p = 0.99$). There were no differences in disease-specific survival which were identified for race when stratified by stage. Sun et al. (2007) analyzed 3952 patients from SEER database of 1973–2002 and found similar results. Chinese patients had lower risks of overall mortality compared with non-Hispanic White patients (hazard ratio = 0.73, 95% CI = 0.64–0.84), but no differences in cause-specific mortality by race. The superior survival of Chinese/Asian-American NPC patients is generally attributed to the much higher prevalence of the favorable nonkeratinizing carcinoma histology diagnosed among Chinese/Asian-American NPC patients (Marks et al. 1998). However, Ou et al. (2007) report statistically significant improved survival of Chinese keratinizing squamous cell carcinoma NPC patients compared with keratinizing squamous cell carcinoma NPC patients from other ethnicities even after adjustment for other prognostic factors. This survival advantage of Chinese NPC patients with keratinizing squamous cell carcinoma largely contributed to the Chinese race being an independent and favorable prognostic factor in the multivariate analyses.

In contrast to the aforementioned studies, the results from some hospital-based studies suggest a different impact of race on survival in NPC (Flores et al. 1986, Bailet et al. 1992, Su and Wang 2002). One large retrospective study from the Massachusetts General Hospital found that the rate of distant metastases was significantly higher for Chinese patients compared with non-Chinese patients by univariate analysis (5-year distant metastasis rate = 33% vs. 16%, $p < 0.01$) and multivariate analysis (relative risk = 4.0, $p = 0.007$). Local control rate at 5-year was similar (70% vs. 68%) between Chinese and non-Chinese patients. In the analysis of overall survival, Chinese patients had worse 5-year rate (49% vs. 56%) and multivariate analysis showed that race was a borderline significant predictor ($p = 0.06$) (Su and Wang 2002). Another large study from the Cancer Control Agency of British Columbia assembled 167 Chinese patients and 119 Caucasian patients. They found no differences in overall survival by race (Flores et al. 1986). A retrospective analysis of 103 NPC patients treated by RT alone at The University of California, Los Angles, from 1955 to 1990 revealed that there was no differences in disease-free survival rates between Asian and non-Asian patients (Bailet et al. 1992).

Only one study outside North America addressed the significance of ethnicity on prognoses in NPC patients (Corry et al. 2006). After excluding 23 patients with WHO Type 1 histology, a total of 158 patients with WHO Type 2/3 histology at the Peter MacCallum Cancer Center, Australia from April 1984 to December 1999 were analyzed. The results demonstrated no significant differences in failure-free survival and overall survival between Asian and non-Asian patients. However, higher rate of late primary failures (offset by a lower rate of distant failure) in the Asian population was established.

9.5.1.4
Performance Status, Weight Loss, and Anemia

Performance status, weight loss, and anemia at presentation have been shown as prognostic factors for some malignancies. However, these are usually rare conditions at the diagnosis of NPC. A recent study containing 59 NPC patients reported that the comorbidity burden did not affect prognosis independent of the TNM staging (Ramakrishnan et al. 2007). A report from Australia failed to demonstrate significant effect of performance status on failure-free survival (Corry et al. 2006). Yi et al. (2006) retrospectively reviewed clinical outcome of 905 NPC patients treated by radiation alone during 1990 to 1999 from Mainland China. Karnofsky performance status, weight loss, and hemoglobin level had no significant effect on overall and disease-free survival by multivariate analysis. Chow et al. (2002) from Canada reported weight loss as a poor prognostic factor on overall and disease-free survival. Johansen et al. (2001) from Denmark demonstrated that patients with higher pretreatment hemoglobin level had higher 5-year local control rate than those with lower hemoglobin level (75% vs. 58%, $p < 0.05$). Chua et al. (2004a) investigated the impact of hemoglobin levels on treatment outcome by retrospectively reviewing the data from a Phase III randomized trial of patients treated with induction chemotherapy followed by radiation or radiation alone, and found no significant difference in treatment outcome according to baseline or preradiotherapy hemoglobin levels. However, a mid-radiation hemoglobin level of <= 11 g/dl was associated with significantly poorer 5-year rates of local recurrence-free (60% vs. 80%, $p = 0.0059$) and disease-specific survival (51% vs. 68%, $p = 0.001$), with no significant effect in distant metastasis-free rates (69% vs. 67%, $p = 0.83$). Multivariate analysis showed that a low mid-radiation hemoglobin level, but not a low baseline or preradiotherapy hemoglobin level, was an independent predictor of local disease recurrence and malignancy-related death.

9.5.2 Pathology

In 1978, the WHO classified NPC into three different histological types: keratinizing squamous cell carcinoma is classified as WHO Type 1, nonkeratinizing carcinoma is classified as WHO Type 2, and undifferentiated carcinoma is classified as WHO Type 3. WHO Types 2 and 3 are the major histological type in endemic areas, whereas WHO Type 1 usually comprises fewer than 5% of the endemic population (Shanmugaratnam and Sobin, 1993). In 1991, WHO classification retained the keratinizing squamous cell carcinoma subtype (original WHO Type 1) and combined WHO Type 2 and 3 histological subtypes into "nonkeratinizing carcinoma." Nonkeratinizing carcinoma was further divided as being "differentiated" and "undifferentiated." The differentiated subtype constituted the original WHO Type 2 and the undifferentiated subtype constituted the original WHO Type 3 (Lo et al. 2004, Barnes et al. 2005).

Data on the prognostic significance of histological types is difficult to interpret. Generally, studies from nonendemic regions always demonstrated that patients with keratinizing carcinoma had a worse prognosis than those with nonkeratinizing or undifferentiated carcinoma. Studies from endemic regions usually consisted of nonkeratinizing or undifferentiated carcinoma (>98% of all patients). Thus it is difficult to validate the findings of nonendemic regions. The distinction between WHO Types 2 and 3 is not clear. NPC is not a surgically treated disease. The specimen by punch biopsy for pathological diagnosis is only a tiny part from a big tumor. In our experience, tumors of most patients showed mixed morphology of Type 2 and 3 in different portions of the same specimen. In addition, some controversy existed between different pathologists to differentiate the Type 2 and 3 because a large variation between the proportions of Type 2 and 3 from different hospitals of the same regions was reported.

Epidemiological studies containing more than 1000 patients from the SEER of the United States or EUROCARE database have identified WHO histological type as an independent prognostic factor for survival in NPC (Levine et al. 1980, Burt et al. 1992; Marks et al. 1998; Lee and Ko 2005; Ou et al. 2007; Jiong et al. 1998). Patients with nonkeratinizing or undifferentiated carcinoma of the nasopharynx have significantly better survival than those with keratinizing carcinoma. Marks et al. (1998) reported that the 5-year rates of overall survival for Type 1, 2, and 3 patients were 37%, 65%, and 64%, respectively ($p < 0.05$). Lee and Ko (2005) found different 5-year survival rates of different histologies- 28.9% for Type 1, 39.1% for Type 2, and 47.0% for Type 3 during 1973–79 period, and 35.7%, 53.3%, and 57.5% during 1980–89, and 41.7%, 56.1%, and 68.5% during 1990–99 period ($p < 0.05$). In a more recent study, Ou et al. (2007) demonstrated the 5-year overall survival rates of Type 1, Type 2, Type 3, and carcinoma not otherwise specified were 45.6%, 57.6%, 55.9%, and 68.1%, respectively ($p < 0.0001$).

Single institute's experience from nonendemic regions showed controversial results. A retrospective study containing 378 NPC patients from the M.D. Anderson Cancer Center revealed poor local control rate (p < 0.0001), poor disease-specific survival (p = 0.006), and higher distant failure rate (p = 0.03) for keratinizing squamous cell carcinoma, compared with other histologies by univariate analyses (Sanguineti et al. 1997). Multivariate analyses also showed that histology (lymphoepithelioma vs. other pathologies) is an independent prognostic factor for local control (relative risk = 0.29, 95% CI = 0.18–0.46), neck control (relative risk = 0.37, 95% CI = 0.20–0.69), and disease-specific survival (relative risk = 0.48, 95% CI = 0.35–0.65). Reddy et al. (1995) investigated the prognostic significance of keratinization in 50 NPC patients and found all evaluated endpoints, including rates of local control, neck control, and distant metastasis, and overall survival were significantly worse for patients with keratinizing squamous cell carcinoma (p = 0.001). The 5-year overall survival rates were 6% for those with keratinizing squamous cell carcinoma and 51% for nonkeratinizing or undifferentiated carcinoma, respectively. Santos et al. (1995) from Spain reported their 30 years experience on 228 NPC patients. They divided patients into two groups—well differentiated squamous cell carcinoma (131 cases) and undifferentiated carcinoma (97 cases). The 5-year rates of overall survival were 39% and 48%, respectively (p = 0.02). However, multivariate analysis revealed that histology was not a significant factor on overall survival. The study from the Mallinckrodt Institute of Radiology consisting 143 NPC patients found no prognostic impact between different histologies (Perez et al. 1992). The p-values by multivariate analyses for locoregional control, disease-free survival, and overall survival were 0.262, 0.789, and 0.824, respectively.

The effect of histology on the prognosis of NPC patients in endemic regions was rarely addressed. One study from the Chinese University of Hong Kong (Chan et al. 1998) tried to focus on and solve this problem. The histological slides of 693 patients treated under a uniform protocol between 1984 and 1989 were standardized reviewed by the same senior pathologist and classified into two distinct groups of WHO Type 1 (n = 13) or WHO Types 2 and 3 (n = 662). The remaining 18 patients were excluded because of difficulty in assignment of the pathological type. The patient characteristics and clinical outcome of the two groups were not statistically or significantly different. After adequate follow-up, they found there were no significant differences between the two groups in terms of actuarial survival, disease-free survival, freedom from local failure rate, and freedom from distant metastasis rate. The hazard ratios were 1.19 (95% CI = 0.53–2.6) for actuarial survival, 1.30 (95% CI = 0.65–2.6) for disease-free survival, 1.81 (95% CI = 0.74–4.3) for freedom from local failure, and 1.05 (95% CI = 0.39–2.8) for freedom from distant failure, respectively. Hsu et al. (1982) collected 1555 NPC patients from the National Taiwan University Hospital and investigated the effect of pathological classification on survival. They only divided patients into two histological types: differentiated squamous cell carcinoma (54 patients, 3.5%) and anaplastic carcinoma (1,501 patients, 96.5%). The 5- and 10-year actuarial survival rates between differentiated squamous cell carcinoma and anaplastic carcinoma were 43% vs. 48% (p = 0.5156) and 37% vs. 40% (p = 0.7872). They concluded that pathological classification in NPC played a minor role in prognosis. A third study from Mainland China which included 1,302 NPC patients also found no statistical difference in 10-year survival rate between patients of undifferentiated type (43 cases, 39.5%), and those of clear vesicular nuclear cell type (96 cases, 40.6%) or poorly differentiated squamous cell carcinoma (1,012 cases, 33.4%) (Zhang et al. 1989). The prognosis of patients with well-differentiated squamous cell carcinoma (21 cases) and adenocarcinoma (1 case) was not better than those of the anaplastic type. Again, the authors concluded that the pathological classification did not affect prognosis.

A unique report by pathologists from the National Taiwan University Hospital (Hsu et al. 1987) analyzed the prognostic impact of different histology. The researchers performed a thorough histological review of 494 NPC patients who received complete course of radiation therapy with a minimal follow-up of 5 years and correlated with patient prognosis. The analyses between outcome and WHO classification was first performed. Seventy-eight patients (15.8%) were WHO Type 1, and their 5-year survival rate was significantly worse than those of WHO Types 2/3 (21.2% vs. 48.3%, p < 0.0000). The 5-year survival rates of WHO Type 2 and 3 were similar (47.3% and 50.4% respectively). The authors further divided patients into four groups according to the main cell types: keratinizing squamous cell carcinoma (KSCC, 78 cases, 15.8%), spindle cell carcinoma (SP, 167 cases, 33.8%), round cell of undifferentiated carcinoma (RC, 84 cases, 17%), and mixed cell carcinoma (Mix, 165 cases, 33.4%). The 5-year survival rate of patients with SP (41%) was significantly better than that of KSCC (21.2%, p < 0.002), but worse than that (53.1%) of other nonkeratinizing variants (RC and Mix), p < 0.002. The 5-year survival rates between RC (51.2%) and Mix (54.1%), however, did not differ significantly. They further defined patients of three nonkeratinizing carcinomas (SP, RC, and Mix) into two subgroups each, according to the degree of anaplasia and/or pleomorphism: Type A (with marked anaplasia and/or pleomorphism), and Type B (with moderate or little anaplasia). They found that Type B had significant better survival than those of Type A in each three nonkeratinizing carcinomas (60.5% vs. 35% for SP, $p < 0.005$; 71.8% vs. 33.3% for RC, $p < 0.0005$; and 60% vs. 38.6% for Mix, $p < 0.02$). Based on these results, the authors proposed that the histology of NPC could be divided into three grades of malignancy: high-grade malignancy (KSCC, 5-year survival rate of 20%), intermediate malignancy (Type A carcinomas, 5-year survival rates of 30%–40%), and low-grade malignancy (Type B carcinomas, 5-year survival rates of 60%–72%).

Cheng et al. (2006a) proposed a prognostic scoring system for locoregional control in NPC following conformal radiation therapy with or without chemotherapy. Histology was found to be one of the four important factors in their model. Among 630 patients included in that study, 17, 131, and 482 patients were justified as WHO Types 1, 2, and 3, respectively. The 5-year locoregional control rates for patients with WHO Type 1, 2, and 3 were 81%, 81%, and 91%, respectively. Multivariate analysis confirmed WHO Type 3 as a favorable independent factor (hazard ratio = 2.3, 95% CI = 1.4–3.8, $p = 0.002$).

In summary, histological type is a significant prognostic factor for NPC patients in nonendemic regions with worse results in keratinizing sqaumous cell carcinoma. Due to the small number of patients with keratinizing squamous cell carcinoma histology in endemic areas, the histological impact on survival is still unknown and deserves to be studied further with multicenter cooperation. In addition, consensus between different pathologists should be reached to set uniform criteria for histological classification.

9.5.3 Factors Associated with Diagnostic Procedures

9.5.3.1 Parapharyngeal Space Invasion or Retropharyngeal Lymphadenopathy

Parapharyngeal space (PPS) invasion and/or retropharyngeal lymph nodes (RPLN) metastasis are two common routes of NPC spreading. Precise definition of the extent of PPS and/or RPLN invasion is not possible until the utilization of CT scan. The use of MRI further improves the discrimination between PPS invasion and RPLN metastasis. Studies exploring the prognostic impact of PPS invasion and RPLN metastasis suggest that both conditions are significant factors affecting various survival endpoints, besides TNM staging.

Sham and Choy (1991) performed a thorough investigation regarding PPS invasion on local control and short-term survival in 262 NPC patients who had pretreatment CT scan. Three reference lines to grade the extent of PPS invasion were proposed: The first line was defined from the free edge of the medial pterygoid plate posterolaterally to the lateral border of the carotid artery, the second line extending from the scaphoid fossa at the base of the medial pterygoid plate posterolaterally to the styloid process, and the third line extending from the free edge of the lateral pterygoid plate posterolaterally to the posterior border of the ascending ramus of the mandible. The tumor is considered confined to the nasopharynx, with no PPS invasion, if the tumor is confined medial to the first line. Tumor on each side extending into the retrostyloid space, prestyloid space, and anterior part of the masticator space, by reaching or extending beyond the first, second, and third lines, respectively, were designated Grade 1, 2, and 3 PPS invasion, respectively. In this study, 84.4% (221/262) patients had PPS invasion and 40.2% (105/262) of patients had bilateral involvement. PPS invasion was shown as one of the significant factors affecting local control and survival by both univariate ($p = 0.0001$ and $p = 0.0001$) and multivariate ($p = 0.0001$ and $p = 0.0335$) analyses. In a subsequent study of another group of 364 NPC patients by the same research team and definition of PPS invasion with a longer follow-up time, PPS invasion was confirmed to be a significantly independent prognostic factor for relapse-free survival, local failure-free survival, and metastasis-free survival by both univariate and multivariate analyses (Chua et al. 1996). The 5-year relapse-free, local failure-free, and metastasis-free survival rates for Grade 0/1 and Grade 2/3 PPSI were 72% vs. 45% ($p < 0.0001$), 86% vs. 72% ($p < 0.0001$), and 87% vs. 68% ($p = 0.0002$), respectively.

Three other studies used the same definition of Sham and Chua grading system to evaluate the prognostic impact of PPS invasion (Heng et al. 1999; Ma et al. 2001a; Kalogera-Fountzila et al. 2006). Kalogera-Fountzila et al. (2006) studied 162 NPC patients with Stage II–IV disease from Greece and observed the same results. PPS invasion has significant effect on overall survival by both univariate

($p = 0.007$) and multivariate ($p = 0.02$) analyses. Two larger series containing more patient numbers from Singapore (677 cases) and Mainland China (621 cases), further divided PPS invasion into two subgroups: paranasopharyngeal space and paraoropharyngeal space invasion with distinction at the C1/C2 interspace (Heng et al. 1999; Ma et al. 2001a). Both studies found that the PPS invasion was not a significant prognostic factor. Whereas, the paraoropharyngeal space invasion itself was an independent variable on overall survival ($p = 0.02$) in Heng's study and on overall ($p = 0.0028$), local failure-free ($p = 0.0116$), and metastasis-free ($p = 0.0050$) survivals in Ma's study. Using similar definition of PPS invasion, several large studies from endemic regions (Xiao et al. 2002; Yeh et al. 2005; Cheng et al. 2005) consistently showed that PPS invasion was an important prognostic factor for various survival analyses. Among series using CT scan as a detection tool for PPS invasion, two studies failed to support the prognostic value of PPS invasion. Teo et al. (1996) from Hong Kong reported that PPS invasion had no survival impact for 903 patients as a whole when a parapharyngeal boost radiation was given, except for the Ho's stage T2N0M0 subgroup. An additional study of 1294 patients by Au et al. (2003) also illustrated that PPS invasion was not a significant factor for survival or failure at any site on multivariate analysis.

Two recent studies used MRI and 3D conformal radiation technique as a diagnostic and therapeutic modality. Of the 364 Stage I–III NPC patients enrolled in the study reported by Cheng et al. (2005), 201 (55.2%) had PPS invasion or skull base involvement. The 5-year distant metastasis-free survival rates in Stage I–IIA (30 cases), Stage II–III without PPS invasion/T3 disease (133 cases), and Stage IIB-III with PPS invasion/T3 disease were 100%, 95.8%, and 83.0%, respectively ($p = 0.004$). They suggest that PPS invasion/T3 is a poor prognostic factor for distant failure in Stage I–III NPC patients. In addition, their data also demonstrate significant improvement of overall ($p = 0.005$) and recurrence-free ($p = 0.01$) survival using adjuvant chemotherapy for Stage II–III NPC patient with PPS invasion/T3 disease. With the advancement of 3D conformal radiation therapy, better dosimetric coverage of the PPS can be achieved. Ng et al. (2008) postulated that the poor clinical outcome of PPS invasion was predominantly related to the suboptimal dose. They retrospectively analyzed the prognostic value of PPS invasion after conformal radiation therapy for 700 NPC patients. In their series, the whole incidence of PPS invasion was high (74%) by MRI detection. On univariate analysis, the degree of PPS invasion seemed to predict for overall, local failure-free, metastasis-free survivals. However, after stratification according to T-Classification, the prognostic value of PPS invasion was lost for local failure-free and metastasis-free survivals, and it only reached statistical significance in predicting overall survival for T3 patients. Multivariate Cox regression analysis revealed that the extent of PPS invasion was not an independent prognostic factor for overall, local failure-free, and metastasis-free survivals. The authors suggested that PPS invasion per se no longer predicts disease outcome.

The significance of RPLN metastasis in clinical staging and prognosis has not been defined clearly for NPC. The current version of AJCC/UICC staging system does not include the status of RPLN. The reasons may be (1) very rare reports addressed the prognostic impact of RPLN metastasis and results were controversial; (2) most previous studies used CT scan for RPLN detection, which was less sensitive than MRI; (3) the criteria of RPLN metastasis differed in different studies. MRI has proven to be superior to CT scan in delineating primary soft tissue invasion, subtle intracranial invasion, and RPLN metastasis and has become more valuable in both staging and treatment planning for NPC management. The reported detection rates of RPLN in NPC were 11.2%–51.8% with CT scan (Chong et al. 1995; Chua et al. 1997a; Xiao et al. 2002; Kalogera-Fountzila et al. 2006; Ma et al. 2007) and 51.8%–89% with MRI (Chong et al. 1995; Lam et al. 1997; Sakata et al. 1999; King et al. 2000; Ng et al. 2004, 2007; Liu et al. 2006; Lu et al. 2006; Tang et al. 2008; Wang et al. 2009). Six studies reported the prognostic value of RPLN metastasis in NPC. Using CT scan and size of 10 mm or more as positive for RPLN metastasis, Chua et al. (1997a) observed no significant difference in treatment outcome between patients with or without RPLN metastasis. Without mention of the cutoff size of positive RPLN metastasis, Kalogera-Fountzila et al. (2006) reported no significant effect of RPLN on overall survival analysis. Using CT scan and nodal size 5 mm or more, Ma et al. (2007) found 51.5% of 749 NPC patients had RPLN metastasis. The 5-year overall survival and metastasis-free survival rates were 58.7% vs. 72.2% ($p < 0.001$) and 75.0% vs. 84.6% ($p < 0.001$) for patient with or without RPLN metastasis. After adjusting for T-calssification and N-calssification, the prognostic value became less significant for overall survival ($p = 0.118$) and metastasis-free survival ($p = 0.079$). One of the three MRI-based studies reported that RPLN metastasis was an independent prognostic factor for metastasis-free survival (Tang et al. 2008). The other two studies failed to show significant effect of RPLN metastasis on treatment outcome (Lu et al. 2006; Ng et al. 2007).

Based on the aforementioned discussion, PPS invasion and RPLN metastasis seem to be a potential prognostic factor in NPC. However, these two factors have been embedded in or associated with existing T- and N-classifications, which are the most important prognostic factor and usually override the effect of other factors. Thus, PPS invasion and RPLN metastasis may become less relevant to treatment outcome in the era using MRI staging and IMRT technique unless both signs themselves have different malignant potential of biological aspect. Table 9.9 summarizes important reports regarding prognostic impact of PPSI and RPLN metastasis.

9.5.3.2 Other Adjacent Structures Involvement

Skull-base erosion/destruction or cranial-nerve palsy was occasionally evaluated as a risk factor besides T-classification for outcome analysis. On univariate analysis, both factors were usually shown as a significant parameter on overall survival (Sham and Choy 1991; Teo et al. 1996; Heng et al. 1999; Ma et al. 2001a; Au et al. 2003, Yeh et al. 2005). Some studies also demonstrated that skull-base erosion/destruction or cranial-nerve palsy could affect local failure-free survival (Sham and Choy 1991) and disease-free survival (Yeh et al. 2005). On multivariate analysis, cranial-nerve palsy still keeps as an independent factor affecting overall survival (Sham and Choy 1991; Teo et al. 1996; Heng et al. 1999; Ma et al. 2001a), local failure-free survival (Sham and Choy 1991; Teo et al. 1996; Ma et al. 2001a, Au et al. 2003), metastasis-free survival (Teo et al. 1996; Ma et al. 2001a; Au et al. 2003; Yeh et al. 2005), and disease-free survival (Teo et al. 1996; Au et al. 2003). But the prognostic impact of skull-base erosion/destruction usually became less significant. Two other studies from the Koo Foundation Sun Yat-Sen Cancer Center, Taiwan reported that infiltration of the clivus by the tumor is an independent and useful prognostic factor on metastasis-free survival (Cheng et al. 1998) and prevertebral muscle involvement is an independent poor prognostic sign for any recurrence (adjusted relative risk = 2.01, $p < 0.001$), locoregional recurrence (adjusted relative risk = 2.69, $p < 0.001$) and distant metastasis (adjusted relative risk = 2.25, $p < 0.01$), and a borderline significant increased risk for overall survival (Feng et al. 2006). One study from Mainland China found that prognosis of patient with skull-base bone abnormality of two or more sites was significantly different from those with none or one site involvement by both univariate and multivariate analyses (Lu et al. 2004). Table 9.10 summarizes some series investigating the prognostic effect of adjacent structures involvement or crania-nerve palsy. Based on the results of these studies, we concluded that cranial-nerve palsy is a definite poor prognostic sign for NPC, the effect of skull-base erosion/destruction is still controversial.

9.5.3.3 Implication of MRI and PET Scan

MRI has become the most preferred imaging modality in NPC staging. It is also a helpful reference for radiation planning. However, the benefit gained by the use of MRI in the clinical practice was rarely analyzed. Two recent studies addressed this problem and consistently demonstrated a significant improvement of tumor control and survival. Chang et al. (2005) investigated the impact of imaging modalities in 330 NPC patients with cranial nerve palsy who were treated during 1979–2000. Imaging modalities varied over the period, and included conventional tomography for 47 patients, CT scan for 195 patients, and MRI for 88 patients. All patients received external radiotherapy with a median dose of 70.2 Gy, 156 patients also received brachytherapy boost, and 139 patients received chemotherapy. Patients who had an MRI had a significantly improved tumor control rate than those evaluated with CT or conventional tomography, with a 15%–30% improvement in local tumor control and survival. Lee et al. (2005b) retrospectively reviewed 2687 consecutive patients from five oncology centers in Hong Kong during 1996–2000. Thirty-two percent patients were imaged by MRI, and 68% by CT scan. Multivariate analysis revealed that the MRI group had significant lower hazard of local failure than the CT-scan group (HR = 0.73, 95% CI = 0.56–0.94, $p = 0.013$). The corresponding data for progression, cancer-specific deaths, and all deaths were [HR = 0.84, 95% CI = 0.72–0.97, $p = 0.018$], [HR = 0.70, 95% CI = 0.56–0.87, $p < 0.001$], and [HR = 0.67, 95% CI = 0.55–0.81, $p < 0.01$] respectively.

Previous studies have shown that (18)F-fluorodeoxyglucose PET scan is a useful technique for early detection and staging in many malignant diseases. It is also more accurate in the differential diagnosis of local recurrence/persistent tumor or distant metastasis than other conventional staging work-up. Studies regarding the prognostic impact of PET scan in NPC were very rare. Yen et al. (2006) evaluated whether PET-scan findings could predict local response in 39 NPC patients with T4 disease treated by concurrent chemoradiotheapy at Chang Gung Memorial Hospital, Taiwan. They found that neither the pretreatment standard uptake value (SUV) nor the changes of SUV between pretreatment and post-treatment were significant predictors for local response. The SUV at three months after treatment for local responders and nonresponders were 2.1 ± 0.8 and 5.5 ± 3.2, respectively ($p = 0.001$). Using an SUV < 4.0 as the criterion for a negative PET result, the negative and positive predictive values were both 100%. They concluded that the cutoff of 4.0 for SUV at three months after treatment could predict patients with recurrent or residual tumor accurately. Another study by the same investigators on 65 NPC patients reported that pretreatment SUV > 12 of the primary tumor was a significant and independent predictor for subsequent distant failure by both univariate ($p = 0.013$) and multivariate ($p = 0.037$) analyses (Chan et al. 2009). Yen et al. (2005) from the National Taiwan University Hospital, Taiwan explored the utility of PET scan in monitoring the tumor response and in predicting prognosis. They collected 50 NPC patients with Stage IVA-IVB disease who received induction chemotherapy followed by concurrent chemoradiation therapy. Results of PET scan performed after first or second cycle induction chemotherapy could predict therapeutic response and final outcome. The recurrence-free survival and overall survival in major responders (56.4 ± 9.2 and 58.1 ± 2.2 months) were significantly better than those in nonmajor responders (33.7 ± 23.2 and 44.7 ± 20.0 months), with $p < 0.0001$ and $p = 0.0024$ respectively.

9.5.4 Treatment-Related Factors

Because of the anatomic location of nasopharynx, invasiveness nature and a high degree of radiosensitivity of the disease, radiation therapy is the standard treatment for nonmetastatic NPC. Several approaches have been demonstrated to increase the therapeutic effect, such as dose escalation by brachytherapy for early-stage disease, stereotactic body radiation therapy (SBRT) boost for advanced-stage disease, altered fractionated radiation schedule, sophisticated IMRT or image-guided IMRT technique, and combined chemo-radiotherapy. These approaches have greatly improved outcome, especially in local control. Thus, significant prognostic factors established under conventional 2D radiotherapy may be changed substantially, and caution must be applied when applying prognostic factors after modern effective treatment modality. For example, the local control rate has approached to 95% using IMRT technique. Any significant prognostic factors affecting local control, even T-stage, will be less important and make no statistical difference. Treatment modality may be the only significant predictor for local control of NPC in the future.

Advances in both chemotherapy and radiation therapy is presented in detail in subsequent chapters. In this section, treatment-related factors relevant to patient's prognosis are discussed briefly.

9.5.4.1 Radiotherapy-Related Factors

Theoretically, higher dose to the target could enhance local control, and a clear dose-response for the local control of NPC has been demonstrated (Vikram et al. 1985; Marks et al. 1982; Flores et al. 1986; Qin et al. 1988; Yan et al. 1990). It was technically difficult to escalate radiation doses in nasopharynx tumors without increasing normal tissue damage by 2D treatment. The recent development of more sophisticated planning and delivery systems have made it possible to effectively differentiate doses to planned treatment volume and organs at risk.

Brachytherapy was first applied for dose escalation in NPC since 1970s, especially for early-stage disease. Five series containing relatively larger patients and control group (no brachytherapy patients in a non-randomized study) unequivocally demonstrated patients with brachytherapy had significantly higher local control rate than those without brachytherapy (Wang 1991; Chang et al. 1996; Levendag et al. 1998; Teo et al. 2000a; Leung et al. 2008). Three of these five reports also performed multivariate analyses and confirmed that brachytherapy was an independent predictor for local control for early-stage NPC (Chang et al. 1996; Levendag et al. 1998; Teo et al. 2000a). One larger series from the Prince of Wales Hospital included 163 patients in brachytherapy group and 346 patients in external-beam alone group for T1–2 NPC (Teo et al. 2000a). The 5-year local control rates were 94.6% vs. 90.0% ($p = 0.016$), respectively. The risk ratio was 0.49 (95% CI = 0.256–0.975) for less local

Table 9.9. Prognostic impact of parapharyngeal space invasion or retropharyngeal lymphadenopathy in nasopharyngeal carcinoma

Series	No. of cases	Stage	Treatment	Image	Risk factor	Univariate analysis	
						OS	LFFS
SHAM and CHOY (1991)	262	I–IV	RT	CT	PPSI	$p = 0.001$	$p = 0.0001$
CHUA et al. (1996)	364	I–IV	RT ± Ch	CT	PPSI	–	$p < 0.0001$
HENG et al. (1999)	677	I–IV	RT	CT	PPSI	$p = 0.07$	–
					PNSI	$p = 0.08$	–
					POSI	$p < 0.0001$	–
MA et al. (2001a)	621	I–IV	RT	CT	PPSI	–	–
					POSI	–	–
KALOGERA-FOUNTZILA et al. (2006)	162	II–IV	RT ± Ch	CT	PPSI	$p = 0.007$	–
TEO et al. (1996)	903	I–IV	RT ± Ch	CT	PPSI	n.s.	n.s.
	102	subgroup (T_2N_0)	RT ± Ch	CT	PPSI	$p < 0.05$	n.s.
XIAO et al.(2002)	197	I–IV	RT	CT	PPSI	$p = 0.0115$	$p = 0.0367$
AU et al. (2003)	1294	I–IV	RT	CT	PPSI	–	–
YEH et al. (2005)	849	I–IV	RT	CT	PPSI	$p = 0.0002$	–
CHENG et al. (2005)	364	I–III	RT ± Ch	MRI	PPSI/SBMI	–	–
NG et al. (2008)	700	I–IV	RT ± Ch	MRI	PPSI	–	–
CHUA et al. (1997a)	364	I–IV	RT ± Ch	CT	RPLN ≥ 10 mm	–	$p = 0.31$
KALOGERA-FOUNTZILA et al. (2006)	162	II–IV	RT ± Ch	CT	RPLN ≥ ?mm	$p = 0.411$	–
MA et al. (2007)	749	I–IV	RT ± Ch	CT	RPLN ≥ 5 mm	$p < 0.001$	$p = 0.173$
LU et al. (2006)	159	I–IV	RT	MRI	RPLN ≥ 5 mm	–	–
NG et al. (2007)	202	I–IV	RT ± Ch	MRI	RPLN ≥ 5 mm	–	–
TANG et al. (2008)	924	I–IV	RT ± Ch	MRI	RPLN ≥ 5 mm	–	–

OS overall survival; *LFFS* local failure-free survival; *NFFS* neck failure-free survival; *MFS* metastasis failure-free survival; *DFS* disease-free survival; *RT* radiotherapy; *CT* computerized tomography scan; *PPSI* parapharyngeal space invasion; *PNSI* paranasopharyngeal space invasion; *POSI* paraoropharyngeal space invasion; *n.s* not statistically significant difference; *Ch* chemotherapy; *SBMI* skull base marrow involvement; *RPLN* retropharyngeal lymph node; *?* not mentioned

failures in brachytherapy group by multivariate analysis ($p = 0.0328$). Another trial from the Queen Mary Hospital and Tuen Mun Hospital (LEUNG et al. 2008) compared 145 patients with brachytherapy boost with 142 patients without brachytherapy boost. The 5-year local failure-free survival, distant metastasis failure-free survival, progression-free survival, cancer-specific survival and overall survival were 95.8% vs. 88.3% ($p = 0.020$), 95.0% vs. 83.2% ($p = 0.0045$), 89.2% vs. 74.8% ($p = 0.0021$), 94.5% vs. 83.4% ($p = 0.0058$), and 91.1% vs. 79.6% ($p = 0.0062$), respectively. Although one study containing T1–T4 diseases from Turkey (OZYAR et al. 2002) revealed no significant difference in local control between patients with (106 cases) or without (38 cases) brachytherapy boost, brachytherapy boost is generally considered to provide significant impact on local control for early-stage NPC.

			Multivariate analysis				
NFFS	MFS	DFS	OS	LFFS	NFFS	MFS	DFS
–	–	–	$p = 0.035$	$p = 0.0001$	–	–	–
–	$p < 0.0001$	$p < 0.0002$	–	$p = 0.0177$	–	$p = 0.0003$	$p = 0.0002$
–	–	–	$p = 0.91$	–	–	–	–
–	–	–	$p = 0.92$	–	–	–	–
–	–	–	$p = 0.02$	–	–	–	–
–	–	–	n.s.	n.s.	–	n.s.	–
–	–	–	$p = 0.0028$	$p = 0.0116$	–	$p = 0.0050$	–
–	–	–	$p = 0.02$	–	–	–	–
n.s.	n.s.	n.s.	n.s.	n.s.	n.s.	n.s.	n.s.
–	$p = 0.0166$	–	$p = 0.0166$	–	–	$p = 0.0499$	–
–	$p = 0.0153$	$p = 0.0035$	$p = 0.0213$	$p = 0.0710$	–	n.s.	$p = 0.0289$
–	–	–	n.s.	n.s.	n.s.	n.s.	n.s.
–	–	$p = 0.0001$	n.s.	–	–	–	n.s.
–	$p = 0.004$	–	–	–	–	–	–
–	–	–	$p = 0.08$	$p = 0.26$	–	$p = 0.73$	–
$p < 0.01$	$p = 0.30$	$p = 0.07$	–	n.s.	n.s.	n.s.	n.s.
–	–	–	n.s.	–	–	–	–
$p = 0.173$	$p < 0.001$	–	$p = 0.118$	–	–	$p = 0.079$	–
–	–	$p = 0.22$	–	–	–	–	–
–	–	–	$p = 0.09$	–	$p = 0.94$	$p = 0.20$	–
–	–	–	–	–	–	$p = 0.040$	n.s.

The SBRT boost could be delivered to early-stage tumors as well as advanced-stage diseases. Two groups used routine SBRT boost after external-beam radiation therapy for newly diagnosed NPC with Stage I–IV and one reported a 3-year local control rate of 93.1% (Chen et al. 2006) and the other 5-year local control rate of 98% (Hara et al. 2008). In addition, IMRT have been shown as an effective technique for dose escalation in NPC. Nearly all studies reported so far were single-arm treatment study with limited case numbers and showed short-term local control rates around 91%–97% for all-stage patients (Kwong et al. 2006; Lee et al. 2002; Kam et al. 2004; Wolden et al. 2006) and 100% for early-stage patients (Kwong et al. 2004a). In 2008 ASTRO meeting, four abstracts reported from the RTOG0225 trial (68 cases); the Koo Foundation SYS Cancer Center, Taiwan (158 cases); National Cancer Center, Singapore (195 cases); and Sun Yat-Sen Cancer Center, Guangzhou, China (419 cases) also provided 91%–94% local control rate. In the same annual meeting, a randomized trial from Queen Mary Hospital enrolled patients with Stage II NPC into IMRT (42

Table 9.10. Prognostic impact of adjacent structures involvement or cranial nerve palsy in nasopharyngeal carcinoma

Series	No. of cases	Stage	Treatment	Image	Risk factor	Univariate analysis
						OS
Sham and Choy (1991)	262	I–IV	RT	CT	SBE CNP	$p = 0.0005$ $p = 0.0001$
Teo et al. (1996)	903	I–IV	RT ± Ch	CT	SBE CNP	– –
Heng et al. (1999)	677	I–IV	RT	CT	SBE CNP	$p < 0.0001$ $p < 0.0001$
Ma et al. (2001a)	621	I–IV	RT	CT	SBE CNP	– –
Au et al. (2003)	1294	I–IV	RT	CT	SBE CNP	– –
Yeh et al. (2005)	849	I–IV	RT	CT	SBE CNP	$p < 0.0001$ $p < 0.0001$
Cheng et al. (1998)	74	III–IV	CCRT	MRI or CT	CI	–
Feng et al. (2006)	521	I–IV	RT ± Ch	MRI	PVMI	$p < 0.001$
Lu et al. (2004)	122	I–IV	RT	MRI	SBE ≥2 sites	$p = 0.0427$

OS overall survival; *LFFS* local failure-free survival; *MFS*, metastasis failure-free survival; *DFS* disease-free survival; *RT* radiotherapy; *CT* computerized tomography scan; *SBE* skull base erosion; *CNP* cranial nerve palsy; *Ch* chemotherapy; *n.s* not statistically significant difference; *CCRT* concurrent chemoradiotherapy; *MRI* magnetic resonance imaging; *CI* clivus infiltration; *PVMI* prevertebral muscle involvement
[a]indicated locoregional recurrence

cases) or 2D radiotherapy (40 cases). The trial was terminated early because preliminary results showed that the 4-year rates of local control were 90.5% vs. 71.7% ($p = 0.019$). Therefore, treatment technique could be a significant prognostic factor for local control.

Altered fractionated radiation schedule has a potential to improve treatment outcome in several malignancies. A recent large meta-analysis demonstrated that altered fractionated radiation enhances survival in patient with head and neck squamous cell carcinoma (Bourhis et al. 2006). Comparison of the different types of altered fractionated radiotherapy suggests that hyperfractionation has the greatest benefit. Altered fractionated radiotherapy for NPC was rare in literature. Wang (1989) first reported increased tumor control by using 1.6 Gy/fraction, two fractions per day for NPC. Ang et al. (1990) created a new altered fractionated protocol, called concomitant boost radiation and illustrated that this schedule was feasible and effective for NPC and oropharyngeal cancer. Two studies from Taiwan showed a 3-year local control rate of 89.1% for 63 Stage III–IV NPC patients using partially hyperfractionated accelerated schedule plus concomitant chemotherapy (Lin et al. 1996) or 3-year locoregional control rate of 93% for 48 T3–T4 patients using hyperfractionated RT plus conconurrent/adjuvant chemotherapy (Jian et al. 2002). So far, there were two studies to compare altered fractionated and conventional radiation in NPC, but inconsistent results were obtained. Teo et al. (2000b) from the Prince of Wales Hospital, Hong Kong randomly assigned 159 patients with Ho's stage N0 or N1 and nodal size < 4 cm into conventional radiation or a mixed conventional and hyperfractionated radiation therapy in the last two-thirds part of treatment. After a median follow-up of 59.2 months, the authors observed significantly increased radiation-induced damage to the central nervous system and no difference in 5-year local control rate (85.3% vs. 88.9%). A retrospective analysis on 325 NPC patients from Pamela Youde Nethersole Eastern Hospital, Hong Kong reported that accelerated fractionation (6 fractions per week) had significantly higher progression-free survival of 74% vs. 63%, $p = 0.02$, than conventional fractionation (5 fractions per week) without increased late toxicity (Lee et al. 2001).

			Multivariate analysis			
LFFS	MFS	DFS	OS	LFFS	MFS	DFS
$p = 0.0001$	–	–	$p = 0.8555$	$p = 0.7107$	–	–
$p = 0.0001$	–	–	$p = 0.0001$	$p = 0.0006$	–	–
–	–	–	$p = 0.0001$	$p = 0.0001$	$p = 0.0001$	$p = 0.0001$
–	–	–	$p = 0.0001$	$p = 0.0001$	$p = 0.0021$	$p = 0.0001$
–	–	–	n.s.	–	–	–
–	–	–	$p = 0.0001$	–	–	–
–	–	–	$p = 0.0001$	$p < 0.0001$	n.s.	–
–	–	–	$p = 0.0001$	$p = 0.0001$	$p < 0.0001$	–
–	–	–	–	$p = 0.014$	n.s.	$p = 0.008$
–	–	–	–	$p = 0.004$	$p = 0.001$	$p < 0.001$
–	–	$p < 0.0001$	n.s.	$p = 0.002$	n.s.	n.s.
–	–	$p < 0.0001$	n.s.	n.s.	$p = 0.023$	n.s.
–	–	–	–	–	$p = 0.0004$	–
$p < 0.001$[a]	$p < 0.001$	$p < 0.001$	$p = 0.10$	$p < 0.001$[a]	$p < 0.001$	$p < 0.001$
–	–	–	$p = 0.0385$	–	–	–

Of note, all studies mentioned earlier used conventional technique. Thus, whether altered fractionated schedule could be a treatment-related prognostic factor for NPC is largely unknown in the modern era of conformal radiation therapy or IMRT.

Tumor regression at the primary site and the involved cervical lymph nodes are usually observed during the radiation course. It is intuitive to postulate the extent of tumor regression during irradiation as proportional to the radiosensitivity, and outcome after the completion of radiation may be favorably associated with more substantial tumor volume regression during treatment. However, the results from the experience of 101 patients with locoregionally advanced NPC indicated otherwise: No statistically significant differences for local/regional control or overall survival rates could be found among patients with slow, moderate, or rapid response to 45 Gy of radiation therapy at the primary or nodal disease (Fang et al. 2001). Furthermore, T-classification was the only significant prognostic factor for locoregional control after multivariate analysis.

Bony destruction of the skull base is frequently seen in NPC and believed to be a significant prognostic factor as discussed in an earlier section. The implication of bony regeneration after radiation therapy on local control was rarely investigated. Fang et al. (1999) retrospectively reviewed 90 patients with skull-base destruction on CT scan. Bony regeneration in postradiation CT scan was noted in 57 patients. The 3-year rates of local control were 77% vs. 21% for patients with or without bony regeneration ($p < 0.0001$). Multivariate analysis also confirmed that bony regeneration is an independent prognostic factor for local control.

9.5.4.2 Chemotherapy-Related Factors

Chemotherapy has been incorporated with radiation therapy in the management of NPC for about 30 years. Currently, combined chemoradiotherapy has been accepted by most oncologists as the standard treatment of advanced NPC. There is still great controversy, however, regarding the optimal drugs, timing, dosage, and duration of chemotherapy.

In general, there are three different ways to incorporate chemotherapy into a curative course of radiation therapy: before (neoadjuvant), during (concurrent), and after (adjuvant) radiation therapy. Each mode of combined therapy has advantages and disadvantages and has been extensively investigated during past years. A major issue of neoadjuvant chemotherapy is that it may trigger the accelerated repopulation and cross-resistance during subsequent radiation therapy. The dose intensity of concurrent chemotherapy that can be delivered safely during 7–8 weeks radiation therapy is usually lower than neoadjuvant or adjuvant chemotherapy. This may compromise its efficacy in eradication of micrometastasis. Poor compliance and compromised blood supply are the two major problems of adjuvant chemotherapy.

So far, there are 17 randomized trials to investigate combined chemoradiotherapy versus radiotherapy alone in NPC (Rossi et al. 1988; Chan et al. 1995, 2002b, 2005; Cvitkovic 1996; Al-Sarraf et al. 1998; Chua et al. 1998; Ma et al. 2001b; Chi et al. 2002; Hareyama et al. 2002; Lin et al. 2003b; Kwong et al. 2004b; Lee et al. 2005a, 2006; Wee et al. 2005; Zhang et al. 2005; Chen et al. 2008; Hui et al. 2009). Summaries of three meta-analyses (Huncharek and Kupelnick 2002; Langendijk et al. 2004; Baujat et al. 2006) from parts of these randomized trials indicate that concurrent chemotherapy has the largest benefit and adjuvant chemotherapy the least. A detailed discussion of the application of chemotherapy in the management of NPC is out of the scope of this chapter, and is detailed in Chaps 11–15, and 21.

Treatment failures in advanced NPC included both high rates of local recurrence and distant metastasis. Because of recent advances in radiation oncology and the combined use of chemotherapy, the patterns of failure have been predominantly due to distant metastasis. Chemotherapy may become an important prognostic factor in the management of NPC. In future trials, researchers may need to differentiate the risk groups of patients and identify the potential mode of treatment failure in different subgroup of patients to guide the designing of chemotherapy strategy (neoadjuvant, concurrent, adjuvant, or their combination). For example, patients with persistently detectable plasma EBV DNA after chemoradiotherapy or radiation therapy alone will have a very high risk of distant failure. Effective adjuvant chemotherapy for micrometastases may be indicated for this group of patients. A Phase III randomized trial to address this problem has been ongoing using adjuvant chemotherapy consists of gemcitabine + cisplatin in Hong Kong. It is important to recognize that a negative result may just indicate an ineffective regimen, and the high incidence of distant metastasis indicates that the strategy of adjuvant therapy using an effective regimen is urgently needed for special subgroup patients.

9.6 Summary

Among all suggested disease-related prognosticators, stage of NPC at diagnosis, plasma/serum EBV DNA, serum LDH, tumor volume, cranial nerve palsy, and the presence of tumor-associated genes in peripheral blood cells are proven significant prognostic factors. PPS invasion, RPLN metastasis, and skull base erosion/destruction are probably significant factors affecting prognosis. Serum anti-EBV antibodies, other serum tumor markers, and tissue biomarkers are potential prognostic factors which need further studies with well-designed and larger patient numbers to validate. Pathological types or features have high potential to affect prognosis, but are hampered by three factors to be verified – consensus of objective classification criteria between different pathologists, representative of sampling (too small specimen by punch biopsy), and the presence of different pathological types or features in different parts of the specimen in the same patients.

Patients' age at diagnosis is a proven and significant patient-related prognosticator, and young age is a definite favorable prognostic factor for patients with nonmetastatic NPC. The significance of gender, race, performance status, weight loss, and anemia at diagnosis or during the course of radiation therapy on prediction of prognosis after treatment is debatable. Among treatment-related prognosticators, MRI-staged patients have a significantly improved outcome than patients staged using CT scan. However, the prevailing use of MRI in the management of NPC makes the diagnosis and staging of NPC more precise. Last but not least, treatment itself is also a determinant prognostic factor for NPC. Advances in radiation therapy technique such as the use of IMRT and brachytherapy, and combined chemoradiotherapy have significantly improved patients' prognoses. Future researches should be oriented to tailor various treatment strategies according to predictive factors of treatment failure to realize individualized management for patients with NPC.

References

Al-Sarraf M, LeBlanc M, Giri PG, Fu KK, Cooper J, Vuong T, Forastiere AA, Adams G, Sakr WA, Schuller DE, Ensley JF (1998) Chemoradiotherapy versus radiotherapy in patients with advanced nasopharyngeal cancer: phase III randomized intergroup study 0099. J Clin Oncol 16:1310–1317

Ang KK, Peters LJ, Weber RS, Maor MH, Morrison WH, Wendt CD, Brown BW (1990) Concomitant boost radiotherapy schedules in the treatment of carcinoma of the oropharynx and nasopharynx. Int J Radiat Oncol Biol Phys 19:1339–1345

Au JS, Law CK, Foo W, Lau WH (2003) In-depth evaluation of the AJCC/UICC 1997 staging system of nasopharyngeal carcinoma: prognostic homogeneity and proposed refinements. Int J Radiat Oncol Biol Phys 56:413–426

August M, Dodson TB, Nastri A, Chuang SK (2001) Nasopharyngeal carcinoma: clinical assessment and review of 176 cases. Oral Surg Oral Med Oral Pathol Oral Radiol Endod 91:205–214

Bailet JW, Mark RJ, Abemayor E, Lee SP, Tran LM, Juillard G, Ward PH (1992) Nasopharyngeal carcinoma: treatment results with primary radiation therapy. Laryngoscope 102:965–972

Barnes L, Eveson JW, Reichart P, Sidransky D (2005) World health organization classification of tumors: pathology and genetics of head and neck tumors. IARC Press, Lyon, France

Bar-Sela G, Ben Arush MW, Sabo E, Kuten A, Minkov I, Ben-Izhak O (2005) Pediatric nasopharyngeal carcinoma: better prognosis and increased c-Kit expression as compared to adults. Pediatr Blood Cancer 45:291–297

Bar-Sela G, Kaplan-Cohen V, Ilan N, Vlodavsky I, Ben-Izhak O (2006) Heparanase expression in nasopharyngeal carcinoma inversely correlates with patient survival. Histopathology 49:188–193

Baujat B, Audry H, Bourhis J, Chan AT, Onat H, Chua DT, Kwong DL, Al-Sarraf M, Chi KH, Hareyama M, Leung SF, Thephamongkhol K, Pignon JP; MAC-NPC Collaborative Group (2006) Chemotherapy in locally advanced nasopharyngeal carcinoma: an individual patient data meta-analysis of eight randomized trials and 1753 patients. Int J Radiat Oncol Biol Phys 64:47–56

Bhattacharyya N (2004) The impact of race on survival in nasopharyngeal carcinoma: a matched analysis. Am J Otolaryngol 25:94–97

Bourhis J, Overgarrd J, Audry H, Ang KK, Saunders M, Bernier J, Horiot JC, Le Maître A, Pajak TF, Poulsen MG, O'Sullivan B, Dobrowsky W, Hliniak A, Skladowski K, Hay JH, Pinto LH, Fallai C, Fu KK, Sylvester R, Pignon JP; Meta-Analysis of Radiotherapy in Carcinomas of Head and neck (MARCH) Collaborative Group (2006) Hyperfractionated or accelerated radiotherapy in head and neck cancer: a meta-analysis. Lancet 68:843–854

Burt RD, Vaughan TL, McKnight B (1992) Descriptive epidemiology and survival analysis of nasopharyngeal carcinoma in the United States. Int J Cancer 52:549–556

Casselman JW (1994) The value of MRI in the diagnosis and staging of nasopharynx tumors. J Belge Radiol 77:67–71

Chan AT, Teo PM, Leung TW, Leung SF, Lee WY, Yeo W, Choi PH, Johnson PJ (1995) A prospective randomized study of chemotherapy adjunctive to definitive radiotherapy in advanced nasopharyngeal carcinoma. Int J Radiat Oncol Biol Phys 33:569–577

Chan AT, Teo ML, Lee WY, Kwan WH, Choi PH, Johnson PJ (1998) The significance of keratinizing squamous cell histology in Chinese patients with nasopharyngeal carcinoma. Clin Oncol (R Coll Radiol) 10:161–164

Chan AT, Lo YM, Zee B, Chan LY, Ma BB, Leung SF, Mo F, Lai M, Ho S, Huang DP, Johnson PJ (2002a) Plasma Epstein–Barr virus DNA and residual disease after radiotherapy for undifferentiated nasopharyngeal carcinoma. J Natl Cancer Inst 94:1614–1619

Chan AT, Teo PM, Ngan RK, et al (2002b) Concurrent chemo-therapy–radiotherapy compared with radiotherapy alone in locoregionally advanced nasopharyngeal carcinoma: progression-free survival analysis of a phase III randomized trial. J Clin Oncol 20:2038–2044

Chan AT, Leung SF, Ngan RK, Teo PM, Lau WH, Kwan WH, Hui EP, Yiu HY, Yeo W, Cheung FY, Yu KH, Chiu KW, Chan DT, Mok TS, Yau S, Yuen KT, Mo FK, Lai MM, Ma BB, Kam MK, Leung TW, Johnson PJ, Choi PH, Zee BC (2005) Overall survival after concurrent cisplatin-radiotherapy compared with radiotherapy alone in locoregionally advanced nasopharyngeal carcinoma. J Natl Cancer Inst 97:536–539

Chan CM, Ma BB, Hui EP, Wong SC, Mo FK, Leung SF, Kam MK, Chan AT (2007) Cyclooxygenase-2 expression in advanced nasopharyngeal carcinoma–a prognostic evaluation and correlation with hypoxia inducible factor 1α and vascular endothelial growth factor. Oral Oncol 43:373–378

Chan KC, Zhang J, Chan AT, Lei KI, Leung SF, Chan LY, Chow KC, Lo YM (2003) Molecular characterization of circulating EBV DNA in the plasma of nasopharyngeal carcinoma and lymphoma patients. Cancer Res 63:2028–2032

Chan SC, Chang JT, Wang HM, Lin CY, Ng SH, Fan KH, Chin SC, Liao CT, Yen TC (2009) Prediction for distant failure in patients with stage M0 nasopharyngeal carcinoma: the role of standardized uptake value. Oral Oncol 45:52–58

Chang CC, Chen MK, Liu MT, Wu HK (2002) The effect of primary tumor volumes in advanced T-staged nasopharyngeal tumors. Head Neck 24:940–946

Chang JT, See LC, Tang SG, Lee SP, Wang CC, Hong JH (1996) The role of brachytherapy in early-stage nasopharyngeal carcinoma. Int J Radiat Oncol Biol Phys 36:1019–1024

Chang JT, Lin CY, Chen TM, Kang CJ, Ng SH, Chen IH, Wang HM, Cheng AJ, Liao CT (2005) Nasopharyngeal carcinoma with cranial nerve palsy: the importance of MRI for radiotherapy. Int J Radiat Oncol Biol Phys 63:1354–1360

Chang KP, Hao SP, Chang JH, Wu CC, Tsang NM, Lee YS, Hsu CL, Ueng SH, Liu SC, Liu YL, Wei PC, Liang Y, Chang YS, Yu JS (2008) Macrophage inflammatory protein-3α is a novel serum marker for nasopharyngeal carcinoma detection and prediction of treatment outcomes. Clin Cancer Res 14:6979–6987

Chang YS, Tyan YS, Liu ST, Tsai MS, Pao CC (1990) Detection of Epstein–Barr virus DNA sequences in nasopharyngeal carcinoma cells by enzymatic DNA amplification. J Clin Microbiol 28:2398–2402

Chen CL, Wen WN, Chen JY, Hsu MM, Hsu HC (1993) Detection of Epstein–Barr virus genome in nasopharyngeal carcinoma by in situ DNA hybridization. Intervirology 36:91–98

Chen HH, Tsai ST, Wang MS, Wu YH, Hsueh WT, Yang MW, Yeh IC, Lin JC (2006) Experience in fractionated stereotactic body radiation therapy boost for newly diagnosed nasopharyngeal carcinoma. Int J Radiat Oncol Biol Phys 66:1408–1414

Chen KW, Lin JF, Jan JS, Chao JY, Lin JC (2009) The effect of primary tumor volume measured by MR imaging on T-stage, local control, and survival in patients with advanced nasopharyngeal carcinoma. Therapeut Radiol Oncol 16:1–13

Chen MK, Chen TH, Liu JP, Chang CC, Chie WC (2004) Better prediction of prognosis for patients with nasopharyngeal carcinoma using primary tumor volume. Cancer 100:2160–2166

Chen Y, Liu MZ, Liang SB, Zong JF, Mao YP, Tang LL, Guo Y, Lin AH, Zeng XF, Ma J (2008) Preliminary results of a prospective randomized trial comparing concurrent chemoradiotherapy plus adjuvant chemotherapy with radiotherapy alone in patients with locoregionally advanced nasopharyngeal carcinoma in endemic regions of China. Int J Radiat Oncol Biol Phys 71:1356–1364

Cheng SH, Jian JJ, Tsai SY, Chan KY, Yen LK, Chu NM, Tan TD, Tsou MH, Huang AT (1998) Prognostic features and treatment outcome in locoregionally advanced nasopharyngeal carcinoma following concurrent chemotherapy and radiotherapy. Int J Radiat Oncol Biol Phys 41:755–762

Cheng SH, Tsai SY, Yen KL, Jian JJ, Feng AC, Chan KY, Hong CF, Chu NM, Lin YC, Lin CY, Tan TD, Hsieh CY, Chong V, Huang AT (2005) Prognostic significance of parapharyngeal space venous plexus and marrow involvement: potential landmarks of dissemination for stage I–III nasopharyngeal carcinoma. Int J Radiat Oncol Biol Phys 61:456–465

Cheng SH, Tsai SY, Horng CF, Yen KL, Jian JJ, Chan KY, Lin CY, Terng SD, Tsou MH, Chu NM, Chen HH, Chen PL, Chung YL, Hsieh CI, Tan TD, Huang AT (2006a) A prognostic scoring system for locoregional control in nasopharyngeal carcinoma following conformal radiotherapy. Int J Radiat Oncol Biol Phys 66:992–1003

Cheng SW, Yang SN, Liang JA, Tsai MH, Shiau AC, Lin FJ (2006b) Value of computed tomography-based tumor volume as a predictor of outcomes in hypopharyngeal cancer after treatment with definitive radiotherapy. Laryngoscope 116: 2012–2017

Chi KH, Chang YC, Guo WY, Leung MJ, Shiau CY, Chen SY, Wang LW, Lai YL, Hsu MM, Lian SL, Chang CH, Liu TW, Chin YH, Yen SH, Perng CH, Chen KY (2002) A phase III study of adjuvant chemotherapy in advanced nasopharyngeal carcinoma patients. Int J Radiat Oncol Biol Phys 52:1238–1244

Chien YC, Chen JY, Liu MY, Yang HI, Hsu MM, Chen CJ, Yang CS (2001) Serologic markers of Epstein–Barr virus infection and nasopharyngeal carcinoma in Taiwanese men. N Engl J Med 345:1877–1882

Chong VF, Fan YF, Khoo JBK (1995) Retropharyngeal lymphadenopathy in nasopharyngeal carcinoma. Eur J Radiol 21:100–105

Chong VF, Mukherji SK, Ng SH, Ginsberg LE, Wee JT, Sham JS, O'Sullivan B (1999) Nasopharyngeal carcinoma: review of how imaging affects staging. J Comput Assist Tomogr 23: 984–993

Chow E, Payne D, O'Sullivan B, Pintilie M, Liu FF, Waldron J, Warde P, Cummings B (2002) Radiotherapy alone in patients with advanced nasopharyngeal cancer: comparison with an intergroup study. Is combined modality treatment really necessary? Radiother Oncol 63:269–274

Chua DT, Sham JS, Kwong DL, Choy DT, Au GK, Wu PM (1996) Prognostic value of parapharyngeal extension of nasopharyngeal carcinoma. A significant factor in local control and distant metastasis. Cancer 78:202–210

Chua DT, Sham JS, Kwong DL, Au GK, Choy DK (1997a) Retropharyngeal lymphadenopathy in patients with nasopharyngeal carcinoma. A computed tomography-based study. Cancer 79:869–877

Chua DT, Sham JS, Kwong DL, Tai KS, Wu PM, Lo M, Yung A, Choy D, Leong L (1997b) Volumetric analysis of tumor extent in nasopharyngeal carcinoma and correlation with treatment outcome. Int J Radiat Oncol Biol Phys 39:711–719

Chua DT, Sham JS, Choy D, Lorvidhaya V, Sumitsawan Y, Thongprasert S, Vootiprux V, Cheirsilpa A, Azhar T, Reksodiputro AH (1998) Preliminary report of the Asian-Oceanian Clinical Oncology Association randomized trial comparing cisplatin and epirubicin followed by radiotherapy versus radiotherapy alone in the treatment of patients with locoregionally advanced nasopharyngeal carcinoma. Cancer 83:2270–2283

Chua DT, Sham JS, Wei WI, Ho WK, Au GK (2001) The predictive value of the 1997 American Joint Committee on Cancer stage classification in determining failure patterns in nasopharyngeal carcinoma. Cancer 92:2845–2855

Chua DT, Sham JS, Choy DT (2004a) Prognostic impact of hemoglobin levels on treatment outcome in patients with nasopharyngeal carcinoma treated with sequential chemoradiotherapy or radiotherapy alone. Cancer 101:307–316

Chua DT, Sham JS, Leung LH, Tai KS, Au GK (2004b) Tumor volume is not a independent prognostic factor in early-stage nasopharyngeal carcinoma treated by radiotherapy alone. Int J Radiat Oncol Biol Phys 58:1437–1444

Chua DT, Nicholls JM, Sham JS, Au GK (2004c) Prognostic value of epidermal growth factor receptor expression in patients with advanced stage nasopharyngeal carcinoma treated with induction chemotherapy and radiotherapy. Int J Radiat Oncol Biol Phys 59:11–20

Chung NN, Ting LL, Hsu WC, Lui LT, Wang PM (2004) Impact of magnetic resonance imaging versus CT on nasopharyngeal carcinoma: primary tumor target delineation for radiotherapy. Head Neck 26:241–246

Cooper JS, Cohen R, Stevens RE (1998) A comparison of staging systems for nasopharyngeal carcinoma. Cancer 83:213–219

Corry J, Fisher R, Rischin D, Peters LJ (2006) Relapse patterns in WHO 2/3 nasopharyngeal cancer: is there a difference between ethnic Asian vs. non-Asian patients? Int J Radiat Oncol Biol Phys 64:63–71

Cvitkovic E; the International Nasopharynx Cancer Study Group (1996) Preliminary results of a randomized trial comparing neoadjuvant chemotherapy (cisplatin, epirubicin, bleomycin) plus radiotherapy vs. radiotherapy alone in stage IV (≥N2, M0) undifferentiated nasopharyngeal carcinoma: a positive effect on progression-free survival. Int J Radiat Oncol Biol Phys 35:463–469

Datta YH, Adams PT, Drobyski WR, Ethier SP, Terry VH, Roth MS (1994) Sensitive detection of occult breast cancer by the reverse-transcriptase polymerase chain reaction. J Clin Oncol 12:475–482

de-Vathaire F, Sancho-Garnier H, de-Thé H, Pieddeloup C, Schwaab G, Ho JH, Ellouz R, Micheau C, Cammoun M, Cachin Y, et al (1988) Prognostic value of EBV markers in the clinical management of nasopharyngeal carcinoma (NPC): a multicenter follow-up study. Int J Cancer 42:176–181

Fan H, Nicholls J, Chua D, Chan KH, Sham J, Lee S, Gulley ML (2004) Laboratory markers of tumor burden in nasopharyngeal carcinoma: a comparison of viral load and serologic tests for Epstein–Barr virus. Int J Cancer 112:1036–1041

Fang FM, Leung SW, Wang CJ, Su CY, Lui CC, Chen HC, Sun M, Lin TM (1999) Computed tomography findings of bony regeneration after radiotherapy for nasopharyngeal carcinoma with skull base destruction: implications for local control. Int J Radiat Oncol Biol Phys 44:305–309

Fang FM, Tsai WL, Go SF, Ho MW, Wu JM, Wang CJ, Su CY, Chen WC, Huang EY (2001) Implications of quantitative tumor and nodal regression rates for nasopharyngeal carcinomas after 45 Gy of radiotherapy. Int J Radiat Oncol Biol Phys 50:961–969

Fang FM, Li CF, Chien CY, Rau KM, Huang HY (2007) Immunohistochemical expression of epidermal growth factor receptor and cyclooxygenase-2 in pediatric nasopharyngeal carcinomas: no significant correlations with clinicopathological variables and treatment outcomes. Int J Pediatr Otorhinolaryngol 71:447–455

Fang FM, Chien CY, Li CF, Shiu WY, Chen CH, Huang HY (2009) Effect of S-phase kinase-associated protein 2 expression on distant metastasis and survival in nasopharyngeal carcinoma patients. Int J Radiat Oncol Biol Phys 73:202–207

Farias TP, Dias FL, Lima RA, Kligerman J, de Sá GM, Barbosa MM, Gonçalves FB Jr (2003) Prognostic factors and outcome for nasopharyngeal carcinoma. Arch Otolaryngol Head Neck Surg 129:794–799

Feng AC, Wu MC, Tsai SY, Chan KY, Cheng SH, Wang A, Chen SS, Jian JJ, Terng SD, Huang AT (2006) Prevertebral muscle involvement in nasopharyngeal carcinoma. Int J Radiat Oncol Biol Phys 65:1026–1035

Flores AD, Dickson RI, Riding K, Coy P (1986) Cancer of the nasopharynx in British Columbia. Am J Clin Oncol 9:281–291

Foote RL, Weidner N, Harris J, Hammond E, Lewis JE, Vuong T, Ang KK, Fu KK (2005) Evaluation of tumor angiogenesis measured with microvessel density (MVD) as a prognostic indicator in nasopharyngeal carcinoma: results of RTOG 9505. Int J Radiat Oncol Biol Phys 61:745–753

Fournié GJ, Courtin JP, Laval F, Chalé JJ, Pourrat JP, Pujazon MC, Lauque D, Carles P (1995) Plasma DNA as a marker of cancerous cell death. Investigations in patients suffering from lung cancer and in nude mice bearing human tumors. Cancer Lett 91:221–227

Fujieda S, Lee K, Sunaga H, Tsuzuki H, Ikawa H, Fan GK, Imanaka M, Takenaka H, Saito H (1999) Staining of interleukin-10 predicts clinical outcome in patients with nasopharyngeal carcinoma. Cancer 85:1439–1445

Fujii M, Yamashita T, Ishiguro R, Tashiro M, Kameyama K (2002) Significance of epidermal growth factor receptor and tumor associated tissue eosinophilia in the prognosis of patients with nasopharyngeal carcinoma. Auris Nasus Larynx 29:175–181

Genç E, Hoşal AS, Gediko lu G, Ozyar E, Sözeri B (2000) Prognostic value of p53, proliferating cell nuclear antigen, and Ki-67 expression in undifferentiated nasopharyngeal carcinomas. Otolaryngol Head Neck Surg 122:868–873

Hamilton S, Venkatesan V, Matthews TW, Lewis C, Assis L (2004) Computed tomographic volumetric analysis as a predictor of local control in laryngeal cancers treated with conventional radiotherapy. J Otolaryngol 33:289–294

Hara W, Loo BW Jr, Goffinet DR, Chang SD, Adler JR, Pinto HA, Fee WE, Kaplan MJ, Fischbein NJ, Le QT (2008) Excellent local control with stereotactic radiotherapy boost after external beam radiotherapy in patients with nasopharyngeal carcinoma. Int J Radiat Oncol Biol Phys 71:393–400

Hareyama M, Sakata K, Shirato H, Nishioka T, Nishio M, Suzuki K, Saitoh A, Oouchi A, Fukuda S, Himi T (2002) A prospective, randomized trial comparing neoadjuvant chemotherapy with radiotherapy alone in patients with advanced nasopharyngeal carcinoma. Cancer 94:2217–2223

Heng DM, Wee J, Fong KW, Lian LG, Sethi VK, Chua ET, Yang TL, Khoo Tan HS, Lee KS, Lee KM, Tan T, Chua EJ (1999) Prognostic factors in 677 patients in Singapore with nondisseminated nasopharyngeal carcinoma. Cancer 86:1912–1920

Henle G, Henle W (1976) Epstein–Barr virus-specific IgA serum antibodies as an outstanding feature of nasopharyngeal carcinoma. Int J Cancer 17:1–7

Henle W, Henle G, Ho HC, Burtin P, Cachin Y, Clifford P, de Schryver A, de-Thé G, Diehl V, Klein G (1970) Antibodies to Epstein–Barr virus in nasopharyngeal carcinoma, other head and neck neoplasms and control groups. J Natl Cancer Inst 44:225–231

Ho HC, Ng MH, Kwan HC, Chau JC (1976) Epstein–Barr virus-specific IgA and IgG serum antibodies in nasopharyngeal carcinoma. Br J Cancer 34:655–660

Ho KY, Kuo WR, Chai CY, Tsai SM, Sheu SH, Wu SC, Juan KH (2001) A prospective study of p53 expression and its correlation with clinical response of radiotherapy in nasopharyngeal carcinoma. Laryngoscope 111:131–136

Hong MH, Mai HQ, Min HQ, Ma J, Zhang EP, Cui NJ (2000) A comparison of the Chinese 1992 and fifth-edition International Union Against Cancer staging systems for staging nasopharyngeal carcinoma. Cancer 89:242–247

Hong RL, Ting LL, Ko JY, Hsu MM, Sheen TS, Lou PJ, Wang CC, Chung NN, Lui LT (2001) Induction chemotherapy with mitomycin, epirubicin, cisplatin, fluorouracil, and leucovorin followed by radiotherapy in the treatment of locoregionally advanced nasopharyngeal carcinoma. J Clin Oncol 19:4305–4313

Hsiao JR, Jin YT, Tsai ST (2002) Detection of cell free Epstein–Barr virus DNA in sera from patients with nasopharyngeal carcinoma. Cancer 94:723–729

Hsu HC, Chen CL, Hsu MM, Lynn TC, Tu SM, Huang SC (1987) Pathology of nasopharyngeal carcinoma. Proposal of a new histologic classification correlated with prognosis. Cancer 59:945–951

Hsu MM, Chen JY, Chen CJ (1988) A prospective study of antibodies to Epstein–Barr virus DNase and viral capsid antigen for prognostication of patients with nasopharyngeal carcinoma. J Formosan Med Assoc 87:984–988

Hsu MM, Huang SC, Lynn TC, Hsieh T, Tu SM (1982) The survival of patients with nasopharyngeal carcinoma. Otolaryngol Head Neck Surg 90:289–295

Hsu MM, Chiou CR, Ko JY, Sheen TS, Hong RL, Ting LL (2000) DNA content of nasopharyngeal carcinoma: an independent prognostic indicator. Cancer Detect Prev 24:119–126

Huang GW, Sunagawa M, Jie-En L, Shimada S, Gang Z, Tokeshi Y, Kosugi T (2000) The relationship between microvessel density, the expression of vascular endothelial growth factor (VEGF), and the extension of nasopharyngeal carcinoma. Laryngoscope 110:2066–2069

Hui EP, Sung FL, Yu BK, Wong CS, Ma BB, Lin X, Chan A, Wong WL, Chan AT (2008) Plasma osteopontin, hypoxia, and response to radiotherapy in nasopharyngeal cancer. Clin Cancer Res 14:7080–7087

Hui EP, Ma BB, Leung SF, King AD, Mo F, Kam MK, Yu BK, Chiu SK, Kwan WH, Ho R, Chan I, Ahuja AT, Zee BC, Chan AT (2009) Randomized phase II trial of concurrent cisplatin-radiotherapy with or without neoadjuvant decetaxel and cisplatin in advanced nasopharyngeal carcinoma. J Clin Oncol 27:242–249

Huncharek M, Kupelnick B (2002) Combined chemoradiation versus radiation therapy alone in locally advanced nasopharyngeal carcinoma: results of a meta-analysis of 1528 patients from six randomized trials. Am J Clin Oncol 25:219–223

Hwang CF, Cho CL, Huang CC, Wang JS, Shih YL, Su CY, Chang HW (2002) Loss of cyclin D1 and p16 expression correlates with local recurrence in nasopharyngeal carcinoma following radiotherapy. Ann Oncol 13:1246–1251

Jahr S, Hentze H, Englisch S, Hardt D, Fackelmayer FO, Hesch RD, Knippers R (2001) DNA fragments in the blood plasma of cancer patients: quantitations and evidence for their origin from apoptotic and necrotic cells. Cancer Res 61:1659–1665

Jian JJ, Cheng SH, Prosnitz LR, Tsai SY, Tsai MJ, Huang AT (1998) T classification and clivus margin as risk factors for determining locoregional control by radiotherapy of nasopharyngeal carcinoma. Cancer 82:261–267

Jian JJ, Cheng SH, Tsai SY, Yen KC, Chu NM, Chan KY, Tan TD, Cheng JC, Lin YC, Leu SY, Hsieh CI, Tsou MH, Lin CY, Huang AT (2002) Improvement of local control of T3 and T4 nasopharyngeal carcinoma by hyperfractionated radiotherapy and concomitant chemotherapy. Int J Radiat Oncol Biol Phys 53:344–352

Jiong L, Berrino F, Coebergh JW (1998) Variation in survival for adults with nasopharyngeal cancer in Europe, 1978–1989. Eur J Cancer 34:2162–2166

Johansen LV, Grau C, Overgaard J (2001) Squamous cell carcinoma of the nasopharynx – an analysis of treatment results in 149 consecutive patients. Acta Oncol 40:801–809

Kalogera-Fountzila A, Karanikolas D, Katodritis N, Samantas E, Sarafopoulos A, Ikonomou I, Zamboglou N, Tselis N, Dimitriadis AS, Fountzila G (2006) Prognostic factors and significance of the revised 6th edition of the AJCC classification in patients with locally advanced nasopharyngeal carcinoma. Strahlenther Onkol 182:458–466

Kam MK, Teo PM, Chau RM, Cheung KY, Choi PH, Kwan WH, Leung SF, Zee B, Chan AT (2004) Treatment of nasopharyngeal carcinoma with Intensity-modulated radiotherapy: the Hong Kong experience. Int J Radiat Oncol Biol Phys 60:1440–1450

Khademi B, Mahmoodi J, Omidvari S, Mohammadianpanah M (2006) Treatment results of nasopharyngeal carcinoma: a 15-year single institutional experience. J Egypt Natl Cancer Inst 18:147–155

Kim JH, Lee JK (2005) Prognostic value of tumor volume in nasopharyngeal carcinoma. Yonsei Med J 46:221–227

King AD, Lam WW, Leung SF, Chan YL, Teo P, Metreweli C (1999) MRI of local disease in nasopharyngeal carcinoma: tumor extent vs tumor stage. Br J Radiol 72:734–741

King AD, Teo P, Lam WW, Leung SF, Metreweli C (2000) Paranasopharyngeal space involvement in nasopharyngeal cancer: detection by CT and MRI. Clin Oncol (R Coll Radiol) 12:397–402

Krishna SM, James S, Balaram P (2006) Expression of VEGF as prognosticator in primary nasopharyngeal cancer and its relation to EBV status. Virus Res 115:85–90

Kwong DL, Pow EH, Sham JS, McMillan AS, Leung LH, Leung WK, Chua DT, Cheng AC, Wu PM, Au GK (2004a) Intensity-modulated radiotherapy for early-stage nasopharyngeal carcinoma: a prospective study on disease control and preservation of salivary function. Cancer 101:1584–1593

Kwong DL, Sham JS, Au GK, Chua DT, Kwong PW, Cheng AC, Wu PM, Law MW, Kwok CC, Yau CC, Wan KY, Chan RT, Choy DD (2004b) Concurrent and adjuvant chemotherapy for nasopharyngeal carcinoma: a factorial study. J Clin Oncol 22:2643–2653

Kwong DL, Sham JS, Leung LH, Cheng AC,Kwong PW, Lui WM, Yau CC, Wu PM, Wei W, Au G (2006) Preliminary results of radiation dose escalation for locally advanced nasopharyngeal carcinoma. Int J Radiat Oncol Biol Phys 64:374–381

Lam WWM, Chan YL, Leung SF, Metreweli C (1997) Retropharyngeal lymphadenopathy in nasopharyngeal carcinoma. Head Neck 19:176–181

Langendijk JA, Leemans CR, Buter J, Berkhof J, Slotman BJ (2004) The additional value of chemotherapy to radiotherapy in locally advanced nasopharyngeal carcinoma: a meta-analysis of the published literature. J Clin Oncol 22:4604–4612

Le QT, Jones CD, Yau TK, Shirazi HA, Wong PH, Thomas EN, Patterson BK, Lee AW, Zehnder JL (2005) A comparison study of different PCR assays in measuring circulating plasma Epstein–Barr virus DNA levels in patients with nasopharyngeal carcinoma. Clin Cancer Res 11:5700–5707

Lee AW, Foo W, Law SC, Poon YF, SK O, Tung SY, Sze WM, Chappell R, Lau WH, Ho JH (1999) Staging of nasopharyngeal carcinoma: from Ho's to the new UICC system. Int J Cancer 84:179–187

Lee AW, Sze WM, Yau TK, Yeung RMW, Chappell R, Fowler JF (2001) Retrospective analysis of treating nasopharyngeal carcinoma with accelerated fractionation (6 fractions per week) in comparison with conventional fractionation (5 fractions per week): report on 3-year tumor control and normal tissue toxicity. Radiother Oncol 58:121–130

Lee AW, Au JS, Teo PM, Leung TW, Chua DT, Sze WM, Zee BC, Law SC, Leung SF, Tung SY, Kwong DL, Lau WH (2004) Staging of nasopharyngeal carcinoma: suggestions for improving the current UICC/AJCC staging system. Clin Oncol 16:269–276

Lee AW, Lau WH, Tung SY, Chua DT, Chappell R, Xu L, Siu L, Sze WM, Leung TW, Sham JS, Ngan RK, Law SC, Yau TK, Au JS, O'Sullivan B, Pang ES, SK O, Au GK, Lau JT; Hong Kong Nasopharyngeal Cancer Study Group (2005a) Preliminary results of a randomized study on therapeutic gain by concurrent chemotherapy for regionally-advanced nasopharyngeal carcinoma: NPC-9901 trial by the Hong Kong Nasopharyngeal Cancer Study Group. J Clin Oncol 23: 6966–6975

Lee AW, Sze WM, Au JS, Leung SF, Leung TW, Chua DT, Zee BC, Law SC, Teo PM, Tung SY, Kwong DL, Lau WH (2005b) Treatment results for nasopharyngeal carcinoma in the modern era: the Hong Kong experience. Int J Radiat Oncol Biol Phys 61:1107–1116

Lee AW, Tung SY, Chan AT, Chappell R, Fu YT, Lu TX, Tan T, Chua DT, O'sullivan B, Xu SL, Pang ES, Sze WM, Leung TW, Kwan WH, Chan PT, Liu XF, Tan EH, Sham JS, Siu L, Lau WH (2006) Preliminary results of a randomized study (NPC-9902 trial) on therapeutic gain by concurrent chemotherapy and/or accelerated fractionation for locally advanced nasopharyngeal carcinoma. Int J Radiat Oncol Biol Phys 66:142–151

Lee CC, Ho HC, Lee MS, Hsiao SH, Hwang JH, Hung SK, Chou P (2008) Primary tumor volume of nasopharyngeal carcinoma: significance for survival. Auris Nasus Larynx 35:376–380

Lee JT, Ko CY (2005) Has survival improved for nasopharyngeal carcinoma in the United States? Otolaryngol Head Neck Surg 132:303–308

Lee N, Xia P, Quivey JM, Sultanem K, Poon I, Akazawa C, Akazawa P, Weinberg V, Fu KK (2002) Intensity-modulated radiotherapy in the treatment of nasopharyngeal carcinoma: an update of the UCSF experience. Int J Radiat Oncol Biol Phys 53:12–22

Lee SW, Cho KJ, Park JH, Kim SY, Nam SY, Lee BJ, Kim SB, Choi SH, Kim JH, Ahn SD, Shin SS, Choi EK, Yu E (2005) Expressions of Ku70 and DNA-PKcs as prognostic indicators of local control in nasopharyngeal carcinoma. Int J Radiat Oncol Biol Phys 62:1451–1457

Leon SA, Shapiro B, Sklaroff DM, Yaros MJ (1977) Free DNA in the serum of cancer patients and the effect of therapy. Cancer Res 37:646–650

Leung SF, Chan AT, Zee B, Ma BB, Chan LY, Johnson PJ, Lo YM (2003) Pretherapy quantitative measurement of circulating Epstein–Barr virus DNA is predictive of posttherapy distant failure in patients with early-stage nasopharyngeal carcinoma of undifferentiated type. Cancer 98:288–291

Leung SF, Zee B, Ma BB, Hui EP, Mo F, Lai M, Chan KC, Chan LY, Kwan W, Lo YM, Chan AT (2006) Plasma Epstein–Barr viral deoxyribonucleic acid quantitation complements tumor-node-metastasis staging prognostication in nasopharyngeal carcinoma. J Clin Oncol 24:5414–5418

Leung TW, Tung SY, Sze WK, Wong FC, Yuen KK, Lui CM, Lo SH, Ng TY, SK O (2005) Treatment results of 1070 patients with nasopharyngeal carcinoma: an analysis of survival and failure patterns. Head Neck 27:555–565

Leung TW, Wong VY, Sze WK, Lui CM, Tung SY (2008) High-dose-rate intracavitary brachytherapy boost for early T stage nasopharyngeal carcinoma. Int J Radiat Oncol Biol Phys 70:361–367

Levendag PC, Schmitz PI, Jansen PP, Eijkenboom WM, Visser AG, Kolkman-Deurloo IK, Sipkema D, Visch LL, Senan S (1998) Fractionated high-dose-rate brachytherapy in primary carcinoma of the nasopharynx. J Clin Oncol 16: 2213–2220

Levine PH, Connelly RR, Easton JM (1980) Demographic patterns for nasopharyngeal carcinoma in the United States. Int J Cancer 26:741–748

Liao WT, Song LB, Zhang HZ, Zhang X, Zhang L, Liu WL, Feng Y, Guo BH, Mai HQ, Cao SM, Li MZ, Qin HD, Zeng YX, Zeng MS (2007) Centromere protein H is a novel prognostic marker for nasopharyngeal carcinoma progression and overall patient survival. Clin Cancer Res 13:508–514

Liaw CC, Wang CH, Huang JS, Kiu MC, Chen JS, Chang HK (1997) Serum lactate dehydrogenase level in patients with nasopharyngeal carcinoma. Acta Oncol 36:159–164

Lin JC, Chen KY, Jan JS, Hsu CY (1996) Partially hyperfractionated accelerated radiotherapy and concurrent chemotherapy for advanced nasopharyngeal carcinoma. Int J Radiat Oncol Biol Phys 36:1127–1136

Lin JC, Chen KY, Wang WY, Jan JS, Liang WM, Tsai CS, Wei YH (2001) Detection of Epstein–Barr virus DNA in the peripheral-blood cells of patients with nasopharyngeal carcinoma: relationship to distant metastasis and survival. J Clin Oncol 19:2607–2615

Lin JC, Chen KY, Wang WY, Jan JS, Liang WM, Wei YH (2002) Evaluation of cytokeratin-19 mRNA as a tumor marker in the peripheral blood of nasopharyngeal carcinoma patients receiving concurrent chemoradiotherapy. Int J Cancer 97: 548–553

Lin JC, Jan JS, Hsu CY, Jiang RS, Wang WY (2003a) Outpatient weekly neoadjuvant chemotherapy followed by radiotherapy for advanced nasopharyngeal carcinoma: high complete response and low toxicity rates. Br J Cancer 88: 187–194

Lin JC, Jan JS, Hsu CY, Liang WM, Jiang RS, Wang WY (2003b) Phase III study of concurrent chemoradiotherapy versus radiotherapy alone for advanced nasopharyngeal carcinoma: positive effect on overall and progression-free survival. J Clin Oncol 21:631–637

Lin JC, Wang WY, Chen KY, Wei YH, Liang WM, Jan JS, Jiang RS (2004) Quantification of plasma Epstein–Barr virus DNA in patients with advanced nasopharyngeal carcinoma. New Engl J Med 350:2461–2470

Lin JC, Wang WY, Liang WM, Chou HY, Jan JS, Jiang RS, Wang JY, Twu CW, Liang KL, Chao J, Shen WC (2007) Long-term prognostic effects of plasma Epstein–Barr Virus DNA by minor groove binder-probe real-time quantitative PCR on nasopharyngeal carcinoma patients receiving concurrent chemoradiotherapy. Int J Radiat Oncol Biol Phys 68:1342–1348

Liu MY, Chang YL, Ma J, Yang HL, Hsu MM, Chen CJ, Chen JY, Yang CS (1997) Evaluation of multiple antibodies to Epstein–Barr virus as markers for detecting patients with nasopharyngeal carcinoma. J Med Virol 52:262–269

Liu MZ, Tang LL, Zong JF, Huang Y, Sun Y, Mao YP, Liu LZ, Lin AH, Ma J (2008) Evaluation of sixth edition of AJCC staging system for nasopharyngeal carcinoma and proposed improvement. Int J Radiat Oncol Biol Phys 70:1115–1123

Liu LZ, Zhang GY, Xie CM, Liu XW, Cui CY, Li L (2006) Magnetic resonance imaging of retropharyngeal lymph node metastasis in nasopharyngeal carcinoma: patterns of spread. Int J Radiat Oncol Biol Phys 66:721–730

Lo KW, To KF, Huang DP (2004) Focus on nasopharyngeal carcinoma. Cancer Cell 5:423–428

Lo YM, Chan LY, Lo KW, Leung SF, Zhang J, Chan AT, Lee JC, Hjelm NM, Johnson PJ, Huang DP (1999a) Quantitative analysis of cell-free Epstein–Barr virus DNA in plasma of patients with nasopharyngeal carcinoma. Cancer Res 59: 1188–1191

Lo YM, Chan LY, Chan AT, Leung SF, Lo KW, Zhang J, Lee JC, Hjelm NM, Johnson PJ, Huang DP (1999b) Quantitative and temporal correlation between circulating cell-free Epstein–Barr virus DNA and tumor recurrence in nasopharyngeal carcinoma. Cancer Res 59:5452–5455

Lo YM, Chan AT, Chan LY, Leung SF, Lam CW, Huang DP, Johnson PJ (2000a) Molecular prognostication of nasopharyngeal carcinoma by quantitative analysis of circulating Epstein–Barr virus DNA. Cancer Res 60:6878–6881

Lo YM, Leung SF, Chan LY, Chan AT, Lo KW, Johnson PJ, Huang DP (2000b) Kinetics of plasma Epstein–Barr virus DNA during radiation therapy for nasopharyngeal carcinoma. Cancer Res 60:2351–2355

Lo YM, Leung SF, Chan LY, Lo KW, Zhang J, Chan AT, Lee JC, Hjelm NM, Johnson PJ, Huang DP (2000c) Plasma cell-free Epstein–Barr virus DNA quantitation in patients with nasopharyngeal carcinoma. Correlation with clinical staging. Ann NY Acad Sci 906:99–101

Lu JC, Wei BQ, Chen WZ, Qian PD, Zhang YQ, Wei Q, Cha WW, Li F, Ni M (2006) Staging of nasopharyngeal carcinoma investigated by magnetic resonance imaging. Radiother Oncol 79:21–26

Lu JC, Wei Q, Zhang YQ, Li F (2004) Influence of MRI abnormality in skull base bone on prognosis of nasopharyngeal carcinoma. Cancer Radiother 8:230–233

Ma BB, Poon TC, To KF, Zee B, Mo FK, Chan CM, Ho S, Teo PM, Johnson PJ, Chan AT (2003) Prognostic significance of tumor angiogenesis, Ki 67, p53 oncoprotein, epidermal growth factor receptor and HER2 receptor protein expression in undifferentiated nasopharyngeal carcinoma – a prospective study. Head Neck 25:864–872

Ma BB, Leung SF, Hui EP, Mo F, Kwan WH, Zee B, Yuen J, Chan AT (2004) Prospective validation of serum CYFRA 21-1, β-2-microglobulin, and ferritin levels as prognostic markers in patients with nonmetastatic nasopharyngeal carcinoma undergoing radiotherapy. Cancer 101:776–781

Ma BB, King A, Lo YM, Yau YY, Zee B, Hui EP, Leung SF, Mo F, Kam MK, Ahuja A, Kwan WH, Chan AT (2006) Relationship between pretreatment level of plasma Epstein–Barr virus DNA, tumor burden, and metabolic activity in advanced nasopharyngeal carcinoma. Int J Radiat Oncol Biol Phys 66:714–720

Ma J, Mai HQ, Hong MH, Cui NJ, Lu TX, Lu LX, Mo HY, Min HQ (2001a) Is the 1997 AJCC staging system for nasopharyngeal carcinoma prognostically useful for Chinese patient populations? Int J Radiat Oncol Biol Phys 50:1181–1189

Ma J, Mai HQ, Hong MH, Min HQ, Mao ZD, Cui NJ, Lu TX, Mo HY (2001b) Results of a prospective randomized trial comparing neoadjuvant chemotherapy plus radiotherapy with radiotherapy alone in patients with locoregionally advanced nasopharyngeal carcinoma. J Clin Oncol 19:1350–1357

Ma J, Liu L, Tang L, Zong J, Lin A, Lu T, Cui N, Cui C, Li L (2007) Retropharyngeal lymph node metastasis in nasopharyngeal carcinoma: prognostic value and staging categories. Clin Cancer Res 13:1445–1452

Mai HQ, Zeng ZY, Zhang CQ, Feng KT, Guo X, Mo HY, Deng MQ, Min HQ, Hong MH (2006) Elevated plasma big ET-1 is associated with distant failure in patients with advanced-stage nasopharyngeal carcinoma. Cancer 106:1548–1553

Mäkitie AA, MacMillan C, Ho J, Shi W, Lee A, O'Sullivan B, Payne D, Pintilie M, Cummings B, Waldron J, Warde P, Irish J, Brown D, Gilbert R, Gullane P, Liu FF, Kamel-Reid S (2003) Loss of p16 expression has prognostic significance in human nasopharyngeal carcinoma. Clin Cancer Res 9:2177–2184

Mao YP, Liang SB, Liu LZ, Chen Y, Sun Y, Tang LL, Tian L, Lin AH, Liu MZ, Ma J (2008) The N staging system in nasopharyngeal carcinoma with Radiation Therapy Oncology Group guidelines for lymph node levels based on magnetic resonance imaging. Clin Cancer Res 14:7497–7503

Mao YP, Xie FY, Liu LZ, Sun Y, Li L, Tang LL, Liao XB, Xu HY, Chen L, Lai SZ, Lin AH, Liu MZ, Ma J (2009) Re-evaluation of 6th edition of AJCC staging system for nasopharyngeal carcinoma and proposed improvement based on magnetic resonance imaging. Int J Radiat Oncol Biol Phys 73:1326–1334

Marks JE, Bedwink JM, Lee F, Purdy JA, Perez CA (1982) Dose-response analysis for nasopharyngeal carcinoma: a historical perspective. Cancer 50:1042–1050

Marks JE, Phillips JL, Menck HR (1998) The national cancer data base report on the relationship of race and national origin to the histology of nasopharyngeal carcinoma. Cancer 83:582–588

Masuda M, Shinokuma A, Hirakawa N, Nakashima T, Komiyama S (1998) Expression of bcl-2-, p53, and Ki-67 and outcome of patients with primary nasopharyngeal carcinomas following DNA-damaging treatment. Head Neck 20:640–644

Moll R, Franke WW, Schiller DL, Geiger B, Krepler R (1982) The catalog of human cytokeratins: patterns of expression in normal epithelia, tumor and cultured cells. Cell 31:11–24

Mutirangura A, Pornthanakasem W, Theamboonlers A, Sriuranpong V, Lertsanguansinchi P, Yenrudi S, Voravud N, Supiyaphun P, Poovorawan Y (1998) Epstein–Barr viral DNA in serum of patients with nasopharyngeal carcinoma. Clin Cancer Res 4:665–669

Neel HB III, Pearson GR, Taylor WF (1984a) Antibody-dependent cellular cytotoxicity: relation to stage and disease course in North American patients with nasopharyngeal carcinoma. Arch Otolaryngol 110:742–747

Neel HB III, Pearson GR, Taylor WF (1984b) Antibodies to Epstein–Barr virus in patients with nasopharyngeal carcinoma and in comparison groups. Ann Otol Rhinol Laryngol 93:477–482

Neel HB III, Taylor WF (1990) Epstein–Barr virus-related antibody. Changes in titers after therapy for nasopharyngeal carcinoma. Arch Otolaryngol Head Neck Surg 116:1287–1290

Ng SH, Chang JT, Chan SC, Ko SF, Wang HM, Liao CT, Chang YC, Yen TC (2004) Nodal metastases of nasopharyngeal carcinoma: patterns of disease on MRI and FDG PET. Eur J Nucl Med Mol Imaging 31:1073–1080

Ng WT, Lee AW, Kan WK, Chan J, Pang ESY, Yau TK, Lau KY (2007) N-staging by magnetic resonance imaging for patients with nasopharyngeal carcinoma: pattern of nodal involvement by radiological levels. Radiother Oncol 82:70–75

Ng WT, Chan SH, Lee AW, Lau KY, Yau TK, Hung WM, Lee MC, Choi CW (2008) Parapharyngeal extension of nasopharyngeal carcinoma: still a significant factor in era of modern radiotherapy? Int J Radiat Oncol Biol Phys 72:1082–1089

Ou SH, Zell JA, Ziogas A, Anton-Culver H (2007) Epidemiology of nasopharyngeal carcinoma in the United States: improved survival of Chinese patients within the keratinizing squamous cell carcinoma histology. Ann Oncol 18:29–35

Ozyar E, Yildz F, Akyol FH, Atahan IL (1999) Comparison of AJCC 1988 and 1997 classifications for nasopharyngeal carcinoma. Int J Radiat Oncol Biol Phys 44:1079–1087

Ozyar E, Yildz F, Akyol FH, Atahan IL (2002) Adjuvant high-dose-rate brachytherapy after external beam radiotherapy in nasopharyngeal carcinoma. Int J Radiat Oncol Biol Phys 52:101–108

Pathmanathan R, Prasad U, Sadler R, Flynn K, Raab-Traub N (1995) Clonal proliferations of cells infected with Epstein–Barr virus in preinvasive lesions related to nasopharyngeal carcinoma. N Engl J Med 333:693–698

Perez CA, Devineni VR, Marcial-Vega V, Marks JE, Simpson JR, Kucik N (1992) Carcinoma of the nasopharynx: factors affecting prognosis. Int J Radiat Oncol Biol Phys 23:271–280

Pignon JP, le Maître A, Bourhis J; MACH-NC Collaborative Group (2007) Meta-analyses of chemotherapy in head and neck cancer (MACH-NC): an update. Int J Radiat Oncol Biol Phys 69:S112–114

Plataniotis GA, Theofanopoulou ME, Kalogera-Fountzila A, Haritanti A, Ciuleanou E, Ghilezan N, Zamboglou N, Dimitriadis A, Sofroniadis I, Fountzilas G (2004) Prognostic impact of tumor volumetry in patients with locally advanced head-and neck carcinoma (non-nasopharyngeal) treated by radiotherapy alone or combined radiochemotherapy in a randomized trial. Int J Radiat Oncol Biol Phys 59:1018–1026

Porter MJ, Field JK, Leung SF, Lo D, Lee JC, Spandidos DA, van Hasselt CA (1994) The detection of the c-myc and ras oncogenes in nasopharyngeal carcinoma by immunohistochemistry. Acta Otolaryngol 114:105–109

Qian CN, Zhang CQ, Guo X, Hong MH, Cao SM, Mai WY, Min HQ, Zeng YX (2000) Elevation of serum vascular endothelial growth factor in male patients with metastatic nasopharyngeal carcinoma. Cancer 88:255–261

Qin DX, Hu YH, Yan JH, Xu GZ, Cai WM, Wu XL, Cao DX, Gu XZ (1988) Analysis of 1379 patients with nasopharyngeal carcinoma treated by radiation. Cancer 61:1117–1124

Raab-Traub N, Flynn K (1986) The structure of the termini of the Epstein–Barr virus as a marker of clonal cellular proliferation. Cell 47:883–889

Ramakrishnan Y, Paleri V, Shah R, Steen IN, Wight RG, Kelly CG (2007) Comorbidity in nasopharyngeal carcinoma: a preliminary communication on the prevalence, descriptive distribution and impact on outcome. Clin Otolaryngol 32:484–488

Reddy SP, Raslan WF, Gooneratne S, Kathuria S, Marks JE (1995) Prognostic significance of keratinization in nasopharyngeal carcinoma. Am J Otolaryngol 16:103–108

Rossi A, Molinari R, Boracchi P, Del Vecchio M, Marubini E, Nava M, Morandi L, Zucali R, Pilotti S, Grandi C, et al (1988) Adjuvant chemotherapy with vincristine, cyclophosphamide, and doxorubicin after radiotherapy in local-regional nasopharyngeal cancer: results of a 4-year multicenter randomized study. J Clin Oncol 6:1401–1410

Roychowdhury DF, Tseng A Jr, Fu KK, Weinburg V, Weidner N (1996) New prognostic factors in nasopharyngeal carcinoma. Tumor angiogenesis and C-erbB2 expression. Cancer 77:1419–1426

Rubio L, Burgos JS, Morera C, Vera-Sempere FJ (2000) Morphometric study of tumor angiogenesis as a new prognostic factor in nasopharyngeal carcinoma patients. Pathol Oncol Res 6:210–216

Sanguineti G, Geara FB, Garden AS, Tucker SL, Ang KK, Morrison WH, Peters LJ (1997) Carcinoma of the nasopharynx treated by radiotherapy alone: determinants of local and regional control. Int J Radiat Oncol Biol Phys 37:985–996

Santos JA, González C, Cuesta P, de la Fuente I, Carrión JR (1995) Impact of changes in the treatment of nasopharyngeal carcinoma: an experience of 30 years. Radiother Oncol 36:121–127

Sakata K, Hareyama M, Tamakawa M, Oouchi A, Sido M, Nagakura H, Akiba H, Koito K, Himi T, Asakura K (1999) Prognostic factors of nasopharynx tumors investigated by MR imaging and the value of MR imaging in the newly published TNM staging. Int J Radiat Oncol Biol Phys 43:273–278

Schoenfeld A, Kruger KH, Gomm J, Sinnett HD, Gazet JC, Sacks N, Bender HG, Luqmani Y, Coombes RC (1997) The detection of micrometastases in the peripheral blood and bone marrow of patients with breast cancer using immunohistochemistry and reverse transcriptase polymerase chain reaction for keratin 19. Eur J Cancer 33:854–861

Sham JS, Choy (1991) Prognostic value of parapharyngeal extension of nasopharyngeal carcinoma on local control and short-term survival. Head Neck 13:298–310

Shanmugaratnam K, Sobin LH (1993) The World Health Organization histological classification of tumors of the upper respiratory tract and ear. A commentary on the second edition. Cancer 71:2689–2697

Shao JY, Li YH, Gao HY, Wu QL, Cui NJ, Zhang L, Cheng G, Hu LF, Ernberg I, Zeng YX (2004) Comparison of plasma Epstein–Barr virus (EBV) DNA levels and serum EBV immunoglobulin A/virus capsid antigen antibody titers in patients with nasopharyngeal carcinoma. Cancer 100:1162–1170

Shen C, Lu JJ, Gu Y, Zhu G, Hu C, He S (2008) Prognostic impact of primary tumor volume in patients with nasopharyngeal carcinoma treated by definitive radiation therapy. Laryngoscope 118:1206–1210

Shotelersuk K, Khorprasert C, Sakdikul S, Pornthanakasem W, Voravud N, Mutirangura A (2000) Epstein–Barr virus DNA in serum/plasma as a tumor marker for nasopharyngeal cancer. Clin Cancer Res 6:1046–1051

Smith B, Selby P, Southgate J, Pittman K, Bradley C, Blair GE (1991) Detection of melanoma cells in peripheral blood by means of reverse transcriptase and polymerase chain reaction. Lancet 338:1227–1229

Sozzi G, Roz L, Conte D, Mariani L, Andriani F, Verderio P, Pastorino U (2005) Effects of prolonged storage of whole plasma or isolated plasma DNA on the results of circulating DNA quantification assays. J Natl Cancer Inst 97:1848–1850

Su CK, Wang CC (2002) Prognostic value of Chinese race in nasopharyngeal cancer. Int J Radiat Oncol Biol Phys 54:752–758

Sun LM, Li CI, Huang EY, Vaughan TL (2007) Survival differences by race in nasopharyngeal carcinoma. Am J Epidemiol 165:271–278

Sundram FX, Aw SE (1986) Tissue polypeptide antigen (TPA) and β2-microglobulin (β2-MG) as tumor markers in nasopharyngeal cancer. Ann Acad Med Singapore 15:507–510

Sze WM, Lee AW, Yau TK, Yeung RM, Lau KY, Leung SK, Hung AW, Lee MC, Chappell R, Chan K (2004) Primary tumor volume of nasopharyngeal carcinoma: prognostic significance of local control. Int J Radiat Oncol Biol Phys 59:21–27

Tang L, Li L, Mao Y, Liu L, Liang S, Chen Y, Sun Y, Liao X, Tian L, Lin A, Liu M, Ma J (2008) Retropharyngeal lymph node metastasis in nasopharyngeal carcinoma detected by magnetic resonance imaging. Cancer 113:347–354

Teo PM, Lee WY, Yu P (1996) The prognostic significance of parapharyngeal tumor involvement in nasopharyngeal carcinoma. Radiother Oncol 39:209–221

Teo PM, Leung SF, Lee WY, Zee B (2000a) Intracavitary brachytherapy significantly enhances local control of early T-stage nasopharyngeal carcinoma: the existence of a dose-tumor-control relationship above conventional tumoricidal dose. Int J Radiat Oncol Biol Phys 46:445–458

Teo PM, Leung SF, Chan AT, Leung TW, Choi PH, Kwan WH, Lee WY, Chay RM, Yu PK, Johnson PJ (2000b) Final report of a randomized trial on altered-fractionated radiotherapy in nasopharyngeal carcinoma prematurely terminated by significant increase in neurologic complications. Int J Radiat Oncol Biol Phys 48:1311–1322

Tsai ST, Jin YT, Su IJ (1996) Expression of EBER1 in primary and metastatic nasopharyngeal carcinoma tissues using in situ hybridization. A correlation with WHO histologic subtypes. Cancer 77:231–236

Turen S, Ozyar E, Altundag K, Gullu I, Atahan IL (2007) Serum lactate dehydrogenase level is a prognostic factor in patients with locoregionally advanced nasopharyngeal carcinoma treated with chemoradiotherapy. Cancer Invest 25:315–321

Twu CW, Wang WY, Liang WM, Jan JS, Jiang RS, Chao J, Jin YT, Lin JC (2007) Comparison the prognostic impact of serum Anti-EBV antibody and plasma EBV DNA assays in nasopharyngeal carcinoma. Int J Radiat Oncol Biol Phys 67:130–137

Uen WC, Luka J, Pearson GR (1988) Development of an enzyme-linked immunosorbent assay (ELISA) for detecting IgA antibodies to the Epstein–Barr virus. Int J Cancer 41:479–482

Vikram B, Mishra UB, Strong EW, Manolatos S (1985) Patterns of failure in carcinoma of the nasopharynx: I. Failure at the primary site. Int J Radiat Oncol Biol Phys 11:1455–1459

Wang CC (1989) Accelerated hyperfractionation radiation therapy for carcinoma of the nasopharynx. Techniques and results. Cancer 63:2461–2467

Wang CC (1991) Improved local control of nasopharyngeal carcinoma after intracavitary brachytherapy boost. Am J Clin Oncol 14:5–8

Wang WY, Chien YC, Jan JS, Chueh CM, Lin JC (2002) Consistent sequence variation of Epstein–Barr virus nuclear antigen 1 in primary tumor and peripheral blood cells of patients with nasopharyngeal carcinoma. Clin Cancer Res 8:2586–2590

Wang XS, Hu CS, Ying HM, Zhou ZR, Ding JH, Feng Y (2009) Patterns of retropharyngeal node metastasis in nasopharyngeal carcinoma. Int J Radiat Oncol Biol Phys 73:194–201

Wee J, Tan EH, Tai BC, Wong HB, Leong SS, Tan T, Chua ET, Yang E, Lee KM, Fong KW, Tan HS, Lee KS, Loong S, Sethi V, Chua EJ, Machin D (2005) Randomized trial of radiotherapy versus concurrent chemoradiotherapy followed by adjuvant chemotherapy in patients with American Joint Committee on Cancer/International Union Against Cancer stage III and IV nasopharyngeal cancer of the endemic variety. J Clin Oncol 23:6730–6738

Willner J, Baier K, Pfreundner L, Flentje M (1999) Tumor volume and local control in primary radiotherapy of nasopharyngeal carcinoma. Acta Oncol 38:1025–1030

Wolden SL, Chen WC, Pfister DG, Kraus DH, Berry SL, Zelefsky MJ (2006) Intensity-modulated radiation therapy (IMRT) for nasopharynx cancer: update of the Memorial Sloan-Kettering experience. Int J Radiat Oncol Biol Phys 64:57–62

Xiao GL, Gao L, Xu GZ (2002) Prognostic influence of parapharyngeal space involvement in nasopharyngeal carcinoma. Int J Radiat Oncol Biol Phys 52:957–963

Yan JH, Xu GZ, Hu YH, Li SY, Lie YZ, Qin DX, Wu XL, Gu XZ (1990) Management of local residual primary lesion of nasopharyngeal carcinoma: II. Results of prospective randomized trial on booster dose. Int J Radiat Oncol Biol Phys 18:295–298

Yeh SA, Tang Y, Lui CC, Huang YJ, Huang EY (2005) Treatment outcomes and late complications of 849 patients with nasopharyngeal carcinoma treated with radiotherapy alone. Int J Radiat Oncol Biol Phys 62:672–679

Yen RF, Chen TH, Ting LL, Tzen KY, Pan MH, Hong RL (2005) Early restaging whole-body ^{18}F-FDG PET during induction chemotherapy predicts clinical outcome in patients with locoregionally advanced nasopharyngeal carcinoma. Eur J Nucl Med Mol Imaging 32:1152–1159

Yen TC, Lin CY, Wang HM, Huang SF, Liao CT, Kang CJ, Ng SH, Chan SC, Fan KH, Chen IH, Lin WJ, Cheng AJ, Chang JT (2006) 18F-FDG-PET for evaluation of the response to concurrent chemoradiation therapy with intensity-modulated radiation technique for stage T4 nasopharyngeal carcinoma. Int J Radiat Oncol Biol Phys 65:1307–1314

Yeung WM, Zong YS, Chiu CT, Chan KH, Sham JS, Choy DT, Ng MH (1993) Epstein–Barr virus carriage by nasopharyngeal carcinoma in situ. Int J Cancer 53:746–750

Yi JL, Gao L, Huang XD, Li SY, Luo JW, Cai WM, Xiao JP, Xu GZ (2006) Nasopharyngeal carcinoma treated by radical radiotherapy alone: Ten-year experience of a single institution. Int J Radiat Oncol Biol Phys 65:161–168

Yip TT, Ngan RK, Lau WH, Poon YF, Joab I, Cochet C, Cheng AK (1994) A possible prognostic role of immunoglobulin-G antibody against recombinant Epstein-Barr virus BZLF-1 transactivator protein ZEBRA in patients with nasopharyngeal carcinoma. Cancer 74:2414–2424

Yip TT, Lau WH, Chan JK, Ngan RK, Poon YF, Lung CW, Lo TY, Ho JH (1998) Prognostic significance of DNA flow cytometric analysis in patients with nasopharyngeal carcinoma. Cancer 83:2284–2292

Zeng Y, Zhong JM, Li LY, Wang PZ, Tang H, Ma YR, Zhu JS, Pan WJ, Liu YX, Wei ZN, et al (1983) Follow-up studies on Epstein–Barr virus IgA/VCA antibody-positive persons in Zangwu County, China. Intervirology 20:190–194

Zhang EP, Lian PG, Cai KL, Chen YF, Cai MD, Zheng XF, Guang XX (1989) Radiation therapy of nasopharyngeal carcinoma: prognostic factors based on a 10-year follow-up of 1302 patients. Int J Radiat Oncol Biol Phys 16: 301–305

Zhang L, Zhao C, Peng PJ, Lu LX, Huang PY, Han F, Wu SX (2005) Phase III study comparing standard radiotherapy with or without weekly oxaliplatin in treatment of locoregionally advanced nasopharyngeal carcinoma: preliminary results. J Clin Oncol 23:8461–8468

Zhou JY, Chong VF, Khoo JB, Chan KL, Huang J (2007) The relationship between nasopharyngeal carcinoma tumor volume and TNM T-classification: a quantitative analysis. Eur Arch Otorhinolaryngol 264:169–174

10

Early Stage Nasopharyngeal Cancer: A Highly Curative Disease with Radiation Therapy

Roger Ove, Ron R. Allison, and Jiade J. Lu

CONTENTS

Roger Ove, MD, PhD
Department of Radiation Oncology, Leo Jenkins Cancer Center, The Brody School of Medicine at ECU, 600 Moye Blvd., Greenville NC, 27834, USA
Ron R. Allison, MD
Department of Radiation Oncology, The Brody School of Medicine at ECU, 600 Moye Blvd., Greenville, NC 27834, USA
Jiade J. Lu, MD, MBA
Department of Radiation Oncology, National University Cancer Institute, National University Health System, National University of Singapore, 5 Lower Kent Ridge Road, Singapore 119074, Republic of Singapore

10.1 Introduction

Historically, surgery and radiotherapy were the mainstays of therapy for nasopharyngeal cancer. Owing to the difficulty of the surgical approach to the nasopharynx, and the difficulty in excising tumors in this location with adequate margins, radiotherapy has been the primary modality since 1950 (Wilson 1950). This was also due in part to the good results obtained with radiotherapy. More recently, phase III data has established the role of concurrent chemotherapy with or without sequential adjuvant chemotherapy as the cornerstone of treatment for the majority of cases. The landmark trial that established this was the Intergroup 0099 trial, more recently supported by larger trials from Asia (Chan et al. 1995, 2002, 2004; Al-Sarraf et al. 1998; Chua et al. 1998; Ma et al. 2001; Lee et al. 2004; Wee et al. 2004). These trials have been limited to advanced stage disease, with the definition of "advanced" varying based on the staging system used.

Nasopharyngeal cancer in the western world is relatively rare and typically presents as advanced stage disease. No randomized data are available to assess the benefit of concurrent chemotherapy for early stage disease in this population, nor is it likely to materialize. As a result, in the community it is common practice to employ chemoradiation for all stages of disease. Even in the much larger Asian trials, early stage disease is not directly addressed. However, the results with radiotherapy as monotherapy have been quite good for early stage disease, and the benefit of adding chemotherapy, either sequential or concurrent, is not at all clear. This issue is confused by the fact that the definition of early stage has migrated over time, and it is important to interpret the results of studies in the context of the staging used.

Another confounding factor in analyzing results of historical series is that the results of modern series show a substantial improvement in survival. This is quite likely due to improvements in imaging and advances in radiotherapy technology (intensity-modulated radiotherapy, IMRT), and increased dose with techniques such as intracavitary brachytherapy. A substantial portion of this improvement is most likely due to stage migration, as more accurate staging secondary to improved imaging and the availability of positron emission tomography (PET) will tend to upstage patients formerly thought to be low risk.

For carefully selected patients, radiotherapy alone can offer excellent results. However, it is important not to neglect the benefits of multidisciplinary management for these patients, as for locally advanced cases. Attention to nutrition, swallowing function, dental issues, social support, and potential complications of therapy remain important. In addition, the multidisciplinary environment provides an appropriate forum for review of pathology in clinical context, and a mechanism for input from all appropriate specialties regarding imaging and staging.

10.2 Evolution of Staging

Staging of nasopharyngeal cancer, as with most malignancies, is a complex issue that evolves over time as prognostic factors become apparent. As the management of the disease tends to be nonsurgical, staging is clinical rather than pathological. Several staging systems have been used over the past 20 years, and the prognostic significance of various risk factors is a complex issue. Early American Joint Committee on Cancer (AJCC) classifications (1977 and 1992) for head and neck cancer typically resulted in a stage III or IV grouping for most nasopharyngeal malignancies, owing to the high incidence of clinically involved neck disease (AJCC 1977, 1992). (A detailed discussion on the staging of NPC is out of the scope of this chapter and is detailed in chapter 24. However, knowledge on evolution of the staging especially for early stage disease is partinent)

In Asia, the Ho staging system (Ho 1972) is commonly used, and may result in superior prognostic separation of patient groups when compared with the 1977 AJCC system or the 1967 Uniform International Committee on Cancer (UICC) system (Ho 1978; Teo et al. 1991). Because of the high incidence of lymph node involvement with nasopharyngeal cancer, the Ho system separates patients based on the level of lymph node involvement (Table 10.1). The 1992 AJCC system, unchanged from AJCC 1977, included some patients with N1 disease in stage III, but the remaining patients with nodal involvement and metastases outside the neck were all grouped together into stage IV. Nodal involvement appears in stage II of the Ho system, and supraclavicular metastases are represented in a separate stage IV (Table 10.1). The AJCC system now incorporates some of the aspects of the Ho system (AJCC 1998). The current AJCC system is superior to both the Ho system and the previous AJCC system (Cooper et al. 1998; Au et al. 2003). Further refinement may lead to improvement in risk stratification. For example, T4 patients with intracranial invasion or involvement of the orbit or cranial nerves have a poor prognosis (Au et al. 2003). However, the benefits of such refinement must be weighed against the benefits of staging stability over time, simplicity, and accuracy of reporting.

In the mid-1990s, data from several investigators indicated that lateral invasion into the parapharyngeal space was associated with higher risk of failure (Chua et al. 1996; Teo et al. 1996; Xiao et al. 2002). Such invasion is of increased prognostic significance in patients without other more significant risk factors, such as cranial nerve invasion or lymph node positivity. Parapharyngeal space invasion predicts for decreased survival, disease-free survival, and local control. The 1997 (and current) AJCC staging system separates T2 into T2a and T2b based on this risk stratification, and subsequent chemoradiation trials have included T2bN0 patients. Between 75 and 90% of patients with T2 disease are stage T2b. Posterior involvement of the parapharyngeal space (posterior to the styloid process) portends a worse prognosis in some series, but this has not been consistently reported (Chua et al. 1996; Xiao et al. 2002). The Chinese staging system adopted in 1992 classifies parapharyngeal involvement posterior to the styloid process as T3, while anterior involvement is T2 (Hong et al. 2000; Ma et al. 2001). Retropharyngeal lymph node involvement does not appear to be an independent risk factor for recurrence (Chua et al. 1997).

In reviewing the various staging systems, with regard to their impact on the definition of early stage disease, one sees that the current AJCC system is similar to the Ho and Chinese system. The older AJCC systems would classify patients with nasal cavity or oropharyngeal involvement as T3, while this is classified as T2 in the other systems. Thus, patients with such involvement treated on older trials using the

Table 10.1. Staging systems

Current and 1997 AJCC	1992 AJCC	Ho	1992 Chinese
T1:confined to nasopharynx	T1:one subsite	T1:confined to nasopharynx	T1:confined to nasopharynx
T2:soft tissue invasion (nasal cavity or oropharynx) a: Without parapharyngeal extension b: With parapharyngeal extension	T2:more than one subsite	T2:nasal fossa, oropharynx, muscle or nerves below base of skull	T2:nasal cavity, oropharynx, soft palate, cervical prevertebral soft tissue, parapharyngeal anterior to the SO[a] line
T3:bony or paranasal sinus extension	T3:nasal cavity and/or oropharynx involvement	T3a:bone involvement below base of skull	T3:posterior to SO[a] line, either anterior or posterior cranial nerves, skull base, pterygoid plates, pterygopalatine fossa.
T4:intercranial extension or cranial nerve or infratemporal fossa, hypopharynx or orbital involvement	T4:invades adjacent structure	T3b:involves base of skull T3c:cranial nerves T3d:orbits, laryngopharynx or infratemporal fossa	T4:both anterior and posterior cranial nerves, paranasal sinuses, cavernous sinus, orbit, infratemporal fossa, C1 or C2
N1:unilateral, ≤6 cm	N1:single ipsilateral ≤3 cm node	N1:upper neck above thyroid notch	N1:mobile nodes <4 cm above hyoid
N2:bilateral, ≤6 cm	N2a:single ipsilateral >3, ≤6 cm	N2:below thyroid notch above line joining end of clavicle and superior margin of trapezius	N2:nodes below hyoid or 4–7 cm
N3a:>6 cm node	N2b:or multiple ipsilateral nodes all ≤6 cm	N3:supraclavicular or skin involvement	N3:supraclavicular, fixed, skin involvement, or >7 cm
N3b:supraclavicular involvement	N2c:bilateral or contralateral nodes all ≤6 cm		
Stage I: T1N0M0	N3:>6 cm node		
Stage IIA: T2aN0M0	M1:metastases	M1:metastases	M1:metastases
Stage IIB T1N1M0 T2N1M0 T2aN1M0 T2bN0M0 T2bN1M0	Stage I: T1 N0M0	Stage I: T1N0	Stage I: T1N0M0
Stage III T1N2M0 T2aN2M0 T2bN2M0 T3N0M0 T3N1M0 T3N2M0	Stage II: T2 N0M0	Stage II: T2 and/or N1	Stage II: T2N0–1M0 or T1–2N1M0
Stage IVA T4N0M0 T4N1M0 T4N2M0	Stage III T3 N0M0 T1N1M0 T1N1M0 T2N1M0 T3N1M0	Stage III: T3 and/or N2 Stage IV: N3 (any T) Stage V: M1	Stage III: T3N0–2M0 or T1–3N2M0 Stage IVA: T4N0–3M0 or T1–4N3M0 Stage IVB: M1
Stage IVB: any T N3M0	Stage IV T4N0M0 T4N1M0 Any T N2M0 Any T N3M0 Any T any N M1		
IVC: any T any N M1			

[a]The SO (stylo-occipital) line extends from the styloid process to posterior edge of the occipital foramen

AJCC system, in particular the Intergroup 0099 trial, included some patients that would be classified as T2 with modern staging. Thus, there may well be a benefit to concurrent chemotherapy for such patients, and it may be reasonable to extrapolate that bulk of disease is an indication to consider more aggressive therapy.

10.3 Management Strategy for Early Stage NPC

10.3.1 Radiotherapy Alone: Historical Data

Historically, radiotherapy alone was used for both early stage and advanced nasopharyngeal carcinoma. Interpreting the results of studies from various parts of the world is difficult, as the prognostic roles of Epstein–Barr Virus (EBV) and histological classifications are incompletely understood. Undifferentiated tumors (WHO type 3) tend to be more prevalent in Southern China and Hong Kong, and there is a higher incidence of EBV positivity, which is poor prognostic factor (YIP et al. 1994). Paradoxically, in nasopharyngeal cancer the better differentiated keratinizing squamous histology (WHO type 1) carries the worst prognosis among histological subtypes (NEEL and TAYLOR 1989). Thus, both western and Asian populations are characterized by differing high-risk factors, with a higher percentage of WHO type 1 than type 2 or 3 disease in the west, but a lower incidence of high EBV titers. Early stage disease is also more common in the Asian population, where nasopharyngeal cancer is more common, screening is practical, and clinicians are more familiar with the disease.

It may be these counteracting factors balance one another. The results of radiation therapy alone series in the United States at MD Anderson Cancer Center (MDACC) (SANGUINETI et al. 1997), Denmark (WILSON 1950), and Hong Kong (LEE et al. 1992) achieved roughly similar 10-year survival of 34, 37, and 43%, respectively. The Hong Kong series somewhat superior results may be due to a higher percentage of node negative disease (39%) and relatively few patients with WHO type 1 histology (0.3%) (LEE et al. 1992).

The MDACC series is a classic western series detailing the long-term outcome in a relatively large population (184) of patients treated with radiotherapy alone (SANGUINETI et al. 1997). The 1992 AJCC staging system was used. T-classification, squamous histology, and cranial nerve deficits were poor prognostic factors for local control. Poorly differentiated or undifferentiated carcinoma, or lymphoepithelioma, experienced only half the local failure rate of better differentiated squamous cell carcinomas. T stage was correlated with local control, but not with neck control, and in general actuarial neck control was better than control at the primary site. Five-year local control for T1, T2, T3, and T4 were 93%, 79%, 68%, and 53%, respectively. Twenty percent of the patients were T1–2N0 or T1–2N1. These results illustrate that radiotherapy alone for early stage lesions can achieve excellent results, but for more advanced lesions the outcome was suboptimal, leading to a series of sequential and concurrent chemoradiotherapy trials.

Other western series are similarly very limited in providing insight into early stage disease, as the disease tends to be diagnosed late, and the overall incidence of nasopharyngeal cancer is low. However, sizeable numbers of early stage patients have been reported in recent years from endemic areas.

10.3.2 Radiotherapy Alone for Early Stage Disease

A large series of 362 early stage patients was recently reported from China, where chemotherapy for stage I and II cases is not routinely used, as it is considered experimental (XIAO et al. 2009). The Chinese staging system was used for these cases, a system that is similar to the AJCC system with respect to early stage disease (HONG et al. 2000; MA et al. 2001). In the Chinese system, N1 refers to small mobile nodes in the high neck. The majority of these patients were treated with external beam radiotherapy alone, with 20% receiving a portion of the dose via an intracavitary brachytherapy boost. Conventional RT was used (not IMRT). The majority of the patients had poorly differentiated squamous cell carcinoma, and three quarters were T2. T2N1 patients were found to have a worse prognosis than the other stage I and II patients (T1–2N0 and T1N1). Distant disease was the primary pattern of failure, particularly in the case of T2N1 patients.

The authors analyzed the failure rates and survival by specific stage, and found 5 year survival of:

T1N0 96.6%
T2N0 91.3%
T1N1 85.8%
T2N1 73.1%

The overall 5-year survival was 85%, and local control was approximately 90% and did not vary among the groups. Roughly 20% of the T2N1 patients suffered a distant failure, while distant metastases free survival

Table 10.2. Survival for stage I patients treated with radiotherapy alone

Reference	Location	Patients	Staging	Brachy	f/u (year)	Survival
CHANG et al. (1996)	Taiwan	183[a]	AJCC77	Yes	5	86%
COOPER et al. (1998)	US	19	AJCC97	No	3	75%
OZYAR et al. (1999)	Turkey	8	AJCC97	No	3	100%
CHENG et al. (2000)	Taiwan	11	AJCC97	No	3	92% DFS
CHUA et al. (2003a, b)	Hong Kong	50	AJCC97	No	10	98% DSS
LEUNG et al. (2005)	Hong Kong	113	AJCC97	No	5	85%
YEN et al. (2005)	Taiwan	51	AJCC97	Yes	5	82%
LU et al. (2005)	China	35	Chinese	No	4	89%
CAO et al. (2007)	China	53	Chinese	Yes	5	91–95%
LU et al. (2004)	Singapore	13	AJCC97	Yes	2	100%
KWONG et al. (2004)	Hong Kong	33	AJCC97	No	3	100%
FANG et al. (2008)	Taiwan	15	AJCC97	No	3	94–100%
THAM et al. (2009)	Singapore	21	AJCC97	Yes	3	93%
XIAO et al. (2009)	China	62	Chinese	Yes	5	95%

Overall survival is given if available. The majority of the references are from endemic areas, due to the relative rarity of early stage nasopharyngeal carcinoma in the western world
DFS disease-free survival; Overall survival not reported; *DSS* disease-specific survival. Overall survival not reported
[a]T1-T2N0 mixed for this publication

was 95% for the other groups. The majority (91%) of the T2 patients has parapharyngeal space invasion, and would be classified as T2b with the current AJCC staging system. The authors conclude that chemotherapy may be helpful for T2N1, and suggest that the topic be explored in a randomized trial.

A similar series from Hong Kong reported on 141 stage I and II patients treated with radiotherapy alone (CHUA et al. 2003a, b). The patients were restaged per the current AJCC system, and all were treated with radiotherapy alone. Fifty seven were node positive. Stage I patients had outstanding results, with 10-year disease specific survival of 98%, recurrence free survival 94%, local control 96%, and 2% distant failure. For stage II patients, the numbers were considerably worse, with 60% disease specific survival and 36% distant metastases, although local control was good at 93%. N1 status was found to be more important than T2 disease, consistent with the recent series from China (XIAO et al. 2009).

In most series that break down stage II into those with or without T2b disease (parapharyngeal involvement), the majority of stage II patients have such progression. Thus, results for stage II disease is often considerably worse than stage I. Table 10.1 shows the overall survival for publications that reported a substantial number of stage I patients treated with radiotherapy alone. Table 10.2 shows the corresponding results for stage II.

10.3.3 Chemotherapy and Early Stage Disease

There have been no randomized studies on the use of concurrent chemotherapy with radiotherapy for early stage (I and II) nasopharyngeal cancer, nor were a substantial number of such patients included in more general trials. Neoadjuvant chemotherapy has been more commonly explored in the past, and some data is available, with inconsistent results.

A retrospective series from Taiwan reported on a subset of 44 early stage (I and II) patients among the 189 nasopharyngeal patients undergoing concurrent chemoradiation or radiotherapy alone (CHENG et al. 2000). These patients were staged per AJCC 1997.

Table 10.3. Survival for stage II patients treated with radiotherapy alone

Reference	Location	Patients	Staging	Brachy	f/u (year)	Survival
Chang et al. (1996)	Taiwan	183[a]	AJCC77	Yes	5	86%
Cooper et al. (1998)	US	33	AJCC97	No	3	65%
Ozyar et al. (1999)	Turkey	21	AJCC97	No	3	72%
Chua et al. (2003a, b)	Hong Kong	91	AJCC97	No	10	60% DSS
Leung et al. (2005)	Hong Kong	398	AJCC97	No	5	92%A,78%B
Yen et al. (2005)	Taiwan	325	AJCC97	Yes	5	72%
Lu et al. (2005)	China	215	Chinese	No	4	91%
Cao et al. (2007)	China	268	Chinese	Yes	5	81–93%
Fang et al. (2008)	Taiwan	78	AJCC97	No	3	80–89%
Tham et al. (2009)	Singapore	52	AJCC97	Yes	3	88%
Xiao et al. (2009)	China	300	Chinese	Yes	5	85%

Two survival numbers appear for one series, which reflects the survival for stage IIA and IIB disease (overall stage II not reported)
DSS disease-specific survival. Overall survival not reported
[a]T1-T2N0 mixed for this publication

Of these 44 patients, 32 received concurrent chemoradiation, to a dose of 70 Gy with standard fractionation and concurrent cisplatin and 5-FU. The patients treated with radiotherapy alone were primarily stage I. The locoregional control rate and disease-free survival at 3 years for the stage II chemoradiotherapy group was no worse than that of the stage I patients treated with radiotherapy alone, with 100% local control for the chemoradiation stage II group. Patient numbers in this retrospective data were relatively low to make firm conclusions (Table 10.3).

Neoadjuvant chemotherapy was employed in multiple trials in endemic areas, with mixed results overall, and some of these included early stage patients. The results of two phase III induction trials performed in Hong Kong were pooled, with the early stage patients combined and analyzed (Chua et al. 2006). The subgroup analysis pooled data from trials incorporating platinum, bleomycin, and 5-FU followed by radiotherapy, compared with radiotherapy alone. The patients were restaged according to the AJCC 1997 system. A total of 784 patients were included. Surprisingly, differences in survival, local control, and metastases were only seen in the stage I/II patients. All the patients in the stage I/II group had stage IIb disease (parapharyngeal space invasion or N1). The 5-year survival rate was 79% in the combined modality arm and 67% in the RT-alone arm ($p = 0.048$). Local control was unchanged, but distant metastasis-free survival was 86% when compared with 74% ($p = 0.0053$). A weakness of this study is the lack of concurrent chemotherapy, and the failure to see any improvement with the addition of chemotherapy for higher stage patients.

A recent analysis from Seoul, Korea, reported on the outcomes of 60 early stage nasopharyngeal cancer patients treated with radiotherapy alone or combination chemotherapy and radiotherapy (Song et al. 2008). Twenty-nine patients received induction chemotherapy, in most cases with cisplatin and 5-FU. Concurrent chemotherapy was not used. One patient received carboplatin, and two received docetaxel as part of the induction regimen. Of the 60 patients, 17 were AJCC 1997 stage I or IIa, and 43 were stage IIb, equally distributed between the groups. There was no significant difference in survival, local control, metastases, or disease-free survival, and results were numerically superior in the radiotherapy alone group. The patients receiving chemotherapy were treated at later dates (after 1996) predominantly, but otherwise the groups were relatively well balanced. In multivariate analysis, delay in the onset of radiotherapy was significantly associated with locoregional failure in the IIb patients ($p = 0.044$). Weaknesses of this study include being retrospective, as selection bias may have favored adding chemotherapy for higher risk patients despite that fact that risk factors appeared balanced, and also the time span over, which these patients were accrued (1986–2004). However, most nasopharyngeal series show improved outcomes for patients treated in more modern times, and the opposite is seen here.

Locally advanced chemoradiation trials for nasopharyngeal cancer show a clear benefit to concurrent chemotherapy, and less certain benefit to sequential chemotherapy. Trials exploring the benefit of concurrent chemotherapy in the setting of a high-risk population of early-stage disease are lacking.

10.4 Radiation Therapy Technique in the Treatment of Early Stage NPC

10.4.1 Altered Fractionation

Altered fractionation regimens, including hyperfractionation and concomitant boost accelerated fractionation, have been explored in multiple head and neck cancer trials, and typically nasopharyngeal primaries are excluded. The U. S. Intergroup Study trial 0099 trial (Al-Sarraf et al. 1998) employed once daily radiation therapy with or without chemotherapy. There has been some activity exploring nasopharyngeal cancer with altered fractionation regimens because they have led to local control improvements in other sites such as the oropharynx (Horiot et al. 1992; Fu et al. 2000).

Few randomized trials addressing the role of twice-a-day irradiation vs. once-a-day irradiation in head and neck cancer have included tumors of the nasopharynx (Sanchiz et al. 1990; Teo et al. 2000). Sanchiz and colleagues' (1990) trial included 892 locally advanced head and neck cancers (UICC stage T3-T4, N0–3, M0). The patients were randomized to daily radiotherapy (Group A), twice-daily irradiation (Group B), and once daily irradiation with 5-fluorouracil (5-FU) (Group C). This study included 92 patients with nasopharyngeal cancer, a practice that stopped once results of the Intergroup 0099 study determined a standard of care for nasopharyngeal cancer. Disease-free survival and survival were improved with both hyperfractionation and chemotherapy (Groups B and C), in comparison with Group A. No difference was seen between the hyperfractionation group and the chemotherapy group. Inadequate details and patient numbers are available to assess the efficacy of hyperfractionation for early stage disease.

A randomized trial specific to the nasopharynx was conducted in Hong Kong and accrued 159 patients, and compared conventional radiotherapy with accelerated hyperfractionated radiotherapy (Teo et al. 2000). All patients in this study were N0 or N1 (Ho stage). Data at 5 years demonstrated no difference in survival or disease control, but there was an increased incidence of neurological injury with the experimental arm, with increased temporal lobe necrosis, optic apparatus injury, and brainstem/cord injury. Conventional two-dimensional radiotherapy technique was employed in this study, and it is possible that with modern technique and increased interfraction interval the results could be improved. An increase in acute and late complications secondary to accelerated fractionation for nasopharyngeal carcinoma, without improvement in disease control, has been reported elsewhere (El-Weshi et al. 2001). The University of Florida employed hyperfractionation in 45 of 82 patients undergoing radiotherapy (with or without chemotherapy) for nasopharyngeal carcinoma, and reported no increase in efficacy or complications (Mendenhall et al. 2006).

10.4.2 Intensity Modulation

IMRT has essentially become standard of care for the majority of head and neck cancer sites. IMRT is a useful technique for the nasopharynx, due to the proximity of critical structures to the target. With conventional therapy, there is considerable risk of late morbidity. Several dosimetric studies have demonstrated an improvement for IMRT over conventional techniques and 3D conformal techniques in the setting of nasopharyngeal cancer (Verhey 1999; Sultanem et al. 2000; Hunt et al. 2001; Munter et al. 2002; Lee et al. 2003). There are several single institution series demonstrating the efficacy of IMRT for head and neck cancer in general (Chao et al. 2003) and for the nasopharynx in particular (Lee et al. 2002), and a phase II multiinstitutional trial has been conducted by the RTOG (RTOG 0225).

RTOG 0225 utilized an integrated boost technique of the boost, with 2.12 Gy delivered to the primary PTV while 1.8 Gy is delivered to an intermediate subclinical PTV, both over 33 fractions. The low neck and regions at lesser risk received lesser doses. The regimen was based on UCSF experience, showing excellent results for 67 nasopharynx patients treated with IMRT (Lee et al. 2002). At 4 years, local control was 97% and regional control 98%. Xerostomia was remarkably mild, considering the need to cover the bilateral neck.

For early stage disease, results with IMRT have been promising, as described in a series of 203 nasopharyngeal patients from Taiwan treated with either IMRT or conformal techniques (Fang et al. 2008). Roughly half were treated with IMRT. Forty-five of the patients were AJCC 1997 stage I or II. Quality of life was superior for the IMRT group, with no significant difference in oncologic measures. Three year survival for the IMRT group was 94 and 89% for stage I and II, respectively. The corresponding survival numbers for conformal radiotherapy were 100 and 80%. A series of 33 T1N0 patients treated in Hong Kong established good results at 3 year follow-up, with 100% overall survival and local control, with one neck failure (Kwong et al. 2004). Mean parotid dose was high, at 38 Gy, but 85% of patients recovered 25% of their baseline parotid function at 2 years. The National Cancer Centre in Singapore published its nasopharyngeal experience, which included 72 stage I and II patients (Tham et al. 2009). Disease-free survival was excellent, at approximately 95% for T1 and 90% for stage II, but detailed morbidity information was not reported. Some patients also received an intracavitary boost.

It has been argued that IMRT should not be used for head and neck cancer if the upper aspects of neck level II require treatment bilaterally, as sparing parotid function will prevent adequate coverage of the upper portions of level II. In the case of nasopharyngeal cancers, early stage or otherwise, it is certainly the case that level II should be treated. At present, it appears that using IMRT in this scenario has important benefits, with a reduction in the risk of CNS complications, improved parotid function, and no unusual incidence of neck failures. Although mean parotid doses tend to be higher than for other ipsilateral head and neck cancers, there does appear to be a clinical reduction in xerostomia and improvement in quality of life (Hsiung et al. 2006; Fang et al. 2008).

10.4.3 Brachytherapy

Intracavitary brachytherapy is often used to boost the primary site. Owing to the limitation of the effective treatment range, brachytherapy is considered more effective in early T-classification disease. Technical details and dosing are often omitted from publications, and the technique has been used selectively. The typical technique utilizes one or two pediatric endotracheal tubes, with sources placed between the posterior wall of the maxillary sinus and the free edge of the soft palate. Dose is then prescribed to a point or surface 0.5 cm deep to the vault mucosa, pending normal tissue tolerance of adjacent structures (Wang et al. 1975). Custom applicators are also commercially available. Both high-dose rate (HDR) and low-dose rate brachytherapy have been used.

Brachytherapy boosts have been associated with improved local control, and allow a higher dose to be delivered than could be safely delivered with conventional external beam techniques (Wang 1991). Retrospective data suggest that early stage patients treated with conventional radiotherapy technique benefit from a brachytherapy boost, with both improvement in local control and survival seen (Chang et al. 1996; Cao et al. 2007). The use of brachytherapy has declined in recent years as the use of IMRT has become more widespread, but HDR has been used with IMRT for nasopharyngeal cancer (Tham et al. 2009). HDR brachytherapy has been studied prospectively, with 100% local control achieved for a series of stage I and II patients (Lu et al. 2004). The regimen used was 5 Gy × 2 delivered 1 week apart, after delivering 66 Gy to the primary site with conventional external beam radiotherapy. Dose was prescribed 1 cm superior to the midpoint of the sources.

HDR brachytherapy is not without risk, particularly late complications, and care must be taken if target tissue is adjacent to the optic apparatus. For early stage disease, normal anatomy will most likely lead to acceptable tolerances with standard technique. Complications have been reported, however. The largest published series employing routine HDR brachytherapy for early stage nasopharyngeal carcinoma treated 133 patients, with 64.8–68.4 Gy external beam RT and 1–3 HDR boosts of 5–5.5 Gy each (Chang et al. 1996). The results were compared to a similar cohort treated with external beam RT alone, dosed slightly higher at 68.4–72 Gy. Brachytherapy use was associated with improved survival and local control. It was also associated with perforation of the sphenoid sinus floor, necrosis of soft tissue, and other complications involving the palate. The authors recommended limiting the fraction size, but limiting the number of fractions to two 5 Gy fractions is very likely safe and effective.

10.4.4 Radiosurgery

Recurrent disease after primary radiotherapy or chemoradiotherapy has been treated with radiosurgery, with promising results (Cmelak et al. 1997; Xiao et al. 2001; Chua et al. 2003a, b; Roh et al. 2008). One of the advantages of this technique over brachytherapy salvage is that inverse planning optimization can be used to spare normal tissues and hopefully reduce complications. This is particularly attractive in the case of bulky locally advanced recurrences with irregular shapes, typically in close proximity to critical structures. Such recurrences are usually not amenable to salvage with brachytherapy. Both single fraction (Cmelak et al. 1997) and fractionated (Xiao et al. 2001; Roh et al. 2008) stereotactic salvage has been reported. For single fraction radiosurgery, the dose to the optic nerve, optic chiasm, brainstem, and cavernous sinus should be kept under 8 Gy when the recurrence does not directly involve these structures. Complications have of course been reported, including cranial nerve palsies, bone and soft tissue necrosis, CSF leaks, and trismus (Cmelak et al. 1997; Roh et al. 2008).

More recently, radiosurgery as a component of primary treatment for nasopharyngeal cancer has been reported (Le et al. 2003; Hara et al. 2008). These patients were locally advanced cases treated at Stanford University with Cyberknife radiosurgery, now totaling 82 cases. Reported local control has been excellent in this series, 98% at 5 years, with 70% survival. Temporal lobe necrosis has occurred in ten patients (nine of which were T4 primaries), and retinopathy occurred in three patients. For early stage disease, radiosurgery has not yet been reported, and presumably the risk of complications would be less.

10.5 Conclusions

Despite the excellent results obtained with combination chemoradiotherapy for locally advanced nasopharyngeal carcinoma, radiation therapy alone remains a viable option for low-risk cases. A review of the literature indicates that including all stage I and II patients in this group is not appropriate, and that there is a subset of stage II patients for which chemotherapy is beneficial. In the US population, it has been common practice to consider T2b patients locally advanced, and candidates for enrollment in concurrent chemoradiotherapy trials. In view of the higher incidence of WHO type 1 histology in the western world, and the poorer prognosis of this subgroup, this is appropriate. Recent evidence suggests that T2N1 patients in endemic areas also benefit from the addition of chemotherapy. In addition, variations in the staging systems used lead to some ambiguity in the definition of high risk, and as a result patients with bulky disease that are not strictly T3 should be considered for more aggressive therapy. Randomized trials to establish the benefit of concurrent chemotherapy and refine an appropriate regimen are needed.

It has long been known that radiation dose plays an important role in achieving optimal results for nasopharyngeal cancer (Marks et al. 1982; Vikram et al. 1985). Brachytherapy and radiosurgery are methods that can be effective in delivering this dose appropriately, if performed with appropriate respect for normal tissue tolerance.

References

AJCC (1977) AJCC Cancer Staging Manual. Philadelphia, Lippincott Raven

AJCC (1992) AJCC Cancer Staging Manual. Philadelphia, Lippincott Raven

AJCC (1998) AJCC Cancer Staging Manual. Philadelphia, Lippencott Raven

Al-Sarraf M, LeBlanc M, et al (1998) Chemoradiotherapy versus radiotherapy in patients with advanced nasopharyngeal cancer: phase III randomized Intergroup study 0099. J Clin Oncol 16(4):1310–1317

Au JS, Law CK, et al (2003) In-depth evaluation of the AJCC/UICC 1997 staging system of nasopharyngeal carcinoma: prognostic homogeneity and proposed refinements. Int J Radiat Oncol Biol Phys 56(2):413–426

Cao XP, Lu TX, et al (2007) Prospective study on long-term efficacy of external plus intracavitary radiotherapy on stage I-II nasopharyngeal carcinoma. Ai Zheng 26(2): 204–207

Chan AT, Ngan RK, et al (2004) Final results of a phase III randomized study of concurrent weekly cisplatin-RT versus RT alone in locoregionally advanced nasopharyngeal carcinoma (NPC). Proceedings of the American Society of Clinical Oncology. J Clin Oncol 22:493a

Chan AT, Teo PM, et al (1995) A prospective randomized study of chemotherapy adjunctive to definitive radiotherapy in advanced nasopharyngeal carcinoma. Int J Radiat Oncol Biol Phys 33(3):569–577

Chan AT, Teo PM, et al (2002) Concurrent chemotherapy-radiotherapy compared with radiotherapy alone in locoregionally advanced nasopharyngeal carcinoma:

progression-free survival analysis of a phase III randomized trial. J Clin Oncol 20(8):2038–2044
Chang JT, See LC, et al (1996) The role of brachytherapy in early-stage nasopharyngeal carcinoma. Int J Radiat Oncol Biol Phys 36(5):1019–1024
Chao KS, Ozyigit G, et al (2003) Patterns of failure in patients receiving definitive and postoperative IMRT for head-and-neck cancer. Int J Radiat Oncol Biol Phys 55(2):312–321
Cheng SH, Tsai SY, et al (2000) Concomitant radiotherapy and chemotherapy for early-stage nasopharyngeal carcinoma. J Clin Oncol 18(10):2040–2045
Chua DT, Ma J, et al (2006) Improvement of survival after addition of induction chemotherapy to radiotherapy in patients with early-stage nasopharyngeal carcinoma: Subgroup analysis of two Phase III trials. Int J Radiat Oncol Biol Phys 65(5):1300–1306
Chua DT, Sham JS, et al (1996) Prognostic value of paranasopharyngeal extension of nasopharyngeal carcinoma. A significant factor in local control and distant metastasis. Cancer 78(2):202–210
Chua DT, Sham JS, et al (1997) Retropharyngeal lymphadenopathy in patients with nasopharyngeal carcinoma: a computed tomography-based study. Cancer 79(5):869–877
Chua DT, Sham JS, et al (1998) Preliminary report of the Asian-Oceanian Clinical Oncology Association randomized trial comparing cisplatin and epirubicin followed by radiotherapy versus radiotherapy alone in the treatment of patients with locoregionally advanced nasopharyngeal carcinoma. Asian-Oceanian Clinical Oncology Association Nasopharynx Cancer Study Group. Cancer 83(11):2270–2283
Chua DT, Sham JS, et al (2003a) Treatment outcome after radiotherapy alone for patients with Stage I-II nasopharyngeal carcinoma. Cancer 98(1):74–80
Chua DT, Sham JS, et al (2003b) Linear accelerator-based stereotactic radiosurgery for limited, locally persistent, and recurrent nasopharyngeal carcinoma: efficacy and complications. Int J Radiat Oncol Biol Phys 56(1):177–183
Cmelak AJ, Cox RS, et al (1997) Radiosurgery for skull base malignancies and nasopharyngeal carcinoma. Int J Radiat Oncol Biol Phys 37(5):997–1003
Cooper JS, Cohen R, et al (1998) A comparison of staging systems for nasopharyngeal carcinoma. Cancer 83(2): 213–219
El-Weshi A, Khafaga Y, et al (2001) Neoadjuvant chemotherapy plus conventional radiotherapy or accelerated hyperfractionation in stage III and IV nasopharyngeal carcinoma—a phase II study. Acta Oncol 40(5):574–581
Fang FM, Chien CY, et al (2008) Quality of life and survival outcome for patients with nasopharyngeal carcinoma receiving three-dimensional conformal radiotherapy vs. intensity-modulated radiotherapy-a longitudinal study. Int J Radiat Oncol Biol Phys 72(2):356–364
Fu KK, Pajak TF, et al (2000) A radiation therapy oncology group (RTOG) phase III randomized study to compare hyperfractionation and two variants of accelerated fractionation to standard fractionation radiotherapy for head and neck squamous cell carcinomas: first report of RTOG 9003. Int J Radiat Oncol Biol Phys 48(1):7–16
Hara W, Loo BW Jr, et al (2008) Excellent local control with stereotactic radiotherapy boost after external beam radiotherapy in patients with nasopharyngeal carcinoma. Int J Radiat Oncol Biol Phys 71(2):393–400
Ho JH (1972) Nasopharyngeal carcinoma (NPC). Adv Cancer Res 15:57–92
Ho JH (1978) Stage classification of nasopharyngeal carcinoma: a review. IARC Sci Publ (20):99–113
Hong MH, Mai HQ, et al (2000) A comparison of the Chinese 1992 and fifth-edition International Union Against Cancer staging systems for staging nasopharyngeal carcinoma. Cancer 89(2):242–247
Horiot JC, Lefur R, et al (1992) Status of the experience of the EORTC cooperative group of radiotherapy with hyperfractionated and accelerated radiotherapy regimen. Semin Radiat Oncol 2:34–37
Hsiung CY, Ting HM, et al (2006) Parotid-sparing intensity-modulated radiotherapy (IMRT) for nasopharyngeal carcinoma: preserved parotid function after IMRT on quantitative salivary scintigraphy, and comparison with historical data after conventional radiotherapy. Int J Radiat Oncol Biol Phys 66(2):454–461
Hunt MA, Zelefsky MJ, et al (2001) Treatment planning and delivery of intensity-modulated radiation therapy for primary nasopharynx cancer. Int J Radiat Oncol Biol Phys 49(3):623–632
Kwong DL, Pow EH, et al (2004) Intensity-modulated radiotherapy for early-stage nasopharyngeal carcinoma: a prospective study on disease control and preservation of salivary function. Cancer 101(7):1584–1593
Lee AW, Lau WH, et al (2004) Prospective randomized study on therapeutic gain achieved by addition of chemotherapy for T1–4N2–3M0 nasopharyngeal carcinoma (NPC). Proceedings of the American Society of Clinical Oncology. J Clin Oncol 22:5506
Lee AW, Poon YF, et al (1992) Retrospective analysis of 5037 patients with nasopharyngeal carcinoma treated during 1976–1985: overall survival and patterns of failure. Int J Radiat Oncol Biol Phys 23(2):261–270
Lee N, Xia P, et al (2002) Intensity-modulated radiotherapy in the treatment of nasopharyngeal carcinoma: an update of the UCSF experience. Int J Radiat Oncol Biol Phys 53(1):12–22
Lee N, Xia P, et al (2003) Intensity-modulated radiation therapy for head-and-neck cancer: the UCSF experience focusing on target volume delineation. Int J Radiat Oncol Biol Phys 57(1):49–60
Le QT, Tate D, et al (2003) Improved local control with stereotactic radiosurgical boost in patients with nasopharyngeal carcinoma. Int J Radiat Oncol Biol Phys 56(4):1046–1054
Leung TW, Tung SY, et al (2005) Treatment results of 1070 patients with nasopharyngeal carcinoma: an analysis of survival and failure patterns. Head Neck 27(7):555–565
Lu JJ, Shakespeare TP, et al (2004) Adjuvant fractionated high-dose-rate intracavitary brachytherapy after external beam radiotherapy in Tl and T2 nasopharyngeal carcinoma. Head Neck 26(5):389–395
Lu TX, Zhao C, et al (2005) Retrospective analysis of 934 nasopharyngeal carcinoma patients treated with conventional external beam radiotherapy alone]. Zhonghua Zhong Liu Za Zhi 27(10):620–622
Ma J, Mai HQ, et al (2001) Results of a prospective randomized trial comparing neoadjuvant chemotherapy plus radiotherapy with radiotherapy alone in patients with locoregionally advanced nasopharyngeal carcinoma. J Clin Oncol 19(5):1350–1357

Marks JE, Bedwinek JM, et al (1982) Dose-response analysis for nasopharyngeal carcinoma: an historical perspective. Cancer 50(6):1042–1050

Mendenhall WM, Morris CG, et al (2006) Definitive radiotherapy for nasopharyngeal carcinoma. Am J Clin Oncol 29(6):622–627

Munter MW, Debus J, et al (2002) Inverse treatment planning and stereotactic intensity-modulated radiation therapy (IMRT) of the tumor and lymph node levels for nasopharyngeal carcinomas. Description of treatment technique, plan comparison, and case study. Strahlenther Onkol 178(9):517–523

Neel HB 3rd, Taylor WF (1989) New staging system for nasopharyngeal carcinoma. Long-term outcome. Arch Otolaryngol Head Neck Surg 115(11):1293–1303

Ozyar E, Yildiz F, et al (1999) Comparison of AJCC 1988 and 1997 classifications for nasopharyngeal carcinoma. American joint committee on cancer. Int J Radiat Oncol Biol Phys 44(5):1079–1087

Roh KW, Jang JS, et al (2008) Fractionated stereotactic radiotherapy as reirradiation for locally recurrent head and neck cancer. Int J Radiat Oncol Biol Phys

Sanchiz F, Milla A, et al (1990) Single fraction per day versus two fractions per day versus radiochemotherapy in the treatment of head and neck cancer. Int J Radiat Oncol Biol Phys 19(6):1347–1350

Sanguineti G, Geara FB, et al (1997) Carcinoma of the nasopharynx treated by radiotherapy alone: determinants of local and regional control. Int J Radiat Oncol Biol Phys 37(5):985–996

Song CH, Wu HG, et al (2008) Treatment outcomes for radiotherapy alone are comparable with neoadjuvant chemotherapy followed by radiotherapy in early-stage nasopharyngeal carcinoma. Laryngoscope 118(4):663–670

Sultanem K, Shu HK, et al (2000) Three-dimensional intensity-modulated radiotherapy in the treatment of nasopharyngeal carcinoma: the University of California-San Francisco experience. Int J Radiat Oncol Biol Phys 48(3):711–722

Teo P, Lee WY, et al (1996) The prognostic significance of parapharyngeal tumour involvement in nasopharyngeal carcinoma. Radiother Oncol 39(3):209–221

Teo PM, Leung SF, et al (1991) A comparison of Ho's, International Union Against Cancer, and American Joint Committee stage classifications for nasopharyngeal carcinoma. Cancer 67(2):434–439

Teo PM, Leung SF, et al (2000) Final report of a randomized trial on altered-fractionated radiotherapy in nasopharyngeal carcinoma prematurely terminated by significant increase in neurologic complications. Int J Radiat Oncol Biol Phys 48(5):1311–1322

Tham IW, Hee SW, et al. (2009) Treatment of Nasopharyngeal Carcinoma Using Intensity-Modulated Radiotherapy-The National Cancer Centre Singapore Experience. Int J Radiat Oncol Biol Phys 2009 Apr 20. [Epub ahead of print]

Verhey LJ (1999) Comparison of three-dimensional conformal radiation therapy and intensity-modulated radiation therapy systems. Semin Radiat Oncol 9(1):78–98

Vikram B, Mishra UB, et al (1985) Patterns of failure in carcinoma of the nasopharynx: I. Failure at the primary site. Int J Radiat Oncol Biol Phys 11(8):1455–1459

Wang CC (1991) Improved local control of nasopharyngeal carcinoma after intracavitary brachytherapy boost. Am J Clin Oncol 14(1):5–8

Wang CC, Busse J, et al (1975) A simple afterloading applicator for intracavitary irradiation of carcinoma of the nasopharynx. Radiology 115(3):737–738

Wee J, Tan EH, et al (2004) Phase III randomized trial of radiotherapy versus concurrent chemotherapy followed by adjuvant chemotherapy in patients with AJCC/UICC (1997) stage 3 and 4 nasopharyngeal cancer of the endemic variety. Proceedings of the American Society of Clinical Oncology. J Clin Oncol 23:487

Wilson CP (1950) The approach to the nasopharynx. Proc Res Soc Med 44:353–358

Xiao GL, Gao L, et al (2002) Prognostic influence of parapharyngeal space involvement in nasopharyngeal carcinoma. Int J Radiat Oncol Biol Phys 52(4):957–963

Xiao J, Xu G, et al (2001) Fractionated stereotactic radiosurgery for 50 patients with recurrent or residual nasopharyngeal carcinoma. Int J Radiat Oncol Biol Phys 51(1): 164–170

Xiao WW, Han F, et al (2009) Treatment outcomes after radiotherapy alone for patients with early-stage nasopharyngeal carcinoma. Int J Radiat Oncol Biol Phys 74:1070–1076

Yeh SA, Tang Y, et al (2005) Treatment outcomes and late complications of 849 patients with nasopharyngeal carcinoma treated with radiotherapy alone. Int J Radiat Oncol Biol Phys 62(3):672–679

Yip TT, Ngan RK, et al (1994) A possible prognostic role of immunoglobulin-G antibody against recombinant Epstein-Barr virus BZLF-1 transactivator protein ZEBRA in patients with nasopharyngeal carcinoma. Cancer 74(9): 2414–2424

Drug Therapy for Nasopharyngeal Carcinoma: Cytotoxic and Targeted Therapy

11

BRIGETTE B. Y. MA and ANTHONY T. C. CHAN

CONTENTS

ANTHONY T. C. CHAN, MD
BRIGETTE B. Y. MA, MD
Department of Clinical Oncology at the Sir YK Pao Centre for Cancer, State Key Laboratory in Oncology in South China, The Chinese University of Hong Kong, Shatin, NT, Hong Kong, SAR, P.R. China

11.1 Introduction

Nasopharyngeal carcinoma (NPC) occurring in endemic areas such as Southern China and Southeast Asia are typically nonkeratinizing, undifferentiated, or poorly differentiated squamous cell carcinoma. These histological subtypes are characterized by their susceptibility to cytotoxic chemotherapy and association with Epstein–Barr virus (EBV) infection. In Hong Kong, where the annual incidence rate of NPC is around 20/100,000 persons, the stage distribution at diagnosis is reportedly 48% for early stage NPC (American Joint Committee for Cancer, AJCC stages I and II (2002)), and 52% for advanced NPC (stages III and IV) (LEE et al. 2005). In a multi-institutional review by the Hong Kong Nasopharyngeal Cancer Study Group of over 2,600 NPC patients treated between 1996 and 2000, the 5-year overall survival rate for stage I and II NPC reached 85% following radiotherapy alone, whereas only 66% of patients with nonmetastatic stage III and IVB NPC remained alive 5 years after radical radiotherapy (LEE et al. 2005). This poor outcome is mainly attributed to the fact that over 30% of patients with stage III to IV NPC relapse at distant sites following radiotherapy, where the median overall survival is only 12–18 months (MA et al. 2008). Cytotoxic chemotherapy plays an important role in the curative and palliative treatment of advanced NPC. This chapter provides an overview of the clinical development of cytotoxic and targeted therapy in endemic NPC, and the impact of drug therapy on the clinical outcome of NPC over the last two decades. Particular attention will be given to the historical development of platinum and nonplatinum chemotherapy, and also targeted therapies against the epidermal growth factor receptor (EGFR), tumor angiogenesis, and epigenetic mechanisms of the control of gene expression in NPC.

11.2 Clinical Indications for Drug Therapy in NPC

11.2.1 Palliative

The most common indication for drug therapy in NPC is in the treatment of patients with locoregional recurrence or metastatic disease that are not amenable to potentially curative local therapies, such as reirradiation and nasopharyngectomy. The survival of patients with metastatic NPC can vary depending on the anatomical site of metastases, and the metastasis-free interval from the time of diagnosis. In general, patients who present with synchronous metastases at diagnosis have worse prognosis than those who developed distant failure after radiotherapy. Patients with only pulmonary metastases have a more favorable outlook than those with hepatic or skeletal metastases (Hui et al. 2004). Isolated reports of prolonged disease-free survival of up to 15 years have also been described in patients with nonpulmonary metastases (Fandi et al. 2000). The impact of chemotherapy on survival in patients with recurrent and metastatic NPC has never been directly compared with supportive care alone in randomized trials, and currently available data are derived mainly from retrospective or phase II studies. Successive phase II studies of platinum-based chemotherapeutic regimens published since the 1990s have reported a median overall survival of 11–19 months for patients with recurrent or metastatic NPC who were treatment-naïve (Al-Kourainy et al. 1988; Bachouchi et al. 1990; Boussen et al. 1991; Wang and Tan 1991; Siu et al. 1998; Yeo et al. 1996; Ma et al. 2009). The median time to disease progression reported between 5 and 10 months in these studies. These regimens have not been directly compared with each other in randomized studies; therefore, there is no universally accepted "standard" regimen. Drug selection is based mainly on patient's performance status, medical comorbidities, toxicity profile, and institutional preference. Nevertheless, platinum-based combinations with either 5-fluorouracil, taxanes, or gemcitabine are popularly used in clinical practice in Hong Kong and other Asian centers.

11.2.2 Concurrent

The use of concurrent chemoradiation therapy in non-metastatic, stage III to IV NPC is based on the rationale that chemotherapy may control micrometastases and can act as a radiosensitizer. To date, at least eight phase III studies comparing radiotherapy alone vs. concurrent chemoradiation have been published from centers in both endemic and non-endemic regions (Al-Sarraf et al. 1998; Chan et al. 2002; Lin et al. 2003; Wee et al. 2005; Lee et al. 2005, 2006; Kwong et al. 2004; Zhang et al. 2005). The concurrent regimens used in these studies varied in terms of the choice of drugs (i.e., platinum (Al-Sarraf et al. 1998; Chan et al. 2002; Lin et al. 2003; Wee et al. 2005; Lee et al. 2005; Zhang et al. 2005) or non-platinum (Kwong et al. 2004)), schedule (e.g., weekly low-dose cisplatin (Chan et al. 2002), 3-weekly high-dose cisplatin (Al-Sarraf et al. 1998; Chan et al. 2002; Wee et al. 2005; Lee et al. 2005, 2006; Kwong et al. 2004; Zhang et al. 2005), or a cisplatin-based two-drug regimen (Lin et al. 2003)). In spite of these differences, these studies unanimously reported a statistically significant improvement in progression-free survival (or failure-free survival) and/or overall survival favoring the chemoradiation arm than the radiotherapy alone. Two meta-analyses have reported that concurrent chemoradiation reduces the risk of death in non-metastatic stage III and IV NPC by around 40%–52%, and reduces the risk of distant failure by 28% (Baujat et al. 2006; Langendijk et al. 2004). It should be noted that concurrent chemoradiation can exacerbate the acute and late toxicities of radiotherapy including radiation mucositis, ototoxicity, and other soft tissue damage (Lee et al. 2005).

Researchers from the Prince of Wales Hospital and Queen Elizabeth Hospital in Hong Kong published the first completed Asian phase III study, where 350 patients with non-metastatic, AJCC stage IIB to IV NPC were randomized to radiotherapy (66 Gy plus a 10–20 Gy parapharyngeal boost) with or without concurrent weekly cisplatin (40 mg/m^2/week) for seven cycles. At a median follow-up of 5.5 years, the concurrent arm was associated with a non-statistically significant trend toward an improved overall ($p = 0.05$) and progression-free survival ($p = 0.06$). However, in a subgroup analysis, a statistically significant improvement in overall ($p = 0.01$) and progression-free ($p = 0.01$) survival was reported in patients with T3–T4 tumors. No difference in distant and local recurrence rates was identified in this study (Chan et al. 2005). Since the mid-1990s, this protocol has been adopted for routine practice at the Department of Clinical Oncology, Prince of Wales Hospital, where the current standard of care for patients with non-metastatic NPC that are stage IIB, stage III or IVB, is to offer intensity-modulated radiotherapy and concurrent weekly low-dose cisplatin for seven cycles. For the territory as a whole, the introduction of concurrent chemoradiation has contributed to the improved clinical outcome of patients with locoregionally advanced NPC over the last decade. In a report by the Hong Kong NPC Study Group (Lee et al. 2005), the survival rates for NPC have improved significantly during the period from 2000 to 2006, compared with historic series reported in the 1970–1980s (Teo et al. 1989; Lee et al. 1992; Hong et al. 2000; Cooper et al. 1998). In the contemporary setting, the 5-year overall and progression-free rates for stage III–IVB NPC are expected to be 66% and 53%, respectively (Lee et al. 2005).

11.2.3 Neoadjuvant

Neoadjuvant chemotherapy with platinum-based regimens has been used in clinical practice since the early 1980s in Hong Kong, for the treatment of bulky primary tumors where adequate radiation dose and coverage cannot be given without a significant risk of damaging the vital structures, such as the optic nerve or brainstem (Teo et al. 1989). Of all the phase III studies published to date, none has conclusively reported a survival benefit of neoadjuvant chemotherapy over radiotherapy alone (Roussy 1996; Ma et al. 1998; Chua et al. 1998; Hareyama et al. 2002). In a pooled analysis of two previously reported negative studies conducted in Hong Kong (Chua et al. 1998) and China (Ma et al. 1998), an absolute 12.9% improvement in overall survival favoring the neoadjuvant arm was reported at 5-year follow-up (Chua et al. 2005).

Since the adoption of concurrent chemoradiation as a standard of care for locoregionally advanced NPC, researchers at the Prince of Wales Hospital evaluated the strategy of combining neoadjuvant therapy with taxane-based regimens with chemoradiation. In a phase II study, the addition of two cycles of carboplatin and paclitaxel were tolerated when given before chemoradiation (Chan et al. 2004). This strategy was subsequently evaluated against chemoradiation with weekly low-dose cisplatin in a randomized phase II study of 60 patients (Hui et al. 2009). The 3-year overall survival for patients who had neoadjuvant cisplatin and taxotere was 94.1%, compared with 67.7% for those who had chemoradiation alone (hazard ratio = 0.24; 95% confidence interval, CI, 0.078–0.73; p = 0.012) (Hui et al. 2009). This strategy is promising and warrants further evaluation in the setting of a well-powered phase III study.

11.2.4 Adjuvant

Based on the U. S. Intergroup protocol, which first demonstrated the superiority of adding 3-weekly high-dose cisplatin during radiotherapy followed by three cycles of cisplatin and 5-fluorouracil (Al-Sarraf et al. 1998), adjuvant chemotherapy has been used routinely in locoregionally advanced NPC in some Asian centers. However, none of the phase III studies published to date have demonstrated a survival benefit of adjuvant chemotherapy over chemoradiation alone (Rossi et al. 1988; Chan et al. 1995; Chi et al. 2002). Similarly, a meta-analysis reported by the MAC–NPC Collaborative group, based on the data derived from 1,753 individual participants from eight clinical trials, did not find any survival benefit with adjuvant chemotherapy (Baujat et al. 2006). Poor patient compliance has been thought to contribute to this lack of benefit, as up to 15% of patients did not receive any planned adjuvant chemotherapy in phase III trials owing to patient refusal or toxicity (Al-Sarraf et al. 1998; Wee et al. 2005).

11.3 Cytotoxic Chemotherapy

11.3.1 Platinum-Based Chemotherapy

Cisplatin and its analogs, carboplatin and oxaliplatin, are alkylating-like agents, which interfere with DNA repair by forming DNA crosslinks and adducts. In preclinical studies on NPC cell lines, cisplatin can enhance cell killing from radiation (Wang et al. 2002), induce apoptosis (Cheung et al. 2005) and sensenescent-like growth arrest in the CNE-1 cells (an EBV-negative NPC cell line) (Wang et al. 1998). A preclinical study in NPC cell lines also suggested that the synergistic effect of cisplatin on radiation was best observed when cisplatin was administered before radiation (Wang et al. 2002).

Cisplatin is the first-generation platinum that was first used in NPC in Hong Kong during the early 1980s for neoadjuvant and palliative indications (Teo et al. 1989). Successive generations of phase II studies have focused on optimizing the clinical response to cisplatin, by combining it with one or more classes of chemotherapy such as the anthracyclines, antimetabolites, alkylating agents, microtubule inhibitors, and cytotoxic antibiotics. The rationale of these combinations was based on tolerability and activity observed in other cancers (e.g., non-NPC squamous cell cancers of the head and neck), rather than preclinical synergism in NPC models. Furthermore, most of these non-platinum agents have single-agent activity against NPC. As will be further discussed in Sect. 11.3.3, although cisplatin-based regimens with three or more drugs appear to induce higher response rates than doublets, the risk of serious toxicities were also increased and the impact on survival has yet to be defined in randomized trials.

Patients with NPC are at risk of long-term sensorineural hearing loss from a variety of reasons, including radiation-related injury to the inner ear (Ho et al. 1999) and the use of adjunctive cisplatin with radiotherapy (Low et al. 2006). The second-generation platinum, carboplatin, was first evaluated in NPC in the late-1990s as a less toxic alternative to cisplatin. It is not nephrotoxic, and is less neurotoxic and ototoxic than cisplatin. In clinical practice, carboplatin is often used to substitute cisplatin in patients with borderline performance status, renal and hearing impairment, despite the paucity of randomized data supporting the therapeutic equivalence of carboplatin and cisplatin. Most of the data concerning the activity of carboplatin are derived from phase II studies in recurrent NPC. Carboplatin has a single-agent response rate of 44% (Chi et al. 1997); 38% when combined with 5-fluorouracil (Yeo et al. 1996); and 58%–78% with combined with paclitaxel (Tan et al. 1999; Yeo et al. 1998). In the radical treatment of NPC, Parliament et al. (2001) has shown that carboplatin was well tolerated when used concurrently with radiotherapy (70 Gy) in a weekly schedule at 100 mg/m^2. In this study, where 90% of patients had stage III–IV NPC, the 3-year progression-free and overall survival were 58% and 56%, respectively. These survival rates seem to be inferior to the rates reported in the phase III study led by the Prince of Wales Hospital, where weekly low-dose cisplatin and radiotherapy was associated with an estimated 3-year progression-free and overall survival of at least 70% (Chan et al. 2002). This observation was supported by a non-randomized study of 75 patients with stage IV NPC who were treated with neoadjuvant chemotherapy followed by chemoradiation, where the respective 3-year progression-free and overall survival were only 39% and 61% in 18 patients who received carboplatin as a substitute of cisplatin (Yau et al. 2006). The only randomized study published was reported by Chitapanarux et al., where 206 patients with locoregionally advanced NPC were randomized to cisplatin or carboplatin at a 3-weekly schedule in combination with radiotherapy (Chitapanarux et al. 2007). The study did not find any differences in survival after a relatively short median follow-up of 2.5 years, except that carboplatin was better tolerated and resulted in less mucosal and renal toxicity than cisplatin. This study may be underpowered if it was intended to demonstrate non-inferiority between the two arms. Also, less than 50% of the patients randomized to the cisplatin arm actually received the planned chemotherapy.

The third-generation platinum, oxaliplatin, has no cross-resistance with cisplatin (Raymond et al. 1999) and can enhance the anticancer effect of gemcitabine in vitro (Louvet et al. 2005). A phase II study led by researchers at the Prince of Wales Hospital evaluated the activity of a bi-weekly regimen of gemcitabine and oxaliplatin (the GEMOX regimen) in 42 previously untreated patients with recurrent and metastatic NPC (Ma et al. 2009). In this cohort where 48% of patients had prior exposure to cisplatin in the curative setting (i.e., adjunctive to radiotherapy), the overall response rate was 56%, with a median time to progression and overall survival of 9 and 19.6 months, respectively. Notably, this median overall survival duration is the longest reported to date in phase II trials of similar setting. Treatment was well tolerated with grade 3 oxaliplatin-related sensory neuropathy occurring in 10% of patients. Oxaliplatin was also tested at a dose of 70 mg/m^2/week in combination with radiation therapy, was compared against radiation alone in a randomized study of 115 patients with locoregionally advanced NPC (Zhang et al. 2005). Although this study might be underpowered, a statistically significant difference in 2-year overall survival, metastasis-free and relapse-free survival were reported favoring the oxaliplatin-radiotherapy arm.

11.3.2 Nonplatinum-Based Chemotherapy

Many different classes of non-platinum agents have activity against NPC alone or in combination with platinum as first-line or subsequent lines of therapy. These include the anti-metabolites (e.g., gemcitabine (Foo et al. 2002; Ngan et al. 2002; Leong et al. 2005), 5-fluorouracil (Fandi et al. 1997), capecitabine (Chua et al. 2008; Li et al. 2008), methotrexate (Molinari 1978)), alkylating agents (e.g., cyclophosphamide (Molinari 1978), ifosfamide (Stein et al. 1996), microtubule inhibitors (e.g., paclitaxel (Tan et al. 1999; Yeo et al. 1998; Au et al. 1998; Airoldi et al. 2002), docetaxel (Hui et al. 2009; Johnson et al. 2004)), anthracyclines (e.g., epirubicin (Azli et al. 1995), doxorubicin (Molinari 1978), mitoxantrone (Dugan et al. 1993)), vinca alkaloids (vinorelbine (Wang et al. 2006)), irinotecan (Poon et al. 2005), bleomycin (Boussen et al. 1991; Molinari 1978), and mitomycin C (Hong et al. 1999) (Table 11.1). Some of these agents, such as gemcitabine (Foo et al. 2002), capecitabine (Chua et al. 2008), and irinotecan (Poon et al. 2005) are active in the second- or third-line treatment of patients who have progressed after platinum-based chemotherapy.

11.3.3 Factors Affecting Response to Drug Therapy

11.3.3.1 Multi-Drug Regimen vs. Doublets

To date, there is no randomized data supporting a therapeutic advantage of multi-drug regimens with three or more agents, over platinum-based doublets. As shown in Table 11.1, although the reported overall response rates of multi-drug regimens (three or more drugs combination: up to 80% [Siu et al. 1998; Leong et al. 2005]) appear to be slightly higher than platinum-based doublets (up to 73% [Ngan et al. 2002]) in phase II studies, the survival rates reported for the first-line palliative setting are comparable, while the incidence of serious toxicities were higher for the multi-drug regimens. For instance, the respective median progression-free and overall survival rates of a cisplatin–gemcitabine combination were 10.6 and 15 months (Ngan et al. 2002), while the corresponding rates reported in another study where paclitaxel (70 mg/m^2, days 1 and 8) was added to a carboplatin–gemcitabine backbone were 8.1 and 18.6 months (Leong et al. 2005). Without growth factor support, the respective incidence rates of grade 3–4 neutropenia and thrombocytopenia were 78% and 41% with the three-drug regimen (Leong et al. 2005), and only 37% and 16% in the two-drug regimen (Ngan et al. 2002). Combinations with four or more older agents such as mitomycin and bleomycin were associated with a higher incidence of toxic deaths in some phase II studies (Siu et al. 1998; Taamma et al. 1999; Hasbini et al. 1999).

11.3.3.2 Dose Intensity and Drug Maintenance

Airoldi and De Crescenzo (2001) was the only group that reported their preliminary experience with autologous peripheral blood stem cell transplantation in the treatment of six patients with predominantly locoregional relapse following radiotherapy. Cisplatin and epirubicin were used for stem cell mobilization, followed by high-dose ifosfamide, etoposide, and carboplatin with stem cell rescue. At 30 months follow-up, two patients remained alive without disease, one was alive with bone metastases, and the rest had died (Airoldi and De Crescenzo 2001). There is a paucity of evidence supporting the role of dose intensification in the treatment of NPC, and the available evidence seems to suggest that such strategy only increased toxicity without therapeutic gain. For instance, two groups have independently published their phase II experience with carboplatin and paclitaxel in metastatic NPC. Both studies used carboplatin at AUC of six without growth factor support, but the study by Tan et al. (1999) used paclitaxel at a modestly higher dose of 175 mg/m^2, while Yeo et al. (1998) used a lower dose at 135 mg/m^2. Although the response rates reported by Tan et al. was higher than Yeo et al. (78% vs. 59%), the neutropenic sepsis rate was much higher (28% vs. 3%), and the median overall survival was only 12 months when compared with 13.9 months as reported by Yeo et al. (1998).

The use of "maintenance" chemotherapy – the continuation of chemotherapy once best response is achieved after neoadjuvant chemotherapy – in the treatment of recurrent and metastatic NPC has not been formally evaluated in randomized studies. The only published report is a phase II study, where responders to four cycles of cisplatin, doxorubicin, and mitomycin C received weekly 5-fluorouracil and leucovorin until disease progression for a median duration of 38 weeks (Hong et al. 1999). The weekly treatment was well tolerated, and the respective median time to progression and overall survival were 11.6 and 18 months, respectively. These data are comparable with those reported with phase II studies of platinum-based doublets discussed in Sect. 11.2.1, and further studies are warranted.

Table 11.1 Selected cytotoxic chemotherapy with known activity against nasopharyngeal carcinoma in the palliative or neoadjuvant setting

Drug	Single agent: RR (%)	Combination with other drugs: RR
Platinum		
Cisplatin	NA	[a]5-FU: 66% (Au and Ang 1994)
		[b]Docetaxel: 76% (Hui et al. 2009)
		[a]Gemcitabine: 73% (Ngan et al. 2002)
Carboplatin	[a]44% (Chi et al. 1997)	[a]5-FU: 38% (Yeo et al. 1996)
		[a]Paclitaxel: 59% (Yeo et al. 1998)
Oxaliplatin	NA	[a]Gemcitabine: 56% (Ma et al. 2009)
Non-platinum		
Bleomycin	[a]28% (Molinari 1978)	[a]Cisplatin, 5-FU: 79% (Boussen et al. 1991)
		[a]Cisplatin, epirubicin: 48% (Azli et al. 1995)
		[b]Cisplatin, epirubicin: 98% (Bachouchi et al. 1990)
Capecitabine	[a]37% (Chua et al. 2008)	[a]Cisplatin: 62% (Li et al. 2008)
Cyclophosphamide	[a]38% (Molinari 1978)	[a]CAPABLE: 80% (Siu et al. 1998)
Docetaxel	NA	[a]Cisplatin: 22% (McCarthy et al. 2002)
		[b]Cisplatin: 76% (Hui et al. 2009)
Doxorubicin	39% (Molinari 1978)	[a]CAPABLE: 80% (Siu et al. 1998)
5-FU (infusional)	25% (Fandi et al. 1997)	See under "cisplatin" and "carboplatin"
Gemcitabine	[a]28% (Foo et al. 2002)	[a]Cisplatin: 73% (Ngan et al. 2002)
		[a]Carboplatin, paclitaxel: 78% (Leong et al. 2005)
Ifosfamide	NA	[a]Cisplatin: 59% (Stein et al. 1996)
Irinotecan	[c]14% (Poon et al. 2005)	NA
Methotrexate	17% (Molinari 1978)	See under "CAPABLE"
Paclitaxel	22% (Au et al. 1998)	See under "carboplatin"
Vinorelbine	NA	[c]Gemcitabine: 36% (Wang et al. 2006)

NA not available; *RR* response rate (partial and complete response); *5-FU* 5-fluorouracil; *CAPABLE* 5-drug regimen with cyclophosphamide, doxorubicin, cisplatin, methotrexate, and bleomycin
[a]Palliative first-line study
[b]Neoadjuvant
[c]Palliative second- or third-line study

11.3.3.3
Molecular Factors Affecting Cellular Response to Chemotherapy in Nasopharyngeal Carcinoma

Altered expression of cell cycle regulators and EBV-related proteins has been implicated as factors affecting cellular response to cisplatin in preclinical studies of NPC. For instance, NPC cells transfected with the oncogenic EBV-encoded latent membrane protein-1 (LMP-1) were up to four times more susceptible to cisplatin-induced cell death than LMP-1 negative NPC cells (Liu et al. 2002).

The cytotoxicity of cisplatin is cell cycle-dependent, such that rapidly proliferating cells are more susceptible to its action. Researchers have evaluated the association between some cell cycle checkpoint regulators and sensitivity to DNA-damaging agents in NPC cells. The mitotic arrest deficient 2 protein (MAD2) regulates the mitotic checkpoint, which ensures the accurate segregation of chromosomes (Wang and Wong 2003).

Increased expression of the *MAD2* gene in *MAD2*-transfected NPC cells resulted in enhanced sensitivity to cisplatin, possibly via induction of mitotic arrest and activation of apoptosis (Cheung et al. 2005). Likewise, MAD2-induced sensitization of CNE2 cells to the vinca alkaloid, vincristine, was associated with G2/M mitotic arrest (Wang and Wong 2003).

The tumor suppressor *p16* gene suppresses cell proliferation primarily by inhibiting G1 cell cycle progression, and is frequently inactivated via promoter methylation in NPC (Lo et al. 1996). Restoration of *p16* function via *p16*-transfection in CNE1 NPC cells resulted in a modest increase in sensitivity to 5-fluorouracil and cisplatin in vitro (Chow et al. 2000).

TWIST (or TWIST-1) is a basic helix–loop–helix (bHLH) protein implicated in carcinogenesis, the function of which is to interfere with p53-mediated apoptosis and cell differentiation. Using an NPC cell line, HNE1-T3, upregulation of the gene encoding TWIST has been associated with increased resistance to microtubule-disrupting agents such as paclitaxel and vincristine (Wang et al. 2004), possibly by suppressing paclitaxel-induced apoptosis (Zhang et al. 2007). Inactivation of the gene encoding TWIST via small RNA interference resulted in sensitization to paclitaxel in HNE1-T3 cells (Zhang et al. 2007).

P-glycoprotein (ABCB1, or MDR1) is a member of the ATP-binding cassette (ABC) superfamily of multidrug transporters, and has been implicated in resistance against platinum, paclitaxel, and anthracyclines in a variety of cancers. MDR1 expression can be found in up to 12% of NPC samples (Chen et al. 2001; Hsu et al. 2002), and has been associated with shorter survival in metastatic NPC in two studies (Chen et al. 2001; Hsu et al. 2002). No association with response to doxorubicin-containing chemotherapy was found in one study (Hsu et al. 2002).

11.4 The Clinical Development of Targeted Therapy for Nasopharyngeal Carcinoma

11.4.1 Molecular Abnormalities in Nasopharyngeal Carcinoma

Advances in the understanding of the molecular pathogenesis of NPC have led to the identification of many genetic and epigenetic aberrations that are common in NPC. Genome-wide microarray studies of NPC tissues have revealed a high frequency of aberrant expression of genes controlling apoptosis, cell cycle progression, cell migration and adhesion, growth, and differentiation (Sriuranpong et al. 2004). Important oncogenes such as *BCL2, CCND1, MDM2, MYC, H-RAS, N-RAS, RAF1, EGFR,* and *PIK3CA* are frequently amplified in NPC tissues and/or cell lines (Hui et al. 2002; Or et al. 2006). Inactivation of tumor suppressor genes (TSGs) are particularly prevalent in NPC, with chromosomal deletions occurring in between 85 and 95% of regions involving 9p21 and 3p (Tao and Chan 2007). These regions contain TSGs such as *p16* (Lo et al. 1995), *p15* (Kwong et al. 2002), *p14ARF* (Kwong et al. 2002), and *RASSF1A* (Lo et al. 2001), which are inactivated via mechanisms including promoter methylation, mutation, or deletions. EBV latent infection and epigenetic silencing of immunodominant EBV genes may also contribute to the evasion of host-derived immunosurveillance, while the production of oncogenic EBV proteins (e.g., latent membrane protein-1, LMP-1) contributes to NPC carcinogenesis (Young and Rickinson 2004). For more comprehensive overview of the genetic and epigenetic abnormalities in NPC, readers may refer to several excellent reviews (Tao and Chan 2007; Young and Rickinson 2004; Lo and Huang 2002).

11.4.2 Targeting Epidermal Growth Factor Receptor-Mediated Signaling

Inhibitors against the epidermal growth factor receptor (EGFR) were the first targeted therapy evaluated clinically in recurrent and metastatic NPC. This is based on the observation that the *EGFR* gene is amplified in 40% (Hui et al. 2002) and EGFR protein is overexpressed in over 80% of NPC tumors. EGFR overexpression is also associated with shorter survival following chemoradiotherapy in locoregionally advanced NPC (Ma et al. 2003). In NPC cells, the anti-EGFR monoclonal antibody, cetuximab (Sung et al. 2005), and the EGFR tyrosine kinase inhibitor, gefitinib (Hsu et al. 2002), have been shown to inhibit cell growth, induce apoptosis, and exert an additive effect when combined with cisplatin. Based on these data, researchers at the Prince of Wales Hospital led a multicenter phase II study of cetuximab and carboplatin in 60 patients with metastatic NPC who had failed previous platinum-based regimens (Chan et al.

2005). There were seven partial responses with an overall response rate of 11.7%, and disease stabilization rate was 48.3%. In this cohort where over 30% of patients had three or more lines of prior therapy, the median time to progression and overall survival were 2.6 and 7.7 months, respectively. Treatment was well tolerated, and grade 3–4 cetuximab-related rash occurred in 12% of patients.

Another EGFR inhibitor, gefitinib, was evaluated in a phase II study at a dose of 500 mg daily in chemotherapy-refractory patients at the Prince of Wales Hospital (Ma et al. 2007). Three patients experienced disease stabilization lasting up to 8 months, and the study was terminated after 15 patients were accrued owing to a lack of response. This is probably due to the absence of activating mutations of the EGFR tyrosine kinase in NPC tumors (Lee et al. 2006).

11.4.3 Targeting Tumor Angiogenesis

Hypoxia-inducible factor-1 alpha (HIF-1α) is a key hypoxia-inducible transcriptional factor, which upregulates the expression of important mediators of angiogenesis such as vascular endothelial growth factor and its ligands, and of glucose metabolism such as carbonic anhydrase 9 (CA-9). Genome-wide expression analysis of NPC cell lines has demonstrated that expression of genes encoding HIF-1α, CA-9, VEGF, and other signaling proteins in NPC are upregulated under hypoxic conditions (Sung et al. 2007). HIF-1α, CA-9, and VEGF are also overexpressed in over 50% of NPC tumors, while co-expression of these hypoxic-angiogenic factors predict shorter survival following radiotherapy in patients with locoregionally advanced NPC (Hui et al. 2002). Therefore, pharmacological inhibition of the downstream signaling mediators of HIF-1α may be useful against NPC. Researchers have evaluated the clinical activity of several inhibitors of VEGF (e.g., bevacizumab) or its receptors (VEGFR-2 and -3), such as sorafenib, sunitinib, and pazopanib in NPC patients. The only reported published to date is a phase II study of sorafenib (400mg bd) in chemo-refractory patients with either advanced NPC and non-NPC head and neck cancer (Elser et al. 2007). No response was reported among the 6 out of 27 who had NPC, and the study was terminated after the first stage of accrual. Phase II studies of sunitinib and pazopanib as single agent in patients with previously treated advanced NPC are either ongoing or completed accrual. Results have not yet been reported. The anti-VEGF antibody, bevacizumab, is currently being evaluated in combination with IMRT in patients with locoregionally advanced NPC in a Radiation Therapy Oncology Group (RTOG)-sponsored study involving both North American and Asian centers.

The use of anti-angiogenesis agents is associated with an increased bleeding tendency. This is of theoretical concern in the clinical evaluation of such agents in NPC; therefore, such agents should be avoided in patients with locally advanced tumors invading major blood vessels or venous plexus, and in those presenting with epistaxis.

11.4.4 Epigenetic Modulation

The EBV exist in a state of latency in undifferentiated NPC cells where it evades the host's immune response by expressing a limited repertoire of EB latent genes, while expression of the more immunodominant EBV nuclear and lytic antigens are silenced. Epigenetic gene silencing via promoter methylation has been found to be one of the key mechanisms of silenced expression of EBV nuclear and lytic antigens, as well as host-derived tumor suppressor genes (Kwong et al. 2002; Ambinder et al. 1999). It has been postulated that pharmacological reversal of promoter methylation may result in re-expression of the EBV immunodominant antigens, thereby attracting host's immune response and/or providing target antigens for cytotoxic T-cell therapy. Researchers of the Chinese University of Hong Kong and Johns Hopkins University (Singapore) were able to demonstrate for the first time in humans that the demethylating agent, azacitadine, could induce expression of silenced EBV genes in NPC tissues (Chan et al. 2004). In this study, patients with recurrent EBV-associated NPC and lymphoma who had exhausted all treatment options had paired tumor biopsies performed before and after treatment with azacitdine. Treatment was well tolerated by the eight NPC patients, and expression of the viral regulatory protein, Zta, was re-expressed in the posttreatment biopsy of a patient. Using methylation-specific polymerase chain reaction and bisulfite genomic sequencing, the postbiopsies of four patients showed partial demethylation at the *Cp* and *Wp* promoter of the EBV genome (Chan et al. 2004). A phase I study of combining azacitidine and a histone deacetylase inhibitor in NPC is ongoing.

11.5 Conclusions

Systemic chemotherapy has contributed significantly to the improved clinical outcome of patients with advanced NPC over the last two decades. The combined use of neoadjuvant chemotherapy and concurrent chemoradiation, and the role of adjuvant chemotherapy following chemoradiation warrant further investigation in a phase III setting. An increasing number of cytotoxic agents have now been shown to be active against NPC, and drugs targeting the EGFR and angiogenesis are shown under phase I and II evaluation. The priorities now are to identify predictive biomarkers for individualizing drug therapy in advanced NPC, to evaluate more effective drugs for the eradication of micrometastases following chemoradiation, and also as maintenance therapy after achieving best response with palliative chemotherapy in advanced NPC.

References

Airoldi M, De Crescenzo A, Pedani F, et al (2001) Feasibility and long-term results of autologous PBSC transplantation in recurrent undifferentiated nasopharyngeal carcinoma. Head Neck 23:799–803

Airoldi M, Pedani F, Marchionatti S, et al (2002) Carboplatin plus taxol is an effective third-line regimen in recurrent undifferentiated nasopharyngeal carcinoma. Tumori 88:273–276

Al-Kourainy K, Crissman J, Ensley J, et al (1988) Excellent response to cis-platinum-based chemotherapy in patients with recurrent or previously untreated advanced nasopharyngeal carcinoma. Am J Clin Oncol 11:427–430

Al-Sarraf M, LeBlanc M, Giri PG, et al (1998) Chemoradiotherapy versus radiotherapy in patients with advanced nasopharyngeal cancer: phase III randomized Intergroup study 0099. J Clin Oncol 16:1310–1317

Ambinder RF, Robertson KD, Tao Q (1999) DNA methylation and the Epstein–Barr virus. Semin Cancer Biol 9: 369–375

American Joint Committee on Cancer. Head and Neck sites (2002) Cancer staging handbook. Springer, New York, 50–52*

Au E, Ang PT (1994) A phase II trial of 5-fluorouracil and cisplatinum in recurrent or metastatic nasopharyngeal carcinoma. Ann Oncol 5:87–89

Au E, Tan EH, Ang PT (1998) Activity of paclitaxel by three-hour infusion in Asian patients with metastatic undifferentiated nasopharyngeal cancer. Ann Oncol 9:327–329

Azli N, Fandi A, Bachouchi M, et al (1995) Final report of a phase II study of chemotherapy with bleomycin, epirubicin, and cisplatin for locally advanced and metastatic/recurrent undifferentiated carcinoma of the nasopharyngeal type. Cancer J Sci Am 1:222

Bachouchi M, Cvitkovic E, Azli N, et al (1990) High complete response in advanced nasopharyngeal carcinoma with bleomycin, epirubicin, and cisplatin before radiotherapy. J Natl Cancer Inst 82:616–620

Baujat B, Audry H, Bourhis J, et al (2006) MAC-NPC Collaborative Group. Chemotherapy in locally advanced nasopharyngeal carcinoma: an individual patient data meta-analysis of eight randomized trials and 1753 patients. Int J Radiat Oncol Biol Phys 64:47–56*

Boussen H, Cvitkovic E, Wendling JL, et al (1991) Chemotherapy of metastatic and/or recurrent undifferentiated nasopharyngeal carcinoma with cisplatin, bleomycin, and fluorouracil. J Clin Oncol 9:1675–1681

Chan A, Tao Q, Keith D, et al (2004) Azacitidine induces demethylation of the Epstein–Barr virus genome in tumors. J Clin Oncol 22:1373–1381

Chan AT, Hsu MM, Goh BC, et al (2005) Multicenter, phase II study of cetuximab in combination with carboplatin in patients with recurrent or metastatic nasopharyngeal carcinoma. J Clin Oncol 23:3568–3576

Chan AT, Leung SF, Ngan RK, et al (2005) Overall survival after concurrent cisplatin-radiotherapy compared with radiotherapy alone in locoregionally advanced nasopharyngeal carcinoma. J Natl Cancer Inst 97:536–539

Chan AT, Ma BB, Lo YM, et al (2004) Phase II study of neoadjuvant carboplatin and paclitaxel followed by radiotherapy and concurrent cisplatin in patients with locoregionally advanced nasopharyngeal carcinoma: therapeutic monitoring with plasma Epstein-Barr virus DNA. J Clin Oncol 22:3053–3060

Chan AT, Teo PM, Leung TW, et al (1995) A prospective randomized study of chemotherapy adjunctive to definitive radiotherapy in advanced nasopharyngeal carcinoma. Int J Radiat Oncol Biol Phys 33:569–577

Chan AT, Teo PM, Ngan RK, et al (2002) Concurrent chemotherapy-radiotherapy compared with radiotherapy alone in locoregionally advanced nasopharyngeal carcinoma: progression-free survival analysis of a phase III ranodmized trial. J Clin Oncol 20:2038–2044

Chen CL, Sheen TS, Lou IU, et al (2001) Expression of multidrug resistance 1 and glutathione-S-transferase-Pi protein in nasopharyngeal carcinoma. Hum Pathol 32:1240–1244

Cheung HW, Jin DY, Ling MT, et al (2005) Mitotic arrest deficient 2 expression induces chemosensitization to a DNA-damaging agent, cisplatin, in nasopharyngeal carcinoma cells. Cancer Res 65:1450–1458

Chi KH, Chang YC, Chan WK, et al (1997) A phase II study of carboplatin in nasopharyngeal carcinoma. Oncology 54: 203–207

Chi KH, Chang YC, Guo WY, et al (2002) A phase III study of adjuvant chemotherapy in advanced nasopharyngeal carcinoma patients. Int J Radiat Oncol Biol Phys 52: 1238–1244

Chitapanarux I, Lorvidhaya V, Kamnerdsupaphon P, et al (2007) Chemoradiation comparing cisplatin versus carboplatin in locally advanced nasopharyngeal cancer: randomised, non-inferiority, open trial. Eur J Cancer 43:1399–1406

Chow LS, Wang X, Kwong DL, et al (2000) Effect of p16INK4a on chemosensitivity in nasopharyngeal carcinoma cells. Int J Oncol 17:135–140

Chua D, Ma J, Sham J (2005) Long-term survival after cisplatin-based induction chemotherapy and radiotherapy for nasopharyngeal carcinoma: a pooled data analysis of two phase III trials. J Clin Oncol 23:1118–1124

Chua DT, Sham JS, Choy D, et al (1998) Preliminary report of the Asian-Oceanian Clinical Oncology Association randomized trial comparing cisplatin and epirubicin followed by radiotherapy versus radiotherapy alone in the treatment of patients with locoregionally advanced nasopharyngeal carcinoma. Asian-Oceanian Clinical Oncology Association Nasopharynx Cancer Study Group. Cancer 83:2270–2283

Chua D, Wei WI, Sham JS, et al (2008) Capecitabine monotherapy for recurrent and metastatic nasopharyngeal cancer. Jpn J Clin Oncol 38:244–249

Cooper JS, Cohen R, Stevens RE (1998) A comparison of staging systems for nasopharyngeal carcinoma. Cancer 83: 213–219

Dugan M, Choy D, Ngai A, et al (1993) Multicenter phase II trial of mitoxantrone in patients with advanced nasopharyngeal carcinoma in Southeast Asia: an Asian-Oceanian Clinical Oncology Association Group study. J Clin Oncol 11:70–76

Elser C, Siu LL, Winquist E, et al (2007) Phase II trial of sorafenib in patients with recurrent or metastatic squamous cell carcinoma of the head and neck or nasopharyngeal carcinoma. J Clin Oncol 25:3766–3773

Fandi A, Bachouchi M, Azli N, et al (2000) Long-term disease-free survivors in metastatic undifferentiated carcinoma of nasopharyngeal type. J Clin Oncol 18:1324–1330

Fandi A, Taamma A, Azli N, et al (1997) Palliative treatment with low-dose continuous infusion 5-fluorouracil in recurrent and/or metastatic undifferentiated nasopharyngeal carcinoma type. Head Neck 19:41–47

Foo KF, Tan EH, Leong SS, et al (2002) Gemcitabine in metastatic nasopharyngeal carcinoma of the undifferentiated type. Ann Oncol 13:150–156

Hareyama M, Sakata K, Shirato H, et al (2002) A prospective, randomized trial comparing neoadjuvant chemotherapy with radiotherapy alone in patients with advanced nasopharyngeal carcinoma. Cancer 94:2217–2223

Hasbini A, Mahjoubi R, Fandi A, et al (1999) Phase II trial combining mitomycin with 5-fluorouracil, epirubicin, and cisplatin in recurrent and metastatic undifferentiated carcinoma of nasopharyngeal type. Ann Oncol 10: 421–425

Hong MH, Min H, Min HQ, et al (2000) A comparison of the Chinese 1992 and fifth-edition International Union Against Cancer staging systems for staging nasopharyngeal carcinoma. Cancer 89:242–247

Hong RL, Sheen TS, Ko JY, et al (1999) Induction with mitomycin C, doxorubicin, cisplatin and maintenance with weekly 5-fluorouracil, leucovorin for treatment of metastatic nasopharyngeal carcinoma: a phase II study. Br J Cancer 80:1962–1967

Ho WK, Kwong DL, Sham JS, et al (1999) Long-term sensorineural hearing deficit following radiotherapy in patients suffering from nasopharyngeal carcinoma: a prospective study. Head Neck 21:547–553

Hsu CH, Chen CL, Hong RL, et al (2002) Prognostic value of multidrug resistance 1, glutathione-S-transferase-pi and p53 in advanced nasopharyngeal carcinoma treated with systemic chemotherapy. Oncology 62:305–312

Hsu CH, Chen CL, Yeh PY, et al (2002) Inhibitors of epidermoid growth factor receptor suppress cell growth and enhance chemosensitivity of nasopharyngeal cancer cells in vitro. Oncology 68:538–547

Hui AB, Lo KW, Teo PM, et al (2002) Genome wide detection of oncogene amplifications in nasopharyngeal carcinoma by array based comparative genomic hybridization. Int J Oncol 20:467–473

Hui EP, Chan AT, Pezzella F, et al (2002) Coexpression of hypoxia-inducible factors 1alpha and 2alpha, carbonic anhydrase IX, and vascular endothelial growth factor in nasopharyngeal carcinoma and relationship to survival. Clin Cancer Res 8:2595–2604

Hui EP, Leung SF, Au JS, et al (2004) Lung metastasis alone in nasopharyngeal carcinoma: a relatively favorable prognostic group. A study by the Hong Kong Nasopharyngeal Carcinoma Study Group. Cancer 101:300–306

Hui EP, Ma BB, Leung SF, et al (2009) Randomized phase II trial of concurrent cisplatin-radiotherapy with or without neoadjuvant docetaxel and cisplatin in advanced nasopharyngeal carcinoma. J Clin Oncol 27:242–249

Johnson FM, Palmer JL, Kies M, et al (2004) A phase II study of docetaxel and carboplatin as neoadjuvant therapy for nasopharyngeal carcinoma with early T status and advanced N status. Cancer 100:991–998

Kwong DL, Sham J, Au GK, et al (2004) Concurrent and adjuvant chemotherapy for nasopharyngeal carcinoma: a factorial study. J Clin Oncol 22:2643–2653

Kwong J, Lo KW, To KF, et al (2002) Promoter hypermethylation of multiple genes in nasopharyngeal carcinoma. Clin Cancer Res 8:131–137

Langendijk JA, Leemans C, Buter J, et al (2004) The additional value of chemotherapy to radiotherapy in locally advanced nasopharyngeal carcinoma: a meta-analysis of the published literature. J Clin Oncol 22:4604–4612

Lee AW, Lau WH, Tung SY, et al (2005) Preliminary results of a randomized study on therapeutic gain by concurrent chemotherapy for regionally-advanced nasopharyngeal carcinoma: NPC-9901 trial by the Hong Kong Nasopharyngeal Cancer Study Group. J Clin Oncol 23:6966–6975

Lee AW, Poon YF, Foo W, et al (1992) Retrospective analysis of 5037 patients with nasopharyngeal carcinoma treated during 1976–1985: overall survival and patterns of failure. Int J Radiat Oncol Biol Phys 23:261–270

Lee AW, Sze WM, Au JS, et al (2005) Treatment results for nasopharyngeal carcinoma in the modern era: the Hong Kong experience. Int J Radiat Oncol Biol Phys 61:1107–1116

Lee AW, Tung S, Chan AT, et al (2006) Preliminary results of a randomized study (NPC-9902 Trial) on therapeutic gain by concurrent chemotherapy and/or accelerated fractionation for locally advanced nasopharyngeal carcinoma. Int J Radiat Oncol Biol Phys 66:142–151

Lee SC, Lim SG, Soo R, et al (2006) Lack of somatic mutations in EGFR tyrosine kinase domain in hepatocellular and nasopharyngeal carcinoma. Pharmacogenet Genomics 16:73–74

Leong SS, Wee J, Tay MH, et al (2005) Paclitaxel, carboplatin, and gemcitabine in metastatic nasopharyngeal carcinoma: a Phase II trial using a triplet combination. Cancer 103: 569–575

Lin JC, Jan JS, Hsu CY, et al (2003) Phase III study of concurrent chemoradiotherapy versus radiotherapy alone for advanced nasopharyngeal carcinoma: positive effect on overall and progression-free survival. J Clin Oncol 21:631–637

Liu Y, Wang X, Lo AK, et al (2002) Latent membrane protein-1 of Epstein–Barr virus inhibits cell growth and induces sensitivity to cisplatin in nasopharyngeal carcinoma cells. J Med Virol 66:63–69

Li YH, Wang FH, Jiang WQ, et al (2008) Phase II study of capecitabine and cisplatin combination as first-line chemotherapy in Chinese patients with metastatic nasopharyngeal carcinoma. Cancer Chemother Pharmacol 62:539–544

Lo KW, Cheung ST, Leung SF, et al (1996) Hypermethylation of the p16 gene in nasopharyngeal carcinoma. Cancer Res 56:2721–2725

Lo KW, Huang DP (2002) Genetic and epigenetic changes in nasopharyngeal carcinoma. Semin Cancer Biol 12:451–462

Lo KW, Huang DP, Lau KM (1995) p16 gene alterations in nasopharyngeal carcinoma. Cancer Res 55:2039–2043

Lo KW, Kwong J, Hui AB, et al (2001) High frequency of promoter hypermethylation of RASSF1A in nasopharyngeal carcinoma. Cancer Res 61:3877–3881

Louvet C, Labianca R, Hammel P, et al (2005) Gemcitabine in combination with oxaliplatin compared with gemcitabine alone in locally advanced or metastatic pancreatic cancer: results of a GERCOR and GISCAD phase III trial. J Clin Oncol 23:3509–3516

Low WK, Toh ST, Wee J, et al (2006) Sensorineural hearing loss after radiotherapy and chemoradiotherapy: a single, blinded, randomized study. J Clin Oncol 24:1904–1909

Ma BB, Hui EP, Chan AT (2008) Systemic approach to improving treatment outcome in nasopharyngeal carcinoma: current and future directions. Cancer Sci 99:1311–1318

Ma BB, Hui EP, Wong SCC, et al (2009) Multicenter phase II study of gemcitabine and oxaliplatin in advanced nasopharyngeal carcinoma - correlation with excision repair cross complementing-1 polymorphisms Ann Oncol.*

Ma B, Hui EP, King A, et al (2007) A phase II study of gefitinib in patients with metastatic or locoregionally recurrent nasopharyngeal carcinoma and evaluation of plasma Epstein–Barr virus DNA as a biomarker of efficacy. Cancer Chemother Pharmacol 62:59–64

Ma B, Poon T, KF To, et al (2003) Expression and prognostic significance of epidermal growth factor receptor and HER2 protein in nasopharyngeal carcinoma. Head Neck 2003; 25:864–872

Ma J, Mai HQ, Hong MH, et al (1998) Results of a prospective randomized trial comparing neoadjuvant chemotherapy plus radiotherapy with radiotherapy alone in patients with locoregionally advanced nasopharyngeal carcinoma. J Clin Oncol 19:1350–1357

McCarthy J, Tannock I, Degendorfer P, et al (2002) A Phase II trial of docetaxel and cisplatin in patients with recurrent or metastatic nasopharyngeal carcinoma. Oral Oncol 38:686

Molinari R (1978) European Organization for Research on Treatment of Cancer (E.O.R.T.C.). Controlled trials of chemotherapy as an adjuvant or palliative treatment of nasopharyngeal carcinoma. IARC Sci Publ 20:565–574

Ngan RK, Yiu HH, Lau WH, et al (2002) Combination gemcitabine and cisplatin chemotherapy for metastatic or recurrent nasopharyngeal carcinoma: report of a phase II study. Ann Oncol 13:1252–1258

Or YY, Hui AB, To KF, et al (2006) PIK3CA mutations in nasopharyngeal carcinoma. Int J Cancer 118:1065–1067

Parliament M, Jha N, Rapp E, et al (2001) Concurrent weekly carboplatin and radiotherapy for nasopharyngeal carcinoma: report of a joint phase II study. Radiother Oncol 58:131–136s

Poon D, Chowbay B, Cheung YB, et al (2005) Phase II study of irinotecan (CPT-11) as salvage therapy for advanced nasopharyngeal carcinoma. Cancer 103:576–581

Raymond E, Faivre S, Woynarowski JM, et al (1999) Oxaliplatin: mechanism of action and antineoplastic activity. Semin Oncol 25:4–12

Rossi A, Molinari R, Boracchi P, et al (1988) Adjuvant chemotherapy with vincristine, cyclophosphamide, and doxorubicin after radiotherapy in local-regional nasopharyngeal cancer: results of a 4-year multicenter randomized study. J Clin Oncol 6:1401–1410

Roussy InstituteGustave (1996) Preliminary results of a randomized trial comparing neoadjuvant chemotherapy (cisplatin, epirubicin, bleomycin) plus radiotherapy vs. radiotherapy alone in stage IV(> or = N2, M0) undifferentiated nasopharyngeal carcinoma: a positive effect on progression-free survival. International Nasopharynx Cancer Study Group. VUMCA I trial. Int J Radiat Oncol Biol Phys 35:463–469

Siu LL, Czaykowski PM, Tannock IF (1998) Phase I-II study of the CAPABLE regimen for patients with poorly differentiated carcinoma of the nasopharynx. J Clin Oncol 16: 2514–2521

Sriuranpong V, Mutirangura A, Gillespie JW, et al (2004) Global gene expression profile of nasopharyngeal carcinoma by laser capture microdissection and complementary DNA microarrays. Clin Cancer Res 10:4944–4958

Stein ME, Ruff P, Weaving A, et al (1996) A phase II study of cisplatin/ifosfamide in recurrent/metastatic undifferentiated nasopharyngeal carcinoma among young blacks in southern Africa. Am J Clin Oncol 19:386–388

Sung FL, Hui EP, Tao Q, et al (2007) Genome-wide expression analysis using microarray identified complex signaling pathways modulated by hypoxia in nasopharyngeal carcinoma. Cancer Lett 253:74–88

Sung FL, Poon TC, Hui EP, et al (2005) Antitumor effect and enhancement of cytotoxic drug activity by cetuximab in nasopharyngeal carcinoma cells. In Vivo 19:237–245

Taamma A, Fandi A, Azli N, et al (1999) Phase II trial of chemotherapy with 5-fluorouracil, bleomycin, epirubicin, and cisplatin for patients with locally advanced, metastatic, or recurrent undifferentiated carcinoma of the nasopharyngeal type. Cancer 86:1101–1108

Tan EH, Khoo KS, Wee J, et al (1999) Phase II trial of a paclitaxel and carboplatin combination in Asian patients with metastatic nasopharyngeal carcinoma. Ann Oncol 10: 235–237

Tao Q, Chan AT (2007) Nasopharyngeal carcinoma: molecular pathogenesis and therapeutic developments. Expert Rev Mol Med 9:1–24

Teo P, Tsao SY, Shiu W, et al (1989) A clinical study of 407 cases of nasopharyngeal carcinoma in Hong Kong. Int J Radiat Oncol Biol Phys 17:515–530

Wang CC, Liu TW, Lin CY, et al (2006) Phase II study of gemcitabine plus vinorelbine in the treatment of cisplatin-resistant nasopharyngeal carcinoma. Head Neck 28: 74–80

Wang TL, Tan YO (1991) Cisplatin and 5-fluorouracil continuous infusion for metastatic nasopharyngeal carcinoma. Ann Acad Med Singapore 20:601–603

Wang X, Chow LS, Nicholls JM, et al (2002) Significance of scheduling on the cytotoxicity of radiation and cisplatin combination treatment in nasopharyngeal carcinoma cells. Anticancer Drugs 13:957–964

Wang X, Ling MT, Guan XY, et al (2004) Identification of a novel function of TWIST, a bHLH protein, in the development of acquired taxol resistance in human cancer cells. Oncogene 23:474–482

Wang X, Wong H, Feng H, et al (2003) MAD2-induced sensitization to vincristine is associated with mitotic arrest and Raf/Bcl-2 phosphorylation in nasopharyngeal carcinoma cells. Oncogene 22:109–116

Wang X, Wong SC, Pan J, et al (1998) Evidence of cisplatin-induced senescent-like growth arrest in nasopharyngeal carcinoma cells. Cancer Res 58:5019–5022

Wee J, Tan EH, Tai BC, et al (2005) Randomized trial of radiotherapy versus concurrent chemoradiotherapy followed by adjuvant chemotherapy in patients with American Joint Committee on Cancer/International Union against cancer stage III and IV nasopharyngeal cancer of the endemic variety. J Clin Oncol 23:6730–6738

Yau TK, Lee AW, Wong DH, et al (2006) Treatment of Stage IV(A-B) nasopharyngeal carcinoma by induction-concurrent chemoradiotherapy and accelerated fractionation: impact of chemotherapy schemes. Int J Radiat Oncol Biol Phys 66:1004–1010

Yeo W, Leung TW, Chan AT, et al (1998) A phase II study of combination paclitaxel and carboplatin in advanced nasopharyngeal carcinoma. Eur J Cancer 34: 2027–2031

Yeo W, Leung TW, Leung SF, et al (1996) Phase II study of the combination of carboplatin and 5-fluorouracil in metastatic nasopharyngeal carcinoma. Cancer Chemother Pharmacol 38:466–470

Young LS, Rickinson A (2004) Epstein–Barr virus: 40 years on. Nat rev Cancer 4:757–768

Zhang L, Peng PJ, Lu LX, et al (2005) Phase III study comparing standard radiotherapy with or without weekly oxaliplatin in treatment of locoregionally advanced nasopharyngeal carcinoma: preliminary results. J Clin Oncol 23:8461–8468

Zhang X, Wang Q, Ling MT, et al (2007) Anti-apoptotic role of TWIST and its association with Akt pathway in mediating taxol resistance in nasopharyngeal carcinoma cells. Int J Cancer 120:1891–1898

The Intergroup 0099 Trial for Nasopharyngeal Cancer: History, Perceptions, and Transitions

12

Jay S. Cooper

"Because the nasopharynx is immediately adjacent to the base of the skull, surgical resection of the neoplasm with an acceptable margin is impossible; hence, radiation therapy has been the sole treatment for carcinoma of the nasopharynx

Carlos Perez (1997) Principles and Practice of Radiation Oncology, 3rd edn, p 909"

CONTENTS

Jay S. Cooper, MD, FACR, FACRO, FASTRO
Department of Radiation Oncology, Maimonides Cancer Center, 6300 Eighth Avenue, Brooklyn, NY 11220, USA

12.1 Introduction

In recent years, the management of locoregionally advanced nasopharyngeal cancer has evolved quickly. Radiation therapy, delivered alone, was generally considered to be the only potentially curative therapy for this tumor only a brief time ago. How times have changed! The volume of data that demonstrates potential contributions of chemotherapy to the management of nasopharyngeal cancer is now substantial; however, many questions about the precise role of chemotherapy remain unanswered. The purpose of this chapter is to look back briefly at the state of clinical practice one to two decades ago, survey the benefits and limitations of radiation therapy as it was administered then, review the essential details of the Intergroup 0099 landmark trial (which provided prospective randomized data supporting the use of chemotherapy), and evaluate critically what we learned and did not learn from that trial.

12.2 Traditional Therapy

Less than two decades ago, following radiation therapy alone, patients who had stage III or IV nasopharyngeal cancer generally had a substantial incidence (50%–80%) of local recurrence (Hoppe et al. 1976; Mesic et al. 1981; Perez et al. 1969; Scanlon et al. 1967; Cooper et al. 1983; Ahmad and Stefani 1986; Dimery et al. 1979) and a relatively high (approximately 30%) risk of distant dissemination of disease. To some degree, the failure of radiation therapy could be attributed to late diagnosis resulting in the discovery of some tumors that were so large or so resistant to radiation that any attempt would fail and to some degree the failure reflected limitations of the techniques then available. Larger tumors of any type are more difficult to control than smaller ones with radiation therapy. And, inadequate radiation therapy certainly has a direct effect on local and regional disease. Perhaps less obvious, there is data to suggest that inadequate radiation therapy, which leads to local recurrence, is also associated with a higher risk of distant dissemination, i.e., suggesting that local recurrences can metastasize (Leibel et al. 1991). It is therefore appropriate to review the previous limitations of radiation therapy as a way of understanding how they influenced outcome in the pre-chemotherapy era.

12.3 Radiotherapy Evolution: From 2½D to 3D to IMRT

Radiation therapy for nasopharyngeal cancer, historically, was delivered from two lateral fields designed to include the primary tumor and upper neck nodes mated to one anterior (low volume tumor) or opposed anterior and posterior (high volume tumor) lower neck portal(s). The margins of the beams were defined by normal anatomy and clinically visible and/or palpable disease. With the availability of CT scanners (and then MRI scanners), a greater appreciation of the extent of disease was possible and by the late-1980s, the 3D information from these diagnostic scans was routinely incorporated into the 2D fluoroscopically designed radiation therapy portals, creating so-called 2½D treatment plans. This was the state of the art when the Intergroup 0099 trial was designed.

Delivering a relatively cancericidal dose to a point in the middle of the nasopharynx has been possible for many years. The lateral diameter of the face poses little challenge to megavoltage beams. Doses of approximately 70Gy, still the current standard, could be delivered once Cobalt-60 machines became widely available one half-century ago. However, that dose was not immediately adopted everywhere and as late as 1988, the journal Cancer considered worthy of publication the results of Wang et al. (1988), which demonstrated superior overall survival (OS) associated with doses greater than 4,000 rad. In fact, some data suggested that some tumors needed to be treated more intensively than 70Gy. In Boston, Wang (1989) used accelerated hyperfractionation to treat 60 patients who had nasopharyngeal cancers and reported better local control than was obtained following conventionally fractionated radiation 5-years earlier at the same institution. He also began (Wang 1991) to add a 10-15Gy intracavitary boost and reported even better local control in some patients. In the same era, the physicians at Stanford University began to investigate the use of stereotactic radiosurgery to boost the dose delivered to the nasopharynx and reported (Cmelak et al. 1997) that 11 of 11 patients who received radiosurgery as a nasopharyngeal boost after standard fractionation radiotherapy remained locally free of disease with follow-up ranging from 2 to 34 months. However, in retrospect, the interpretation of these findings may have been partially incorrect.

More important than the 2½D mid-plane dose delivered in the nasopharynx, the proximity of the brainstem and the spinal cord sometimes limited the dose that could be delivered homogeneously to the entire tumor when the tumor approached these relatively radiosensitive structures. The technology to do true 3D, CT-simulator-based planning and 3D conformal treatment delivery was not commonly available when the Intergroup study was conducted. This raises the possibility that the reported effectiveness of techniques to make radiation therapy more effective than 2½D planned, 70Gy delivered once daily over 7 weeks reflects (a) true resistance to that dose, (b) serendipitously bringing the dose in "cold spots" within the tumor to at least 70Gy equivalent, or (c) a combination of (a) and (b).

12.3.1 Target Localization Limitations

The quality of the CT scans (and when available MRI scans) of the late-1980s also was not equal to those commonly available today. The number of detectors per machine was fewer, the scan times longer (and therefore more susceptible to patient movement) and the clarity of the scans worse. Yet, that was the best information available.

12.3.2 State of the Art Circa 1980

Hampered by the limitations of the technology (both for detection and treatment) that was available, the prospect for locoregionally advanced nasopharyngeal carcinoma treated solely by radiation therapy was "set up" to fail to reach the levels that radiation therapy alone could achieve today. Five year OS approximated 45% for stage III and 30% for stage IV. Five-year disease-free survival approximated 40% for T3 or T4 tumors and 35% for N2 or N3 tumors and as little as 20% for patients who were unlucky enough to have both T3–4 and N2–3 tumors (FREZZA et al. 1986). In part, this reflected limitations of local control (approximately 70% for T3 and T4 tumors), in part of regional control (approximately 80% for N3 disease) and in part of distant control (approximately 70%) (MESIC et al. 1981). But, we truly do not know how much better results would be without these limitations.

12.4 Chemotherapy: A Potential Ally

Against this backdrop, it was appropriate to wonder if the addition of a spatially nontargeted agent, such as cytotoxic chemotherapy, to radiation therapy likely would be of benefit. To be useful, the addition of chemotherapy would need to (a) be inherently cancericidal (i.e., it would need to be able to kill locoregional disease that could survive radiation therapy and/or kill subclinical-size, hematogeneously borne emboli of tumor that would otherwise give rise to distant metastases), (b) sensitize tumor to the effects of radiation therapy (i.e., augment the biologic effect of radiation therapy to the point that additional irradiated tumor cells were killed) or (c) both and it would need to do so without being unacceptably toxic. And, there was evidence that chemotherapy might be able to do so.

By the time that the Intergroup 0099 study was launched, there was substantial evidence that chemotherapy produced a beneficial response in patients who had metastatic or locoregionally recurrent nasopharyngeal cancer (AL-KOURAINY et al. 1988; BOUSSEN et al. 1991; CHOO and TANNOCK 1991; DECKER et al. 1983). Salutary response rates (approximately 20%–25% complete response and 55%–75% total response) were reported. The common denominator of these chemotherapy trials appeared to be cisplatin, often in combination with 5-FU. This logically led to a desire to try to combine either cisplatin alone or cisplatin and 5-FU with radiation therapy, giving the chemotherapy before, during, and/or after radiation therapy. Several phase II trials (ATICHARTAKAN et al. 1988; BACHOUCHI et al. 1990; DIMERY et al. 1993) began to suggest that chemotherapy and radiation therapy could safely be combined and further suggested that the concurrent administration of the two agents was the most effective strategy.

Furthermore, in vitro, there was evidence of benefit when cisplatin was combined with radiation therapy (RICHMOND et al. 1977; DOUPLE et al. 1977; SOLOWAY et al. 1979; SZUMIEL and NIAZ 1976).

12.4.1 Suggestive Evidence of Chemotherapy Effect

But, the most exciting data came from a phase II RTOG study (RTOG 8117) (AL-SARRAF et al. 1990). Between December 1981 and December 1984, the RTOG conducted a nonrandomized, phase II trial of concurrent cisplatin (100 mg/m^2 i.v. bolus administered every 3–4 weeks for a total of three courses) and radiation therapy (1.8-2Gy per day 5 days a week for a total dose of up to 73.8Gy to the primary tumor site) in patients who had stage III or IV head and neck cancer. Of the 134 patients enrolled in this trial, 28 had nasopharyngeal cancer. One patient had inadequate data submitted and the published report is based on the 27 patients who had nasopharyngeal cancer (26 of the 27 had stage IV disease) with a median follow-up of 17.5 months and a range between less than 1 and 95 months. Complete response to treatment was observed in 24 of the 27 (89%) with 4 of the 24 patients experiencing grade 3 or 4 toxicity. All the patients were able to receive at least 90% of their planned radiation therapy dose; six patients did not receive their third dose of chemotherapy because of prohibitive toxicity and another two patients refused their third dose. With the typical caveats of the limitations of comparison with other historical groups, the authors concluded "superior results are obtained with chemo-radiotherapy as compared with radiotherapy alone in patients with stage IV" nasopharyngeal cancer. A prospective phase III trial just for locoregionally advanced nasopharyngeal cancer clearly appeared to be justified and the RTOG, SWOG, and ECOG asked the American National Cancer Institute for permission to do so.

Design of the prospective trial had to reflect reality. In the United States, there are a limited number of patients who are found to have nasopharyngeal cancer annually and the number needed for a prospective trial would most likely require the combined resources of the RTOG, SWOG, and ECOG. Even then, only a two-arm trial would likely be completed in a "reasonable" timeframe. Therefore, the proposed trial could test radiation therapy alone vs. concurrent chemoradiotherapy or concurrent chemoradiotherapy followed by adjuvant chemotherapy, but not both. Several proposals were considered and the NCI designated SWOG as the lead group and concurrent chemoradiotherapy followed by adjuvant chemotherapy as the experimental arm. The hope was that the experimental arm would prove better than the standard and questions about the relative contributions of concurrent vs. adjuvant chemotherapy could be investigated later.

12.5 Intergroup 0099: The Details

Designated Intergroup #0099, eligibility for the trial (Al-Sarraf et al. 1998) included biopsy-proven stage III or IV cancers (AJCC 4th edition) of the nasopharynx that were bi-dimensionally measurable on a CT or MRI scan and without evidence of systemic metastasis. Progression-free survival (PFS) and OS were the primary end points of the study with PFS being defined as the time from registration to the date progressive disease or death due to any cause was first known. The study planned to accrue a total of 270 patients, but interim analyses were planned after 56 and 78% of the patients were accrued in case the results strongly favored one arm of the trial.

Radiation therapy was relatively crude by current standards. CT-based treatment planning was required, but that implies only that all diseases visible on a diagnostic CT scan was included in one or more treatment portals; 3D conformal treatment planning simply was not commonly available. Similarly, treatment equipment did not meet today's standards. Any unit with beam energy equal to cobalt-60 (approximately 1.25 million volts and more penumbra of the beam edge than current linacs have) or higher and a minimum source skin distance of at least 80 cm (and therefore greater divergence of the beam than current typical 100 cm linacs) could be used. The nasopharynx and upper neck were expected to be treated by two opposed lateral fields and all detectable tumor plus a 2-cm margin was intended to receive at least 90% of the mid-plane central axis dose. A separate anterior treatment portal, with spinal cord shielding, was used to treat the lymph node beds caudad (inferior) to the thyroid notch. Total doses of 70Gy were prescribed for the primary tumor and lymph nodes greater than 2 cm in size. The suggested minimum total dose was 66Gy for nodes up to 2 cm and 50Gy for clinically uninvolved (but presumed to be microscopically at risk) nodes.

Concurrent chemotherapy was prescribed as cisplatin every 3 weeks (and when toxicity did not prevent it) ideally on days 1, 22, and 43 of radiotherapy, given at 100 mg/m^2 as a rapid intravenous infusion over 15–20 min. Subsequent adjuvant chemotherapy, beginning 4 weeks after radiotherapy or the last dose of cisplatin, was prescribed as cisplatin 80 mg/m^2 intravenously on days 71, 99, and 127 and 5-FU 1,000 mg/m^2/d by 96 h infusion on days 71–74, 99–102, and 127–130.

12.5.1 Intergroup 0099: The Good News

Between May 1989 and December 1995, 193 patients were enrolled in the study, 103 by RTOG, 60 by SWOG, and 30 by ECOG. Of these, 147 could be analyzed at the time of the first planned interim analysis in October 1995, when the null-hypothesis test of no difference in survival for radiotherapy vs. chemoradiotherapy was rejected at the 0.001 level. The median survival of patients treated by radiation therapy alone was 30 months, but had not been reached for patients treated by chemoradiotherapy. Similarly, the PFS of patients treated by radiation therapy alone was 15 months, but had not been reached for patients treated by chemoradiotherapy. The corresponding 3-year actuarial OS rates (47% and 78%, $p = 0.005$) and progression-free survival (24% and 69%, $p < 0.001$) also significantly favored chemoradiotherapy. The SWOG Data and Safety Monitoring Committee therefore recommended that the study be closed and reported immediately.

The Intergroup 0099 study thereby became the first prospectively randomized study to demonstrate an improvement in OS from the addition of concurrent chemotherapy and adjuvant chemotherapy to radiation therapy (when compared with radiation therapy alone). Furthermore, it did so without unacceptably increasing the toxicity of treatment. While a significantly greater incidence of grade 3 or 4 leukopenia and vomiting was observed in patients treated with chemoradiotherapy ($p < 0.05$), 63% of patients were able to tolerate all three planned courses of concurrent chemoradiotherapy and 55% were able to tolerate all three planned courses of subsequent adjuvant chemotherapy. While it must be recognized that *p*-values are not proof and that any one trial can produce misleading results, in the absence of data to contradict the findings of 0099, the trial needs to be viewed as the defining data that changed the paradigm of treatment of locoregionally advanced nasopharyngeal carcinoma from radiation therapy alone to combined radiation therapy and chemotherapy. As a proof of the principle that chemotherapy could augment the effectiveness of radiation therapy (at least radiation therapy of the quality that could be delivered in the late 1980s – early 1990s), the trial justified exploration of other combinations in the treatment of nasopharyngeal cancer and, by extension of the principle, the treatment of other malignancies.

12.5.2 Intergroup 0099: The Limitations

However, the trial did not answer many questions. By design, it could not address the relative importance/contribution of the concurrent application of cisplatin chemotherapy with radiation therapy vs. the sequential provision of two drug adjuvant chemotherapy after radiation therapy. Furthermore, the leadership of SWOG made the decision not to perform any subgroup analyses and therefore there is no publically accessible 0099-related data from which hypotheses about the relative merits of the treatment in different cohorts of patients (e.g., T-category, N-category, histologic grade, age, etc.) could be derived.

We are also left to ponder the potential influence of the 2½ D radiation therapy technique that was used in the trial. Did chemotherapy merely compensate for inadequate radiation therapy? Would routine MRI assessment of the extent of tumor have mattered? Would coverage of tumors that spread into the parapharyngeal regions have improved and PFS with it? Would CT-based simulation, 3D conformal, or intensity-modulated radiation therapy have influenced the results? As radiation therapy does a better job of eliminating tumor in a greater proportion of patients, does the presumably added benefit of chemotherapy become more or less important?

Similarly, what was the influence of the specific manner in which chemotherapy was administered in the trial? Would other schedules (weekly, daily) have improved or worsened the outcome? Would the inclusion of other drugs that work by different mechanisms, such as bleomycin or tirapazamine, have mattered? Could 5-FU have been omitted? Would the radiation therapy coverage of tumors have been better if chemotherapy was used in a neo-adjuvant fashion before irradiation, or would the added toxicity have precluded subsequent concurrent chemoradiation in an unacceptable number of patients?

These remaining questions form the framework of the following chapters. Some of the answers will be found there, but some remain as yet unknown.

References

Ahmad A, Stefani S (1986) Distant metastases of nasopharyngeal carcinoma: a study of 256 male patients. J Surg Oncol 33:184–197

Al-Kourainy K, Crissman J, Ensley J, et al (1988) Excellent response to cisplatinum-based chemotherapy in patients with recurrent or previously untreated advanced nasopharyngeal carcinoma. Am J Clin Oncol 11:427–430

Al-Sarraf M, LeBlanc M, Giri PG, et al (1998) Chemoradiotherapy versus radiotherapy in patients with advanced nasopharyngeal cancer: phase III randomized Intergroup study 0099. J Clin Oncol 16(4):1310–1317

Al-Sarraf M, Pajak TF, Cooper JS, et al (1990) Chemoradiotherapy in patients with locally advanced nasopharyngeal carcinoma: a Radiation Therapy Oncology Group Study. J Clin Oncol 8(8):1342–1351

Atichartakan V, Kraiphibul P, Clongsusuek P, et al (1988) Nasopharyngeal carcinoma: result of treatment with cis-diamminedichloroplatinum II, 5 fluorouracil, and radiation therapy. Int J Radiat Oncol Biol Phys 14:461–469

Bachouchi M, Cvitkovic E, Azli N, et al (1990) High complete response in advanced nasopharyngeal carcinoma with bleomycin, epirubicin, and cisplatin before radiotherapy. J Natl Cancer Inst 82:616–620

Boussen H, Cvitkovic E, Wendling JL, et al (1991) Chemotherapy of metastatic and/or recurrent undifferentiated nasopharyngeal carcinoma with cisplatin, bleomycin and fluorouracil. J Clin Oncol 9:1675–1681

Choo R, Tannock I (1991) Chemotherapy for recurrent or metastatic carcinoma of the nasopharynx; a review of the Princess Margaret Hospital experience. Cancer 68:2120–2124

Cmelak AJ, Cox RS, Adler JR, et al (1997) Radiosurgery for skull base malignancies and nasopharyngeal carcinoma. Int J Radiat Oncol Biol Phys 37(5):997–1003

Cooper JS, DelRowe J, Newall J (1983) Regional stage IV carcinoma of the nasopharynx treated by aggressive radiotherapy. Int J Radiat Oncol Biol Phys 9:1737–1745

Decker DA, Drelichman A, Al-Sarraf M, et al (1983) Chemotherapy for nasopharyngeal carcinoma. A 10 year experience. Cancer 52:602–605

Dimery IW, Legha SS, Peters LJ, et al (1979) Adjuvant chemotherapy for advanced nasopharyngeal carcinoma. Cancer 60:943–949

Dimery IW, Peters LJ, Goepfert H, et al (1993) Effectiveness of combined induction chemotherapy and radiotherapy in advanced nasopharyngeal carcinoma. J Clin Oncol 11:1919–1928

Douple EB, Richmond RC, Logan ME (1977) Therapeutic potentiation in a mouse mammary tumor and an intracerebral rat brain tumor by combined treatment with cisdichlorodiammineplatinum (II) and radiation. J Clin Hematol Oncol 7:585–603

Frezza G, Barbieri E, Emiliani E, et al (1986) Patterns of failure in nasopharyngeal cancer treated with megavoltage irradiation. Radiother Oncol 5(4):287–294

Hoppe RI, Goffinet DR, Bagshaw MA (1976) Carcinoma of the nasopharynx. Eighteen years experience with megavoltage radiation therapy. Cancer 37:2605–2612

Leibel SA, Scott CB, Mohiuddin M, et al (1991) The effect of local-regional control on distant metastatic dissemination in carcinoma of the head and neck: results of an analysis from the RTOG head and neck database. Int J Radiat Oncol Biol Phys 21(3):549–556

Mesic JB, Fletcher GH, Goepfert H (1981) Megavoltage irradiation of epithelial tumors of the nasopharynx. Int J Radiat Oncol Biol Phys 7:447–453

Perez CA, Ackerman LV, Mill WB, et al (1969) Cancer of the nasopharynx. Factors influencing prognosis. Cancer 24:1–17

Richmond RC, Zimbrick JD, Hykes DL (1977) Radiation induced DNA damage and lethality in *E coli* as modified by the antitumor agent cis-dichlorodiammineplatinum (II). Radiat Res 71:447–460

Scanlon PW, Rhodes RE, Woolner LB, et al (1967) Cancer of the nasopharynx. Am J Roentgenol 99:313–325

Soloway MS, Morris CR, Sudderth B (1979) Radiation therapy and cis-diamminedichloroplatinum (II) in transplantable and primary murine bladder cancer. Int J Radiat Oncol Biol Phys 5:1355–1360

Szumiel I, Nias AHW (1976) The effect of combined treatment with a platinum complex and ionizing radiation on Chinese hamster ovary cells in vitro. Br J Cancer 33:450–458

Wang CC (1989) Accelerated hyperfractionation radiation therapy for carcinoma of the nasopharynx. Techniques and results. Cancer 63(12):2461–2467

Wang CC (1991) Improved local control of nasopharyngeal carcinoma after intracavitary brachytherapy boost. Am J Clin Oncol 14(1):5–8

Wang DC, Cai WM, Hu YH, et al (1988) Long-term survival of 1035 cases of nasopharyngeal carcinoma. Cancer 61:2338–2341

Concurrent Chemotherapy-Enhanced Radiation: Trials and Conclusions

13

Joseph Wee

CONTENTS

Joseph Wee, MD, FRCR
Department of Radiation Oncology, Division of Clinical Trials and Epidemiological Sciences, The Humphrey Oei Institute of Cancer Research, National Cancer Center, 11 Hospital Drive, Singapore 169610 , Republic of Singapore

13.1 Introduction

When Al-Sarraf et al. (1996) presented the preliminary results of the U. S. Intergroup 0099 Trial at the plenary session of the 1996 Annual Meeting of the American Society of Clinical Oncology (ASCO), it signaled the advent of a new era in head and neck oncology and a paradigm shift in the role of chemotherapy as an adjunct to radiation therapy (RT) in the curative management of head and neck cancer, nasopharyngeal cancer (NPC) in particular. Today, concurrent chemoradiation therapy is considered a standard of care for all patients with locally advanced NPC worldwide (NCCN 2008; Chan and Felip 2008).

Radiation therapy has been used to treat head and neck cancers since the early twentieth century, when the first patient with laryngeal cancer was successfully treated with radiation. New (1922) first described the use of radium for the treatment of NPC, but it was not until the advent of cobalt teletherapy and the linear accelerator that the treatment of NPC improved dramatically. Fletcher and Million (1965) recognized the better radiosensitivity of NPC when compared with the other squamous cell carcinomas of the head and neck (SCCHN).

Chemotherapy has been used in conjunction with radiation to improve local control or to reduce distant failure. As the nasopharynx lies in proximity to many critical organs, there may be a limit to the tolerance of normal tissue to radiation therapy. But the addition of chemotherapy with a different toxicity profile may overcome this limitation and the combination may also enhance the radiation response. Chemoradiation therapy may also reduce long-term treatment morbidity, by reducing the dose of radiation required for local control or the use of mutilating surgery. On the other hand, chemoradiation therapy may also be associated with enhanced treatment morbidity such as reduced swallowing function. Furthermore, chemotherapy may also have an effect on microscopic distant metastases, thus improving the distant control rates (ADELSTEIN et al. 1997; WEE et al. 2005).

13.2 Historical Perspective

NPC is a very radiosensitive tumor. Radiation therapy alone can produce high cure rates for those with early stage (stage I and II) disease. However, for those with locoregionally advanced stage III and IV NPC, many still suffer local and distant failure.

NPC is also sensitive to chemotherapy. Patients for whom the tumor recurs after radiation therapy can still achieve high response rates with systemic chemotherapy. Cisplatin-containing regimens appear to be superior to noncisplatin regimens. The Wayne State regimen of cisplatin and 5-FU (KISH et al. 1982) achieved a 90% response rate when used in a group of patients with advanced SCCHN and quickly became the gold standard regimen for head and neck cancers. In a subsequent trial on NPC patients, AL-KOURAINY et al. (1988) reported a 75% overall response rate (with 50% being complete responders) with an induction regimen of cisplatin and 5-FU. Similar results have also been achieved in patients with recurrent or metastatic NPC in the East (WANG and TAN 1991; AU and ANG 1994).

In the 1970s, cisplatin was also found to be synergistic with radiation (ZÁK and DROBNÍK 1971; WODINSKY et al. 1974; RICHMOND et al. 1977; DOUPLE and RICHMOND 1979). In a trial of head and neck cancers, the Radiation Therapy Oncology Group (RTOG) found that cisplatin when given concurrent with radiotherapy resulted in an overall response rate of 76% for all head and neck sites, but had a complete response rate of 98% in cancers that were nonkeratinizing (including NPC) (CRISSMAN et al. 1987).

These results prompted the RTOG to perform a Phase II trial of cisplatin concurrent with radiotherapy (RTOG 8117) (AL-SARRAF et al. 1990). Twenty-seven patients with stage III and IV NPC were treated with standard radiotherapy and cisplatin at a dose of 100 mg/m^2 was administered on Day 1 and repeated every 3 weeks for three cycles. All patients completed their radiotherapy (>64.5 Gy); 70% received the full three cycles of concurrent chemotherapy and 30% received two cycles. Twenty-four patients (89%) achieved a complete response (it was 100% for those with the undifferentiated histology). Twenty-six patients with stage IV disease were compared with 78 patients treated with radiotherapy alone in the RTOG database. The disease-free survival, overall survival, and distant metastases rates all appeared to be improved with the addition of chemotherapy; and it was concluded that a Phase III trial of chemoradiotherapy vs. radiaton therapy alone was warranted.

13.3 The US Intergroup 0099 Trial

As discussed in greater detail in Chapter 12, on 15 May, 1989, the Southwest Oncology Group (SWOG) together with the Eastern Cooperative Oncology Group (ECOG) and the RTOG in the United States activated a Phase III study of radiotherapy with or without concurrent cisplatin in patients with NPC (US Intergroup 0099).

At the first planned interim analysis, the Data and Safety Monitoring Committee reviewed the interim analysis and recommended that the trial be stopped and reported early. After elimination of ineligible patients, 147 (69 radiation therapy and 78 chemoradiation therapy) patients were considered for survival and toxicity analysis. The 3-year overall survival rate (OS) was 47% (radiation) vs. 78%, (chemoradiation) ($p = 0.005$) (AL-SARRAF et al. 1998). This difference was held up at 5 years when a subsequent report gave the 5-year overall survival rate as 37% vs. 67%, respectively ($p = 0.001$) (AL-SARRAF et al. 2001). The 3-year progression-free survival (PFS) was similarly improved and estimated at 26% (radiation) and 66% (chemoradiation), respectively ($p < 0.001$). There was also significant improvement in local, regional, and distant failure with chemoradiotherapy.

The percentage of patients who completed treatment was 73% in the chemoradiation therapy and 91% in the radiation therapy alone arm. Sixty-three percent of patients received all three cycles of cisplatin concurrent with radiotherapy and 55% received all three cycles of adjuvant chemotherapy. Half of those in the radiotherapy arm and 76% in the chemoradiotherapy arm developed severe (Grade 3 and 4) toxicity during the initial treatment. During the adjuvant phase, 53% developed severe (Grade 3 and 4) toxicity.

However, Intergroup 0099 was only one trial. In addition, concerns were rightly raised because of the large number of patients who were deemed "ineligible" because of "protocol violations" and the relatively high percentage of patients having keratinized lesions (Fu 1998).

13.4 Singapore, Hong Kong, and Guangzhou Trials

Based solely on the results of Intergroup 0099 study, there was hesitancy in adopting chemoradiation therapy as the standard of care in the endemic NPC regions of East Asia. Chan et al. (1998) summarized well the reservations. First, about a third of the patients in the Intergroup 0099 trial had WHO Type I histology, a subtype that had previously been shown to confer a worse prognosis (Hoppe et al. 1978; Shanmugaratnam et al. 1979); whereas in the East over 90% of patients have the endemic non-keratinizing form of NPC (i.e., WHO Types II and III). Second, the radiation technique used was relatively less aggressive with parapharyngeal boosts (Teo et al. 1989a) and brachytherapy (Teo et al. 1989b) being commonly administered as adjuncts for selected patients in the East. Third, the results observed in the radiotherapy alone arm of the 0099 study appeared inferior to those observed in Singapore (Heng et al. 1999) and Hong Kong patients (Lee et al. 1992).

Nevertheless, one could not ignore the remarkable results that the Intergroup 0099 trial had achieved. This resulted in several Phase III trials using the Al-Sarraf regimen being initiated in the endemic regions of East and Southeast Asia. The Singapore group conducted a Phase II trial of the Al-Sarraf regimen to observe the tolerability of this regimen in an Asian population (TAN et al. 1999). Fifty-seven patients were treated, 75% received all three cycles of cisplatin during the radiotherapy phase, and 63% received all three cycles of adjuvant chemotherapy. The protocol had acceptable tolerability and the group proceeded to a Phase III trial.

13.4.1 The Singapore Trial

The *Singapore trial*, SQNP01 (Wee et al. 2005) was activated in September 1997 and accrued 221 patients over the following 5½ years. The aim of the trial was to confirm the results of the Intergroup 0099 study and the applicability of that regimen to the endemic form of NPC. While the trial was essentially modeled after the Intergroup 0099 study there were some differences. Patients were staged according to the new American Joint Committee on Cancer/International Union Against Cancer (1997) Staging System (AJCC 1997). That meant that some tumors that would have been previously considered as stage III for the Intergroup 0099 trial, would now be labeled stage II disease and would thus not be considered eligible for this new study (e.g., patients with N1 disease). Patients also had to have the endemic, non-keratinizing histology (WHO Type II or III) and patients with WHO Type I were specifically excluded. Cisplatin was administered on a divided dose basis of 25 mg/m²/day over 4 days or at 30/30/40 mg/m²/day over 3 days on the first, fourth, and seventh weeks of radiation therapy. During the adjuvant phase, cisplatin was similarly given on a divided dose of 20 mg/m² over 4 days concurrent with 5-FU, which was given at a dose of 1,000 mg/m²/day for 4 days.

Seventy-nine (71%) of the 111 patients on the chemoradiation therapy arm received all three cycles of concurrent cisplatin. Six patients on this arm received less then 62 Gy to their primary tumor. Fifty-seven percent of patients received all three cycles of adjuvant chemotherapy and 35 patients (32%) did not receive any adjuvant treatment. The incidence of Grade 3 and 4 toxicity was higher in the chemoradiation arm, especially with respect to oropharyngeal mucositis, anorexia, emesis, and neutropenia. The 2-year distant metastases rate was 30% for the radiation therapy arm and 13% for the chemoradiotherapy arm. The 3-year disease-free survival (DFS) was also improved from 53% to 72% in the experimental arm. Similarly, the 3-year overall survival was also significantly improved from 65% (radiation therapy) to 80% with chemoradiation therapy. ($p = 0.0061$). Wee (2008) updated the results recently and with a median follow-up of 6.6 years, the distant metastases rate, DFS, and overall survival rates of the chemoradiotherapy arm all remain statistically significantly improved over the radiotherapy alone arm. The 5-year OS was 49% vs. 67% with a hazard ratio of 0.60 and p value of 0.0077 – all in favor of combined treatment..

13.4.2 The Hong Kong Trials

The Hong Kong Nasopharyngeal Cancer Study Group (HKNPCSG) took a slightly different approach in their trials. While their primary objective was to confirm the findings of the Intergroup 0099 study, they also took the opportunity to study the role of accelerated radiation therapy in improving local control in patients with T3–4 disease, but with early or no neck disease (N0–1), where local control was expected to be the major problem. Thus two parallel trials were conducted, the HK 99-01 trial for patients with T1-4N2-3M0 disease, and HK 99-02 for patients with T3-4N0-1M0 disease. This group also used the 1997 version of TNM (AJCC 1997) as their basis of staging and eligibility. The dose of radiation therapy dose was in general higher, as it was routine in Hong Kong to add a "parapharyngeal boost" when there was tumor extension laterally into the parapharyngeal space.

HK 99-01 (Lee et al. 2005a) accrued 348 patients from March 1999 to January 2004, 176 in the radiation therapy arm and 172 in the chemoradiation arm. About 40% of patients on both arms received a boost radiotherapy dose, and about half the patients on both arms were treated using 3D radiation techniques. Fifty-two percent of patients on the chemoradiation therapy arm received all three cycles of concurrent cisplatin and 76% received all three cycles of adjuvant chemotherapy. Patients on the chemoradiation arm suffered more severe acute toxicities (84% vs. 53%; $p < 0.001$) as well as late toxicities (28% vs. 13%; $p = 0.024$). The chemoradiation arm achieved significantly higher failure-free survival (FFS) (72% vs. 62% at 3-year, $p = 0.027$), mostly as a result of an improvement in locoregional control (92% vs. 82%, $p = 0.005$). However, distant control did not improve significantly (76% vs. 73%, $p = 0.47$), and the overall survival rates were almost identical (78% vs. 78%, $p = 0.97$).

The HKNPCSG subsequently published the results of over 2,500 consecutive patients (Lee et al. 2005b) treated with radiation therapy alone at all public oncology centers in Hong Kong during the period 1996–2000 and found similar 3-year overall survival rate (74%) to that achieved in the radiation therapy alone arm of the HK 99-01 trial (78%). The group concluded by questioning if the difference in the result of the HK 99-01 trial, compared with the results from both the Intergroup and Singapore trials, could be explained by improved radiation technology, which could have negated any potential benefit of chemotherapy.

HK 99-02 (Lee et al. 2006) the sister trial to HK 99-01 was a four arm study comparing radiation therapy vs. chemoradiation therapy and standard 5-fractions per week radiation vs. accelerated 6-fractions per week for patients who had T3-4N0-1M0 disease. A blocked randomization scheme was used to allocate patients in equal proportions to the four treatment arms. The accelerated fractionation scheme of 6-fractions per week was based on the Danish Head and Neck Cancer Study Group (DAHANCA) 6–7 Trials (Overgaard et al. 2003). One hundred and eighty-nine patients were accrued to this trial between 1999 and 2004 and the trial was terminated early because of slower than expected accrual. Prolongation of overall treatment time by more than 7 days occurred in 2% of the accelerated 6-fraction/week radiation alone arm and 5% of the accelerated 6-fraction/week chemoradiation arm. There was no difference in the proportion of patients who received all six cycles of chemotherapy (55% vs. 57%) in both the conventional and accelerated fractionation chemoradiation arms. Late toxicity, which just reached statistical significance, was greater in the accelerated fractionation chemo-RT arm when compared with the conventional fractionation RT alone arm (34% vs. 14%; $p = 0.05$). The majority of the toxicities were of Grade 3 severity and only 2% of late toxicities in the accelerated fractionation chemoradiation therapy arm were Grade 4.

At a median follow-up period was 2.9 years, significant improvement in FFS was achieved by the accelerated 6-fraction/week chemoradiation threapy regimen when compared with the conventional 5-fraction/week RT alone regimen (94% vs. 70% at 3 years, $p = 0.008$). Accelerated radiation therapy alone and conventional fractionation chemoradiation therapy did not produce any improvement in FFS when compared with the conventional fractionation radiation alone arm.

13.4.3 The Guangzhou Trial

The *Guangzhou Trial* was the fourth trial to test the Al-Sarraf regimen in an endemic NPC population. It accrued 316 patients between 2002 and 2005 (Chen et al. 2008). Similar to the other three trials, patients were staged according to the 1997 AJCC/TNM staging system (AJCC 1997), and only patients with the endemic form of NPC (WHO Type II and III) were eligible. Like the Hong Kong cohort, selected patients in this study were also routinely treated with a parapharyngeal boost. Unlike the other trials, cisplatin was given weekly at a dose of 40 mg/m^2 for 7 weeks during the radiotherapy phase and the adjuvant chemotherapy consisted of a combination of cisplatin (80 mg/m^2 intravenously) on Day 1 and 5-FU (800 mg/m^2 intravenously) on Days 1–5 by a 120-h infusion. Although the chemoradiotherapy group experienced significantly more acute toxicity (62.6% vs. 32%, $p = 0.000$), most patients completed therapy; a total of 107 patients (68%) and 97 patients (61%) completed all cycles of concurrent chemotherapy and adjuvant chemotherapy, respectively.

With a median follow-up time of 29 months, the 2-year overall survival rate (OS), FFS rate, distant failure-free survival rate (DFFS), and locoregional failure-free survival rate (LRFFS) for the chemoradiotherapy vs. radiotherapy alone groups significantly favored combined therapy: 89.8% vs. 79.7% ($p = 0.003$) for OS, 84.6% vs. 72.5% ($p = 0.001$) for FFS, 86.5% vs. 78.7% ($p = 0.024$) for DFFS, and 98.0% vs. 91.9% ($p = 0.007$) for LRFFS, respectively.

13.5 Other Asian Trials

13.5.1 The Chinese University of Hong Kong Trial

The Chinese University of Hong Kong (CUHK) group embarked on its chemoradiotherapy trial (Chan et al. 2002) on the basis of the significantly improved outcome observed in the French trial (Bachaud et al. 1991) of adjuvant postoperative concurrent weekly cisplatin-radiotherapy in patients with stage III and IV squamous cell head and neck cancer as well as the promising results from the RTOG Phase II trial of concurrent cisplatin-RT in NPC patients (RTOG 8117) (Al-Sarraf et al. 1990). The weekly cisplatin-RT regimen was chosen over the 3 weekly Al-Sarraf protocol because of the perceived better tolerance of the former. Three hundred and fifty patients were accrued between April 1994 and November 1999. Patients were accrued on the basis of their having advanced neck nodal disease by Ho's staging criteria (Ho 1978) (Ho's N2-3 or Ho's N1 with a node >4 cm). The primary tumor was treated to a dose of 66 Gy followed by a parapharyngeal boost in approximately 70% of patients on both arms. Systemic toxicity was more frequent in the chemoradiotherapy arm, but 78% of patients still completed at least four cycles of concurrent cisplatin during radiotherapy and there were no treatment-related deaths.

The 5-year overall survival rate was 58.6% (95% CI = 50.9%–66.2%) for the radiotherapy arm and 70.3% (95% CI = 63.4%–77.3%) for the chemoradiation therapy arm (Chan et al. 2005a). There was, however, no statistically significant difference in local-regional control or distant failure between the two groups.

13.5.2 The Guangzhou Oxaliplatin Trial

Oxaliplatin, a platinum analog, has less renal and GI toxicity than cisplatin and a better myelosuppressive profile when compared with carboplatin. The main dose-limiting toxicity of oxaliplatin is sensory neuropathy. There is also some clinical evidence of synergism between oxaliplatin and radiation (Freyer et al. 2001; McMullen and Blackstock 2002). In this trial reported by investigators from Guangzhou, China, oxaliplatin, which was administered at a dose of 70 mg/m^2 weekly for six doses from the first day of radiation therapy , was used to substitute cisplatin (Zhang et al. 2005). A total of 115 patients were randomized between January 2001 to January 2003 (56 to chemoradiation therapy and 59 to chemoradiation therapy). Patients with AJCC 1997 Stage III and IV (M0) NPC were deemed eligible. Radiation therapy to the primary was intended to be 70–74 Gy with an optional boost for selected patients. All patients had the endemic form (WHO Type II or III) of NPC. Compliance with the protocol was excellent and 97% of patients completed all planned doses of radiotherapy and chemotherapy. Of significance, there was no Grade 4 toxicity in either arm on this regimen. Grade 3 toxicity that occurred in the chemoradiotherapy arm (about 39% overall) was mainly skin or mucosal associated toxicity. The peripheral neuropathy in the combined chemoradiation arm was reversible. With a median follow-up time of 24 months, the overall survival, relapse-free survival, and metastases-free survival were all significantly improved in favor of the chemoradiation arm. The 2-year overall survival rate was 100% (chemoradiation) vs. 77% (radiation alone) ($p = 0.01$); 2-year metastases-free survival was 92 (chemoradiation) vs. 80% (radiation alone) ($p = 0.02$), and the 2-year relapse-free survival was 96% (chemoradiation) vs. 83% (radiation alone) ($p = 0.02$).

13.5.3 The Taiwan: Veterans General Hospital Trial

The Taiwan Veterans General group chose a combination of cisplatin and 5-FU to be administered concurrently with radiotherapy. The two drugs were selected because both drugs had chemotherapeutic as well as radiosensitizing properties. An initial pilot study involving 19 patients with Stage 4 NPC achieved a 100% complete response rate and 3-year overall and disease-free survival rates of 89.5% and 83.3%, respectively (Lin et al. 1997). This spurred the team on to embark on a Phase III trial (Lin et al. 2003). This trial accrued 284 patients between December 1993 and April 1999. Patients were staged according to the 1988 AJCC/TNM staging system (AJCC 1988) and were eligible if they had stage III or IV and M0 disease. Radiotherapy to a dose of 70–74 Gy in 7–8 weeks was administered in both arms. Chemotherapy consisted of cisplatin at 20 mg/m^2/day and 5-FU at 400 mg/m^2/day as a 96-h infusion for 4 days on weeks 1 and 5 of radiotherapy in the experimental arm. Nine patients did not receive the second cycle of chemotherapy and another nine had their chemotherapy delayed by >1 week. The toxicity in the chemoradiotherapy arm was more severe than that of the radiotherapy alone arm, but was less than that of the chemoradiotherapy arm of Intergroup 0099 trial.

The 5-year overall survival rate was significantly improved from 54.2% in the radiotherapy alone arm to 72.3% in the chemoradiation therapy arm ($p = 0.0022$). Similarly, the 5-year progression-free survival rates were 71.6% for the chemoradiation group when compared with 53.0% for the radiation-only group ($p = 0.0012$). Chemoradiation therapy had also appeared to improve local-regional control and distant control, although the differences just failed to achieve statistical significance.

13.5.4 The Hong Kong Queen Mary Hospital Trial

The Queen Mary group launched a 2 × 2 factorial study based on the hypothesis that concurrent chemotherapy would improve local control and that adjuvant chemotherapy would tackle microscopic distant metastases. Patients were first randomized to receive radiation therapy alone or concurrent chemoradiation therapy and then a second randomization after completion of radiation therapy or chemoradiation therapy to determine if adjuvant chemotherapy would or would not be given. The drug used during the radiation phase was the 5-FU prodrug UFT (uracil and tegafur in a 4:1 molar ratio) at a dose of 200 mg three times a day, 7 days a week for the duration of radiation therapy. Previous studies had shown that UFT can simulate continuous infusion 5-FU and enhance the antineoplastic effect of 5-FU while reducing the side effects attributed to 5-FU catabolism (Taguchi 1997). Although there was not a lot of data about the use of UFT in NPC when the study was first conceived, 5-FU was well known to have chemotherapeutic effects on NPC and was also known to have radiosensitization properties. Oral administration also made UFT an attractive alternative to cisplatin radiosensitization. During the adjuvant phase, an alternating regimen of cisplatin-5-FU (PF) and VBM (vincristine, bleomycin, and methotrexate) was given every 3 weeks for a total of six cycles. Both combinations (Al-Kourainy et al. 1988, Hill et al. 1987) are known to have activity in NPC and the group was following the principles of the Goldie Coldman hypothesis (Goldie and Coldman 1979) and aimed to reduce the development of drug resistance and toxicity of individual chemotherapeutic agents, as well as to maximize the additive effects of different effective cytotoxic drugs. Patients accrued had Ho's staging T3 or N2–3 or N1 with LN >4 cm. The primary tumor received at least 68 Gy and selected patients received a 10 Gy boost.

Between May 1995 and October 2001, a total of 222 patients were recruited of whom 219 were included in the final analysis. The preliminary results were published in 2004 (Kwong et al. 2004) and the final 7-year results were presented at ASCO in 2008 (Kwong et al. 2008). Concurrent chemoradiation therapy using UFT significantly reduced distant metastases and disease failure. The 7-year distant metastases-free survival was 68.6% (radiation) vs. 82.9% (chemoradiation) ($p = 0.014$) and the 7-year failure-free survival was 52.4% (radiation) vs. 66.6% (chemoradiation) ($p = 0.016$). The 7-year disease-specific survival was 68.9% (radiation) vs. 78.6% (chemoradiation), but this just missed statistical significance ($p = 0.057$). Local control was not improved with concurrent chemoradiation therapy. None of these parameters were improved with adjuvant chemotherapy. The group postulated that a potential action of concurrent UFT could be the antiangiogenic effect from its metronomic scheduling resulting in a reduction in distant metastases. One potential reason why adjuvant chemotherapy did not work in this study could be attributed to alternating the chemotherapy drug such that their relative dose intensity was compromised.

13.5.5 The Thai Noninferiority Trial of Cisplatin vs. Carboplatin

The Thai group (Chitapanarux et al. 2007) randomized 206 locally advanced NPC tumors to receive either cisplatin or carboplatin concurrent with radiotherapy in their Phase III non-inferiority trial. In the cisplatin arm, 59% of patients completed concurrent chemoradiotherapy and 42% completed three cycles of adjuvant chemotherapy. On the carboplatin arm, 73% completed concurrent treatment and 70% adjuvant therapy. As expected, there was more renal toxicity, leucopenia, and anemia in the cisplatin group, and more thrombocytopenia in the carboplatin arm. The 3-year DFS rates were 63.4% for the cisplatin group and 60.9% for the carboplatin group ($p = 0.9613$) (HR 0.70, 95% confidence interval (CI): 0.50–0.98). The 3-year overall survival rates were 77.7% and 79.2% for cisplatin and carboplatin groups, respectively ($p = 0.9884$) (HR 0.83, 95% CI: 0.63–1.010). It would thus appear from this trial that carboplatin was not significantly worse than cisplatin when used in conjunction with radiotherapy in the curative treatment of NPC. This result must, however, be viewed with some caution as they appear to differ from the results of most other trials comparing cisplatin and carboplatin in other malignancies. A small retrospective study from Hong Kong of stage IVb NPC patients receiving platinum analogs undergoing induction-concurrent accelerated chemoradiation therapy had also reported a poorer outcome with the use of carboplatin (Yau et al. 2006).

13.6 Unresolved Issues

To date, there are six trials for patients with locally advanced NPC (Table 13.1), which have demonstrated a statistically significant overall survival benefit asso ciated with the addition of chemotherapy to radiationtherapy. All six trials have a concurrent chemotherapy component and all use a platinum analog as one of the chemotherapy drugs. There have also been four meta-analysis examining the addition of chemotherapy to radiation therapy for NPC (Huncharek and Kupelnick 2002; Langendijk et al. 2004; Baujat et al. 2006; Yang et al. 2008). All four meta-analyses showed that the beneficial effect of chemotherapy occurred when chemotherapy was administered concurrent with radiation. Today, concurrent chemoradiation therapy needs to be considered the standard of care for the treatment of locally advanced NPC all over the world (NCCN 2008; Chan and Felip 2008). Yet, a few outstanding issues remain.

13.6.1 Stage II Nasopharyngeal Cancer

When both the U. S. Intergroup 0099 and Taiwan Veterans General Trials were being conducted, the AJCC TNM system in use was that of the fourth edition (AJCC 1988). By the time the Singapore, Hong Kong, and Guangzhou trials were conceived, the TNM staging system for NPC had evolved and the AJCC had come out with a fifth edition. Some patients who would be classified as "stage III" (for example – those with N1 nodes) in the fourth edition AJCC would now become classified as "stage II" under the fourth edition AJCC. The current U. S. National Comprehensive Cancer Network (NCCN) guidelines (NCCN 2008) recommend that patients with N1 disease should be treated with chemoradiation therapy, whereas in many centers in the endemic regions, patients with stage II NPC continue to receive radiation therapy alone. stage I (T1N0) NPC patients have 5-year survival rates approaching 90% or better. stage II (T2a-2bN1) patients have a poorer survival of approximately 75% (Heng et al. 1999; Chua et al. 2001). The Singapore group also found that patients with T2b NPC receiving intensity modulated radiation therapy (IMRT) alone appeared to do worse when compared with patients with T3 NPC who received chemotherapy in concurrent with IMRT (Tham et al. 2009). This group represents 30%–39% of all endemic NPC patients. Several workers believe that the cure rate of this group can be improved with the addition of systemic therapy (Cheng et al. 2000; Chua et al. 2006). A 12% improvement at 5 years in overall survival was observed in a Hong Kong study (Chua et al. 2006). However, current cisplatin-containing regimens exact a significant toxicity cost, with nearly 50% of patients experiencing greater than Grade 3 acute toxicity.

One strategy some groups are considering in this cohort of patients is the use of "metronomic" scheduling of chemotherapy concurrent with radiation therapy. Experimental studies have suggested that frequent administration of certain cytotoxic agents at low doses, known as "metronomic" chemotherapy, increases the antiangiogenic activity of the drugs (Browder et al. 2000; Klement et al. 2000). As a therapeutic strategy, antiangiogenesis appears to be gaining in popularity and bevacizumab, an anti-angiogenic agent, has been successfully tested in colon, lung, and breast cancers (Hurwitz et al. 2004; Sandler et al. 2006; Millver et al. 2007). Most of the newer multi-targeted agents also have anti-angiogenesis as one of their therapeutic targets. Willett et al. (2004) has also shown that bevacizumab combined with chemoradiation therapy was feasible and had acceptable toxicity.

While there have been no randomized trials of metronomic chemotherapy, previous experiences with metronomic-like scheduling of drugs have been shown

Table 13.1. Randomized trials of concurrent chemo-radiotherapy for nasopharyngeal cancer

Trial	Duration	Eligibility	Regimen	No
Intergroup 0099	May 89–Dec 95	Fourth AJCC	RT	69
		Stage3, 4	ddp-RT→ ddp/5-FU	78
SQNP01 (Singapore)	Sept 97–May 03	Fifth AJCC	RT	110
		Stage 3, 4	ddp-RT→ ddp/5-FU	111
HK9901 (Hong Kong)	March 99–Jan 04	Fifth AJCC	RT	176
		Any T, N2-3	ddp-RT→ ddp/5-FU	172
HK9902 (Hong Kong)	July 99–Apr 04	Fifth AJCC	RT	
		T3,4; N0-1	ddp-RT→ ddp/5-FU	
			accel-RT	
			ddp-accel-RT→ ddp/5-FU	
Guangzhou	July 02–Sept 05	Fifth AJCC	RT	158
		Stage III, IV	Weekly ddp-RT→ ddp/5-FU	158
VGH(Taiwan)	Dec 93–April 99	Fourth AJCC	RT	143
			ddp/5-FU-RT	141
CUHK	Apr 94–Nov 99	Ho's	RT	176
			Weekly-ddp-RT	174
Guangzhou	Jan 01–Jan 03		RT	56
			Weekly-oxa-RT	59
Queen Mary (HK)	May 95–Oct 01	Ho's	RT	109
			CRT	110
			No AC	108
			AC	111

RT radiation therapy; CRT chemoradiation therapy; AC accelerated radiation therapy; ddp cisplatin; oxa oxaliplatin

to be superior to conventional scheduling. The European Organisation for Research and Treatment of Cancer (EORTC) trial of Classical CMF vs. bolus CMF is one such example (Engelsman et al. 1991), and meta-analyses has shown that 5-FU by continuous infusion is superior to bolus administration (Meta-Analysis Group in Cancer 1998). There have also been previous reported trials utilizing a "metronomic-like" scheduling with daily cisplatin at 6 mg/m² concurrent with standard and hyperfractionation radiotherapy,

Overall survival			Disease-free survival			Distant metastasis		
2 year	3year	5year	2 year	3year	5year	2 year	3year	5year
	47	37		26	29			
	78	67		66	58			
	$p = 0.005$	$p = 0.001$		$p < 0.001$	$p < 0.001$			
78	65	49	57	53	46			
85	80	67	75	72	59			
		$p = 0.0077$			$p = 0.0318$			
	78			62			73	
	78			72			76	
	$p = 0.97$			$p = 0.027$			$p = 0.47$	
	83			68			81	
	87			73			89	
	73			63			77	
	88			88			97	
	$p = 0.65$			$p = 0.061$			$p = 0.029$	
79.7			72.5			78.7		
89.8			84.6			86.5		
$p = 0.003$			$p = 0.001$			$p = 0.024$		
		54.2			53			69.9
		72.3			71.6			78.7
		$p = 0.0022$			$p = 0.0012$			$p = 0.0577$
		58.6	69		52.1			
		70.3	76		60.2			
		$p = 0.049$	$p = 0.1$		$p = 0.16$			
77			83			80		
100			96			92		
$p = 0.01$			$p = 0.02$			$p = 0.02$		
		72.5			54.3			70.7
		80.5			67.7			84.1
		78.5			61.3			78.5
		74.6			60.8			74.6

and all with reported success in both non-small cell lung (Schaake-Koning et al. 1992) and squamous cell carcinoma of the head and neck (Jeremic et al. 1997, 2000). Fu et al. (1987) also reported improved local control as well as relapse-free survival in a trial of twice weekly low-dose bleomycin (5 mg twice weekly to a total of 70 mg) concurrent with standard radiotherapy in SCCHN. Kwong et al. (2008) from Hong Kong have also reported that administering daily oral UFT concurrent with RT has resulted in statistically significant improvements in overall disease-specific and DFSs in patients with locally advanced NPC.

The Singapore group has thus launched a Phase I-II trial looking at the potential role of metronomic oral cyclophosphamide concurrent with IMRT, while the Hong Kong group is considering using UFT concurrent with IMRT in their patients with stage II NPC.

13.6.2 The Difference in Outcomes Between the Hong Kong (HK 99-01) and Singapore (SQNP01) Trials

While both the Hong Kong (HK 99-01) and Singapore Trials appear superficially to be similar – similar types of patients, similar chemotherapy regimen – there are some fundamental differences between the two studies. The Singapore trial, which started earlier, used 2D radiation therapy techniques, whereas more than half of the Hong Kong patients were planned using 3D techniques; a sizable proportion received a parapharyngeal boost, whereas the boost was specifically prohibited in the Singapore protocol for fear of late morbidity, especially with the addition of chemotherapy. With further evidence of the reproducibility of their RT results in non-trial patients (Lee et al. 2005b), the HKNPCSG thus postulated that the reason for the difference could be attributed to the advent of improved radiotherapy technology, which might have negated the impact of chemotherapy.

A second possibility for the difference in outcomes could also be the shorter period of follow-up time for the cohort in the HK 99-01 trial, which was activated only in 1999. A similar situation occurred in the CUHK Trial, which also did not show any survival benefit when it was first reported in 2002 (Chan et al. 2002).

A third reason that might be advanced is related to the type of patients accrued in the trial. By restricting the eligibility criteria to only patients with the highest probability of distant failure, i.e., advanced N disease, the patients on the HK 99-01 trial might inevitably also have had the highest distant tumor burden for which the chemotherapy regimen being used may well be inadequate to handle. Evidence to support this hypothesis comes from two reports. The first by Lin et al. (2004), reanalyzing the data from the Taiwan Veteran's General Hospital Trial (see Sect. 13.5.3) – concluded that concurrent chemoradiotherapy was only effective in patients with early-stage disease and by definition – an expected lower distant tumor burden. The second report was by Chua et al. (2006) who performed subgroup analysis on two previous Phase III trials according to the T and N classifications, came to the same conclusion – that the induction chemotherapy in those two trials made a difference in only patients with early stage disease. The logical conclusion from these findings would suggest that more effective regimens would be required, and may have to be administered either before or after chemoradiotherapy, as it is unlikely that we can further increase the intensity of chemotherapy during the concurrent phase.

13.7 The Future

13.7.1 Multi-Agent Induction Chemotherapy Followed by Chemoradiotherapy

Recent trials in squamous cell head and neck cancers suggest that multiagent induction chemotherapy is superior to the standard cisplatin-5-FU doublet (Posner et al. 2007; Vermorken et al. 2007). Several trials in metastatic NPC also suggest that multiagent regimens may be superior to standard doublets (Siu et al. 1998; Hong et al. 1999; Fandi et al. 2000; Leong et al. 2005, 2008). However, most of these studies were Phase II trials with small sample sizes. Nevertheless, the findings previously that more intensive chemotherapy may be needed to tackle patients with higher distant tumor burden supports this line of investigation. Both the Taiwan and Singapore groups are currently conducting Phase III trials using multi-agent induction regimens followed by chemoradiotherapy ("MEPFL" [Mitomycin, Epirubicin, Platinum, 5-Flourouracil, Leucovorin] in Taiwan; and "GPC" [Gemcitabine, Paclitaxel, Carboplatin] in Singapore).

13.7.2 The Concurrent Use of Biological and Molecular Targeted Therapy

Preclinical studies have demonstrated that recombinant adenovirus-*p53* (rAd-*p53*) gene transduction restores *P53* function in cancer cells, and increases radiosensitivity of NPC cells in vitro and in vivo (Li et al. 1999, 2002). Clinical trials of adenoviral administration in squamous cell head and neck cancers have previously shown feasibility, tolerability, and potential for efficacy (Clayman et al. 1998, 1999). A small-randomized study of recombinant Adenovirus-*p53* (rAd-*p53*) combined with radiotherapy was performed in 42 NPC patients in China and compared with a control group of 40 patients treated with radiation therapy alone (Pan et al. 2009). Patients in this study received an intratumoral injection of rAd-*p53* at 1×10^{12} virus particles/mL once a week (on Friday) for 8 weeks per tumor via naso-endoscopic guidance or through an ultrasound-guided injection for neck nodes. Patients on both arms were treated to a tumor dose of 70 Gy. Adverse effects of the rAd-*p53* administration were minimal. Eighty-one percent of patients in the experimental arm developed a mild and transient fever. At 2 months post radiation therapy, the complete response rate of the group receiving rAd-*p53* combined with radiation was 2.73 times that of the group receiving radiation alone (66.7% vs. 24.4%; $p = 0.01$). After 6 years of follow-up, there was statistically significant difference in 5-year local-regional failure rate (2.7% vs. 28% $p = 0.002$), but there was no difference in overall or disease-free survivals or distant metastases rates.

NPC is known to overexpress EGFR, COX-2, VEGF, and iNOS (Soo et al. 2005). Newer agents specifically target these molecular markers and some of these agents have already made their way to the clinic.

Cetuximab, a monoclonal antibody that targets the EGFR receptor, has been shown to improve survival when administered in conjunction with radiotherapy in squamous cell head and neck cancer (Bonner et al. 2006). In NPC, one study has demonstrated that cetuximab inhibits the growth of NPC cell-lines HK1 and HONE-1 (Sung et al. 2005). The CUHK group then proceeded to perform a Phase II trial of cetuximab–cisplatin concurrent with IMRT in patients with locally advanced NPC in a curative setting (Ma et al. 2008a). Grade 3 mucosal toxicities were common but manageable, and the cohort had an 83% complete response rate and a 17% partial response rate when evaluated 3 months post radiotherapy.

A small Phase II randomized trial of a humanized anti-EGFR monoclonal antibody h-R3 administered concurrent with radiotherapy vs. radiotherapy alone was performed in China. While the initial complete response rate was significantly higher in the experimental arm, longer follow-up did not reveal any significant differences in 3-year locoregional control, distant metastasis-free survival, and overall survival rates between the two groups (Wu et al. 2007).

The tyrosine kinase inhibitor, Gefitinib, was investigated in a group of heavily pretreated recurrent NPC patients (Ma et al. 2008b). No objective response was seen, and three patients had stable disease for up to 8.5 months. The study was terminated prematurely at the first stage after 15 patients were accrued. Another trial of sorafinib (Elser et al. 2007), a multi-targeted agent, also did not reveal any activity in recurrent or metastatic NPC patients

In head and neck squamous cell carcinoma, meta-analysis has shown that positive VEGF staining was associated with an almost twofold higher risk of death at 2 years (Kyzas et al. 2005). In NPC, VEGF has been shown to play an important role in lymph node metastasis through the induction of angiogenesis (Wakisaka et al. 1999). Overexpression of VEGF was seen in 67% of nasopharyngeal cases and the higher expression of VEGF related to higher rate of recurrence, nodal positivity, and lower survival (Krishna et al. 2006). A recent pilot study by Druzgal et al (2005). analyzed the pre- and post-treatment serum levels of angiogenesis factors as markers for outcome in patients with head and neck cancer. With a median follow-up of 37 months, patients were more likely to remain disease-free when the VEGF level decreased post-treatment vs. those who continued to have increased VEGF levels after treatment. In this study, 7% of the patients had nasopharyngeal carcinoma. The RTOG is currently evaluating the current use of bevacizumab with chemoradiotherapy in a Phase II setting.

13.8 Conclusion

The growing number of trials that have been conducted in a wide variety of locations, including a considerable variation in patient selection, precise details of therapy delivered and selection of endpoints measured leave little doubt that the addition of chemotherapy concurrent with radiation therapy has improved the outcomes of patients with NPC. Improvements in radiation treatment technology and the adoption of IMRT has also improved local control and reduced morbidity. The incorporation of new drugs as well as the new targeted agents is currently under intense investigation and there is reason to believe that it will further improve treatment outcomes. In the horizon are immunotherapeutic strategies, and other treatments targeting the Epstein–Barr virus and the NPC epigenome (Tao and Chan 2007). With this proliferation of treatment possibilities, there is potential that NPC will become a highly curable malignancy in the near future.

References

Adelstein DJ, Saxton JP, Lavertu P, et al (1997) A phase III randomized trial comparing concurrent chemotherapy and radiotherapy with radiotherapy alone in resectable stage III and IV squamous cell head and neck cancer: preliminary results. Head Neck 19(7):567–575

American Joint Committee on Cancer (AJCC) (1988) Manual for staging cancer, 4th edn. JP Lippincott, Philadelphia

American Joint Committee on Cancer (AJCC) (1997) Manual for staging cancer, 5th edn. JP Lippincott, Philadelphia

Al-Kourainy K, Crissman J, Ensley J, et al (1988) Excellent response to cis-platinum-based chemotherapy in patients with recurrent or previously untreated advanced nasopharyngeal carcinoma. Am J Clin Oncol 11(4):427–430

Al-Sarraf M, Pajak TF, Cooper JS, et al (1990) Chemoradiotherapy in patients with locally advanced nasopharyngeal carcinoma: a Radiation Therapy Oncology Group study. J Clin Oncol 8(8):1342–1351

Al-Sarraf M, LeBlanc M, Giri PG, et al (1996) Superiority of chemoradiotherapy (CT-radiotherapy) vs radiotherapy (radiotherapy) in patients (pts) with locally advanced nasopharyngeal cancer (NPC). Preliminary results of intergroup (0099) (SWOG 8892, RTOG 8817, ECOG 2388) randomized study. Proc Am Soc Clin Oncol 15: Abstract 882

Al-Sarraf M, LeBlanc M, Giri PG, et al (1998) Chemoradiotherapy versus radiotherapy in patients with advanced nasopharyngeal cancer: phase III randomized intergroup study 0099. J Clin Oncol 16(4):1310–1317

Al-Sarraf M, LeBlanc M, Giri PG, et al (2001) Superiority of five year survival with chemoradiotherapy (CT-radiotherapy) vs radiotherapy in patients (Pts) with locally advanced nasopharyngeal cancer (NPC). Intergroup (0099) (SWOG 8892, RTOG 8817, ECOG 2388) phase III study: final report. Proc Am Soc Clin Oncol 20:Abstract 905

Au E, Ang PT (1994) A phase II trial of 5-fluorouracil and cisplatinum in recurrent or metastatic nasopharyngeal carcinoma. Ann Oncol 5(1):87–89

Bachaud JM, David JM, Boussin G, et al (1991) Combined postoperative radiotherapy and weekly cisplatin infusion for locally advanced squamous cell carcinoma of the head and neck: preliminary report of a randomized trial. Int J Radiat Oncol Biol Phys 20(2):243–246

Baujat B, Audry H, Bourhis J, et al;MAC-NPC Collaborative Group (2006) Chemotherapy in locally advanced nasopharyngeal carcinoma: an individual patient data meta-analysis of eight randomized trials and 1753 patients. Int J Radiat Oncol Biol Phys 64(1):47–56

Bonner JA, Harari PM, Giralt J, et al (2006 Feb) Radiotherapy plus cetuximab for squamous-cell carcinoma of the head and neck. N Engl J Med. 9;354(6):567–78

Browder T, Butterfield CE, Kräling BM, et al (2000) Antiangiogenic scheduling of chemotherapy improves efficacy against experimental drug-resistant cancer. Cancer Res 60(7):1878–1886

Chan AT, Teo PM, Johnson PJ (1998) Controversies in the management of locoregionally advanced nasopharyngeal carcinoma. Curr Opin Oncol 10:219–225

Chan AT, Teo PM, Ngan RK, et al (2002) Concurrent chemotherapy-radiotherapy compared with radiotherapy alone in locoregionally advanced nasopharyngeal carcinoma: progression-free survival analysis of a phase III randomized trial. J Clin Oncol 20(8):2038–2044

Chan AT, Leung SF, Ngan RK, et al (2005a) Overall survival after concurrent cisplatin-radiotherapy compared with radiotherapy alone in locoregionally advanced nasopharyngeal carcinoma. J Natl Cancer Inst 97(7):536–539

Chan AT, Hsu MM, Goh BC, et al (2005b) Multicenter, phase II study of cetuximab in combination with carboplatin in patients with recurrent or metastatic nasopharyngeal. J Clin Oncol 23(15):3568–3576

Chan AT, Felip E; ESMO Guidelines Working Group (2008) Nasopharyngeal cancer: ESMO clinical recommendations for diagnosis, treatment and follow-up. Ann Oncol 19(Suppl 2): ii81–2

Chen Y, Liu MZ, Liang SB, et al (2008) Preliminary results of a prospective randomized trial comparing concurrent chemoradiotherapy plus adjuvant chemotherapy with radiotherapy alone in patients with locoregionally advanced nasopharyngeal carcinoma in endemic regions of China. Int J Radiat Oncol Biol Phys 71(5):1356–1364

Cheng SH, Tsai SY, Yen KL, et al (2000) Concomitant radiotherapy and chemotherapy for early-stage nasopharyngeal carcinoma. J Clin Oncol 18(10):2040–2045

Chitapanarux I, Lorvidhaya V, Kamnerdsupaphon P, et al (2007) Chemoradiation comparing cisplatin versus carboplatin in locally advanced nasopharyngeal cancer: randomised, non-inferiority, open trial. Eur J Cancer 43(9): 1399–1406

Chua DT, Sham JS, Wei WI, et al (2001) The predictive value of the 1997 American Joint Committee on Cancer Stage Classification in determining failure patterns in nasopharyngeal carcinoma. Cancer 92(11):2845–2855

Chua DT, Ma J, Sham JS, et al (2006) Improvement of survival after addition of induction chemotherapy to radiotherapy in patients with early-stage nasopharyngeal carcinoma: subgroup analysis of two phase III trials. Int J Radiat Oncol Biol Phys 65(5):1300–1306

Clayman GL, El-Naggar AK, Lippman SM, et al (1998) Adenovirus-mediated p53 gene transfer in patients with advanced recurrent head and neck squamous cell carcinoma. J Clin Oncol 16:2221–2232

Clayman GL, Frank DK, Bruso PA, et al (1999) Adenovirus-mediated wild-type p53 gene transfer as a surgical adjuvant in advanced head and neck cancers. Clin Cancer Res 5:1715–1722

Crissman JD, Pajak TF, Zarbo RJ, et al (1987) Improved response and survival to combined cisplatin and radiation in non-keratinizing squamous cell carcinomas of the head and neck. An RTOG study of 114 advanced stage tumors. Cancer 59(8):1391–1397

Douple EB, Richmond RC (1979) A review of platinum complex biochemistry suggests a rationale for combined platinum-radiotherapy. Int J Radiat Oncol Biol Phys 5(8): 1335–1339

Druzgal CH, Chen Z, Yeh NT, et al (2005) A pilot study of longitudinal serum cytokine and angiogenesis factor levels as markers of therapeutic response and survival in patients with head and neck squamous cell carcinoma. Head Neck 27(9):771–784

Elser C, Siu LL, Winquist E, et al (2007) Phase II trial of sorafenib in patients with recurrent or metastatic squamous cell carcinoma of the head and neck or nasopharyngeal carcinoma. J Clin Oncol 25(24):3766–3773

Engelsman E, Klijn JC, Rubens RD, et al (1991) "Classical" CMF versus a 3-weekly intravenous CMF schedule in postmenopausal patients with advanced breast cancer. An EORTC Breast Cancer Co-operative Group Phase III Trial (10808). Eur J Cancer 27(8):966–970

Fandi A, Bachouchi M, Azli N, et al (2000) Long-term disease-free survivors in metastatic undifferentiated carcinoma of nasopharyngeal type. J Clin Oncol 18(6):1324–1330

Fletcher GH, Million RR (1965) Malignant tumours of the nasopharynx. Am J Roentgenol Radium Ther Nucl Med 93:44–55

Freyer G, Bossard N, Romestaing P, et al (2001) Addition of oxaliplatin to continuous fluorouracil, l-folinic acid, and concomitant radiotherapy in rectal cancer: the Lyon R 97-03 phase I trial. J Clin Oncol 19(9):2433–2438

Fu KK, Phillips TL, Silverberg IJ, et al (1987) Combined radiotherapy and chemotherapy with bleomycin and methotrexate for advanced inoperable head and neck cancer: update of a Northern California Oncology Group randomized trial. J Clin Oncol 5(9):1410–1418

Fu KK (1998) Combined radiotherapy and chemotherapy for nasopharyngeal carcinoma. Semin Radiat Oncol 8(4): 247–253

Goldie JH, Coldman AJ (1979) A mathematic model for relating the drug sensitivity of tumors to their spontaneous mutation rate. Cancer Treat Rep 63(11–12):1727–1733

Heng DM, Wee J, Fong KW, et al (1999) Prognostic factors in 677 patients in Singapore with nondisseminated nasopharyngeal carcinoma. Cancer 86(10):1912–1920

Hill BT, Price LA, MacRae KD (1987) The promising role of safe initial non-cisplatin-containing combination chemotherapy in nasopharyngeal tumors. Cancer Invest 5(6): 517–522

Ho JH (1978) An epidemiologic and clinical study of nasopharyngeal carcinoma. Int J Radiat Oncol Biol Phys 4(3–4): 182–198

Hong RL, Sheen TS, Ko JY, et al (1999) Induction with mitomycin C, doxorubicin, cisplatin and maintenance with weekly 5-fluorouracil, leucovorin for treatment of metastatic nasopharyngeal carcinoma: a phase II study. Br J Cancer 80(12):1962–1967

Hoppe RT, Williams J, Warnke R, et al (1978) Carcinoma of the nasopharynx – the significance of histology. Int J Radiat Oncol Biol Phys 4(3–4):199–205

Huncharek M, Kupelnick B (2002) Combined chemoradiation versus radiation therapy alone in locally advanced nasopharyngeal carcinoma: results of a meta-analysis of 1,528 patients from six randomized trials. Am J Clin Oncol 25(3): 219–223

Hurwitz H, Fehrenbacher L, Novotny W, et al (2004) Bevacizumab plus irinotecan, fluorouracil, and leucovorin for metastatic colorectal cancer. N Engl J Med 350(23): 2335–2342

International NPC Study Group (1996) Preliminary results of a randomized trial comparing neoadjuvant chemotherapy (cisplatin, epirubicin, bleomycin) plus radiotherapy vs. radiotherapy alone in stage IV(> or = N2, M0) undifferentiated nasopharyngeal carcinoma: a positive effect on progression-free survival. International Nasopharynx Cancer Study Group. VUMCA I trial. Int J Radiat Oncol Biol Phys 35(3):463–469

Jeremic B, Shibamoto Y, Stanisavljevic B, et al (1997) Radiation therapy alone or with concurrent low-dose daily either cisplatin or carboplatin in locally advanced unresectable squamous cell carcinoma of the head and neck: a prospective randomized trial. Radiother Oncol 43(1):29–37

Jeremic B, Shibamoto Y, Milicic B, et al (2000) Hyperfractionated radiation therapy with or without concurrent low-dose daily cisplatin in locally advanced squamous cell carcinoma of the head and neck: a prospective randomized trial. J Clin Oncol 18(7):1458–1464

Kish J, Drelichman A, Jacobs J, et al (1982) Clinical trial of cisplatin and 5-FU infusion as initial treatment for advanced squamous cell carcinoma of the head and neck. Cancer Treat Rep 66(3):471–474

Klement G, Baruchel S, Rak J, et al (2000) Continuous low-dose therapy with vinblastine and VEGF receptor-2 antibody induces sustained tumor regression without overt toxicity. J Clin Invest 105(8):R15–24

Krishna SM, James S, Balaram P (2006) Expression of VEGF as prognosticator in primary nasopharyngeal cancer and its relation to EBV status. Virus Res 115(1):85–90

Kwong DL, Sham JS, Au GK, et al (2004) Concurrent and adjuvant chemotherapy for nasopharyngeal carcinoma: a factorial study. J Clin Oncol 22(14):2643–2653

Kwong DL, Sham JS, Au GK, et al (2008) Long-term results of concurrent and adjuvant chemotherapy for advanced nasopharyngeal carcinoma. J Clin Oncol 26:Abstract 6056

Kyzas PA, Cunha IW, Ionnidis JPA (2005) Prognostic significance of vascular endothelial growth factor immunohistochemical expression in head and neck squamous cell carcinoma: a meta-analysis. Clin Cancer Res 11(4): 1434–1440

Langendijk JA, Leemans CR, Buter J, et al (2004) The additional value of chemotherapy to radiotherapy in locally advanced nasopharyngeal carcinoma: a meta-analysis of the published literature. J Clin Oncol 22(22):4604–4612

Lee AW, Poon YF, Foo W, et al (1992) Retrospective analysis of 5037 patients with nasopharyngeal carcinoma treated during 1976–1985: overall survival and patterns of failure. Int J Radiat Oncol Biol Phys 23(2):261–270

Lee AW, Lau WH, Tung SY, et al; Hong Kong Nasopharyngeal Cancer Study Group (2005a) Preliminary results of a randomized study on therapeutic gain by concurrent chemotherapy for regionally-advanced nasopharyngeal carcinoma: NPC-9901 Trial by the Hong Kong Nasopharyngeal Cancer Study Group. J Clin Oncol 23(28): 6966–6975

Lee AW, Sze WM, Au JS, et al (2005b) Treatment results for nasopharyngeal carcinoma in the modern era: the Hong Kong experience. Int J Radiat Oncol Biol Phys 61(4): 1107–1116

Lee AW, Tung SY, Chan AT, et al (2006) Preliminary results of a randomized study (NPC-9902 trial) on therapeutic gain by concurrent chemotherapy and/or accelerated fractionation for locally advanced nasopharyngeal carcinoma. Int J Radiat Oncol Biol Phys 66(1):142–151

Leong SS, Wee J, Tay MH, et al (2005) Paclitaxel, carboplatin, and gemcitabine in metastatic nasopharyngeal carcinoma: a phase II trial using a triplet combination. Cancer 103(3): 569–575

Leong SS, Wee J, Rajan S, et al (2008) Triplet combination of gemcitabine, paclitaxel, and carboplatin followed by maintenance 5-fluorouracil and folinic acid in patients with metastatic nasopharyngeal carcinoma. Cancer 114(6): 1332–1337

Li JH, Lax SA, Kim J, et al (1999) The effects of combining ionizing radiation and adenoviral p53 therapy in nasopharyngeal carcinoma. Int J Radiat Oncol Biol Phys 43(3): 607–616

Li JH, Chia M, Shi W, et al (2002) Tumor-targeted gene therapy for nasopharyngeal carcinoma. Cancer Res 62(1):171–178

Lin JC, Jan JS, Hsu CY (1997) Pilot study of concurrent chemotherapy and radiotherapy for stage IV nasopharyngeal cancer. Am J Clin Oncol 20(1):6–10

Lin JC, Jan JS, Hsu CY, et al (2003) Phase III study of concurrent chemoradiotherapy versus radiotherapy alone for advanced nasopharyngeal carcinoma: positive effect on overall and progression-free survival. J Clin Oncol 21(4): 631–637

Lin JC, Liang WM, Jan JS, et al (2004) Another way to estimate outcome of advanced nasopharyngeal carcinoma – is concurrent chemoradiotherapy adequate? Int J Radiat Oncol Biol Phys 60(1):156–164

Ma B, Leung SF, Kam MK, et al (2008a) A phase II study of concurrent cetuximab-cisplatin and intensity-modulated radiotherapy (IMRT) in locoregionally advanced nasopharyngeal carcinoma (NPC) with correlation using dynamic contrast-enhanced magnetic resonance imaging (DCE-MRI). J Clin Oncol 26:Abstract 6055

Ma B, Hui EP, King A, et al (2008b) A phase II study of patients with metastatic or locoregionally recurrent nasopharyngeal carcinoma and evaluation of plasma Epstein–Barr virus DNA as a biomarker of efficacy. Cancer Chemother Pharmacol 62(1):59–64

McMullen KP, Blackstock AW (2002) Chemoradiation with novel agents for rectal cancer. Clin Colorectal Cancer 2(1): 24–30

Meta-analysis Group In Cancer (1998) Efficacy of intravenous continuous infusion of fluorouracil compared with bolus administration in advanced colorectal cancer. Meta-analysis group in cancer. J Clin Oncol 16(1):301–308

Miller K, Wang M, Gralow J, et al (2007) Paclitaxel plus bevacizumab versus paclitaxel alone for metastatic breast cancer. N Engl J Med 357(26):2666–2676

NCCN (2008) Clinical practice guidelines in oncology: head and neck cancers. v.2.2008, National Comprehensive Cancer Network, Washington

New GB (1922) Syndrome of malignant tumours of the nasopharynx, a report of 79 cases. JAMA 79(1):10–14

Overgaard J, Hansen HS, Specht L, et al (2003) Five compared with six fractions per week of conventional radiotherapy of squamous cell carcinoma of head and neck: DAHANCA 6&7 randomized controlled trial. Lancet 362:933–940

Pan JJ, Zhang SW, Chen CB, et al (2009) Effect of recombinant adenovirus-p53 combined with radiotherapy on long-term prognosis of advanced nasopharyngeal carcinoma. J Clin Oncol 27(5):799–804

Posner MR, Hershock DM, Blajman CR, et al; TAX 324 Study Group (2007) Cisplatin and fluorouracil alone or with docetaxel in head and neck cancer. N Engl J Med 357(17): 1705–1715

Richmond RC, Zimbrick JD, Hykes DL (1977) Radiation-induced DNA damage and lethality in *E. coli* as modified by the antitumor agent cis-dichlorodiammineplatinum (II). Radiat Res 71(2):447–460

Sandler A, Gray R, Perry MC, et al (2006) Paclitaxel-carboplatin alone or with bevacizumab for non-small-cell lung cancer. N Engl J Med 355(24):2542–2550

Schaake-Koning C, van den Bogaert W, Dalesio O, et al (1992) Effects of concomitant cisplatin and radiotherapy on inoperable non-small-cell lung cancer. N Engl J Med 326(8): 524–530

Shanmugaratnam K, Chan SH, de-Thé G, et al (1979) Histopathology of nasopharyngeal carcinoma: correlations with epidemiology, survival rates and other biological characteristics. Cancer 44(3):1029–1044

Siu LL, Czaykowski PM, Tannock IF (1998) Phase I-II study of the CAPABLE regimen for patients with poorly differentiated carcinoma of the nasopharynx. J Clin Oncol 16(7): 2514–2521

Soo R, Putti T, Tao Q, et al (2005) Overexpression of cyclooxygenase-2 in nasopharyngeal carcinoma and association with epidermal growth factor receptor expression. Arch Otolaryngol Head Neck Surg 131(2):147–152

Sung FL, Poon TC, Hui EP, et al (2005) Antitumor effect and enhancement of cytotoxic drug activity by cetuximab in nasopharyngeal carcinoma cells. In Vivo 19(1):237–245

Taguchi T (1997) Clinical application of biochemical modulation in cancer chemotherapy: biochemical modulation for 5-FU. Oncology 54(Suppl 1):12–18

Tan EH, Chua ET, Wee J, et al (1999) Concurrent chemoradiotherapy followed by adjuvant chemotherapy in Asian patients with nasopharyngeal carcinoma: toxicities and preliminary results. Int J Radiat Oncol Biol Phys 45(3): 597–601

Teo P, Tsao SY, Shiu W, et al (1989a) A clinical study of 407 cases of nasopharyngeal carcinoma in Hong Kong. Int J Radiat Oncol Biol Phys 17(3):515–530

Teo P, Tsao SY, Leung SF (1989b) Afterloading intracavitary radiation treatment of nasopharyngeal carcinoma. Description of a technique and preliminary treatment results. Acta Oncol 28(4):525–527

Tham IW, Hee SW, Yeo RM, et al (2009 Apr 20) Treatment of Nasopharyngeal Carcinoma Using Intensity-Modulated Radiotherapy-The National Cancer Centre Singapore Experience. Int J Radiat Oncol Biol Phys. [Epub ahead of print]

Tao Q, Chan AT (2007) Nasopharyngeal carcinoma: molecular pathogenesis and therapeutic developments. Expert Rev Mol Med 9(12):1–24

Vermorken JB, Remenar E, van Herpen C, et al; EORTC 24971/TAX 323 Study Group (2007) Cisplatin, fluorouracil, and docetaxel in unresectable head and neck cancer. N Engl J Med 357(17):1695–1704

Wakisaka N, Wen QH, Yoshizaki T, et al (1999) Association of vascular endothelial growth factor expression with angiogenesis and lymph node metastasis in nasopharyngeal carcinoma. Laryngoscope 109(5):810–814

Wang TL, Tan YO (1991) Cisplatin and 5-fluorouracil continuous infusion for metastatic nasopharyngeal carcinoma. Ann Acad Med Singapore 20(5):601–603

Wee J, Tan EH, Tai BC, et al (2005) Randomized trial of radiotherapy versus concurrent chemoradiotherapy followed by adjuvant chemotherapy in patients with American Joint Committee on Cancer/International Union against cancer stage III and IV nasopharyngeal cancer of the endemic variety. J Clin Oncol 23(27):6730–6738

Wee J (2008) 4th FY Khoo Memorial Lecture 2008: Nasopharyngeal Cancer Workgroup--the past, the present and the future. Ann Acad Med Singapore 37(7):606–614

Willett CG, Boucher Y, di Tomaso E, et al (2004) Direct evidence that the VEGF-specific antibody bevacizumab has antivascular effects in human rectal cancer. Nat Med 10(2): 145–147

Wodinsky I, Swiniarski J, Kensler CJ, et al (1974) Combination radiotherapy and chemotherapy for P388 lymphocytic leukemia in vivo. Cancer Chemother Rep 2 4(1):73–97

Wu RR, Wu SX, Zhao C, et al (2007) [Phase II clinical trial of h-R3 combined radiotherapy for locoregionally advanced nasopharyngeal carcinoma]. Ai Zheng 26(8):874–879 [Chinese]

Yang AK, Liu TR, Guo X, et al (2008) [Concurrent chemoradiotherapy versus radiotherapy alone for locoregionally advanced nasopharyngeal carcinoma: a meta-analysis]. Zhonghua Er Bi Yan Hou Tou Jing Wai Ke Za Zhi 43(3):218–223 [Chinese]

Yau TK, Lee AW, Wong DH, et al (2006) Treatment of stage IV(A–B) nasopharyngeal carcinoma by induction-concurrent chemoradiotherapy and accelerated fractionation: impact of chemotherapy schemes. Int J Radiat Oncol Biol Phys 66(4):1004–1010

Zák M, Drobník J (1971) Effect of cis-dichlorodiamine platinum (II) on the post-irradiation lethality in mice after irradiation with X-rays. Strahlentherapie 142(1): 112–115

Zhang L, Zhao C, Peng PJ, et al (2005) Phase III study comparing standard radiotherapy with or without weekly oxaliplatin in treatment of locoregionally advanced nasopharyngeal carcinoma: preliminary results. J Clin Oncol 23(33): 8461–8468

Neoadjuvant Chemotherapy: Trials and Conclusions

14

Anne W. M. Lee

CONTENTS

Anne W. M. Lee, MD
Department of Clinical Oncology, Pamela Youde Nethersole Eastern Hospital, 3 Lok Man Road, Chai Wan, Hong Kong, SAR, P.R. China

14.1 Introduction

Megavoltage radiation therapy (RT) has been the primary treatment modality for nasopharyngeal carcinoma (NPC). With improving technology and optimization of dose fractionation, the treatment outcome has been steadily improving. However, while excellent control can be achieved for patients with early disease, further improvements of results for the majority of patients presenting with advanced locoregional diseases are still needed.

Retrospective analyses of 2,070 patients treated by RT alone (90% using 2D technique) from 1996 to 2000 in Hong Kong showed that the 5-year overall survival (OS) was 85% for stages I–II and 66% for stages III–IVB NPC (Lee et al. 2005b). In particular, the 5-year distant failure-free rate (D-FFR) ranged from 93% for stage I to 67% for stage IV. Achievement of locoregional control was associated with improved distant control (D-FFR being 82 vs. 71%; $p < 0.001$). However, even for patients who achieved locoregional control, the metastatic rate remained high (25% at 5-year) for patients presenting with stages III–IV disease. Incorporation of effective systemic treatment is clearly needed.

Clinical observation that NPC is highly responsive to systemic chemotherapy was first reported in the mid-1970s. Of 6 patients with NPC included as part of a trial on head and neck cancers, 3 complete responses (CR) and 2 partial responses (PR) were achieved using bleomycin (BLEO)-containing regimen (Richman et al. 1976). The first study specific for NPC by Decker et al. (1983) showed regression in 53% (9/14) patients; the most effective chemotherapy regimens contained cisplatin (Cisplatin). These data kindled the interests in integrating chemotherapy into a combined modality approach.

14.2 Nonrandomized Studies on Sequential Induction Chemotherapy

The effectiveness of induction chemotherapy followed by radiotherapy was first reported in the 1980s. The initial results showed conflicting conclusions. Tannock et al. (1987) using two cycles of cisplatin (60 mg/m^2) in combination with BLEO and metrotrexate demonstrated that high overall response rate (ORR) of 75% could be achieved, but the OS rate in 51 patients thus treated (48% at 3-year) was almost identical to 140 historical controls of similar stage distribution treated by RT alone ($p = 0.8$).

More promising results were reported by other centers. In a retrospective review reported by Khoury and Paterson (1987), a high ORR of 86% was achieved in 14 patients treated with two cycles of cisplatin-based induction chemotherapy [(3 combined with BLEO and 11 with 5-fluorouracil (FU)]; furthermore, they showed a substantially higher survival rate when compared with 52 historical controls treated by RT alone (86% vs. 35% at 3-year).

Among the various cisplatin-based chemotherapy regimens tested, promising response rates have been reported using cisplatin (100 mg/m^2) in combination with FU (Dimery et al. 1993), cisplatin (100 mg/m^2) in combination with BLEO and epirubicin (EPI) (Bachouchi et al. 1990), cisplatin (60 mg/m^2) in combination with FU, leucovorin, EPI, and mitomycin (Hong et al. 2001).

The most widely used regimen prior to definitive radiation for NPC is cisplatin (100 mg/m^2) in combination with FU (1,000 mg/m^2 continuous infusion per day for 5 days) every 3-weeks for three cycles. A prospective study of 47 patients with stage IV disease (as classified by the American Joint Committee on Cancer [1983]) showed ORR as high as 93% (21% CR and 73% PR), and a 6-year survival rate of 67% (Dimery et al. 1993).

A matched cohort study reported by Geara et al. (1997) showed that 61 patients treated with the above-mentioned cisplatin/FU induction regimen achieved significantly higher 5-year OS than matched controls treated by radiation alone (69% vs. 48%; $p = 0.012$). The 5-year cumulative incidence of Grade 3 or higher late toxicities was similar in both groups (5% vs. 8%; $p = 0.72$). This suggestion of significant improvement in OS was supported by Hong et al. (1999) comparing 55 patients treated by similar regimen when compared with 117 historical controls by RT alone (71% vs. 59% at 5-year; $p = 0.04$). Both studies showed significant reduction of distant metastases (16%–19% vs. 34%; $p < 0.019$), but the reduction of locoregional failure did not reach statistical significance ($p > 0.09$).

A subsequent study from M.D. Anderson Cancer Center tried to use a combination of docetaxel (80 mg/m^2) and carboplatin (to an area under the time–concentration curve of 6) as induction chemotherapy in 18 patients with T1–2N2–3M0 disease (Johnson et al. 2004). The ORR rate was 89%, but the CR rate was only 11% and the relapse rate was 39% (with a median follow-up of 2 years). Compared with the results previously reported by the same institute (Dimery et al. 1993; Geara et al. 1997), it seemed unlikely that this regimen will be superior to the cisplatin/FU regimen. In addition, neutropenia was very common: of 53 treatment courses given, 51% incurred Grade 4 and 21% Grade 3 neutropenia.

14.3 Randomized Trials on Sequential Induction Chemotherapy

Thus far, five randomized trials comparing the efficacy of cisplatin-based induction chemotherapy combined with radiation therapy vs. radiation alone have been published in the English literature. Table 14.1 summarizes the patient characteristics, the regimens used, and the treatment outcome.

The trial by Hareyama et al. (2002) included patients of all stages, while the other four trials (Chan et al. 1995; Cvitkovic et al. 1996; Chua et al. 1998; Ma et al. 2001) included patients with stages II–IVB by the current staging systems of American Joint Committee on Cancer and International Union Against Cancer (AJCC/UICC 2002). The histological type in more than 90% of the patients accrued was the nonkeratinizing type. Conventional 2D radiation technique and conventional fractionation were used in all trials. The total dose given ranged from 65 to 74 Gy.

The chemotherapy cycles were scheduled at 3-weekly interval in all trials. Four trials focused on induction chemotherapy, only Chan et al. 1995 scheduled four more cycles of adjuvant chemotherapy following completion of RT.

Table 14.1. Randomized trials comparing induction chemoradiotherapy vs. radiation therapy alone for NPC

	Chan et al. (1995)	Cvitkovic et al. (1996)	Chua et al. (1998)	Hareyama et al. (2002)	Ma et al. (2001)
Patient characteristics					
Number enrolled	82	339	334	80	456
Treatment period	1988–1992	1989–1993	1989–1993	1991–1998	1993–1994
Stage (AJCC 6th)	II–IVB	II–IVB	II–IVB	I–IVB	II–IVB
Nonkeratinizing type (%)	All	94 vs. 90	All	97 vs. 95	96 vs. 97
Radiotherapy					
Total dose (Gy)	66	65–70	66–74	66–68	68–72
Chemotherapy schedule					
No. of cycles	2 + 4 adjuvant	3	2–3	2	2–3
Cisplatin dose (mg/m^2)	100 q3week	100 q3week	60 q3week	80 q3week	100 q3week
Other drugs	FU	BLEO, EPI	EPI	FU	FU, BLEO
Tumor control (%): chemoradiotherapy vs. radiotherapy alone					
Time point (year)	2	5	3	5	5
Locoregional control	L: 90 vs. 98 NS	S	NS	65 vs. 68 NS	L: 82 vs. 74 $p = 0.04$
Distant control	78 vs. 76 NS	S	NS	74 vs. 56 NS	79 vs. 75 Ns
Event-free survival	68 vs. 72 NS	40 vs.30 $p < 0.01$	48 vs. 42 NS	55 vs. 43 NS	59 vs. 49 $p = 0.05$
Overall survival	80 vs. 81 NS	40 vs. 46 NS	78 vs. 70 NS	60 vs. 48 NS	63 vs. 56 NS

AJCC 6th American Joint Committee on Cancer 6th Edition; *FU* 5-fluorouracil; *BLEO* bleomycin; *EPI* epirubicin; *L* local; *S* significant but no detailed data; *NS* no statistical significance

Two trials aimed to give two cycles of induction chemotherapy (Chan et al. 1995; Hareyama et al. 2002), the sample sizes were small (n = 80–82); both used cisplatin/FU combination, but the doses of cisplatin scheduled per cycle and/or FU were lower than the common schedule mentioned above. The trial by Chua et al. (1998) on behalf of the Asian-Oceanian Clinical Oncology Association aimed to give 2–3 cycles, but the doses of cisplatin scheduled per cycle was only 60 mg/m^2. All three trials failed to achieve significant benefit for all endpoints.

The first randomized trial that achieved significant improvement in event-free survival (EFS) was that by Cvitkovic et al. (1996) on behalf of the International Nasopharynx Cancer Study Group. From 1989 to 1993, 339 patients were accrued from multiple centers in Europe, Asia, Middle East, and North Africa. Three cycles of cisplatin (100 mg/m^2) in combination with EPI and BLEO were scheduled. With a median follow-up of 49 months, they showed significant reduction in both locoregional and distant failure leading to 10% increase in 5-year EFS (40% vs. 30%; $p < 0.01$). However, an excess of treatment-related deaths was observed in the induction chemoradiotherapy (CRT) arm (8% vs. 1%), resulting in no benefit for OS (40% vs. 46%).

The trial by Ma et al. (2001) studied 456 patients from 1993 to 1994. Two to three cycles of cisplatin (100 mg/m^2) in combination with FU and BLEO were scheduled. With a median follow-up of 62 months, they showed significant improvement in local failure-free rate (L-FFR: 82% vs. 74%; $p = 0.04$), but no significant difference in D-FFR (79% vs. 75%; $p = 0.40$). Again a 10% increase in 5-year EFS was observed, this improvement almost reached statistical significance (59% vs. 49%; $p = 0.05$). No excess of treatment-related deaths was observed, but the improvement in OS was still statistically nonsignificant (63% vs. 56%; $p = 0.11$).

Subsequent analyses (Chua et al. 2005) of data on 784 patients pooled from the trials by Chua et al. (1998) and Ma et al. (2001) revealed that with a median follow-up of 67 months, significant improvement was observed in locoregional failure-free rate (LR-FFR: 67% vs. 60% at 5-year; $p = 0.037$), but no significant difference in D-FFR (74% vs. 70%; $p = 0.088$). Significant improvement was shown not only for EFS (51% vs. 43% $p = 0.014$), but also for cancer-specific survival (64% vs. 58%; $p = 0.029$). Although no excess of treatment-related deaths was observed, increase in intercurrent deaths in the induction CRT arm was noted (2.6% vs. 0.5%), the improvement in OS remained statistically nonsignificant (62% vs. 58%; $p = 0.092$).

Further subgroup analyses (Chua et al. 2006) of these pooled data showed that only 208 patients with early-stage disease (T1–2N0–1M0) as classified by the current AJCC/UICC staging system (2002) achieved significant improvement in D-FFR (86% vs. 71%; $p = 0.005$) and OS (79% vs. 67%; $p = 0.048$).

The meta-analysis by Baujat et al. (2006) included four trials on induction chemotherapy (Chan et al. 1995; Chua et al. 1998; Cvitkovic et al. 1996; Hareyama et al. 2002), and the trial by Ma et al. (2001) was excluded because of concern about the randomness of treatment allocation. Together with four other trials (Al-Sarraf et al. 1998a; Chan et al. 2005; Kwong et al. 2004; Chi et al. 2002), 11 comparisons based on updated patient data of 1,753 patients were reported. The results confirmed that significant survival benefit could be achieved by adding chemotherapy: the absolute gain for 5-year EFS was 10% (52% vs. 42%) and OS was 6% (62% vs. 56%). The treatment effect was heterogeneous because of significant interaction with the timing of chemotherapy ($p = 0.03$). Concurrent chemotherapy was the most potent combination, and the only sequence that achieved significant benefit in OS: hazard ratio (HR) = 0.71; 95% confidence interval (CI), 0.53–094; whereas adjuvant chemotherapy *per se* failed to achieve significant benefit in any endpoints. Induction chemotherapy *per se*, based on 830 patients included, could significantly reduce the risk of locoregional failures by 24% and distant failures by 35%. This resulted in significant improvement in EFS (HR = 0.82; 95% CI, 0.68–0.97), but this did not translate into significant benefit in OS (HR = 0.99; 95% CI, 0.80–1.21).

14.4 Phase II Clinical Studies on Induction–Concurrent Chemotherapy

Of the three trials on concurrent chemotherapy valid for inclusion in the meta-analyses by Baujat et al. (2006), only the Intergroup 0099 Study (Al-Sarraf et al. 1998a, b) using concurrent cisplatin plus adjuvant cisplatin/FU combination achieved significant benefit in both EFS and OS. In contrast, the trial by Chan et al. (2005) using concurrent cisplatin alone and that by Kwong et al. (2004) using concurrent uracil and tegafur with or without adjuvant cisplatin-based combination only demonstrated borderline improvement in OS ($p > 0.06$) and no significant improvement in EFS ($p > 0.14$).

In addition, preliminary reports of three subsequent randomized trials (Wee et al. 2005; Lee et al. 2005a; Chen et al. 2008) using concurrent cisplatin plus adjuvant cisplatin/FU regimens confirmed that this strategy could significantly improve EFS, and two of these trials (Wee et al. 2005; Chen et al. 2008) also showed significant benefit in OS. Hence, concurrent–adjuvant CRT is currently recommended for patients with advanced locoregional disease; the Intergroup 0099 regimen (cisplatin 100 mg/m^2 every 3 weeks for three cycles in concurrence with RT, followed by cisplatin 80 mg/m^2 and FU 1,000 mg/m^2/day for 96 h every 4 weeks for three cycles), in particular, was most widely used.

However, the usefulness of the adjuvant phase is questionable and chemotherapy during the immediate post-RT period is often poorly tolerated. Furthermore, there are serious concerns about the efficacy of the Intergroup 0099 regimen for distant control. Preliminary results of the NPC-9901 Trial by Lee et al. (2005a) on behalf of the Hong Kong Nasopharyngeal Cancer Study Group showed little improvement in distant control for patients with N2 or N3 disease (76% vs. 73% at 3-year; $p = 0.47$). Reports from Stanford University (Hara et al. 2008) and University of California, San Francisco (Lee et al. 2002) also showed that despite achievement of excellent locoregional control by new technologies and extensive use of the Intergroup 0099 regimen (>75% of the series), the incidence of distant failure remained high (>30%). Exploration for a more potent strategy is needed.

One logical strategy is to change the sequence of the Intergroup 0099 regimen from concurrent–adjuvant to induction–concurrent because the induction sequence is potent for reduction of failures; substantially better tolerance and patient compliance is often achievable during this phase. Theoretically, early use of potent combination of cytotoxic drugs at full dose would be more effective for eradicating micrometastases. Another possible advantage is that this could shrink the primary tumor to give wider margin for irradiation, an advantage that is particularly needed for patients with extensive locoregional infiltration infiltrating/abutting critical neurological structures.

The first study by Rischin et al. (2002) scheduled three cycles of cisplatin (75 mg/m^2) in combination with FU and EPI followed by two cycles cisplatin (100 mg/m^2) in concurrence with RT at conventional fractionation. Even though the total radiation dose used was only 60 Gy, excellent 4-year OS rate of 90%, D-FFR of 94%, and LR-FFR of 97% was achieved in 35 patients with stages III–IVB by the AJCC 1983 system. However, as only 40% of the series were stage IV with the current staging AJCC/UICC criteria (2002), more intensive RT is probably needed to maximize the chance of cure for more advanced group.

Thus far, eight Phase II studies on induction–concurrent CRT have been reported in the English literature. Table 14.2 summarizes the patient characteristics, the regimens used, and the treatment outcome. All except that the study by Rischin et al. (2002) aimed at a total radiation dose of 66–70 Gy; six studies used conventional fractionation, while two studies that focused on patients with stage IVA–B disease (Lee et al. 2005c; Yau et al. 2006a) used accelerated fractionation. Incorporation of acceleration was attempted because preliminary results from the NPC-9902 Trial (Lee et al. 2006) and other studies testing accelerated fractionation plus concurrent–adjuvant CRT (Lin et al. 1996; Wolden et al. 2001; Jian et al. 2002) suggested encouraging results.

Different chemotherapy regimens have been tested, all except that by Chan et al. (2004) used cisplatin-based combinations for induction chemotherapy, and all except that by Oh et al. (2003) used cisplatin for concurrent chemotherapy. Incorporation of newer cytotoxic drugs has been attempted, for instance, paclitaxel (Chan et al. 2004), gemcitabine (GEM) (Yau et al. 2006a), and docetaxel (Hui et al. 2009). Cross-series comparison is not possible because of marked variation in patient characteristics, particularly regarding the stage distribution. There are no solid data to suggest, which is more likely to be the most cost-effective regimen.

In the first study from our center (Lee et al. 2005c), we changed the sequence of the Intergroup 0099 regimen to give three cycles of cisplatin/FU as induction instead of adjuvant chemotherapy. All 49 patients studied had stage IVA–B disease with extensive locoregional infiltration infiltrating/abutting critical neurological structures. The scheduled dose intensity of cisplatin and FU were increased to 100 and 5,000 mg/m^2, respectively, per cycle every 3 weeks (instead of 80 and 4,000 mg/m^2, respectively, per cycle every 4 weeks in the adjuvant schedule of the Intergroup 0099 regimen). This was followed by cisplatin 100 mg/m^2 every 3 weeks in concurrence with RT. 3D conformal technique was used in this series. A moderate acceleration schedule of 2 Gy per fraction, 6 daily fractions per week to a total dose of 70 Gy was used. Only 2 cycles of concurrent chemotherapy were scheduled unless the patient has prolongation. Given the grave prognosis of patients with such extensive disease, 3-year LR-FFR of 77% and OS of 71% was encouraging.

Patients did indeed show substantially better tolerance and compliance to induction chemotherapy: 98% of patients could complete three cycles of induction chemotherapy, despite a 20% increase in scheduled doses, whereas only 55% of patients in the Intergroup 0099 Trial (Al-Sarraf et al. 1998s) completed three cycles of adjuvant chemotherapy. Only 2% of patients had early termination of induction chemotherapy because of poor response.

The induction treatment did not substantially jeopardize the tolerance during the concurrent phase, 96% of patients could complete the whole course of RT with a median overall treatment time of 41 days, only 7% failed to complete two cycles of concurrent chemotherapy, and altogether 92% had five or more cycles of chemotherapy.

This aggressive treatment did incur a high incidence of acute toxicities (67% grade 3, 22% grade 4, and 2% grade 5). With the exception of one patient who died of neutropenic sepsis, the great majority of toxicities were uneventful and most patients recovered rapidly. With a median follow-up of 3.1 years, the incidence of late toxicities Grade 3 was 22% and Grade 4 was 4%. Hearing loss was the main toxicity (12 of 13 affected patients). Except for neuroendocrine dysfunction (2%), none of the series had radiation-induced neurological damage. However, it must be cautioned that the current fol-

Table 14.2. Phase II studies on induction-concurrent chemoradiotherapy for NPC

	Rischin et al. (2002)	Oh et al. (2003)	Chan et al. (2004)	Al-Amro et al. (2005)	Johnson et al. (2005)	Lee et al. (2005c)	Yau et al. (2006a)	HUI et al. (2009)
Patient characteristics								
Number enrolled	35	27	31	110	44	49	37	34
Stage Group (AJCC-6)	II–IVB	II–IVB	III–IVB	II–IVB	II–IVB	IVA–B	IVA–B	III–IVB
Stage IVA–B (%)	40	NR	39	74	NR	100	100	44
Radiotherapy								
Total dose (Gy)	60	70	66	66	70	70	70	66
Fractionation	CF	Split[a]	CF	CF	CF	AF	AF	CF
Chemotherapy schedule								
Induction phase								
No. of cycles	3	3	2	2	3	3	3	2
Cisplatin dose (mg/m²)	75 q3week	100 q3week	-	100 q3week	100 q3week	100 q3week	100 q3week	75 q3week
Other drugs	EPI, FU	FU, L, I	J, T	EPI	FU	FU	G	D
Concurrent phase								
No. of cycles	2	7	6–8	3	2[b]	2–3	2–3	6–8
Cisplatin dose (mg/m²)	100 q5week	-	40 q1week	100 q3week	330 q1week	100 q3week	100 q3week	40 q1week
Other drugs	-	H, FU	-	-	FU	-	-	
Tumor control (%)								
Time point (year)	4	5	2	3	3	3	3	3
Locoregional control	97	93	90[c]	68	75[c]	77	78	NR
Distant control	94	92	81[c]	74	89[c]	75	76	NR
Overall survival	90	77	92	71	78	71	76	94

AJCC 6th American Joint Committee on Cancer 6th Edition; *FU* 5-fluorouracil; *EPI* epirubicin; *J* carboplatin; *T* paclitaxel; *I* interferon-α; *H* hydroxyurea; *G* gemcitabine; *D* docetaxel; *NR* not reported; *CF* conventional fractionation; *AF* accelerated fractionation

[a]Split fractionation (2 Gy/fraction daily × 5 fraction, q 2 week)

[b]Last 2 weeks of RT course

[c]Crude incidence

low-up is still relatively short for a full assessment of late toxicities.

In a subsequent study (Lee et al. 2008) on another 20 patients treated by intensity-modulated radiotherapy, we further showed that induction chemotherapy using the cisplatin/FU regimen could achieve significant down-staging of T-category ($p = 0.016$): 25% of T3–T4 tumors became T1–T2, and another 10% decreased from T4 to T3. Furthermore, this could achieve significant reduction of tumor volume ($p < 0.001$): 70% of patients had more than 50% reduction in primary tumor

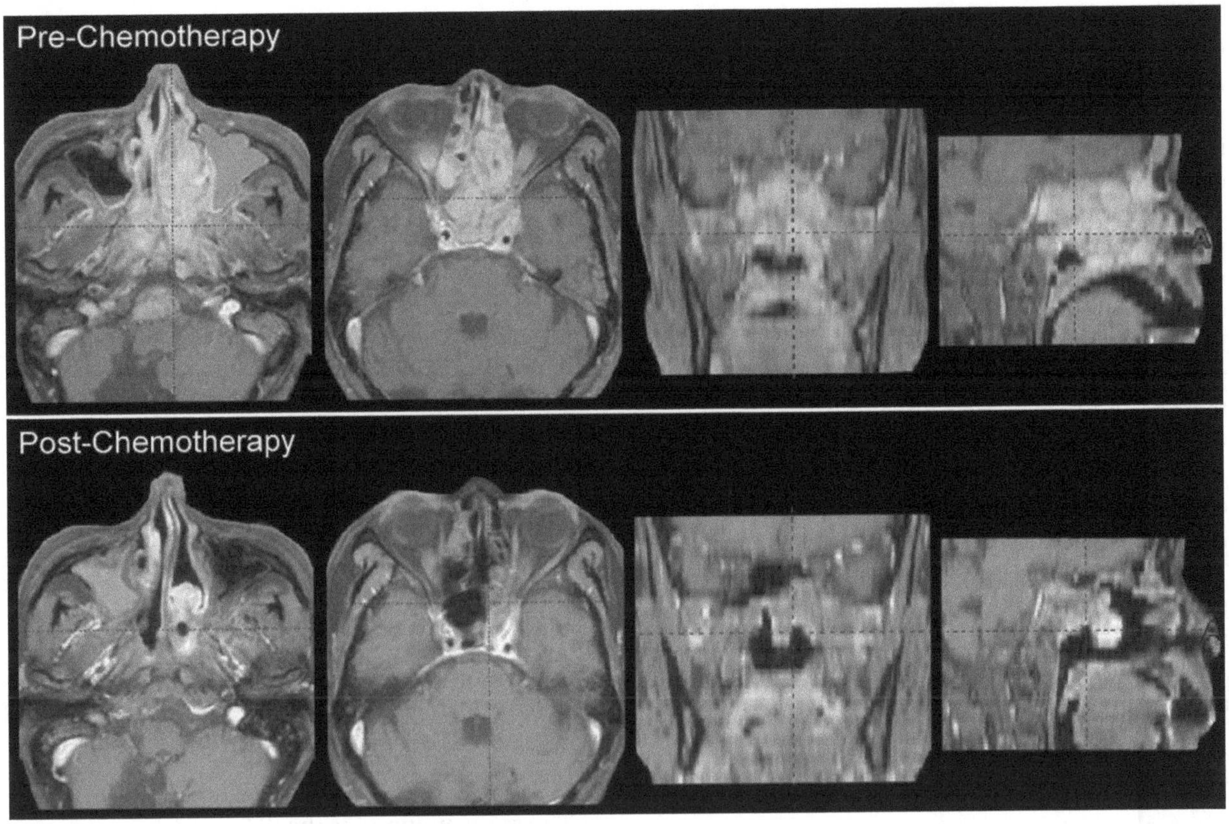

Fig. 14.1. A patient with nasopharyngeal carcinoma T4 category (with extensive infiltration of bilateral nasal fossae, ethmoid sinuses, left inferior orbital fissure, sphenoid sinus, skull base, left cavernous sinus and pre-pontine cistern at presentation (*above*), and substantial regression following three cycles of induction chemotherapy using cisplatin and fluorouracil (*below*)

volume (GTV-P), the average reduction in GTV-P was 61% (Fig. 14.1).

This significant reduction in GTV-P before RT resulted in fewer clonogenic tumor cells and hence a higher chance of complete eradication. In addition, this led to significant improvement in target dose coverage: minimum dose to GTV-P on average increased from 62.3– to 64.5 Gy ($p = 0.020$), and the volume within GTV-P that failed to reach 70 Gy decreased from 10.2% to 3.8% ($p = 0.017$). The estimated tumor control probability (mean value) increased from 0.83 to 0.89 ($p = 0.002$). With a median follow-up of 14 months, only one patient had died of distant failure, while the remaining 95% were alive without locoregional failure (though longer follow-up is needed to confirm the long-term treatment efficacy).

Although this strategy using cisplatin/FU is promising and the treatment toxicity is acceptable, continuous infusion of FU for 120 hours is very inconvenient, requiring frequent hospitalization or central access with insertion of infusion pump for administration. Hence, an effective regimen that is more convenient and less toxic will be desirable. Among the potential drugs, GEM, a novel nucleoside antimetabolite with broad spectrum of activity against various solid cancers, is an attractive alternative. Studies using cisplatin/GEM regimens on patients with metastatic NPC achieved high ORR of 64% (Ma et al. 2002) to 73% (Ngan et al. 2002).

By replacing cisplatin/FU with cisplatin (80 mg/m^2) in combination with GEM as induction chemotherapy and using the same accelerated CRT schedule as above, Yau et al. (2006a) showed encouraging 3-year OS of 76% in 37 patients with stage IVA–B disease. The quality of life as scored by the Functional Assessment of Cancer Therapy - Head and Neck Questionnaires Version 4 (Webster et al. 2003) was maintained up to the end of induction chemotherapy; these scores showed a general worsening at the end of CRT, but recovered gradually afterward.

Subsequent retrospective comparison (Yau et al. 2006b) of the efficacy of the two induction regimens (cisplatinGEM vs. cisplatin/FU) in 75 patients treated in our center showed no significant differences in all tumor control endpoints: the 3-year EFS were almost identical (61% vs. 66%, $p = 0.997$); although the

LR-FFR was slightly higher in the cisplatinGEM Group (85% vs. 76%, $p = 0.310$), no improvements in D-FFR (78% vs. 83%, $p = 0.310$) and OS (70% vs. 85%, $p = 0.310$) were achieved. It seemed that this regimen is likely to be equally effective, but not superior to the cisplatin/FU regimen.

A randomized Phase II trial (Hui et al. 2009) compared a regimen with two cycles of cisplatin (75 mg/m^2) in combination with docetaxel as induction chemotherapy followed by cisplatin (40 mg/m^2) weekly in concurrence with RT vs. concurrent CRT alone on patients with stage III–IVB disease. They showed that the 34 patients treated by induction–concurrent CRT achieved significantly higher OS (94% vs. 68%; $p = 0.012$) than the 31 patients treated by concurrent CRT alone, though the improvement in EFS did not reach statistical significance (88% vs. 60%; $p = 0.12$). This induction regimen incurred Grade 3–4 neutropenia in 97% of patients, the rate of febrile neutropenia was 12%, but no treatment-related death occurred. There were no significant differences in quality of life and late toxicities between the two treatment arms.

14.5 Ongoing Clinical Trials

Induction–concurrent CRT is hence a promising strategy for improving tumor control and further confirmation is warranted. There are two ongoing randomized trials to evaluate this important strategy for patients with nonkeratinizing NPC.

The NPC-0501 Trial by the Hong Kong Nasopharyngeal Cancer Study Group focuses on patients with stage III–IVB disease. The standard arm is the Intergroup 0099 regimen using concurrent cisplatin plus adjuvant cisplatin/FU with RT at conventional fractionation. The aims are to compare the therapeutic benefits achieved by changing the chemotherapy sequence from concurrent–adjuvant to induction–concurrent and changing the RT schedule from conventional to accelerated fractionation. In addition, this trial attempts to study the possibility of replacing FU with the oral pro-drug capecitabine (XE).

Eligible patients are randomly assigned to:

Arm 1A: Concurrent cisplatin plus adjuvant cisplatin/FU with RT at conventional fractionation;
Arm 1B: Concurrent cisplatin plus adjuvant cisplatin/FU with RT at accelerated fractionation;
Arm 2A: Induction cisplatin/FU plus concurrent cisplatin with RT at conventional fractionation;
Arm 2B: Induction cisplatin/FU plus concurrent cisplatin with RT at accelerated fractionation;
Arm 3A: Induction cisplatin/XE plus concurrent cisplatin with RT at conventional fractionation;
Arm 3B: Induction cisplatin/XE plus concurrent cisplatin with RT at accelerated fractionation

The primary endpoints for evaluation of treatment efficacy include EFS (both preliminary and final reports) and OS (final report). Secondary endpoints include evaluation of acute and late toxicities.

The GORTEC-NPC2006 Trial by Groupe Oncologie Radiothérapie Tête et Cou focuses on patients with stage II–IVB disease. The standard arm is cisplatin (40 mg/m^2) weekly in concurrence with radiation at conventional fractionation. The aim is to compare the therapeutic benefits achieved by adding cisplatin (75 mg/m^2) in combination with docetaxel and FU (TPF regimen) as induction chemotherapy.

Eligible patients are randomly assigned to:

Arm 1: Concurrent cisplatin alone (40 mg/m2) weekly during 7 weeks of RT;
Arm 2: Induction chemotherapy using TPF regimen plus concurrent cisplatin.

The main endpoint is the EFS.

14.6 Summary

Nasopharyngeal carcinoma is a chemo sensitive malignancy, and systemic chemotherapy plays an important role in the management of nonmetastatic disease. Induction chemotherapy *per se* using cisplatin-based regimen with adequate dosage can achieve modest but significant improvement in tumor control. Adding induction chemotherapy to concurrent chemoradiation therapy is a promising strategy for NPC; however, confirmation for such strategy by randomized trials is awaited. Optimal balance of cost-effectiveness and toxicities is important, and more accurate prognostication for better tailoring of treatment strategy for individual patient is vital.

References

Al-Amro A, Al-Rajhi N, Khafaga Y, et al (2005) Neoadjuvant chemotherapy followed by concurrent chemo-radiation therapy in locally advanced nasopharyngeal carcinoma. Int J Radiat Oncol Biol Phys 62:508–513

Al-Sarraf M, LeBlanc M, Giri PG, et al (1998a) Chemoradiotherapy versus radiotherapy in patients with advanced nasopharyngeal cancer: phase III randomized Intergroup study 0099. J Clin Oncol 16(4):1310–1317

Al-Sarraf M, LeBlanc M, Giri PG, et al (1998b) Chemoradiotherapy (CT-RT) vs radiotherapy (RT) in patients (PTS) with advanced nasopharyngeal cancer (NPC). Intergroup (0099) (SWOG 8892, RTOG 8817, ECOG 2388) Phase III Study: progress report. J Clin Oncol 17:385a

American Joint Committee on Cancer (AJCC) (1983) Manual for staging of cancer, 2nd edn. JB Lippincott, Philadelphia, pp 25–38

Bachouchi M, Cvitkovic E, Azli N, et al (1990) High complete response in advanced nasopharyngeal carcinoma with bleomycin, epirubicin, and cisplatin before radiotherapy. J Natl Cancer Inst 82(7):616–620

Baujat B, Audry H, Bourhis J, et al (2006) Chemotherapy in locally advanced nasopharyngeal carcinoma: an individual patient data meta-analysis of eight randomized trials and 1753 patients. Int J Radiat Oncol Biol Phys 64(1):47–56

Chan AT, Leung SF, Ngan RK, et al (2005) Overall survival after concurrent cisplatin-radiotherapy compared with radiotherapy alone in locoregionally advanced nasopharyngeal carcinoma. J Natl Cancer Inst 97(7):536–539

Chan AT, Ma BY, Lo YM, et al (2004) Phase II study of neoadjuvant carboplatin and paclitaxel followed by radiotherapy and concurrent cisplatin in patients with locoregionally advanced nasopharyngeal carcinoma: therapeutic monitoring with plasma Epstein–Barr virus DNA. J Clin Oncol 22:3053–3060

Chan AT, Teo PM, Leung TW, et al (1995) A prospective randomized study of chemotherapy adjunctive to definitive radiotherapy in advanced nasopharyngeal carcinoma. Int J Radiat Oncol Biol Phys 33(3):569–577

Chen Y, Liu MZ, Liang SB, et al (2008) Preliminary results of a prospective randomized trial comparing concurrent chemoradiotherapy plus adjuvant chemotherapy with radiotherapy alone in patients with locoregionally advanced nasopharyngeal carcinoma in endemic regions of China. Int J Radiat Oncol Biol Phys 71(5):1356–1364

Chi KH, Chang YC, Guo WY, et al (2002) A phase III study of adjuvant chemotherapy in advanced nasopharyngeal carcinoma patients. Int J Radiat Oncol Biol Phys 52(5): 1238–1244

Chua DT, Ma J, Sham JS, et al (2005) Long-term survival after cisplatin-based induction chemotherapy and radiotherapy for nasopharyngeal carcinoma: a pooled data analysis of two phase III trials. J Clin Oncol 23(6):1118–1124

Chua DT, Ma J, Sham JS, et al (2006) Improvement of survival after addition of induction chemotherapy to radiotherapy in patients with early-stage nasopharyngeal carcinoma: subgroup analysis of two phase III trials. Int J Radiat Oncol Biol Phys 65(5):1300–1306

Chua DT, Sham JS, Choy D, et al (1998) Preliminary report of the Asian-Oceanian Clinical Oncology Association randomized trial comparing cisplatin and epirubicin followed by radiotherapy versus radiotherapy alone in the treatment of patients with locoregionally advanced nasopharyngeal carcinoma. Asian-Oceanian Clinical Oncology Association Nasopharynx Cancer Study Group. Cancer 83(11): 2270–2283

Cvitkovic E, Eschwege F, Rahal M, et al (1996) Preliminary results of trial comparing neoadjuvant chemotherapy (cisplatin, epirubicin, bleomycin) plus radiotherapy vs radiotherapy alone in stage IV (≥N2, M0) undifferentiated nasopharyngeal carcinoma: a positive effect on progression free survival. Int J Radiat Oncol Biol Phys 35:463–469

Decker DA, Drelichman A, Al-Sarraf M, et al (1983) Chemotherapy for nasopharyngeal carcinoma. A ten-year experience. Cancer 52:602–605

Dimery IW, Goepfert JP, Morrison WH, et al (1993) Effectiveness of combined induction chemotherapy and radiotherapy in advanced nasopharyngeal carcinoma. J Clin Oncol 11(10): 1919–1928

Geara FB, Glisson BS, Sanguineti G, et al (1997) Induction chemotherapy followed by radiotherapy versus radiotherapy alone in patients with advanced nasopharyngeal carcinoma. Cancer 79(7):1279–1286

Greene F, Page D, Fleming I (eds) (2002) AJCC cancer staging manual, 6th edn. Springer, New York

Hara W, Loo BW, Goffinet DR, et al (2008) Excellent local control with stereotactic radiotherapy boost after external beam radiotherapy in patients with nasopharyngeal carcinoma. Int J Radiat Oncol Biol Phys 71(2):393–400

Hareyama M, Sakata K, Shirato H, et al (2002) A prospective, randomized trial comparing neoadjuvant chemotherapy with radiotherapy alone in patients with advanced nasopharyngeal carcinoma. Cancer 94(8):2217–2223

Hong RL, Ting LL, Ko JY, et al (2001) Induction chemotherapy with mitomycin, epirubicin, cisplatin, fluorouracil, and leucovorin followed by radiotherapy in the treatment of locoregionally advanced nasopharyngeal carcinoma. J Clin Oncol 19(23):4305–4313

Hong S, Wu HG, Chie EK, et al (1999) Neoadjuvant chemotherapy and radiation therapy compared with radiation therapy alone in advanced nasopharyngeal carcinoma. Int J Radiat Oncol Biol Phys 45(4):901–905

Hui EP, Ma BB, Leung SF, et al (2009) Randomized phase II trial of cisplatin-radiotherapy with and without neoadjuvant docetaxel and cisplatin in advanced nasopharyngeal carcinoma. J Clin Oncol 27(2):242–249

Jian JJ, Cheng SH, Tsai SY, et al (2002) Improvement of local control of T3 and T4 nasopharyngeal carcinoma by hyperfractionated radiotherapy and concomitant chemotherapy. Int J Radiat Oncol Biol Phys 53:344–352

Johnson FM, Garden A, Palmer JL, et al (2004) A phase II study of docetaxel and carboplatin as neoadjuvant therapy for nasopharyngeal carcinoma with early T status and advanced N status. Cancer 100(5):991–998

Johnson FM, Garden AS, Palmer JL, et al (2005) A phase I-II study of neoadjuvant chemotherapy followed by radiation with boost chemotherapy for advanced T-classification nasopharyngeal carcinoma. Int J Radiat Oncol Biol Phys 63: 717–724

Khoury GG, Paterson ICM (1987) Nasopharyngeal carcinoma: a review of cases treated by radiotherapy and chemotherapy. Clin Radiol 38:17–20

Kwong DL, Sham JS, Au GK, et al (2004) Concurrent and adjuvant chemotherapy for nasopharyngeal carcinoma: a factorial study. J Clin Oncol 22(13):2643–2653

Lee AW, Lau KY, Hung WM, et al (2008) Potential improvement of tumor control probability by induction chemotherapy for advanced nasopharyngeal carcinoma. Radiother Oncol 87:204–210

Lee AW, Lau WH, Tung SY, et al (2005a) Preliminary results of a randomized study on therapeutic gain by concurrent chemotherapy for regionally-advanced nasopharyngeal carcinoma: NPC-9901 Trial by the Hong Kong Nasopharyngeal Cancer Study Group. J Clin Oncol 23: 6966–6975

Lee AW, Sze WM, Au SK, et al (2005b) Treatment results for nasopharyngeal carcinoma in the modern era: the Hong Kong experience. Int J Radiat Oncol Biol Phys 61:1107–1116

Lee AW, Tung SY, Chan AT, et al (2006) Preliminary results of a randomized study (NPC-9902 Trial) on therapeutic gain by concurrent chemotherapy and/or accelerated fractionation for locally-advanced nasopharyngeal carcinoma. Int J Radiat Oncol Biol Phys 66:142–151

Lee AW, Yau TK, Wong HM, et al (2005c) Treatment of stage IV(A–B) nasopharyngeal carcinoma by induction-concurrent chemoradiotherapy and accelerated fractionation. Int J Radiat Oncol Biol Phys 63:1331–1338

Lee N, Xia P, Quivey JM, et al (2002) Intensity-modulated radiotherapy in the treatment of nasopharyngeal carcinoma: an update of the UCSF experience. Int J Radiat Oncol Biol Phys 53(1):12–22

Lin JC, Chen KY, Jan JS, et al (1996) Partially hyperfractionated accelerated radiotherapy and concurrent chemotherapy for advanced nasopharyngeal carcinoma. Int J Radiat Oncol Biol Phys 36:1127–1136

Ma BB, Tannock IF, Pond GR, et al (2002) Chemotherapy with gemcitabine-containing regimens for locally recurrent or metastatic nasopharyngeal carcinoma. Cancer 95: 2516–2523

Ma J, Mai HG, Hong MH, et al (2001) Results of a prospective randomized trial comparing neoadjuvant chemotherapy plus radiotherapy versus radiotherapy alone in patients with locoregionally advanced nasopharyngeal carcinoma. J Clin Oncol 19:1350–1357

Ngan RK, Yiu HH, Lau WH, et al (2002) Combination gemcitabine and cisplatin chemotherapy for metastatic or recurrent nasopharyngeal carcinoma: report of a phase II study. Ann Oncol 13:1252–1258

Oh JL, Vokes EE, Kies MS, et al (2003) Induction chemotherapy followed by concomitant chemoradiotherapy in the treatment of locoregionally advanced nasopharyngeal cancer. Ann Oncol 14:564–569

Richman SP, Livingston RB, Gutterman JU, et al (1976) Chemotherapy versus chemoimmunotherapy of head and neck cancer: report of a randomized study. Cancer Treat Rep 60:535–539

Rischin D, Corry J, Smith J, et al (2002) Excellent disease control and survival in patients with advanced nasopharyngeal cancer treated with chemoradiation. J Clin Oncol 20: 1845–1852

Sobin L (2002) International Union Against Cancer (UICC): TNM classification of malignant tumors, 6th edn. Wiley, New York

Tannock I, Payne D, Cummings B, et al (1987) Sequential chemotherapy and radiation for nasopharyngeal cancer: absence of long-term benefit despite a high rate of tumor response to chemotherapy. J Clin Oncol 5(4):629–634

Webster K, Cella D, Yost K (2003) The Functional Assessment of Chronic Illness Therapy (FACIT) Measurement System: properties, applications, and interpretation. Health Qual Life Outcomes 1:79–85

Wee J, Tan EH, Tai BC, et al (2005) Randomized trial of radiotherapy versus concurrent chemoradiotherapy followed by adjuvant chemotherapy in patients with American Joint Committee on Cancer/International Union Against Cancer Stage III and IV nasopharyngeal cancer of the endemic variety. J Clin Oncol 23:6730–6738

Wolden SL, Zelefsky MJ, Kraus DH, et al (2001) Accelerated concomitant boost radiotherapy and chemotherapy for advanced nasopharyngeal carcinoma. J Clin Oncol 19: 1105–1110

Yau TK, Lee AW, Wong DH, et al (2006b) Treatment of stage IV(A–B) nasopharyngeal carcinoma by induction-concurrent chemoradiotherapy and accelerated fractionation: impact of chemotherapy schemes. Int J Radiat Oncol Biol Phys 66:1004–1010

Yau TK, Lee AW, Wong HM, et al (2006a) Induction chemotherapy with cisplatin and gemcitabine followed by accelerated radiotherapy and concurrent cisplatin in patients with stage IV(A–B) nasopharyngeal carcinoma. Head Neck 28:880–887

Adjuvant Chemotherapy for Nasopharyngeal Carcinoma

15

Boon Cher Goh

CONTENTS

15.1 Introduction

Despite the advances in the treatment of locally advanced undifferentiated nasopharyngeal cancer, up to 30% of patients with nodal N2-3 disease and 25%–50% of T3–T4 disease ultimately develop relapse either in the radiation field or in distant sites like the liver, lungs, and bone after radiation therapy alone. Advanced local disease and nodal metastases, including bulky nodal disease or supraclavicular disease, are more likely to relapse after concurrent chemotherapy and radiation therapy using the current protocols (Chua et al. 2001).

The success of concomitant chemotherapy and radiation therapy in the treatment of nasopharyngeal carcinoma (NPC) may improve the local control, but whether distant control is improved remains controversial, given the conflicting results currently reported in phase III trials (Wei and Sham 2005; Lee et al. 2005; Al-Sarraf et al. 1998; Wee et al. 2005). Distant metastasis is believed to arise from micrometastases that have already been present at the diagnosis of the disease or from dissemination due to the failure of locoregional control of the disease.

Therefore, despite advances in radiation techniques and disease management strategy such as concurrent chemoradiation, distant disease remains an issue for patients with locally advanced nasopharyngeal cancer. Efforts have been made to intensify the use of chemotherapy during the radiation phase of treatment, but these have not allowed deployment of full systemic doses of chemotherapy, which potentially limits the systemic control of micrometastases. Therefore, adjuvant therapy with full doses of systemic chemotherapy after definitive radiation therapy or chemoradiation therapy has been studied with an attempt to control micrometastatic disease, thus reducing the risk of relapse. The potential attractiveness of this strategy is supported by the sensitivity of nasopharyngeal cancer to chemotherapy and the proven benefits for adjuvant therapy for other cancers including breast, colorectal, and nonsmall cell lung cancer. The most commonly used regimen is cisplatin and 5-fluorouracil, which has good activity against nasopharyngeal cancer (Al-Kourainy et al. 1988; Au and Ang 1994; Wang and Tan 1991).

In the Intergroup 0099 study, Al-Sarraf et al. (1998) compared standard radiotherapy to standard radiotherapy with concomitant single agent cisplatin chemotherapy followed by three cycles of adjuvant cisplatin with 5-fluorouracil chemotherapy. The results demonstrated a significant improvement in median survival, disease-free survival, and overall survival rates in favor of the experimental arm. However, 45% of patients in the experimental arm did not complete the planned chemotherapy owing to toxicities and other reasons. This, together with

Boon Cher Goh, MD
Department of Medical Oncology, National University Cancer Institute, National University Health System, 5 Lower Kent Ridge Road, Singapore, 119074, Republic of Singapore

the similarly favorable results of concurrent chemoradiotherapy over single modality radiation therapy, suggests that the main benefit of multimodality therapy derives mainly from the concomitant use of chemotherapy with radiation. Subsequent studies with concomitant chemotherapy and radiotherapy without adjuvant chemotherapy compared with radiotherapy alone have shown similar survival benefit for concurrent chemoradiotherapy, further questioning the impact of adjuvant chemotherapy (Chan et al. 2005; Zhang et al. 2005). The advantage of the utilization of adjuvant chemotherapy after definitive radiation therapy or chemoradiation therapy is not clear. The aim of this chapter is to discuss the available clinical evidences and interpret their results, with an attempt to provide insight for future research direction.

15.2 Prospective Randomized Studies

Two prospective studies have examined the role of adjuvant chemotherapy after radiation therapy, specifically in the treatment of NPC (Rossi et al. 1988; Chi et al. 2002). The results of both trials did not demonstrate improved clinical outcome with the addition of chemotherapy in this treatment strategy. The first study was an Italian study conducted between 1979 and1983. A total of 229 patients with NPC were randomized between radiotherapy alone and radiotherapy followed by 6–12 cycles of adriamycin, vincristine, and cyclophosphamide chemotherapy (Rossi et al. 1988). Seventy percent of patients presented with undifferentiated histological subtype, and stage of patients ranged from T2N0 to T4N3 using Ho's staging classification. The relapse-free survival and overall survival were similar in both study arms, as were the patterns of relapse of disease. In the light of currently known efficacy of platinum-containing regimens when compared with the regimen studied, and more proper selection of high-risk patients for additional therapy, as well as the application of concomitant chemoradiotherapy, the results of this study are certainly not applicable to current practice. In addition, there was significant delay between the end of radiation therapy and start of adjuvant chemotherapy of 65 days.

The second study conducted by the Taiwanese Cooperative Oncology Group (TCOG) accrued patients with T4 or N2-3 using AJCC 1992 NPC (Chi et al. 2002). The randomized clinical trial compared radiotherapy alone with radiotherapy followed by 9 weekly cycles of cisplatin, 5-fluorouracil, and leucovorin. Despite this relatively well-tolerated chemotherapy regimen, only 22% of the patients scheduled to receive chemotherapy completed nine cycles of treatment. Furthermore, 34% of patients randomized to receive adjuvant chemotherapy changed their minds after completion of radiotherapy. These reflect the difficulty in achieving compliance with adjuvant chemotherapy after radiotherapy. There was no difference in 5-year overall survival, which were 54.5% and 60.5% ($p = 0.5$) for adjuvant chemotherapy and no adjuvant chemotherapy, respectively. Similarly, median relapse-free survival was no different between the two groups (39 months for radiotherapy alone and 40 months for radiotherapy with adjuvant chemotherapy).

In a 2 × 2 factorial design study conducted in Hong Kong, patients with Ho's stage T3 or N2/3 or patients with cervical lymph nodes equal or larger than 4 cm without distant metastases were randomized to receive radiotherapy alone or with adjuvant chemotherapy, chemoradiotherapy alone or with chemotherapy. Adjuvant chemotherapy consisted of alternating cisplatin/5-FU with vincristine, bleomycin, methotrexate (VBM) for a total of six cycles (Kwong et al. 2004). Comparison of 111 with adjuvant chemotherapy with 108 without adjuvant chemotherapy showed no difference in the 3-year overall survival (80.4% adjuvant chemotherapy vs. 83.1% no adjuvant chemotherapy, $p = 0.69$), failure-free survival (62.5% adjuvant chemotherapy vs. 65% no adjuvant chemotherapy, $p = 0.83$), 3-year local relapse (19.1% for adjuvant chemotherapy vs. 28.6% for no adjuvant chemotherapy, $p = 0.15$), or 3-year distant relapse (24.7% for adjuvant chemotherapy vs. 19.1% for no adjuvant chemotherapy, $p = 0.34$) rates between both arms. The nonconventional use of VBM chemotherapy adds to the difficulty in interpretation of this study.

15.3 Meta-Analysis and Ongoing Studies

A meta-analysis examining the role of chemotherapy on improving event-free survival and overall survival when combined with radiotherapy for NPC included eight studies with updated individual data for 1,753 patients. Chemotherapy was found to lead to improvement of overall survival and event-free survival, but this benefit was contributed mainly by the timing of chemotherapy with concomitant chemotherapy being most contributory (Baujat et al. 2006). This further questions the value of adjuvant chemotherapy for managing locally advanced NPC after concurrent use of chemotherapy and radiotherapy. To address this, currently a study of concurrent chemoradiotherapy alone with or without three cycles of adjuvant chemotherapy with cisplatin at 80 mg/m^2 day 1 with infusional 5-FU at 800 mg/m^2/day for 5 days every 4 weeks is in progress at the Sun Yat-sen University in Mainland China.

15.4 Difficulty in Applying Adjuvant Chemotherapy After Concurrent Chemotherapy and Radiotherapy

The application of chemotherapy post chemoradiotherapy is difficult, and this is highlighted by the poor compliance to planned adjuvant chemotherapy in the various studies, and has been the experience of many groups in managing locally advanced NPC. In the Italian and TCOG studies, similar difficulties were encountered. This reflects the substantial and prolonged toxicities of concurrent chemoradiotherapy for NPC and is perhaps the greatest drawback of this strategy. Concurrent chemoradiotherapy, which carried a higher rate of toxicities than radiotherapy, often leaves significant local mucositis and skin reactions in the radiotherapy field, as well as nutritional problems at the end of the radiotherapy, requiring significant delay to the start of any planned adjuvant chemotherapy. In the phase III studies evaluating the role of concurrent chemotherapy followed by adjuvant chemotherapy against radiotherapy alone, a common observation was that a significant proportion of patients in the combined therapy arm did not receive all scheduled adjuvant chemotherapy (Al-Sarraf et al. 1998; Wee et al. 2005).

One possible clinical situation that has received little attention is the role of adjuvant chemotherapy after nasopharyngectomy or radical neck dissection for locoregional relapse of nasopharyngeal cancer. This is relatively uncommon in the era of concomitant chemoradiotherapy, but may be considered in this situation where further radiotherapy carries a high risk of toxicity.

15.5 Summary

The available clinical evidence indicated a limited role for adjuvant chemotherapy in addition to definitive radiotherapy or concurrent chemoradiotherapy at this point. This is partly contributed by the difficulty in applying chemotherapy after intensive radiotherapy to the head and neck region. Additional investigations using more tolerable, noncytotoxic agents may improve the therapeutic window of such an adjuvant strategy. Other areas of progress may be identification of patients at higher risk of relapse based on biomarkers-like plasma EBV DNA copy number, which would help one to select patients for further adjuvant therapy to reduce local and distant failure.

References

Al-Kourainy K, Crissman J, Ensley J, et al (1988) Excellent response to cis-platinum-based chemotherapy in patients with recurrent or previously untreated advanced nasopharyngeal carcinoma. Am J Clin Oncol 11(4):427–430

Al-Sarraf M, LeBlanc M, Giri PG, et al (1998) Chemoradiotherapy versus radiotherapy in patients with advanced nasopharyngeal cancer: phase III randomized intergroup study 0099. J Clin Oncol 16(4):1310–1317

Au E, Ang PT (1994) A phase II trial of 5-fluorouracil and cisplatinum in recurrent or metastatic nasopharyngeal carcinoma. Ann Oncol 5(1):87–89

Baujat B, Audry H, Bourhis J, et al (2006) Chemotherapy in locally advanced nasopharyngeal carcinoma: an individual patient data meta-analysis of eight randomized trials and 1753 patients. Int J Radiat Oncol Biol Phys 64(1):47–56

Chan AT, Leung SF, Ngan RK, et al (2005) Overall survival after concurrent cisplatin-radiotherapy compared with radiotherapy alone in locoregionally advanced nasopharyngeal carcinoma. J Natl Cancer Inst 97(7):536–539

Chi KH, Chang YC, Guo WY, et al (2002) A phase III study of adjuvant chemotherapy in advanced nasopharyngeal carcinoma patients. Int J Radiat Oncol Biol Phys 52(5): 1238–1244

Chua DT, Sham JS, Wei WI, et al (2001) The predictive value of the 1997 American Joint Committee on Cancer Stage Classification in determining failure pattern in nasopharyngeal carcinoma. Cancer 92:2845–2855

Kwong DL, Sham JS, Au GK, et al (2004) Concurrent and adjuvant chemotherapy for nasopharyngeal carcinoma: a factorial study. J Clin Oncol 22(13):2643–2653

Lee AW, Lau WH, Tung SY, et al (2005) Preliminary results of a randomized study on therapeutic gain by concurrent chemotherapy for regionally-advanced nasopharyngeal carcinoma: NPC-9901 Trial by the Hong Kong Nasopharyngeal Cancer Study Group. J Clin Oncol 23:6966–6975

Li Zhang, Chong Zhao, Pei-Jian Peng, et al (2005) Phase III study comparing standard radiotherapy with or without weekly oxaliplatin in treatment of locoregionally advanced nasopharyngeal carcinoma: preliminary results. J Clin Oncol 23:8461–8468

Rossi A, Molinari R, Boracchi P, et al (1988) Adjuvant chemotherapy with vincristine, cyclophosphamide, and doxorubicin after radiotherapy in local-regional nasopharyngeal cancer: results of a 4-year multicenter randomized study. J Clin Oncol 6(9):1401–1410

Wang TL, Tan YO (1991) Cisplatin and 5-fluorouracil continuous infusion for metastatic nasopharyngeal carcinoma. Ann Acad Med Singapore 20(5):601–603

Wee J, Tan EH, Tai BC, et al (2005) Randomized trial of radiotherapy versus concurrent chemoradiotherapy followed by adjuvant chemotherapy in patients with American Joint Committee on Cancer/International Union Against Cancer Stage III and IV nasopharyngeal cancer of the endemic variety. J Clin Oncol 23: 6730–6738

Wei WI, Sham JS (2005) Nasopharyngeal carcinoma. Lancet 365:2041–2054

Advances in the Technology of Radiation Therapy for Nasopharyngeal Carcinoma

16

Lin Kong, Jiade J. Lu, and Nancy Lee

CONTENTS

16.1 Introduction

Nasopharyngeal carcinoma (NPC) is highly sensitive to ionizing radiation, and radiation therapy is the mainstay treatment modality for nonmetastatic disease. For decades, NPC radiation therapy utilizes conventional treatment using two-dimentional and lately three-dimentional techniques. Both techniques mainly utilize opposed lateral fields with or without a supplement anterior field focused to the primary tumor to deliver tumoricidal doses of radiation. Disease control using conventional radiotherapy techniques has been acceptable; however, insufficient dose to parts of the targets owing to the proximity of the primary disease to critical structures such as optic chiasm, spinal cord, and/or brainstem may result in reduced disease control in locally advanced NPC. Although the local control of T1 and T2 NPC ranges between 76.6% and 93%, the reported overall local control rates were between 58% and 79% in patients with locally advanced NPC treated with conventional radiation (Ma et al. 2001; Leung et al. 2005; Au et al. 2003; Chua et al. 2001; Lee et al. 2005).

Furthermore, high-dose irradiation using conventional radiation has been associated with high probability of treatment-induced toxicities. While acute side effects such as mucositis and skin reaction are usually self-limited and may subside spontaneously with supportive care, late-effects such as xerostomia, trismus, hearing loss, and more severely, temporal lobe necrosis and spinal cord damage are usually permanent with devastating symptoms to patients.

The introduction of intensity-modulated radiation therapy (IMRT) has excited the profession of radiation oncology more than any other new technology since the introduction of the linear accelerator. IMRT is of particular importance for the treatment of head

Lin Kong, MD
Department of Radiation Oncology, Fudan University Shanghai Cancer Center, 270 Dong An Road, Shanghai 200032, P.R. China
Jiade J. Lu, MD, MBA
Department of Radiation Oncology, National University Cancer Institute, National University Health System,National University of Singapore, 5 Lower Kent Ridge Road, Singapore 119074, Republic of Singapore
Nancy Lee, MD
Department of Radiation Oncology, Memorial Sloan Kettering Cancer Center, 1275 York Avenue, Box 22, New York, NY 10021, USA

and neck cancers, especially nasopharyngeal carcinoma. As differentiation of dose distribution towards treatment targets and normal critical tissues/organs adjacent to the nasopharynx significantly improves, IMRT is generally accepted as a more advanced radiation technique for NPC. Results from retrospective and prospective studies have confirmed the efficacy of IMRT in disease control as well as a benefit in treatment toxicity profile. However, a number of issues related to IMRT such as the optimal treatment targets, timing and frequency of replanning during the course of radiation, and the significance of target volume change during treatment remain to be addressed.

The aim of this chapter is to discuss the rationale of utilization, planning, and delivery of IMRT in the treatment of NPC, as well as to review the clinical outcome reported in the literature.

16.2 Technical Advantages of IMRT

Radiation beams delivered in conventional radiation therapy provide universal intensity within each beam. Therefore, dose distribution generated from each radiation beam is largely determined by the density and depth of the tissue. In IMRT, each radiation beam is subdivided into numerous small segments of beams (pencil beams). And the intensities of the neighboring pencil beams have different intensity. Collectively, the beams composed of segments with different intensity produce dose distributions that conform to the required shape of the targets. Generally, IMRT is considered as a more advantageous radiation treatment technique as it can deliver high-dose irradiation to defined tumor targets while minimizing the dose delivered to the surrounding normal organs and tissues, thereby improving the therapeutic ratio of radiation therapy.

The utilization of IMRT is of particular importance in nasopharyngeal carcinoma. As detailed below, a number of critical normal structures are in close proximity to the nasopharynx. Furthermore, the propensity of disease extension to the parapharynx, base of skull, and intracranially makes irradiation of cochlea, spinal cord, brainstem, pituitary, or optic chiasm inevident. IMRT has been shown to offer superior dose conformity to the tumor target and better sparing of critical organs in the treatment of NPC in several studies. And the advantage of IMRT has been demonstrated in patients with all stages (Wu et al. 2004; Hunt et al. 2001; Xia et al. 2000; Kam et al. 2003). IMRT offers the potential for improved tumor control through dose escalating to the tumor targets and high-risk subclinical disease regions, while spares normal structures such as parotid glands with sharp dose gradients.

16.3 Implementation of IMRT in NPC

16.3.1 Patient Setup and Planning CT

Although physiologic movement is usually not a substantial issue in radiation therapy for NPC, patients' immobilization and setup accuracy are important factors influencing the definition of the planning target volumes (PTV). The patient's head position should be extended position, and immobilization device should include neck and shoulder (Fig. 16.1). A thermoplastic mask that covers head only may not be sufficient for neck immobilization. In a report by Gilbeau et al. (2001), the setup accuracy of three different thermoplastic masks used for immobilization of patients with brain or head and neck tumors was compared. Total displacements were in the range of 2–5 mm (1 SD). At the shoulder level, setup variations are reduced when head and shoulder masks are used. For isocenters in the head and in the neck, head mask is as good as head and shoulder mask, while the setup reproducibility was found to be significantly worse at the level of the shoulders with the head mask. Therefore, a thermoplastic head and shoulder mask is strongly recommended for head and neck immobilization to ensure accurate patient daily set-up in IMRT for NPC.

Treatment planning CT scan is required to define gross target volume(s) (GTV) and clinical target volumes (CTV), as well as determining the planning target volumes. All regions to be irradiated must be included in the CT scan. CT scan thickness should be 0.3 cm or smaller slices through the region that contains the primary target volumes. The regions above and below the target volume may be scanned with slice thickness of 0.5cm (Lee et al. 2006). As MRI is superior to CT to demonstrate the extension of primary tumor, especially when targets extend near the base of skull and/or intracranially, MRI fusion with a treatment planning CT is highly recommended during target delineation. Emami et al. (2003) compared CT and MRI target volumes for NPC using CT, MRI, and fused CT/MRI for defining various target volumes (GTV, CTV and PTV) for eight patients. The

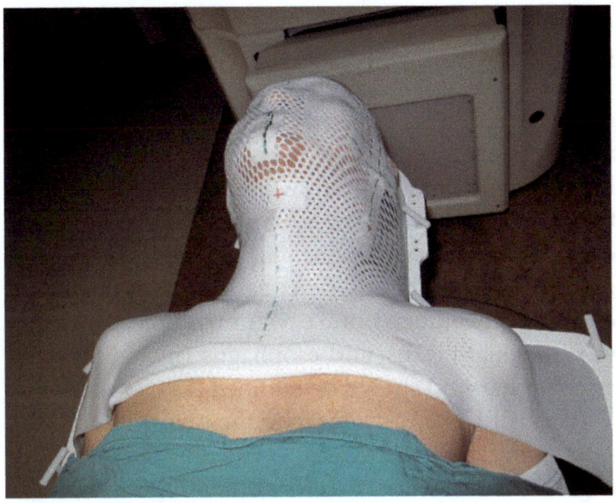

Fig. 16.1. Thermoplastic mask system extending from vertex of scalp to shoulder for immobilization of the patient in the treatment of nasopharyngeal carcinoma

results revealed that MRI-based targets were 74% larger, more irregularly shaped, and did not always include the CT targets when compared with CT-based contouring. CT/MRI fusion improved the determination of target volumes in NPC. If possible, the patient immobilization device should also be used for the MRI scan.

16.3.2 Definition and Dose Specifications of Target Volumes

IMRT offers superior dose conformity to the tumor targets with relative sparing of critical organs and tissues in the treatment of all stage NPC (Wu et al. 2004; Hunt et al. 2001; Xia et al. 2000; Kam et al. 2003). However, as IMRT provides sharp dose fall-off gradient between the tumor targets and surrounding normal tissues/organs, adequate and accurate target volume delineation is absolutely essential. Incorrect or insufficient delineation can result in tumor recurrence.

A detailed description of delineation of GTV, the selection and delineation of CTV, and the definition of PTV is beyond the scope of this chapter, and is detailed in chapter 17.

Briefly, GTV is defined as all detectable tumor tissue observed on imaging studies and physical examination.

CTV is defined as a tissue volume that contains a demonstrable GTV and/or subclinical malignant disease that must be eliminated. The CTVs of NPC include the subclinical disease surrounding the GTV and regional lymphatics. At present, CTV is very much based on our clinical knowledge for potential spread of NPC and pattern of failure after treatment; however, no universal agreed guideline is available for clinical use. The RTOG has set guidelines to use in multiinstitutional protocols. GTV-P (for primary tumor) and GTV-N (for nodal disease) with a margin of >=5mm are called CTV 70-P and CTV 70-N, respectively. This margin can be reduced to as low as 1 mm for tumors in close proximity to critical structures, e.g., tumors abutting the brainstem.

Certain regions are at high risk for microscopic disease. These regions include the areas in close proximity to the GTV(s) and the more direct draining lymph nodal regions from nasopharynx: The entire nasopharynx, anterior 1/2 to 2/3 of the clivus (entire clivus, if involved), skull base (including bilateral foramen ovale and rotundum in all cases), pterygoid fossae, parapharyngeal space, inferior sphenoid sinus (in T3–T4 disease, the entire sphenoid sinus), and posterior fourth to third of the nasal cavity and maxillary sinuses (to ensure pterygopalatine fossae coverage). The cavernous sinus should be included in high-risk patients (T3, T4, bulky disease involving the roof of the nasopharynx). Lymph nodal drainage in NPC usually follows an orderly pattern. Therefore, the high-risk lymph nodal regions (CTV 59.4-N) include level II, III, V, and retropharyngeal nodes. Level IB nodes are at higher risk if ipsilateral level II nodes are clinically involved. Once level III nodes are involved, the low jugular (level IV) and supraclavicular lymph nodes should be considered at high risk.

As higher radiation dose in the range around 59.4 Gy is recommended to treat these subclinical regions, it is known as CTV for high-risk subclinical disease or CTV 59.4. The outermost boundary of CTV 59.4 of the primary tumor should be at least 10 mm from the GTV. The low-risk CTV (CTV 54) includes bilateral uninvolved lower neck nodal regions for patients with N0 disease or with Level II node adenopathy only.

The PTV should provide a margin around the CTVs to compensate for the variabilities of treatment set up and internal organ motion. Studies should be implemented by each institution to define the appropriate magnitude of the uncertain components of the PTV. A minimum of 3–5 mm around the CTVs is usually required in all directions to define each respective PTV.

Although GTVs and CTVs form the most clinically relevant target volumes, radiation doses are prescribed to PTVs. Various dosing regimens have been used and reported. Although outcomes reported in literatures cannot be directly compared, no substantial differences regarding tumor control and treatment-induced toxicities have been observed with intermediate-term follow-up (ranging 30–36 months) (Lee et al. 2002; Kam et al. 2004; Wolden et al. 2006; Lin et al. 2009; Tham et al. 2009). Currently, the RTOG recommended dose to the PTV 70 (i.e., CTV 70 with margin) is ~70 Gy in 33 fractions at 2.12 Gy per fraction; the high risk PTV 59.4 (CTV 59.4 + margin) should receive 59.4 Gy in 33 fractions at 1.7–1.8 Gy per fraction; the PTV 54 (CTV54 + margin) should receive 54 Gy at 1.64 Gy per fraction. If the split beam technique is considered, the low neck or supraclavicular field may be treated with conventional AP or AP/PA fields for a total of 50 Gy at 2.0 Gy per fraction.

Treatment should be delivered once daily, five fractions per week. And all targets should be treated simultaneously using the simultaneous integrated boost (SIB) technique.

16.3.3 Delineation and Dose Limitations of Organs at Risk

One of the most important reasons that head and neck cancers particularly NPC is an ideal target for IMRT is that sufficient sparing of critical normal structures could be achieved. Unlike in other types of head and neck malignancies, radiation therapy for NPC usually involves a larger and far more superior situated treatment portal, which could include brain, pituitary, temporomandibular joints (TMJ), and optic chiasms. Furthermore, encompassing the entire neck lymph nodal chain down to supraclavicular fossa is usually recommended, especially in patients with cervical lymph adenopathy. Therefore, organs at risk including the bilateral temporal lobes, optic nerves and chiasm, eyes, lens, pituitary, brainstem, spinal cord, parotid glands, TMJ, middle and inner ears, skin (in the region of the target volumes), oral cavity, mandible, glottic larynx, brachial plexus, and esophagus (including postcricoid pharynx) should be outlined (Lee et al. 2006).

The ICRU Report 62 recommended the use of a safety margin around the OARs for the planning organ at risk volumes (PRVs). For NPC treatment using IMRT, the PRVs of particular importance include spinal cord, brainstem, and optic apparatus, especially when a high-dose gradient around these tissues is expected (McKenzie et al. 2002). The PRV of spinal cord is determined by adding a 3D margin of at least 5 mm to the delineated spinal cord to ensure sufficient (i.e., 5 mm) margins around the entire cord. The PRVs of the brainstem and optic chiasm are defined by adding a 3D margin of at least 1 mm around the delineated structures. The dose constraints to the OARs and PRVs are provided in Table 16.1.

Dose limitations to the salivary glands warrant further attention, as xerostomia is the most commonly observed late treatment-induced toxicity after

Table 16.1. Dose constraints to the OARs (organs at risk) and planning organ at risk volumes (PRVs) in IMRT for NPC

Structure	True structure constraint	PRV constraint
Brainstem	54 Gy max dose	No more than 1% to exceed 60 Gy
Spinal cord	45 Gy max dose	No more than 1% to exceed 50 Gy
Optic nerves, chiasm	50 Gy max dose	54 Gy max dose
Mandible, TM joint	70 Gy, if not possible then no more than 1 cc to exceed 75 Gy	
Brachial plexus	66 Gy max dose	
Oral cavity (excluding planning target volume (PTV))	Mean dose less than 40 Gy	
Each cochlea	No more than 5% receives 55 Gy or more	
Eyes	Max dose less than 50 Gy	
Lens	Max dose less than 25 Gy	
Glottic larynx	Mean dose less than 45 Gy	
Esophagus, postcricoid pharynx	Mean dose less than 45 Gy	

conventional radiation for NPC. As IMRT has the ability to minimize the dose received by the normal surrounding tissues and organs, parotid gland sparing is of particular importance in the treatment of NPC with IMRT. Approximately 70% of the saliva are produced by the parotid glands in a healthy individual. Xerostomia can be observed after 1–2 weeks of conventional radiation therapy with a minimal dose of 20 Gy or less (Wescott et al. 1978). And permanent salivary dysfunction is common after a mean dose of 26–30 Gy if the entire gland is encompassed in the treatment volume (Eisbruch et al. 2001). Therefore, the dose constraints of the parotid glands should be limited to 26 Gy or less, which should be achieved in at least one parotid gland. Alternatively, at least 20 cc of the combined volume of both parotid glands should receive 20 Gy or less, or at least 50% of one gland should receive 30 Gy or less.

While submental glands are usually spared in most portals of IMRT definitive treatment of NPC, the submandibular glands are at risk in patients with positive cervical lymph adenopathy. Submandibular glands are in close proximity to the level II neck nodes, which are the most frequently involved neck nodal group. For patients with involved level II neck nodes, encompassing the submandibular gland(s) are recommended to ensure sufficient treatment margins to the gross diseases in the neck. However, it is recommended that irradiation to the submandibular glands are kept at minimal if possible to reduce the symptoms of xerostomia.

16.4 Treatment Planning and Delivery

16.4.1 Treatment Planning

Various methods of beam intensity modulation have been used in an attempt to differentiate the dose between tumor targets and the adjacent normal tissues and organs. Prior to the introduction of inverse planning (IP), beam modulation using wedge filters to variably attenuate the radiation beam was used. In addition, the use of field-in-field technique to deliver multiple levels of intensity has also been tried. These two samples represent the simple forms of beam modulation and "forward planning" intensity-modulated radiation techniques. The planning initiates with actively defining the beam directions and shapes, beam weights, wedges, blocks, and margins, followed by dose calculation, and lastly the display, evaluation, and modification of the dose distributions (Lee et al. 2004). A thoroughly prepared "forward planning" treatment plan could provide a relative optimal dose distribution for the treatment of NPC (Fig. 16.2). However, owing to the complexity of the anatomy in the head and neck area, particularly adjacent to the nasopharynx, the workload associated with an optimal treatment planning is usually insurmountable.

To fully use the potential of IMRT in nasopharyngeal cancer, IP is required (Chui et al. 2001a, b; Nutting 2003). The process of IP initiates with clinical objectives that are specified mathematically. It is a result-oriented paradigm, which is based on the desired dose distributions to the tumor targets, subclinical regions, as well as normal organs and tissues at risk. According to the defined targets and the desired dose distribution, the computerized optimization algorithm subdivides each of the radiation beams into a number of segments with different intensity (thus modulates the intensity of radiation). The combined radiation beams composed of segments with various intensities then produce a 3D dose distribution that tailors the irregular shapes of the targets (Fig. 16.3 and 16.4).

Although forward planning IMRT could provide acceptable dose coverage and normal tissue sparing in

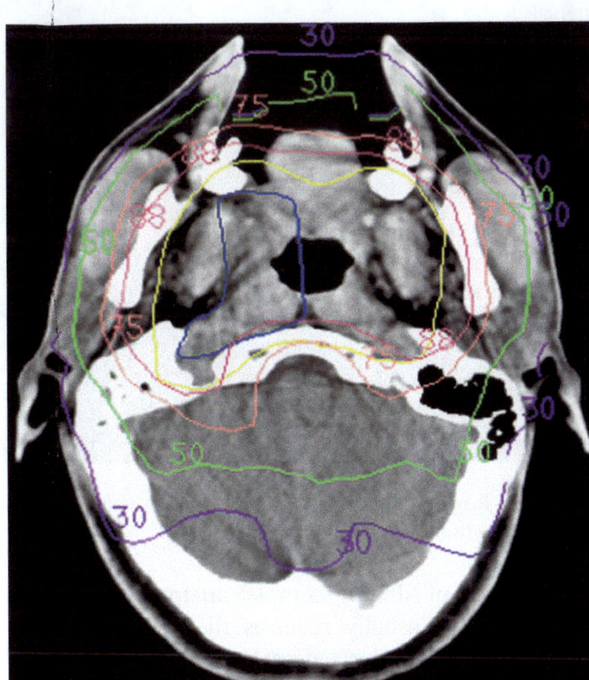

Fig. 16.2. A representative slice of a forward plan for a patient with NPC. (From Poon et al. [2007]. Used with permission from Elsevier)

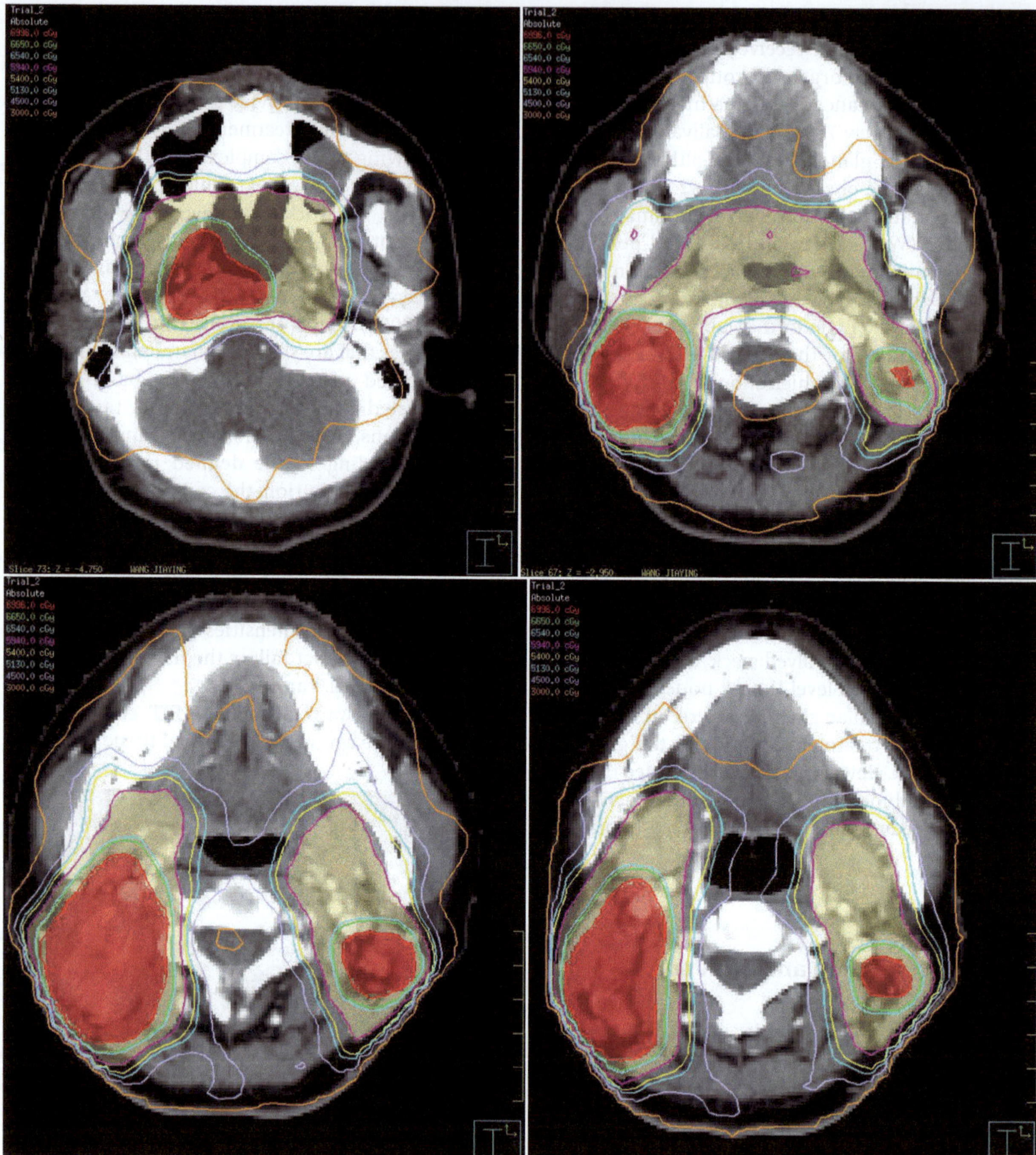

Fig. 16.3. Target volumes and radiation dose distribution of a patient with T2N2M0 NPC. GTV, CTV, and PTC delineated according to the RTOG 0615 protocol.

the treatment of NPC, the complex anatomy of the head and neck area usually requires the utilization of a sophisticated computerized optimization algorithm for better dose distribution. Poon et al. (2007) compared dose–volume histograms of target volumes and organs at risk in 57 patients with NPC using inverse- or forward-planned IMRT. The results revealed that both planning methods provided excellent target coverage with no statistically significant differences; however, the inverse planning IMRT provided improved sparing to a number of organs at risk including parotid glands, temporomandibular joint, brainstem, and spinal cord (Fig. 16.5). Furthermore, inverse planning led to a dose reduction to the middle/inner ear in the T1/T2 subgroup.

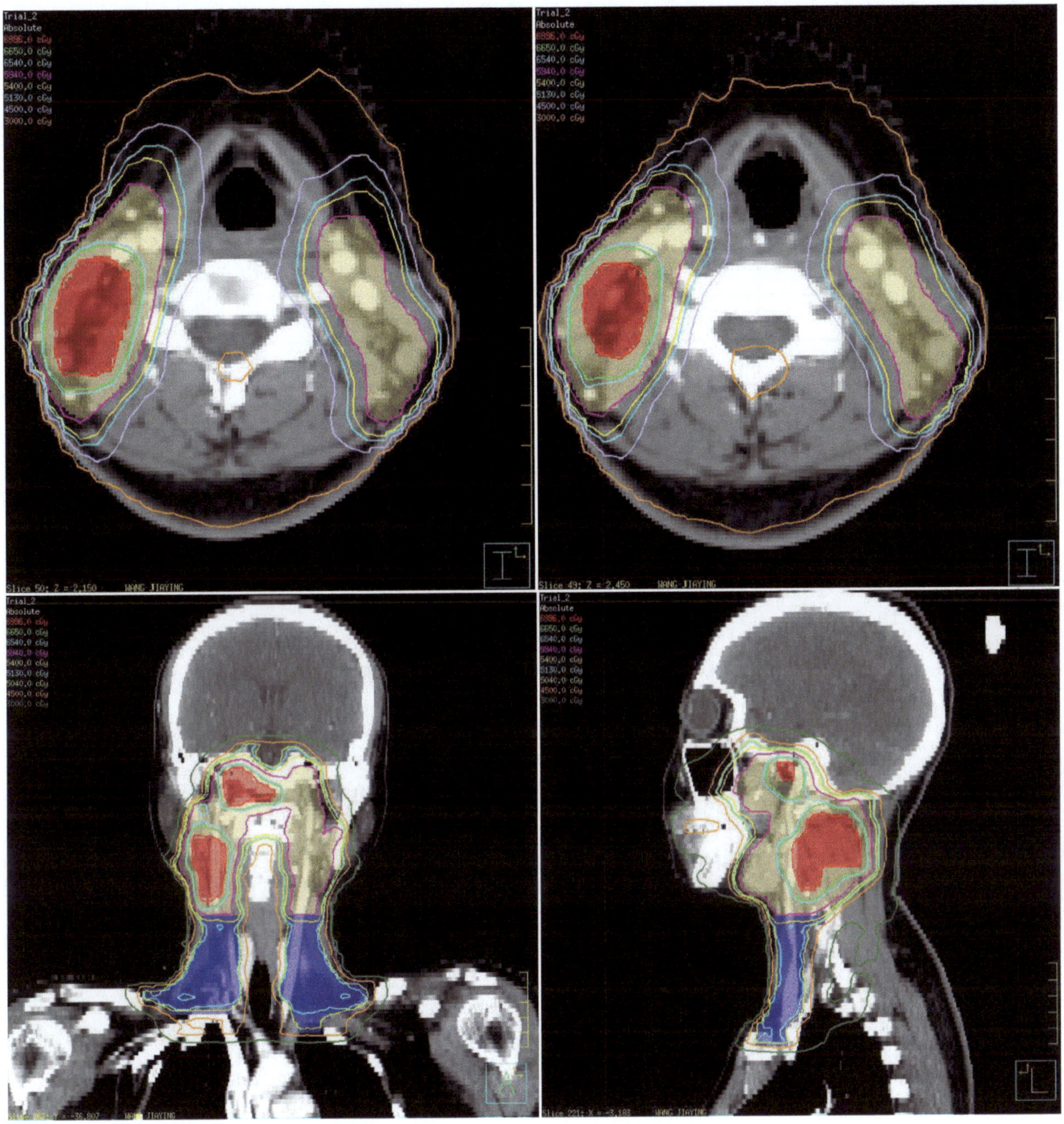

Fig. 16.3. Continued

16.4.2 IMRT Delivery

Two methods of IMRT dose delivery have been used. In the 2-phase plan IMRT, subclinical dose to the entire treatment volume including primary disease (of nasopharynx and involved neck adenopathy) and adjacent regions to the primary disease at risk and clinical negative neck nodal areas is delivered first, followed by a sequential boost dose delivered to the boost volume including gross diseases and high-risk regions. Both phases of treatment use IMRT. In the SIB technique, all planned tumor volumes may be simultaneously treated by IMRT. Different target regions receive differentiated doses per fraction daily.

Results from a number of dosimetry studies have demonstrated that IMRT dose distributions are more

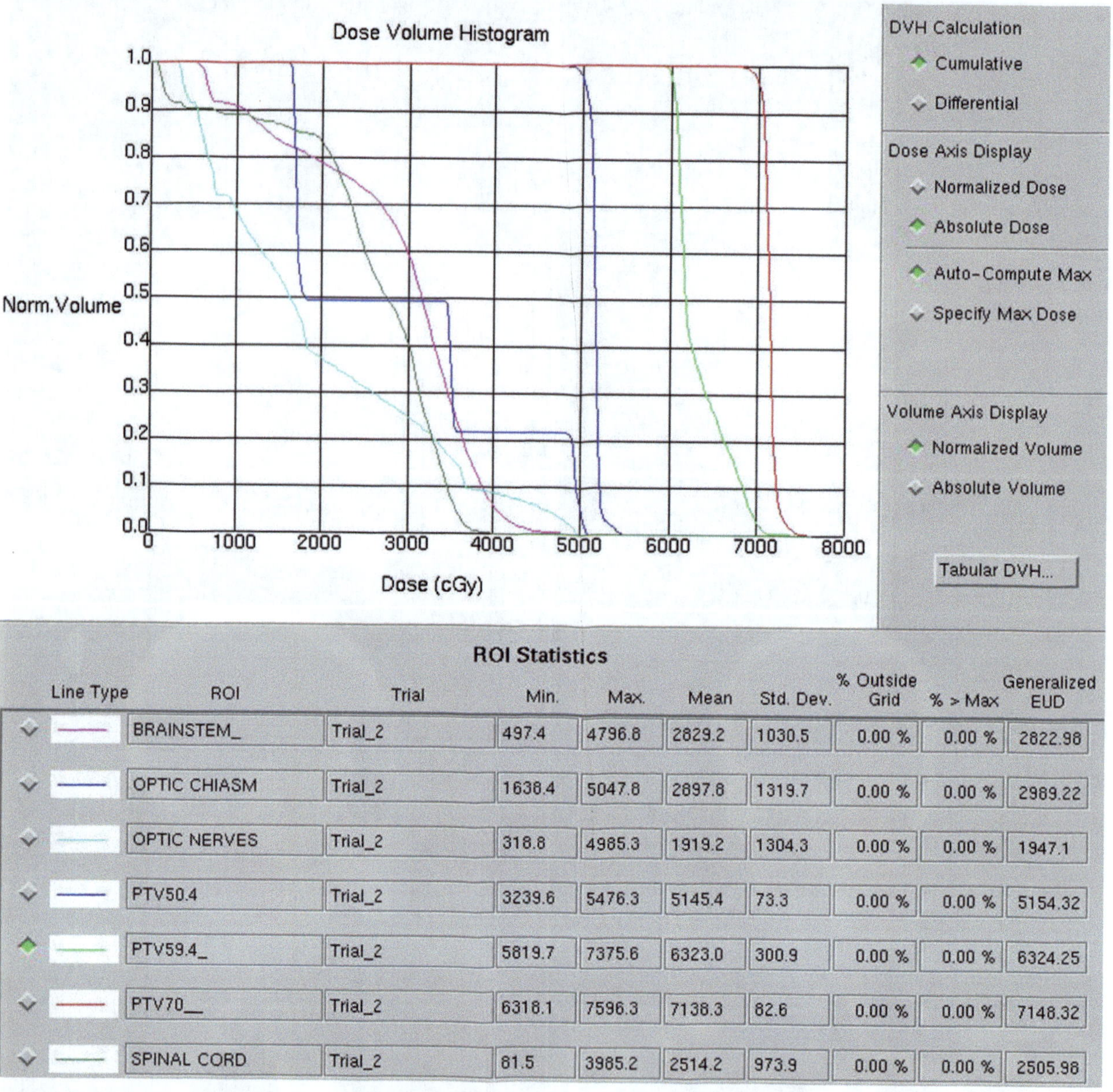

ROI Statistics

Line Type	ROI	Trial	Min.	Max.	Mean	Std. Dev.	% Outside Grid	% > Max	Generalized EUD
	BRAINSTEM_	Trial_2	497.4	4796.8	2829.2	1030.5	0.00 %	0.00 %	2822.98
	OPTIC CHIASM	Trial_2	1638.4	5047.8	2897.8	1319.7	0.00 %	0.00 %	2989.22
	OPTIC NERVES	Trial_2	318.8	4985.3	1919.2	1304.3	0.00 %	0.00 %	1947.1
	PTV50.4	Trial_2	3239.6	5476.3	5145.4	73.3	0.00 %	0.00 %	5154.32
	PTV59.4_	Trial_2	5819.7	7375.6	6323.0	300.9	0.00 %	0.00 %	6324.25
	PTV70__	Trial_2	6318.1	7596.3	7138.3	82.6	0.00 %	0.00 %	7148.32
	SPINAL CORD	Trial_2	81.5	3985.2	2514.2	973.9	0.00 %	0.00 %	2505.98

Fig. 16.4. Dose-volume histogram on target volumes and OARs of the same patient with T2N2M0 NPC

conformal using the simultaneous in-field boost SIB technique (Dogan et al. 2003; Mohan et al. 2000; Wu et al. 2003; Chen 2005). Chen et al. (2005) compared the target volume coverage and normal tissues sparing of the simultaneous in-field boost SIB IMRT technique, and the 2-phase sequential IMRT technique in 14 NPC patients. Although similar target coverages of the primary disease and neck adenopathy were found, the dose distribution in the elective nodal area (i.e., the subclinical regions) with SIB was superior to that with sequential-IMRT. Furthermore, SIB-IMRT provides better sparing of parotid gland and inner ear structures: The mean dose to the right/left parotids was 28.65 ±3.2Gy/29.03 ± 4.29 Gy and 35.67 ± 5.34 Gy/34.76 ±4.89 Gy for SIB and sequential-IMRT, respectively ($p = 0.0001$). In addi-

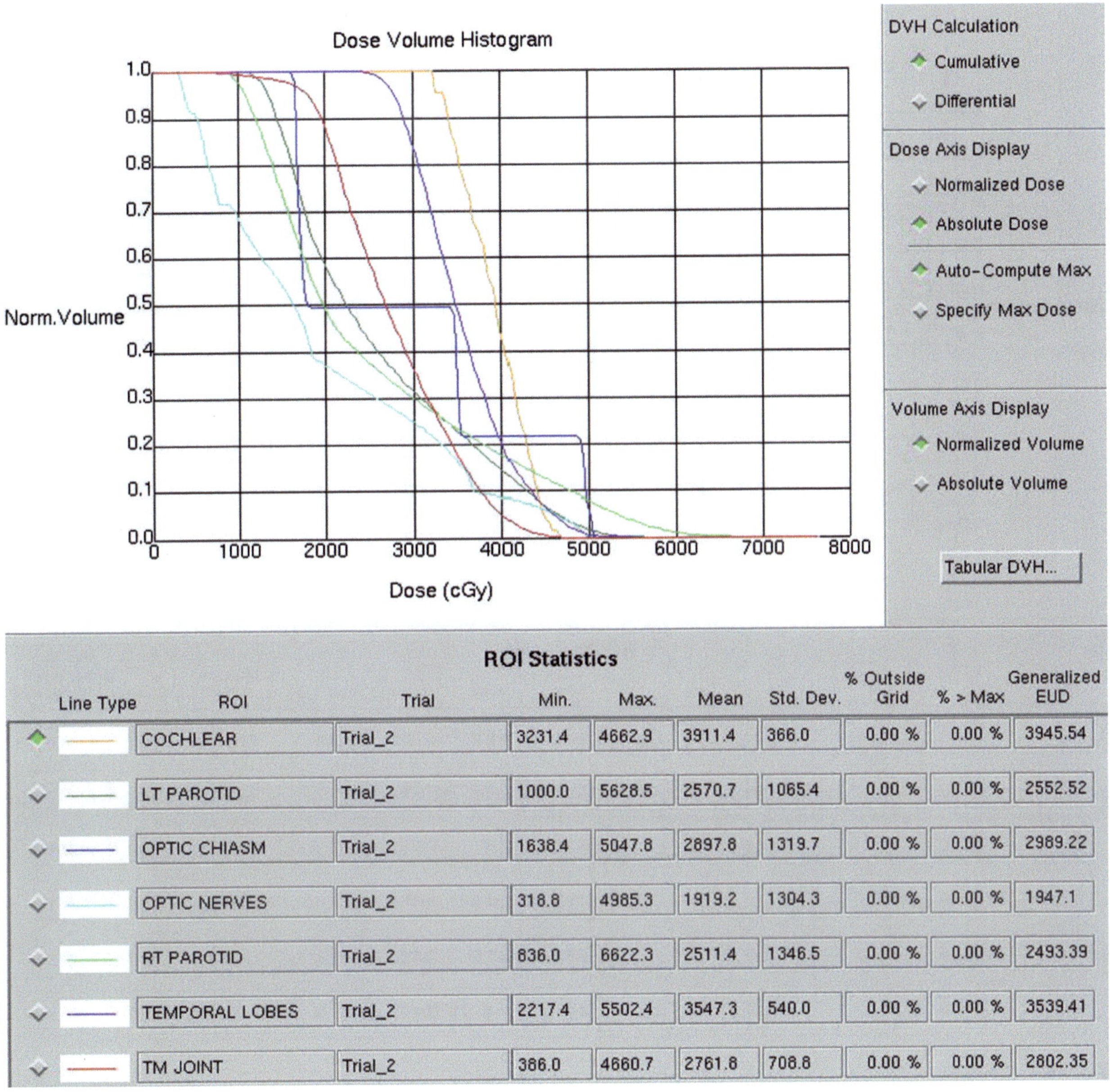

ROI Statistics

Line Type	ROI	Trial	Min.	Max.	Mean	Std. Dev.	% Outside Grid	% > Max	Generalized EUD
	COCHLEAR	Trial_2	3231.4	4662.9	3911.4	366.0	0.00 %	0.00 %	3945.54
	LT PAROTID	Trial_2	1000.0	5628.5	2570.7	1065.4	0.00 %	0.00 %	2552.52
	OPTIC CHIASM	Trial_2	1638.4	5047.8	2897.8	1319.7	0.00 %	0.00 %	2989.22
	OPTIC NERVES	Trial_2	318.8	4985.3	1919.2	1304.3	0.00 %	0.00 %	1947.1
	RT PAROTID	Trial_2	836.0	6622.3	2511.4	1346.5	0.00 %	0.00 %	2493.39
	TEMPORAL LOBES	Trial_2	2217.4	5502.4	3547.3	540.0	0.00 %	0.00 %	3539.41
	TM JOINT	Trial_2	386.0	4660.7	2761.8	708.8	0.00 %	0.00 %	2802.35

Fig. 16.4. Continued

tion, SIB-IMRT enables an escalated dose to be delivered per daily fraction, with as much as 2.12–2.4 Gy for GTV, conventional dose (1.8–2.0 Gy) to the CTV, and lower dose to nontarget tissues. Such dosing regimen has the advantage of compressing the treatment duration, which may further increase the biological effectiveness to the tumor while sparing the normal tissues and organs. The SIB technique in IMRT is a more popular technique in clinical practice for the treatment of head and neck cancers.

A number of IMRT delivery systems are available (Xia et al. 2001). The two commonly used systems include segmental (also called "step-and-shoot") and dynamic IMRT systems. The multileaf collimator (MLC) is the most common hardware used in IMRT delivery. Segmental mode MLC is used in the

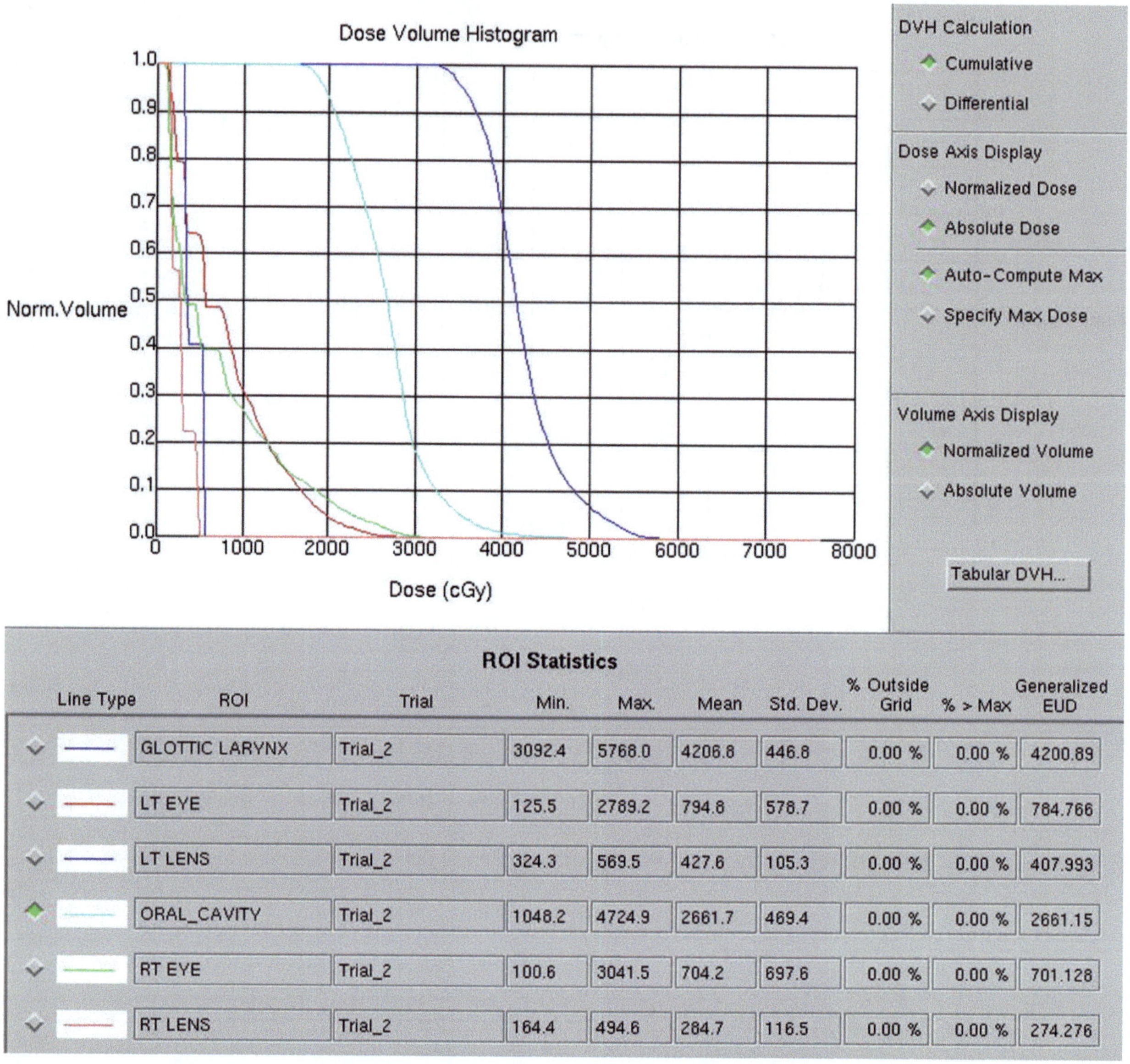

Fig. 16.4. Continued

"step-and-shoot" technique, and intensity-modulated beams are carried out by superimposing many small pencil beams using the MLC. The MLC steps to a predesigned configuration then shoots the pencil beams, the process is repeated using a different configuration until the completion of the treatment. The dynamic IMRT requires dynamic sliding window method (or dynamic MLC). A detailed technical comparison is beyond the scope of this chapter. In general, the clinical outcome assimilates each other using either IMRT delivery system in the treatment of NPC (Alaei et al. 2004; Fogliata et al. 2003).

16.5 Clinical Outcomes

The effectiveness of IMRT in the treatment of NPC has been repeatedly reported in retrospective studies. Results from recently published single institutional experiences are encouraging. IMRT has been demonstrated to improve toxicity profile, especially in preserving parotid function (Lee et al. 2002; Kam et al. 2004; Liu et al. 2006; Kwong et al. 2004, 2006; Wolden et al. 2006; Lin et al. 2009). Furthermore, treatment

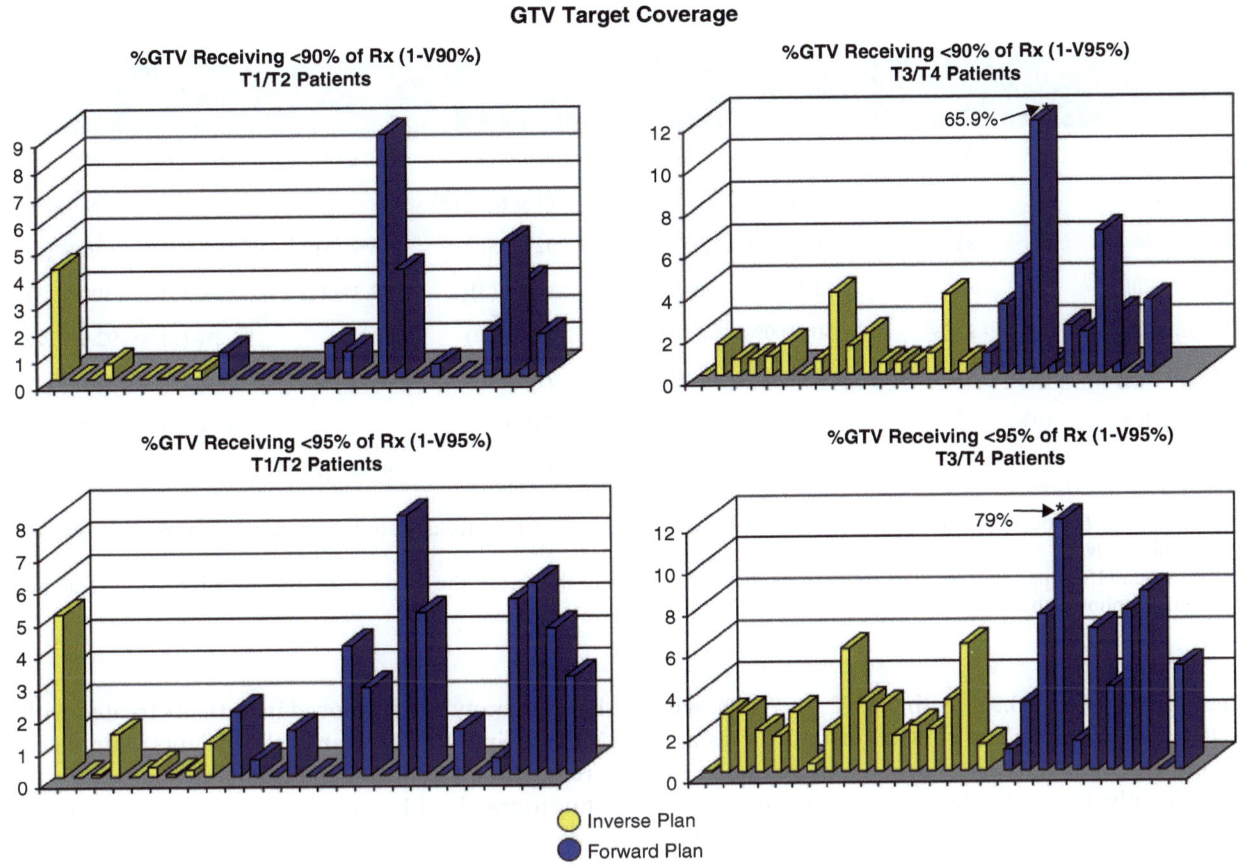

Fig. 16.5. Comparison of dose coverage to the GTV using forward- and inverse-planning intensity-modulated radiation therapy (IMRT) for NPC. (From Poon et al. [2007]. Used with permission from Elsevier)

outcome regarding locoregional control and survival rates are reportedly improved when compared with historic data. In 2002, Lee et al. reported the USCF experience of treating 67 NPC patients using IMRT. Approximately, 70% of all patients had stages III and IV diseases. The prescribed dose was 65–70 Gy (2.12–2.25 Gy/fraction/day) to the GTV and positive neck nodes, 60 Gy (1.8–2.0 Gy/fraction/day) to the CTV, 50–60 Gy to the clinically negative neck. Fifty patients received concomitant cisplatin and adjuvant cisplatin and 5-fluorouracil chemotherapy according to Intergroup 0099 trial. With a median follow-up of 31 months, the 4-year estimates of local progression-free, local-regional progression-free, and distant metastases-free rates were 97%, 98%, and 66%, respectively. The 4-year estimate of overall survival was 88%. This was one of the first studies that demonstrated an improved tumor control by improved tumor target coverage using IMRT.

The above-mentioned favorable outcome has been repeatedly confirmed in other single institutional experiences (Kam et al. 2004; Liu et al. 2003; Kwong et al. 2004, 2006; Wolden et al. 2006; Lin et al. 2009). Furthermore, in a prospective series of 323 patients, Lin et al. (2009) reported that the local and regional control, metastatic-free and overall survival rates reached 98%, 90%, and 90% at 3 years after treatment, respectively. In addition, less than 8% of patients experienced grade II xerostomia, and no patient had grade III or IV parotid dysfunction. The majority of patients with locoregionally advanced disease received neoadjuvant chemotherapy followed by IMRT, and less than 15% received concurrent chemoradiation therapy. Nevertheless, these findings were exceedingly similar to those reported by the team from UCSF. The excellent results of IMRT with or without chemotherapy in the treatment of NPC from the above-mentioned institutions have also been reproduced in a prospective multiinstitutional setting (Lee et al. 2008).

In a randomized trial from Hong Kong, Kwong et al. (2008) compared the disease control and salivary function in stage II NPC patients treated with IMRT vs. two-dimensional radiotherapy (2DRT). The 4-year

Table 16.2. Treatment outcomes of patients with nonmetastatic NPC after IMRT

Author (year)	No.	FU (months)	Stages III + IV	Chemo-therapy	LC(years)	RC(years)	DMFS (years)	OS (years)
Lee 2002	67	31	47 (70%)	50 (75%)	976% (4)	98% (4)	66% (4)	88% (4)
Liu 2003	83	17	52 (63%)	63 (76%)	PFS: 61% (3)			88% (3)
Kam 2004	63	29	36 (57%)	19 (30%)	92% (3)	98% (3)	79% (3)	90% (3)
Kwong 2004	33	24	1 (3%)	0	100% (3)	92.3% (3)	100% (3)	100% (3)
Kwong 2006	50	25	50 (100%)	39 (78%)	95.7% (2)		94.2% (2)	92.1% (2)
Wolden 2006	74	35	57 (77%)	69 (93%)	91% (3)	93% (3)	78% (3)	83% (3)
Tham 2009	195	37	123 (63%)	112 (57%)	90% (3)	–	89% (3)	94% (3)
Lin 2009	323	30	260 (80%)	295 (91%)[a]	95% (3)	98% (3)	90% (3)	90% (3)

FU Follow-up; *LC* local control;*PFS* progression free survival;*RC* regional control;*DMFS* distant metastasis free survival; *OS* overall survival

[a]Forty-seven (15%) patients received concurrent chemotherapy, and the rest of the group were treated with neoadjuvant chemotherapy followed by IMRT

local control was 90.5% with IMRT vs. 71.7% with 2DRT ($p = 0.019$). Neck control, distant metastasis, failure-free, and disease-specific survival were not significantly different between the two arms. Because of the improved treatment outcome and toxicity profile, IMRT is recommended for definitive treatment for all patients with nasopharyngeal cancer in many regions including United States, Singapore, and many institutions in Hong Kong and Mainland China. Table 16.2 summarizes treatment outcomes of IMRT in the management of NPC.

16.6 Treatment-Related Toxicity and Quality of Life

16.6.1 Acute Toxicity

The most commonly observed acute toxicity in IMRT for NPC is radiation-induced mucositis and dermatitis. Owing to the reduction of dose in the nontarget tissues, a reduction in acute toxicity during IMRT is expected and has been observed. Lee et al. (2002) reported a lower incidence of acute toxicity in NPC patients treated with IMRT. RTOG grade 3 mucositis and pharyngitis were observed in 22% patients. Furthermore, compared with the Intergroup 0099 Trial (Al-Sarraf et al. 1998), compliance to adjuvant chemotherapy was improved in patients treated with IMRT. Using IMRT, nearly all patients completed three cycles of adjuvant chemotherapy consisting of 5-fluorouracil and cisplatinum in addition to the three cycles of cisplatinum during radiotherapy, whereas in the Intergroup trial, only 55% of the patients completed three courses of the adjuvant chemotherapy and 45% of the patients received two cycles or less adjuvant chemotherapy due to toxicity. However, in Kwong's series (2006), IMRT does not reduce acute mucositis rates, grade 3 mucositis and skin reaction were observed in 39 patients (78%) and 23 patients (46%), respectively.

16.6.2 Late Toxicity

One of the major complaints from patients treated with conventional external beam radiation therapy to the nasopharynx is xerostomia because of a high-dose irradiation to parotid glands bilaterally. As mentioned above, the probability and severity of xerostomia is largely dependent on the radiation dose and the volume of the parotid gland. IMRT is capable of reducing the dose to the parotid glands while simultaneously delivering high doses to the tumor targets. Reported studies of IMRT for NPC have demonstrated a clear advantage for preserving salivary functions with IMRT (Lee et al. 2002; Kam et al. 2004; Wolden et al. 2006; Lin et al. 2009; Tham et al. 2009).

Most patients complained of xerostomia experienced mild symptoms (grade 2 or less). Furthermore, patients treated with IMRT recover their salivary flow faster and more completely than those treated with conventional radiotherapy. KAM et al (2007) has performed a randomized trial to compare the rates of delayed xerostomia between two-dimensional radiation therapy (2DRT) and IMRT in the treatment of early-stage NPC. At 1 year after treatment, patients in IMRT arm had lower incidence of observer-rated severe xerostomia than patients in the 2DRT arm (39.3 vs. 82.1%; $p = 001$), parallel with a higher fractional stimulated parotid flow rate (0.90 vs. 0.05; $p < 0001$), and higher fractional stimulated whole saliva flow rate (0.41 vs. 0.20; $p = 001$).

In NPC patients treated with IMRT, the dose limitations for parotid glands mentioned above is not always achievable. The mean dose to the parotids ranged from 32 to 46.1 Gy (average, 38.8 Gy) for early-stage NPC patients treated with IMRT in the serials of KWONG et al. (2004). In the study of HSIUNG et al. (2006), the mean parotid ranged from 33.2 to 58.8 Gy (average, 43.9 Gy). However, recovery of salivary flow was observed despite a higher mean dose to the parotid glands.

Anatomically, the nasopharynx is in close proximity to several vital normal structures, such as temporal lobes, brainstem, cranial nerves, pituitary gland, and ear, and they may receive high radiation dose when 2DRT is applied. Thus, radiation injury to these structures may not be avoided (LEE et al. 1992). With IMRT's capability in decreasing radiation doses to these critical structures, damage to these structures can be minimized.

16.6.3 Quality of Life

FANG et al. (2007) analyzed quality of life (QOL) data from 237 NPC patients using the European Organization for the Research and Treatment of Cancer (EORTC) Core QOL questionnaire and the EORTC head and neck QOL questionnaire and found that patients who received conformal radiation therapy (RT) (either 3D-CRT or IMRT) had both statistically and clinically significant improvements in the scales of global QOL, pain, appetite loss, senses, speech, social eating, teeth, opening mouth, xerostomia, sticky saliva, and feeling ill, compared with 2DRT technique. Survivors who received conformal RT had a higher probability of reporting good global QOL and a lower probability of reporting a high-level xerostomia than those who received CRT.

16.7 Unresolved Issues

NPC is highly sensitive to radiation therapy. During the course of radiation, tumor volume reduction is usually expected, especially in patients with large neck adenopathy. In addition, acute treatment-induced toxicities such as xerostomia and mucositis may cause odynophagia and dysphagia, and may induce substantial weight loss. Both tumor shrinkage and weight loss may cause significant alteration of body contour; thus planned dose distribution during the course of IMRT for NPC further change the expected clinical outcome. In a retrospective study using 13 patients with locally advanced head and neck cancers (including six cases of NPC), HANSEN et al. (2006) found that dose to the tumor targets was reduced while doses to the critical organs were increased if replanning is not exercised. The authors concluded that repeat imaging and planning during the course of IMRT for selected patient may be essential to identify dosimetric changes and to ensure appropriate dose coverage to both tumor targets and normal tissues/organs. Whether repeated delineation and planning is indeed required is one of the most pertinent questions for IMRT, for NPC awaits prospective evaluation, especially for patients with locoregionally advanced disease. Furthermore, the optimal frequency of replanning should be addressed.

NPC is endemic in Southeast Asia. IMRT has become a common treatment modality for NPC in those areas; however, resources including treatment facility are always a limiting factor for its prevailing use. A shortened course IMRT may provide substantial saving to the treatment time, thus relieve some constrains on resources. Therefore, whether further reduction of treatment time by dose escalation to the GTV while sparing the organs at risk is possible using an accelerated SIB IMRT technique is of interest. Such measure may also improve the biological effectiveness of radiation therapy.

The optimal definition of CTV is another interesting issue to be addressed in the treatment of NPC using IMRT. The results from a number of retrospective studies indicated that the recurrence in the lower neck areas, especially supraclavicular regions, is limited in patients with N0 NPC (GAO et al. 2009; TANG et al. 2009). Furthermore, NPC treated using a limited volume IMRT technique especially in the neck region seems to produce similar clinical outcome regarding local and regional control (Lin et al. 2009). However, as most reports on IMRT for NPC are of retrospective nature and short of long-term follow-up, coverage to the entire neck lymph nodal drainage regions including the lower neck and supraclavicular areas should be considered until further clinical evidence is available.

16.8 Summary

Radiotherapy techniques for NPC have substantially changed over the past decade. The introduction of intensity-modulated radiation therapy (IMRT) resulted in superior coverage of the tumor while not exceeding the tolerance of nearby normal tissues. IMRT is an ideal radiation modality for NPC. Dosimetry studies showed that IMRT have significant dosimetric advantages in all stages of NPC. Adequate and correct target volume delineation is absolutely essential to control the tumor. IP is required to get better use of IMRT, and IMRT dose distributions are most conformal when designed to be delivered as SIB technique. The published data demonstrated that IMRT has much improved locaregional control, overall survival, and toxicity profile, especially in preserving parotid function.

References

Alaei P, Higgins PD, Weaver R, et al (2004) Comparison of dynamic and step-and-shoot intensity-modulated radiation therapy planning and delivery. Med Dosim Spring;29(1):1–6

Al-Sarraf M, LeBlanc M, Giri PG, et al (1998) Chemoradiotherapy versus radiotherapy in patients with advanced nasopharyngeal cancer: phase III randomized Intergroup study 0099. J Clin Oncol 16:1310–1317

Au JS, Law CK, Foo W, et al (2003) In-depth evaluation of the AJCC/UICC 1997 staging system of nasopharyngeal carcinoma: prognostic homogeneity and proposed refinements. Int J Radiat Oncol Biol Phys 56(2):413–426

Chen SW, Yang SN, Liang JA (2005) Comparative dosimetric study of two strategies of intensity-modulated radiotherapy in nasopharyngeal cancer. Med Dosim 30(4):219–227

Chua DT, Sham JS, Wei WI, et al (2001) The predictive value of the 1997 American Joint Committee on Cancer stage classification in determining failure patterns in nasopharyngeal carcinoma. Cancer 92:2845–2855

Chui CS, Spirou SV (2001a) Inverse planning algorithms for external beam radiation therapy. Med Dosimetry 26:189–197

Chui CS, Chan MF, Yorke E, et al (2001b) Delivery of intensity-modulated radiation therapy with a conventional multileaf collimator: comparison of dynamic and segmental methods. Med Phys 28:2441–2449

Dogan N, King S, Emami B, et al (2003) Assessment of different IMRT boost delivery methods on target coverage and normal-tissue sparing. Int J Radiat Oncol Biol Phys 57(5): 1480–1491

Eisbruch A, Kim HM, Terrell JE. et al (2001) Xerostomia and its predictors following parotid-sparing irradiation of head-and-neck cancer. Int J Radiat Oncol Biol Phys 50(3):695–704

Emami B, Sethi A, Petruzzelli GJ (2003) Influence of MRI on target volume delineation and IMRT planning in nasopharyngeal carcinoma. Int J Radiat Oncol Biol Phys 57(2):481–488

Fang FM, Tsai WL, Chen HC, et al (2007) Intensity-modulated or conformal radiotherapy improves the quality of life of patients with nasopharyngeal carcinoma. Cancer 109:313–321

Fogliata A, Bolsi A, Cozzi L (2003) Comparative analysis of intensity modulation inverse planning modules of three commercial treatment planning systems applied to head and neck tumour model. Radiother Oncol 66(1):29–40

Gao Y, Zhu G, Lu JJ, et al (2009) Is elective irradiation to the lower neck necessary for N0 nasopharyngeal carcinoma? Int J Radiat Oncol Biol Phys: Accepted

Gilbeau L, Octave-Prignot M, Loncol T, et al (2001) Comparison of setup accuracy of three different thermoplastic masks for the treatment of brain and head and neck tumors. Radiother Oncol 58(2):155–162

Hansen EK, Bucci MK, Quivey JM, et al (2006) Repeat CT imaging and replanning during the course of IMRT for head-and-neck cancer. Int J Radiat Oncol Biol Phys 64(2): 355–362

Hsiung CH, Ting HM, Huang HY, et al (2006) Parotid-sparing intensity-modulated radiotherapy (IMRT) for nasopharyngeal carcinoma: preserved parotid function after IMRT on quantitative salivary scintigraphy and comparison with historical data after conventional radiotherapy. Int J Radiat Oncol Biol Phys 66:454–461

Hunt MA, Zelefsky MJ, Wolden S, et al (2001) Treatment planning and delivery of intensity-modulated radiation therapy for primary nasopharynx cancer. Int J Radiat Oncol Biol Phys 49:623–632

Kam MK, Chau RM, Suen J, et al (2003) Intensity-modulated radiotherapy in nasopharyngeal carcinoma: dosimetric advantage over conventional plans and feasibility of dose escalation. Int J Radiat Oncol Biol Phys 56:145–157

Kam MK, Teo PM, Chau RM, et al (2004) Treatment of nasopharyngeal carcinoma with intensity-modulated radiotherapy: the Hong Kong experience.(pwh) Int J Radiat Oncol Biol Phys 60:1440–1450

Kam MK, Leung SF, Zee B, et al (2007) Prospective randomized study of intensity-modulated radiotherapy on salivary gland function in early-stage nasopharyngeal carcinoma patients. J Clin Oncol 25(31):4873–4879

Kwong DL, Pow EH, Sham JS, et al (2004) Intensity-modulated radiotherapy for early-stage nasopharyngeal carcinoma: a prospective study on disease control and preservation of salivary function. Cancer 101:1584–1593

Kwong DL, Sham JS, Leung LH, et al (2006) Preliminary results of radiation dose escalation for locally advanced nasopharyngeal carcinoma. Int J Radiat Oncol Biol Phys 64:374–381

Kwong DL, McMillan A, Pow E, et al (2008) A randomized trial comparing intensity modulated radiotherapy versus 2-dimensional radiotherapy for stage II nasopharyngeal carcinoma. Int J Radiat Oncol Biol Phys 72(Suppl):S98

Lee AW, Law SC, Ng SH, et al (1992) Retrospective analysis of nasopharyngeal carcinoma treated during 1976–1985: late complications following megavoltage irradiation. Br J Radiol 65(778):918–928

Lee AW, Sze WM, Au JS, et al (2005) Treatment results for nasopharyngeal carcinoma in the modern era: the Hong Kong experience. Int J Radiat Oncol Biol Phys 61(4):1107–1116

Lee N, Xia P, Quivey JM, et al (2002) Intensity-modulated radiotherapy in the treatment of nasopharyngeal carcinoma: an update of the UCSF experience. Int J Radiat Oncol Biol Phys 53:12–22

Lee N, Akazawa C, Akazawa P, et al (2004) A forward-planned treatment technique using multisegments in the treatment of head-and-neck cancer. Int J Radiat Oncol Biol Phys 59: 584–594

Lee N, Pfister DG, Garden A, et al (2006) RTOG 0615, A phase II study of concurrent chemoradiotherapy using three-dimentional conformal radiotherapy (3D-CRT) or intensity-modulated radiation therapy (IMRT) + bevacizumab (BV) for locally or regionally advanced nasopharyngeal cancer. http://www.rtog.org/members/protocols/0615/0615.pdf Accessed on August 19 2009

Lee N, Harris J, Garden AS et al (2008) Phase II multi-institutional study of intensity modulated radiation therapy (IMRT) +/− chemotherapy for nasopharyngeal (NPC) carcinoma: preliminary clinical results of RTOG 0225. Int J Radiat Oncol Biol Phys 72(Suppl):S98

Leung TW, Tung SY, Sze WK, et al (2005) Treatment results of 1070 patients with nasopharyngeal carcinoma: an analysis of survival and failure patterns. Head Neck 27(7):555–565

Lin S, Pan J, Lu H, et al (2009) Apr 11. Nasopharyngeal carcinoma treated with reduced-volume intensity-modulated radiation therapy: report on the 3-year outcome of a prospective series. Int J Radiat Oncol Biol Phys. 2009 Apr 11 [Epub ahead of print]

Liu MT, Hsieh CY, Chang TH, et al (2003) Prognostic factors affecting the outcome of nasopharyngeal carcinoma. Jpn J Clin Oncol 33:501–508

Liu WS, Lee SP, Lee JK, et al (2006) Factors influencing the parotid function in nasopharyngeal carcinoma treated with parotid-sparing radiotherapy. Jpn J Clin Oncol 36: 626–631

Ma J, Mai HQ, Hong MH, et al (2001) Is the 1997 AJCC staging system for nasopharyngeal carcinoma prognostically useful for Chinese patient populations? Int J Radiat Oncol Biol Phys 50(5):1181–1189

McKenzie A, van Herk M, Mijnheer B (2002) Margins for geometric uncertainty around organs at risk in radiotherapy. Radiother Oncol 62:299–307

Mohan R, Wu Q, Manning M, et al (2000) Radiobiological considerations in the design of fractionation strategies for intensity modulated radiation therapy of head and neck cancers. Int J Radiat Oncol Biol Phys 46:619–630

Nutting C (2003) Intensity-modulated radiotherapy (IMRT): the most important advance in radiotherapy since the linear accelerator? Br J Radiol 76:673

Poon I, Xia P, Weinberg V, et al (2007) A treatment planning analysis of inverse-planned and forward-planned intensity-modulated radiation therapy in nasopharyngeal carcinoma. Int J Radiat Oncol Biol Phys 69(5):1625–1633

Tham IW, Hee SW, Yeo RM, et al. (2009) Treatment of nasopharyngeal carcinoma using intensity-modulated radiothreapy – The National Cancer Center Singapore Experience. Int J Radiat Oncol Biol Phys. 2009 Apr 20. [Epub ahead of print]

Wescott WB, Mira JG, Starcke EN, et al (1978) Alterations in whole saliva flow rate induced by fractionated radiotherapy. AJR Am J Roentgenol 130(1):145–149

Wolden SL, Chen WC, Pfister DG, et al (2006) Intensity-modulated radiation therapy (IMRT) for nasopharynx cancer: update of the Memorial Sloan-Kettering experience. Int J Radiat Oncol Biol Phys 64:57–62

Wu Q, Mohan R, Morris M, et al (2003) Simultaneous integrated boost intensity-modulated radiotherapy for locally advanced head-and-neck squamous cell carcinomas. I: dosimetric results. Int J Radiat Oncol Biol Phys 56(2): 573–585

Wu VW, Kwong DL, Sham JS (2004) Target dose conformity in 3-dimensional conformal radiotherapy and intensity modulated radiotherapy. Radiother Oncol 71:201–206

Xia P, Fu KK, Wong GW, et al (2000) Comparison of treatment plans involving intensity-modulated radiotherapy for nasopharyngeal carcinoma. Int J Radiat Oncol Biol Phys 48:329–337

Xia P, Verhey LJ (2001) Delivery systems of intensity-modulated radiotherapy using conventional multileaf collimators. Med Dosimetry 26:169–177

Selection and Delineation of Target Volumes in Intensity-Modulated Radiation Therapy for Nasopharyngeal Cancer

17

Jiade J. Lu, Vincent Grégoire, and Shaojun Lin

CONTENTS

Jiade J. Lu, MD, MBA
Department of Radiation Oncology, National University Cancer Institute, National University Health System, National University of Singapore, 5 Lower Kent Ridge Road, Singapore 119074, Republic of Singapore

Vincent Grégoire, MD, PhD
Radiation Oncology Department and Center for Molecular Imaging and Experimental Radiotherapy, Université Catholique de Louvain, St-Luc University Hospital, 10 Avenue Hippocrate, 1200 Bruxelles, Belgium

Shaojun Lin, MD
Department of Radiation Oncology, Cancer Hospital of Fujian Medical University, 91, Fumalu Maluding Road, Fuzhou, Fujian 350014, PR China

17.1 Introduction

Radiation therapy is the mainstay therapeutic modality for nasopharyngeal cancer (NPC), and high-dose radiation is required for curative treatment of the disease. Nasopharynx is in close proximity to the critical structures such as brainstem and brain (temporal lobes), parotid glands, and spinal cord. Irradiating structures close to the nasopharynx may cause symptoms that substantially affect the quality of life of patients after treatment; precise radiation therapy for this malignancy has always been the focus of technology development.

The implementation of intensity-modulated radiation therapy (IMRT) allows a significant improvement in the control of radiation dose distribution and is considered more advantageous for definitive therapy for nonmetastatic NPC. However, the utilization of IMRT in the treatment of NPC requires a different mindset when compared with conventional radiotherapy. One of the most important differences is the selective treatment of structures surrounding the primary disease and neck nodes required with IMRT. Target volumes harbor gross and subclinical diseases that need to be accurately determined and delineated before the planning of IMRT can be initiated. Therefore, the utilization of IMRT in the treatment of NPC requires full understanding of the criteria of radiological diagnosis of the primary disease and cervical lymph adenopathy, the anatomy of the nasopharynx and its adjacent structures, as well as the pattern of lymph node metastases so that the gross tumor volumes (GTV) and clinical target volumes (CTV) for subclinical disease can be selected.

In this framework, this chapter reviews the anatomy of the head and neck area with a focus on nasopharynx, its surrounding structures, and its draining cervical lymph nodes, and discusses the selection and delineation of both GTVs and CTVs in the treatment of NPC.

17.2 Anatomy

Direct extension of the disease to the tissues and organs close to the primary lesion is one of the most important modes of disease spread, and lymph node metastases follow certain specific patterns in NPC. A detailed discussion of imaging-based anatomy is out of the scope of this chapter. However, as the malignancy including its primary lesion and gross or subclinical lymph node metastasis is primarily treated with radiation therapy, a thorough understanding of the computer tomography (CT) or magnetic resonance imaging (MRI) based anatomy of the head and neck area including cervical lymph node distribution is crucial for the accurate selection and delineation of the target volumes in IMRT for NPC.

17.2.1 Anatomy of the Nasopharynx and its Surrounding Structures

The nasopharynx is a roughly cuboidal structure and is located below the central skull base. The roof of the nasopharynx is made of the sphenoid sinus and the basisphenoid. The posterior part of the roof slopes inferiorly and is contiguous with the posterior wall of the nasopharynx, which is made of the clivus, together with the C1 and C2 vertebrae. The nasopharynx is contiguous with the nasal cavity anteriorly and oropharynx inferiorly. The anterior border of the nasopharynx is the posterior nasal apertures and nasal septum, and the soft palate separates the nasopharynx from oropharynx inferiorly. The lateral walls of the nasopharynx are formed by the medial pterygoid plate, the palatal muscle, the torus tubarius, and the pharyngeal fossa (also called the fossa of Rosenmüller). The lateral walls harbor the pharyngeal opening of the eustachian tube, and the cartilaginous extension of the opening with its mucosa coverage, which forms the torus tubarius. The pharyngeal fossa lies just posterior to the torus tubarius and is formed by the junction of the lateral and posterior wall of the nasopharynx (Figs. 17.1–17.3).

One of the clinically important features of the anatomy of nasopharynx and its surrounding structures pertinent to NPC is the foramina and fissures located at the base of skull. Many of the foramina provide the passage to the blood vessels and cranial nerves, and NPC may cause damage of the fossa of Rosenmüller structures located in these passages at its locally

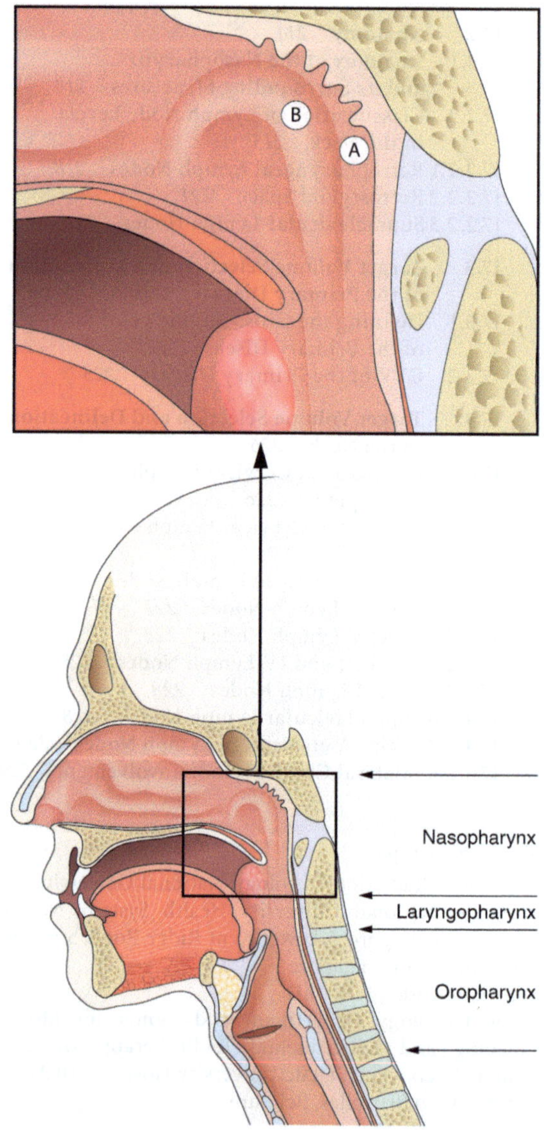

Fig. 17.1. The lateral wall of nasopharynx. (A. Fossa of Rosenmüller; B. torus tubarius;

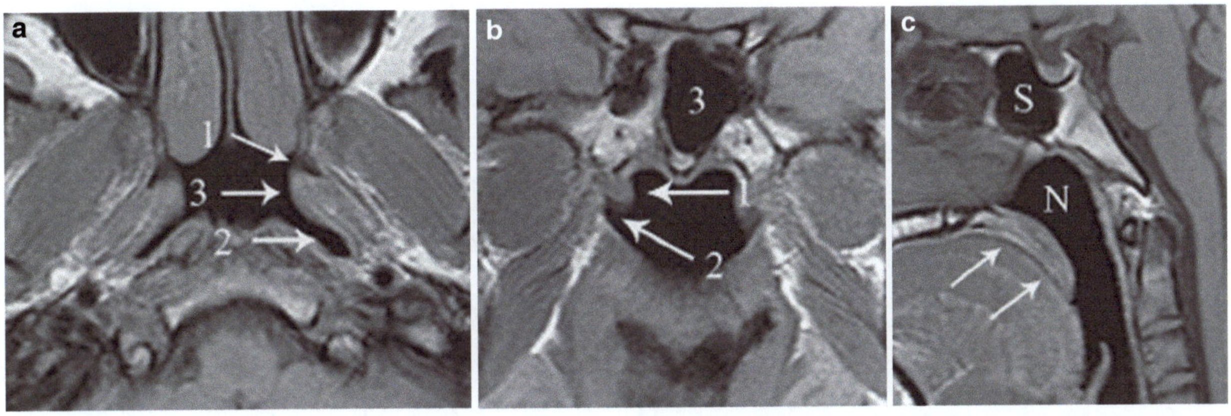

Fig. 17.2. Normal anatomy of the nasopharynx. (**a**) Axial T1-weighted magnetic resonance imaging (MRI) demonstrates the *left* eustachian tumor opening (*arrow 1*), fossa of Rosenmüller (*arrow 2*), and torus tubarius (*arrow 3*). (**b**) Coronal T1-weighted MRI demonstrates *right* torus tubarius (*arrow 1*), eustachian tube opening (*arrow 2*), and sphenoid sinus (3). (**c**) Sagittal T1-weighted MRI demonstrates the nasopharynx (*N*), sphenoid sinus (*S*), and soft palate (*arrows*). (Adopted from Chong and Ong [2008]. Used with permission from Elsevier)

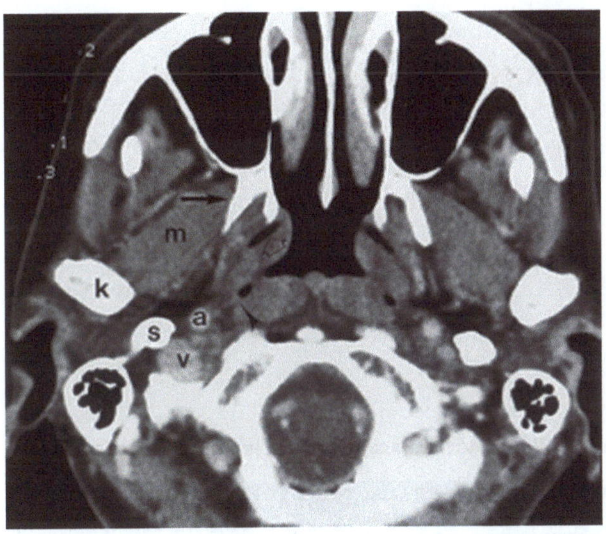

Fig. 17.3. Transverse section of computer tomography (CT) through the nasopharynx at the level of the mandibular condyle (k). The lateral pterygoid muscle (m) runs from the lateral pterygoid plate (*black arrow*) to the insertion along the medial aspects of the mandibular neck. Air is seen in the eustachian tube close to the opening in torus tubarius (*open arrow*). The fossa of Rosenmüller is partly collapsed (*arrowhead*). (*a* internal carotid artery; *v* internal jugular vein; *s* styloid process) (Used with permission from Medcyclopaedia™)

advanced stage. The foramina and fissures also provide potential routes of intracranial extension. Of all the foramina and fissures, the foramen lacerum and foramen ovale are the two important routes of intracranial extension from the primary disease. Foramen lacerum is located superolateral to the fossa of Rosenmüller, and is formed by the posterior margin of the petrous apex and the superior part of the clivus. Foramen ovale is positioned lateral to the foramen lacerum (Fig. 17.4).

17.2.2
Classification of Lymph Node Levels in the Neck

The head and neck region has a rich network of lymphatic vessels, and squamous cell carcinomas originated from the head and neck area including NPC can metastasize to regional cervical neck lymph nodes even in its early stages. Therefore, understanding of the normal anatomy of the neck lymph nodes is crucial for the treatment of head and neck cancers. To ensure effective communication, a standard terminology is needed in the discussion of the complex lymph node regions. Various classifications have been developed for this purpose. Table 17.1 listed two of the more commonly used terminologies/classification. For the purpose of radiation therapy for head and neck malignancies, the recommendation advocated by the Committee for Head and Neck Surgery and American Academy for Otolaryngology-Head and Neck Surgery (AAO-HNS) is one of the most widely utilized systems that is pertinent to radiation therapy for NPC. This classification of the neck lymph nodes (also called the "Robbins classification") was originally proposed by the Memorial Sloan-Kettering Cancer Group, and was adopted by the AAO-HNS in 1991 and lately revised in 1998. It systematically classifies the neck nodes into six levels according to visible structures including bone, muscle,

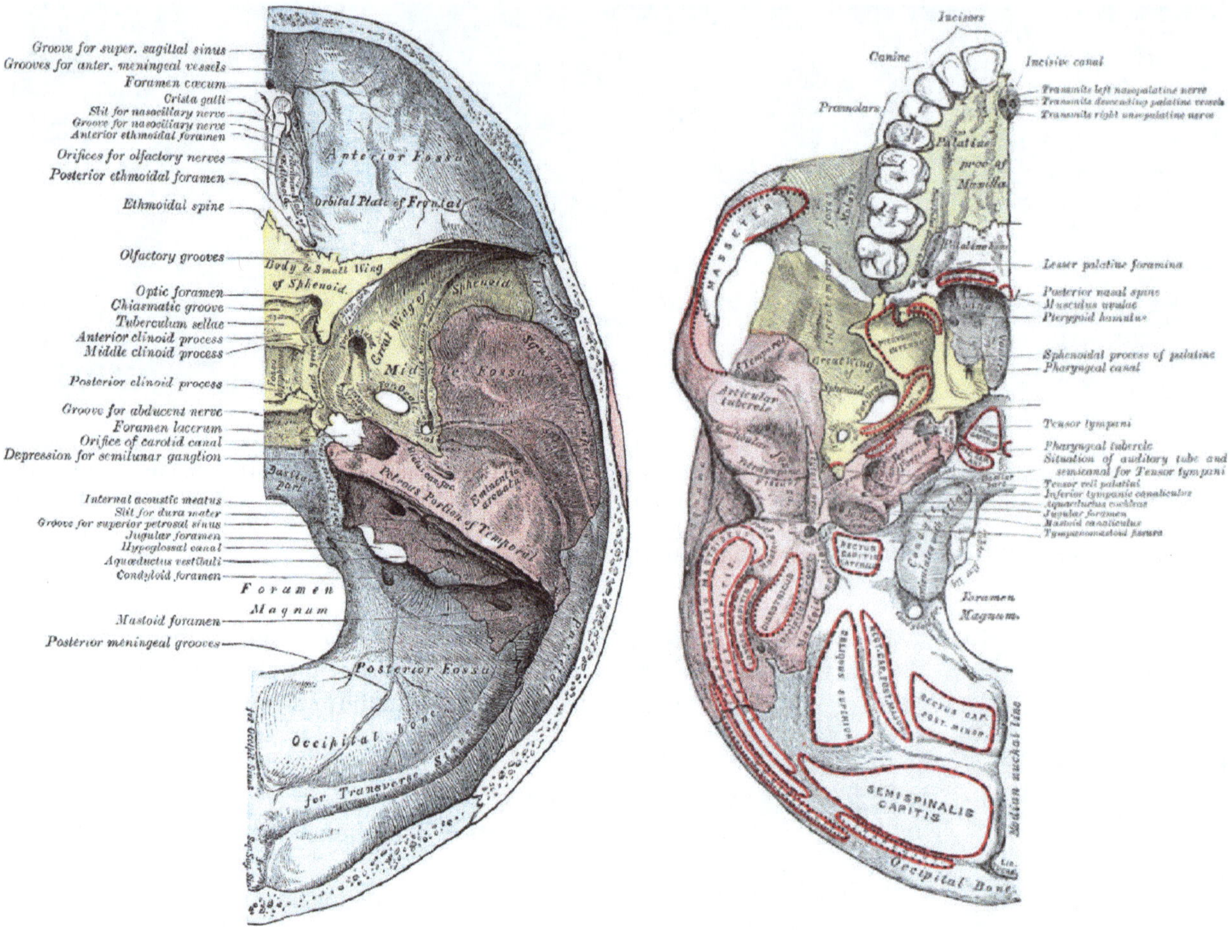

Fig. 17.4. Internal and external view of the base of skull

Table 17.1. Comparison between the TNM atlas terminology and the Robbins' classification of the lymph nodes of the neck

TNM atlas for lymph nodes of the neck		Robbins' classification	
Group number	Terminology	Level	Terminology
1	Submental nodes	Ia	Submental group
2	Submandibular nodes	Ib	Submandibular group
3	Cranial jugular nodes	II	Upper jugular group
4	Medial jugular nodes	III	Middle jugular group
5	Caudal jugular nodes	IV	Lower jugular group
6	Dorsal cervical nodes along the spinal accessory nerve	V	Posterior triangle group
7	Supraclavicular nodes	V	Posterior triangle group
8	Prelaryngeal and paratracheal nodes	VI	Anterior compartment group
9	Retropharyngeal nodes		
10	Parotid nodes		
11	Buccal nodes		
12	Retroauricular and occipital nodes		

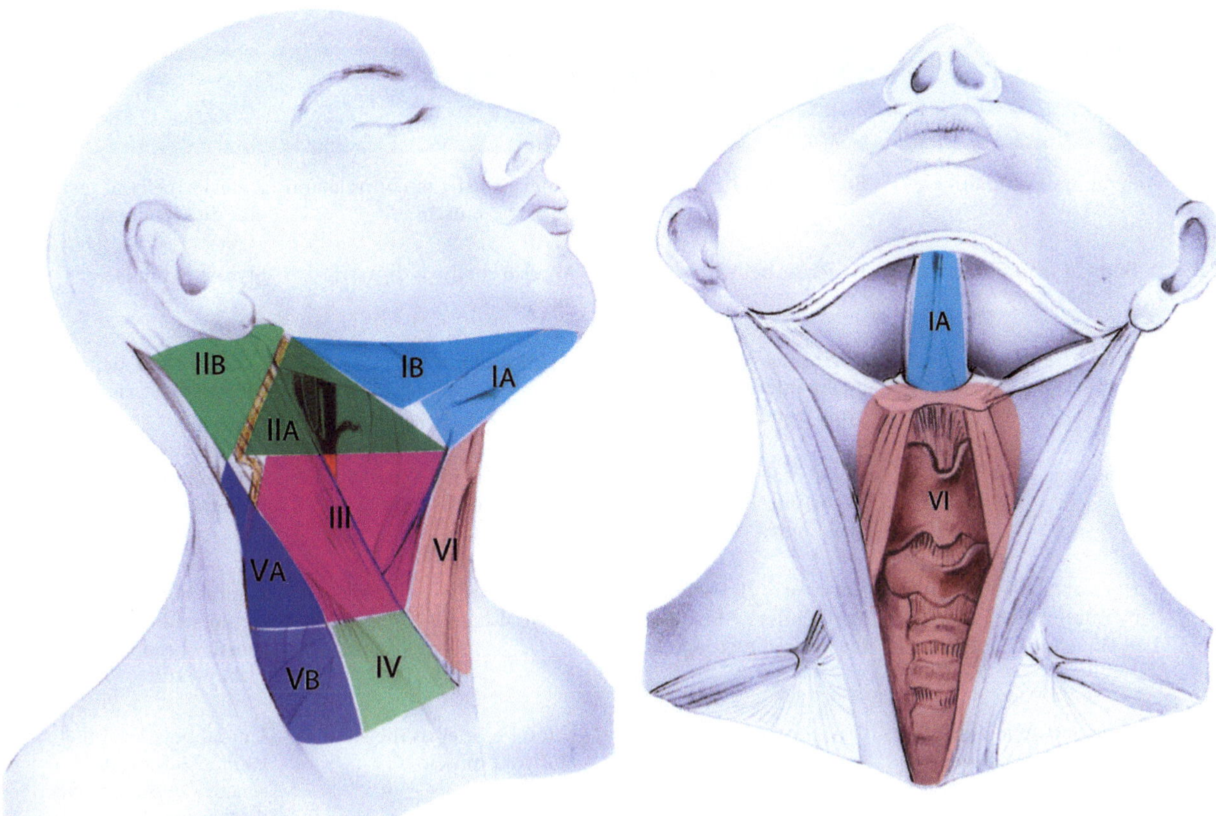

Fig. 17.5. Schematic representation of the various neck node groups: submental (*Ia*) and submandibular (*Ib*); upper jugular (*II*); mid jugular (*III*); lower jugular (*IV*); posterior triangle (*V*); anterior compartment (*VI*)

blood vessels, and nerves during neck dissection (Fig. 17.5, Table 17.2) (Robbins et al. 1991).

The Robbins Classification has been widely accepted by radiation oncologists for management of head and neck malignancies; nevertheless, it was originally developed for neck dissection, and some of the structures including blood vessels and nerves are not readily visible in CT or MRI of the head and neck. Therefore, translation of the anatomic boundaries of the neck node levels on CT or MRI was needed, so accurate identification, selection, and delineation of lymph nodes for the purpose of radiation planning can be achieved. In 2003, a CT-based neck node classification guideline proposal originally advocated by scholars from Brussels was reviewed and discussed by representatives of major cooperative groups in Europe and North America including DAHANCA, EORTC, GORTC, RTOG, and NCIC, and a common set of recommendations for delineation of neck node levels were concluded (the Consensus, Fig. 17.6, Table 17.3) (Grégoire et al. 2003). This consensus has been accepted in most major research organizations including EORTC and RTOG for cervical lymph node classification in their research protocols.

It is important to note that neck extension of patients treated with NPC may or may not be in the same position (anatomical position) used in the delineation of the lymph node groups in the consensus. In addition, lymph adenopathy in the neck may further complicate the delineation of the CTV in the neck area.

The original Robbins Classification provide a clear common nomenclature for most of the lymph node areas in the cervical neck; however, only lymph node groups routinely removed during neck dissection were considered, and several regions harbor lymph nodes pertinent to NPC were not covered by the Robbins Classification and the Consensus, i.e., CT-based cervical node classification. These regions include the retropharyngeal space, the retrostyloid space, and the supraclavicular fossa. However, a clear understanding of the positions of these lymph nodes in CT or MRI is of particular importance in definitive radiation therapy for NPC. As such, in a subsequent supplement to the Consensus for patients with

Table 17.2. Anatomical structures defining the boundaries of the neck levels and sub-levels

Level	Boundary			
	Superior	Interior	Anterior (Medial)	Posterior (Lateral)
IA	Symphysis of mandible	Body of hyoid	Anterior bally of contralateral digastric muscle	Anterior belly of jpsilateral digastric muscia
IB	Body of mandible	Posterior belly of muscle	Anterior belly of digastric muscle	Stylohyoid muscle
IIA	Skull base	Horizontal plane defined by the inferior body of the hyoid bone	Stylohyoid muscle	Vertical plane defined by the spinal accessory nerve
IIB	Skull base	Horizontal plane defined by the inferior body of the hyoid bone	Vertical plane defined by the spinal accessory nerve	Lateral border of the stemodeidomastoid muscle
III	Horizontal plane defined by inferior body of hyoid	Horizontal plane defined by the inferior border of the pricoid cartilage	Lateral border of the sternohyoid muscle	Lateral border of the stemocleidomastoid of sensory branches of cervical plexus
IV	Horizontal plane defined by the inferior border of the cricoid cartilage	Clavicle	Lateral border of the stemohyoid muscle	Lateral border of the stemocleidomastoid or sensory branches of cervical plexus
VA	Apex of the convergence of the sternocleidomastoid and trapezius muscles	Horizontal plane defined by the lower border of the cricoid cartilage	Posterior border of the sternoclaidomastoid muscle or sansory branches of cervical plexus	Anterior border of the trapexius muscle
VB	Horizontal plane defined by the lower border of the cricoid cartilage	Clavicle	Posterior border of the stemocleidomastoid muscle or sansory branches of cervical plexus	Anterior border of the trapezius muscle
VI	Hyoid bone	Suprasternal	Common carolid artery	Common carolid altery

positive neck lymph adenopathy, Grégoire et al. (2006) addressed these nodal regions.

17.2.2.1 Retropharyngeal Lymph Nodes

Retropharyngeal lymph nodes (RLNs) lie within the retropharyngeal space, which is bounded anteriorly by the pharyngeal constrictor muscles and posteriorly by the prevertebral fascia and extends cranially from the base of the skull to the level of C3 caudally (Rouvière 1948). Retropharyngeal nodes can be divided into medial and lateral groups according to their anatomical positions. The medial group lies in or near the midline, and consists of 1–2 lymph nodes, and is usually not visible on image studies in physiological condition. The lateral group of retropharyngeal nodes lies medial to the carotid artery, and can be found at any level within the retropharyngeal space (i.e., skull of base to the level of C3). The most superior lymph node of the lateral group is called the lymph node of Rouvière.

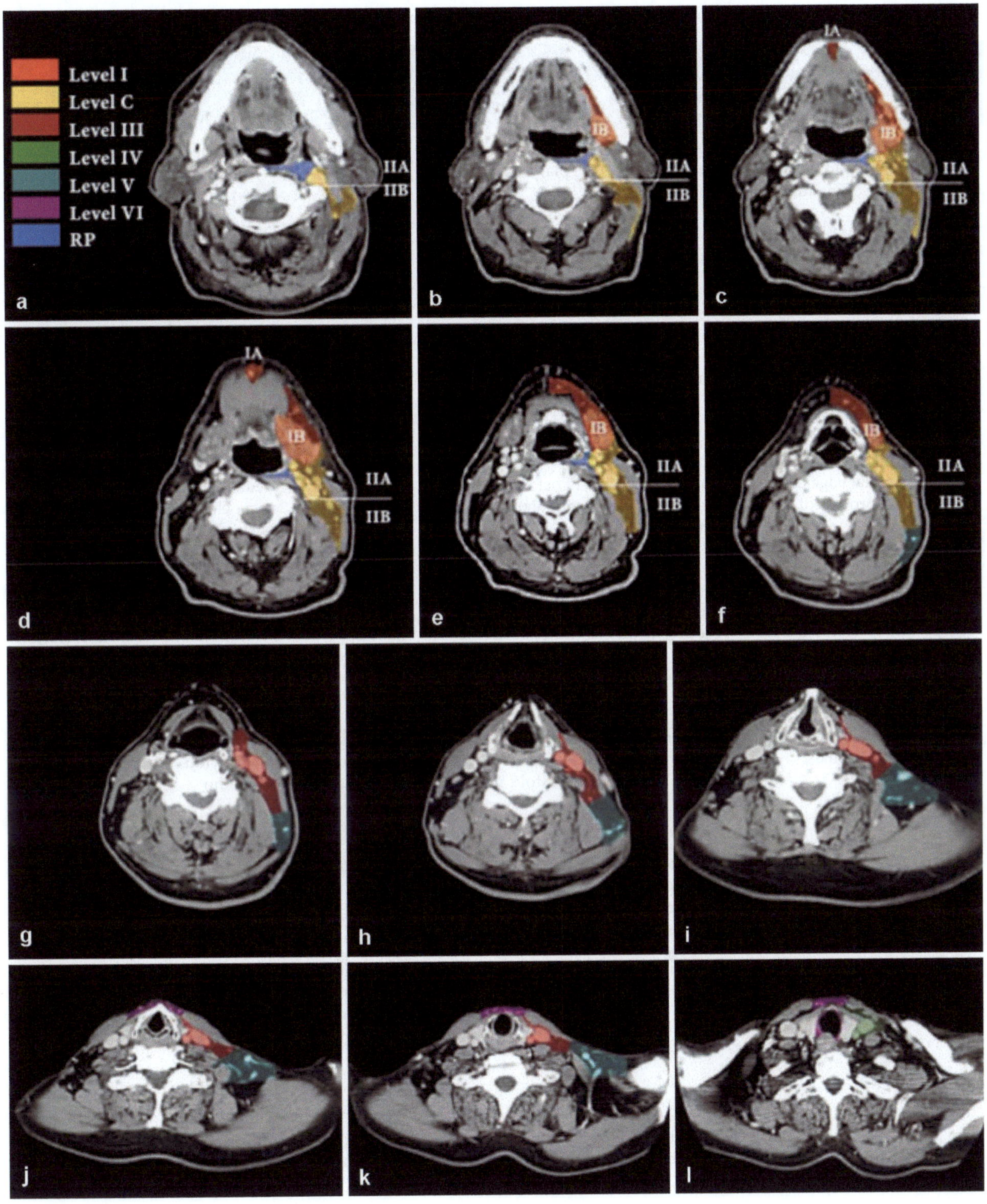

Fig. 17.6. Clinical target volume (CTV) of neck nodes of various levels delineated on the image of a laryngeal cancer patient with T1N0M0 disease

Table 17.3. Consensus guidelines for the radiological boundaries of the neck node levels

Level	Anstomical boundaries					
	Cranial	Caudal	Anterior	Posterior	Lateral	Medial
Ia	Geniohyoid m., plane tangent to basilar edge of mandible	Plane tangent to body of hyoid bone	Symphysis menti. platysma m.	Body of hyoid bone	Medial edge of ant. belly of digastric m.	n.a.[a]
Ib	Mylohyoid m., cranial edge of submandibular gland	Plane through central part of hyoid bone	Symphysis menti, platysma m.	Posterior edge of submandibular gland	Basilar edge/ innerside of mandible, platysma m., skin	Lateral edge of ant. belly of digastric m.
IIa	Caudal edge of lateral process of CI	Caudal edge of the body of hyoid bone	Post edge of submandibular gland: ant. edge of int. carotid artery: post. edge of post. belly of digastric m.	Post border of int. jugular vein	Medial edge of sternocleidomastoidm	Medial edge of int. carouid artery, paraspinal (levator seapulae) m.
IIb	Caudal edge of Internal process of CI	Caudal edge of the body of hyoid bone	Post. border of int. jugular vein	Post. border of the sternocleidomastoid m.	Medial edge of sternocleidomastoidm	Medial edge of int. carotid artery, paraspinal (levator scapulae) m.
III	Caudal edge of the body of hyoid bone	Caudal edge of cricoid cartilage	Postero-lateral edge of the sternohyoid m.: ant. edge of sternocleidomastoid m.	Post. edge of the sternocleidomastoid m.	Medial edge of sternocleidomastoidm	Int. edge of caroid artery, paraspinal (scalenins) m.
IV	Caudal edge of ericoid cartilage	2 cm eranial to sternoclavicular joint	Anteromedial edge of sternocleidomastoid m	Post. edge of the sternocleidomastoid m.	Medial edge of sternocleidomastoidm	Medial edge of Internal carotid artery, paraspinal (scalenius) m.
V	Cranial edge of body of hyoid bone	CT slice encompassing the transverse cervical vessels[b]	Post. edge of the sternocleidomastoid m.	Ant-lateral border of the trapezius m.	Platysma m., skin	Paraspinal (levator scapulae, splenius capitis) m.
VI	Caudal edge of body of thyroid cartilage[c]	Sternal manubrium	Skin; platysma m.	Separation between unchea and esophagus[d]	Medial edges of thyroid gland, skin and antmedial edge of sternocleidomastoid m.	n.a.
Retropharyngeal	Base of skull	Cranial edge of the body of hyoid bone	Fascia under the pharyngeal mucosa	Prevertebral m. (longus colli, longus capitis)	Medial edge of the internal carotid artery	Midline

[a]Midline structure lying between the medial borders of the anterior bellies of the digastric muscles
[b]For NPC, the reader is referred to the original description of the UICC/AJCC 1997 edition of the Ho's triangle. In essence, the fatty planes below and around the evavicle down to the trapezius muscle
[c]For paratraeheal and recurrent nodes, the cranial border is the caudal edge of the cricoid cartilage
[d]For pretracheal nodes, trachea and anterior edge of cricoid cartilage

Table 17.4. Radiological boundaries of the retrostyloid space and supraclavicular fossa

Space	Cranial	Caudal	Anterior	Posterior	Lateral	Medial
Retrostyoid	Base of skull (jugular foramen)	Upper limit of level II	Parapharyngeal space	Vertebral body/ base of skull	Parotid space	Lateral edge of RP notes
Supraclavicular fossa	Lower border of level IV/Vb	Sternoclavicular joint	SCM m.; skin; clavicle	Anterior edge of posterior scalenus m.	Lateral edge of posterior scalenus m.	Thyroid gland/ tracties

SCM sternocleidomastoid; *RP* retropharyngeal

17.2.2.2
Retrostyloid Space

According to the Consensus, the cranial border of the level II lymph nodes is set at the lateral process of C1. However, the lymph nodes lie in the fatty space around the jugulocarotid vessels up to the jugular foramen, i.e., the retrostyloid space (Table 17.4, Fig. 17.7) may receive a retrograde lymph flow from the level II nodes. In addition, direct extension of disease from an infected RLN to the retrostyloid space is not uncommon in NPC. In view of the high probability of disease metastasis to the retropharyngeal and level II lymph nodes in NPC, it is reasonable to consider the retrostyloid space a high-risk region, although the significance of direct drainage from nasopharynx to these nodes is unknown.

17.2.2.3
Supraclavicular Lymph Nodes

The supraclavicular fossa in NPC was originally proposed by Ho et al. and is defined by three points: (1) the superior margin of the sternal end of the clavicle, (2) the superior margin of the lateral end of the clavicle, and (3) the point where the neck meets the shoulder (Ho 1978). This definition was adopted by the latest version of the AJCC/UICC staging system of NPC (Greene 2002). Metastases to the supraclavicular lymph nodes in NPC is a strong indicator for distant failure and poor prognosis, and is currently classified as N3 disease in the AJCC staging system for NPC. Ho's definition of the supraclavicular fossa is clinical and depends on the clinical examination. In an attempt to improve the reliability of detecting the supraclavicular lymph adenopathy, Ng et al. (2007) replaced the clinical boundaries of the supraclavicular fossa with radiological landmarks, and included only level IV and Vb as the supraclavicular nodal region. Such a simplification remained predictive for both distant control and overall survival. However, in the Robbins Classification of cervical lymph node groups and in the Consensus, the supraclavicular fossa is not one of the neck levels (Grégoire et al. 2003). Grégoire et al. (2006) supplemented the Consensus in the lymph node positive and the postoperative neck by proposing criteria for the supraclavicular fossa, which is bounded by the lower border of Level IV/Vb cranially, the sternoclavicular joint caudally, thyroid gland/trachea medially, lateral edge of the posterior scalenus muscle laterally, anterior edge of posterior scalenus muscle posteriorly, and sterno-clado-mastoid muscle, skin, or clavicle anteriorly (Table 17.3, Fig. 17.8).

17.3
Target Volume Selection and Delineation of the Primary Disease

The International Commission on Radiation Units and Measurement (ICRU) Report No. 50 differentiated treatment planning volumes to GTV, CTV, and planning target volume (PTV) (Fig. 17.9):

GTV: all known gross disease, including abnormally enlarged regional lymph nodes. To determine GTV, appropriate radiology examination must be used that give the maximum dimension of what is considered potential gross disease.

CTV: encompass GTV plus regions considered to harbor potential microscopic disease.

PTV: provides margin around CTV to allow for variation in treatment setup and other anatomic motion during treatment, such as respiration, does not account for treatment machine beam characteristics.

The ICRU Report 62 introduced the internal target volume (ITV) to cover the physiological movement of the GTV and/or CTV. Since physiological motion in the head and neck area is usually not

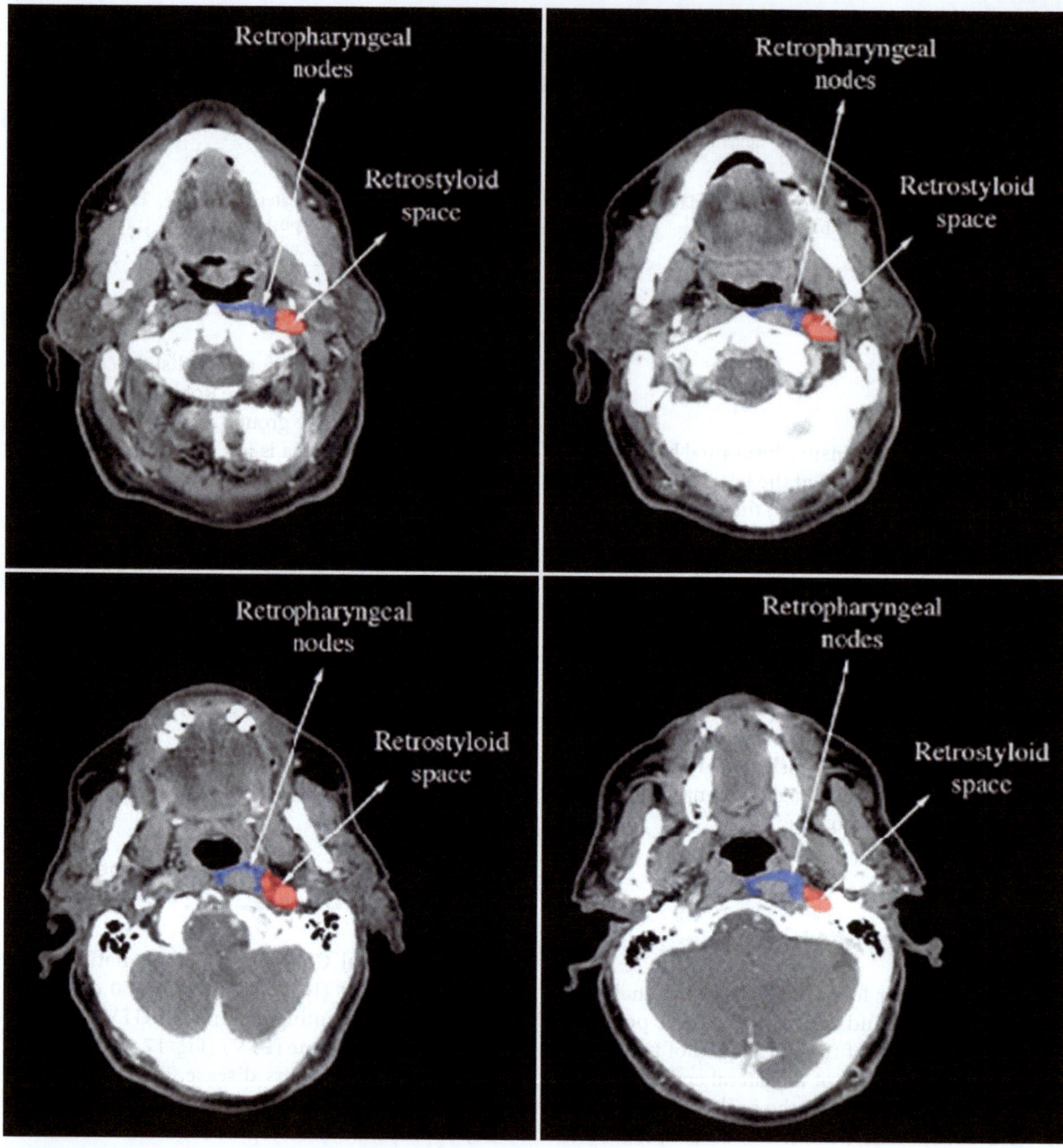

Fig. 17.7. Axial CT images of a patient with N0 neck with retropharyngeal and retrostyloid space delineated. The delineated areas correspond to the CTV, thus no margins for set-up error was included. (Adopted from Grégoire et al. (2006). Used with permission from Elsevier)

substantial after immobilization using thermoplastic mask, the significance of ITV in the radiation therapy of NPC is largely unknown.

Accurate definition and delineation of the target volumes in the precise radiation therapy including IMRT for the treatment of NPC is the single most critical factor for disease control. As the dose distribution becomes more precise, underdosed irradiation of the diseased areas is detrimental to the disease control and thus patients' survival. On the other hand, the nasopharynx is located adjacent to the critical normal organs and tissues such as brain, brainstem, spinal cord, pituitary, optic chiasm, parotid glands, etc. Unnecessary irradiation to these organs at risk

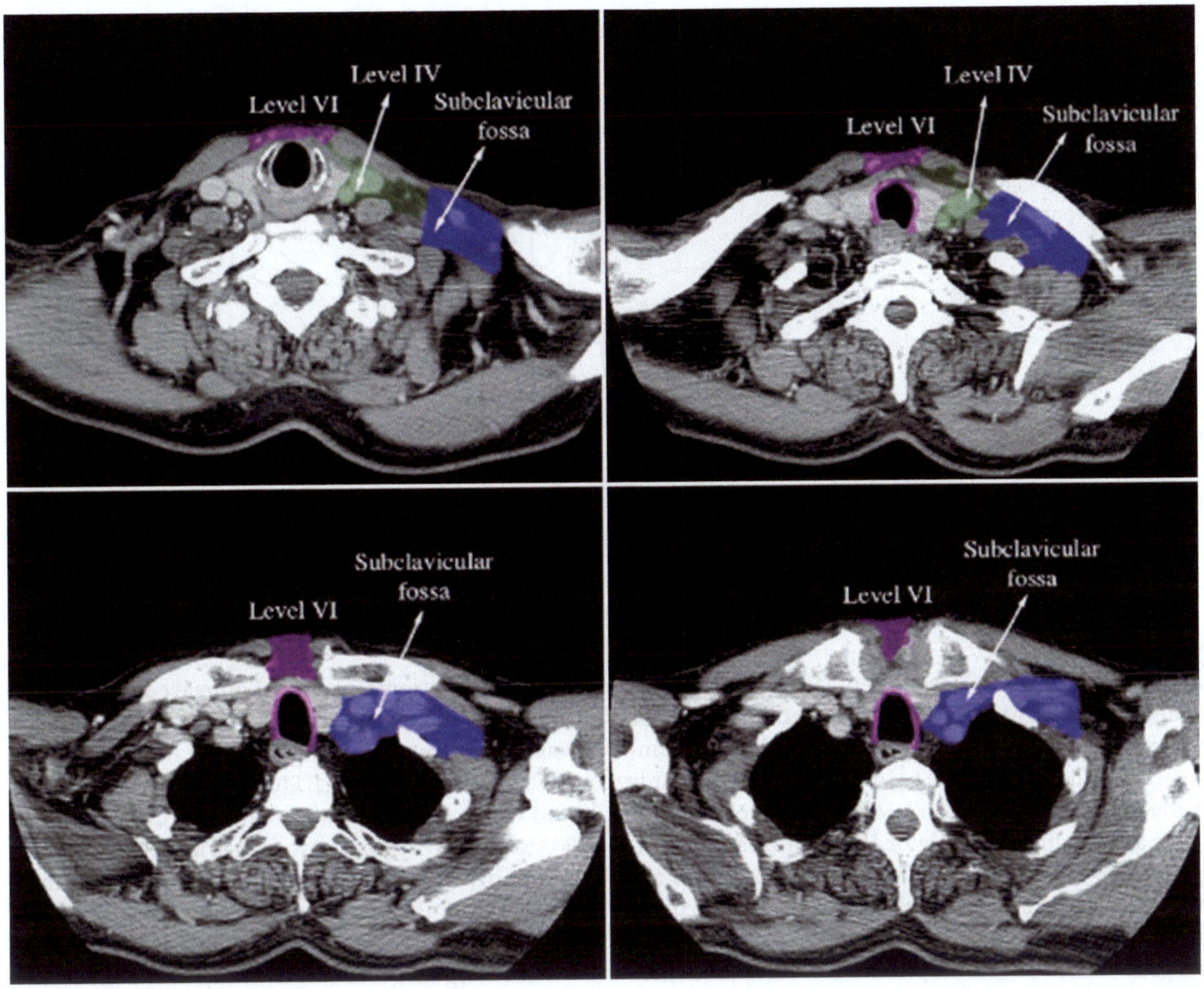

Fig. 17.8. Axial CT images of a patient with N0 neck with supraclavicular fossa delineated. The delineated areas correspond to the CTV, thus no margins for set-up error was included. (Adopted from Grégoire et al. (2006). Used with permission from Elsevier)

(OARs) may cause substantial long-term complications, which may significantly affect the quality of life of survivors, and in severe cases their lives.

17.3.1 Defining the Gross Tumor Volume of the Primary Disease

Although examination through direct or indirect nasopharyngoscopy provides important clinical information by direct visualization of the lesion originated from the nasopharynx, evaluation of the extent of the GTV in NPC cannot be completed without radiological imaging studies. The diagnosis and staging of NPC relies heavily on studies such as CT scan and/or MRI of the head and neck area, and recently the addition of FDG-PET/CT provided further improvement in the sensitivity and specificity in pretreatment evaluation of NPC.

CT has been the mainstay radiological modality for diagnosis and staging of NPC. However, numerous studies comparing MRI and CT for NPC diagnosis and staging have reported a more superior sensitivity and specificity of MRI in evaluating the local and regional extent of disease in NPC. The utilization of MRI and CT in the diagnosis and staging of NPC is detailed in Chapter 8.

The AJCC staging system recommends MRI as the primary radiological study for patients with NPC,

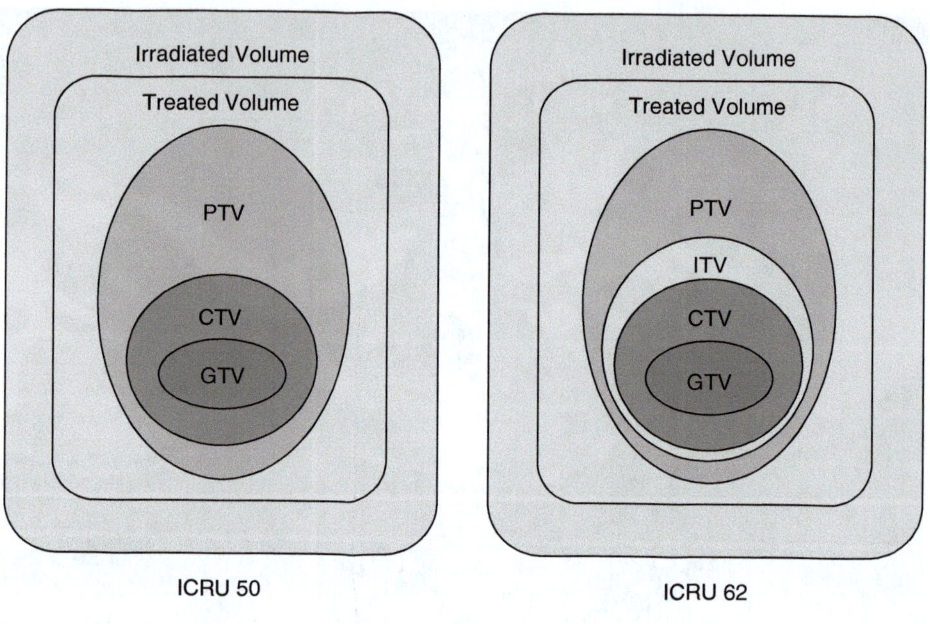

Fig. 17.9. Illustration of the gross tumor volume (*GTV*), clinical target volume (*CTV*), planning target volume (*PTV*), and internal target volume (*ITV*) defined by ICRU Report 50 and ICRU Report 62.

and CT scan can be used when MRI is not readily available. In addition, MRI images should be used (through fusion with planning CT) for better defining and delineation of the primary disease. In a study aimed to compare CT and MRI target volumes for NPC and evaluate the role of IMRT in treating composite CT + MRI targets, Emami et al. (2003) found that that MRI-based targets were 74% larger, more irregularly shaped, and did not always include the CT targets. When CT-based plans were compared with those based on CT + MRI targets, 14% underdosing was found, and doses to the OARs were significantly suboptimal. Approximately 20% of dose reduction could be achieved using targets delineated based on CT and MRI fusion.

Functional imaging, especially FDG-PET/CT, has been studied in the diagnosis and staging of nasopharyngeal carcinoma. However, whether FDG-PET/CT is more superior to MRI or enhancing CT in detecting and staging of NPC is pending for further investigation. In a study of 52 patients with stage III and IV NPC, King et al. (2008) found that MRI demonstrated more extensive disease in nasopharynx, skull base, brain, and/or orbit when compared with FDG-PET/CT. The addition of FDG-PET/CT to MRI did not change the overall stage or management strategy in any patient. Similar findings were reported in a series of 111 patients with histologically confirmed NPC. PET/CT showed a discrepancy with head-and-neck MRI in nearly one-third of the patients, and MRI appeared to be superior to PET/CT for the assessment of locoregional invasion and retropharyngeal nodal metastasis (Ng et al. 2009). Whether PET/CT in addition to MRI could facilitate the definition and delineation of the GTV in NPC treatment planning is largely unknown. Further investigation is needed to study the optimal utilization of PET/CT in the delineation of tumor volumes and radiation planning in NPC treatment.

One intriguing issue in defining and delineation of the primary disease in IMRT is whether the entire mucosa of nasopharynx should be included as the GTV for high-dose irradiation. Because of the invasive nature of the disease and its high probability of submucosal extension, the entire nasopharynx with a safety margin is usually encompassed in the definitive dose region in radiotherapy. However, whether to include the mucosa as part of the GTV, or defining the disease area visualized on enhanced CT, MRI, or FDG-PET/CT as GTV but include the "normal" nasopharyngeal mucosa as a high-risk region to be irradiated in high-dose coverage in IMRT is debatable, and probably possesses no clinical significance. Either method of GTV definition and delineation has been reported in studies on IMRT for NPC. It seems that substantial differences in treatment outcome is unlikely after high-dose radiation therapy using IMRT (Lee et al. 2002; Kam et al. 2004; Lin et al. 2009; Wolden et al. 2006; Tham et al. 2009a).

Table 17.5. Differences of delineation of CTV between the "recuded-volume" technique and the RTOG protocols

	"Reduced-volume" technique	RTOG-0225	RTOG-0615
Sphenoid sinus	Inferior part (in sphenoid sinus involved disease, the entire sphenoid sinus)	Inferior part	Inferior part (in T3 and T4 diseases, the entire sphenoid sinus)
Ethmoid sinus	Posterior	Not included	Not included
Nasal cavity	5 mm anterior to posterior nasal aperture	Posterior 1/3	Posterior 1/4 to 1/3
Maxillary sinus	5 mm anterior to maxillary mucosa	Posterior 1/3	Posterior 1/4 to 1/3
Clivis	Anterior 1/3	Entire	Anterior 1/2 to 2/3
Retropharyngeal nodes	From base of skull to cranial edge of the second cervical vertebra	From base of skull to cranial edge of the hyoid	From base of skull to cranial edge of the hyoid
Upper deep jugular nodes (retrostyloid space)	Not included unless involved	Included	Included
Level Ib	Not included unless involved	Included	Included in node positive patients

17.3.2 CTV of the Primary Disease

In the reported series of NPC treated with IMRT, methods of CTV delineation varied; however, most series reported a superb local control of 90% or above in the primary disease (Lee et al. 2002; Lin et al. 2009; Wolden et al. 2006; Kam et al. 2004; Tham et al. 2009a). The CTV delineated in IMRT for NPC is largely derived from our experience of conventional radiation therapy planning. Although local control is reportedly superb using the current arrangements of CTV, whether such an arrangement is necessary and can be reduced has not been fully addressed.

According to the RTOG 0615 protocol, the CTV of the primary disease should include the entire nasopharynx, anterior 1/2 to 2/3 of the clivus (entire clivus, if involved), skull base (foramen ovale and rotundum bilaterally must be included for all cases), pterygoid fossae, parapharyngeal space, inferior sphenoid sinus, and posterior fourth to third of the nasal cavity and maxillary sinuses to ensure pterygopalatine fossae coverage. The entire sphenoid sinus and cavernous sinus should be included in patients with T3, T4, bulky disease involving the roof of the nasopharynx (Lee et al. 2006). The outermost boundary of the above-mentioned CTV should be at least 10 mm from the GTV of the primary disease. Currently, the RTOG protocol recommends 59.4 Gy to the CTVs listed above.

Such coverage is largely derived from our previous experience of conventional radiation therapy for NPC, and typically encompasses a large volume. Although outcomes from such CTV arrangements produced superb local and regional control rates, whether it is necessary to encompass all normal adjacent structures as described above in radiation therapy for NPC, even in T1 and T2 diseases, is debatable. Isolated marginal local recurrence in the periphery of conventional treatment portal is minimal in any reports even in patients with T3 or T4 diseases (Chau et al. 2001, 2007). In a prospective series that included 323 NPC patients treated with IMRT, Lin et al. (2009) utilized a "reduced-volume" technique and included a limited volume in target delineation in both the primary disease area and to a lesser extent, in the neck lymph node area. The CTVs delineated in the study reported by Lin et al. and required by the RTOG 0225 and 0615 are listed in Table 17.5. At 30 months follow-up, the treatment outcome including local and regional control, as well as disease-free survival and overall survival rates were similar to historical data, and were 95%, 98%, 85%, and 90%, respectively (Lin et al. 2009). Ten patients experienced local recurrence within the delineated GTV, and two patients had marginal local recurrence with a component of recurrent foci in the GTV. Isolated recurrence at the edge of the delineated PTV was not seen. Reduced-CTV described above seems to be acceptable for radiation therapy for NPC using IMRT. However, whether this strategy of CTV delineation was truly sufficient or the superb local control rate was due to high collateral dose encompassing the tissues next to delineated CTV is unknown.

17.4 Target Volume Selection and Delineation in the Neck

17.4.1 Diagnosis of Cervical Lymph Adenopathy

Unlike the primary lesion, cervical lymph nodes involvement is largely determined based on the size (shortest axis) of the lymph node(s) in head and neck cancers, and nodes are considered metastatic if their shortest axis is ≥11 mm in the jugulodigastric regions, or >10 mm in other cervical regions. In addition, a group of three or more lymph nodes of borderline is considered metastatic (van der Brekel et al. 1990). Furthermore, a lymph node is considered involved if there is evidence of central necrosis or extracapsular extension (ECE) (van der Brekel et al. 1990; Som et al. 1992).

The diagnosis of retropharyngeal lymphadenopathy warrant additional discussion. RLNs can be divided into medial and lateral groups, and are exclusively examined through image studies, and pathological confirmation of its status is usually not feasible. The diagnostic criteria of an involved lateral RLN also depends on the presence of central necrosis, extracapsular disease extension, and the size of the lymph node. However, RLNs atrophy with age and are usually obliterated after 20 (Ogura et al. 2004). The short axis of normal RLNs on MRI is usually shorter than 4.5 mm, according to large series of patients with NPC, and the authors recommended that lateral RLN should be considered as involved if the shortest axis is 5 mm or more (Lam et al. 1997; King et al. 2000). Literatures addressing medial RLN in NPC are limited, and medial retropharyngeal lymphadenopathy are reported sporadically (Lam et al. 1997; Ng et al. 2006). As a medial RLN is usually not visible on CT or MRI in a normal individual, it is reasonable to consider any visible medial RLN on CT or MRI abnormal.

Although CT or MRI of the head and neck area can both be used for diagnosis and staging for NPC, MRI provides more superior sensitivity and specificity for detecting cervical lymph adenopathy, include those in the retropharyngeal region (Olmi et al. 1995; Ng et al. 1997).

The accuracy of FDG-PET/CT in detecting cervical lymph adenopathy has been studied in a number of clinical trials. Earlier reports indicated slight improvements regarding sensitivity and specificity of FDG-PET over enhanced CT and MRI (Adams et al. 1998; Kau et al. 1999). However, the results of a meta-analysis recently reported by Kyzas et al. (2008) indicated that the sensitivity and specificity of FDG-PET/CT were 50% and 87% in head and neck cancer patients with clinically negative neck. In addition, the utilization of FDG-PET/CT in the diagnosis and staging specifically for nasopharyngeal carcinoma has not been fully addressed. Convincing results that demonstrate the additive value of PET/CT on top of CT and MRI are needed before PET/CT can be routinely recommended for nasopharyngeal cancer.

17.4.2 Patterns of Cervical Lymph Node Metastases

Nasopharynx is a centrally located structure with extensive submucosal capillary lymphatic plexus. Partly due to this extensive lymphatic existence, NPC has a propensity of lymph node involvement in its early stages. Clinical evident cervical lymph adenopathy is seen in more than 85% of the patients with NPC (Tang 2009; Ng 2000). As a centrally located structure, there is a high probability of bilateral neck node metastases, and up to 50% of the patients with cervical lymph node metastasis have bilateral involvement (Sham et al. 1990; Tang et al. 2009).

Lymph node metastasis in NPC usually follows an orderly pattern, though three specific routes of lymphatic drainage: the retropharyngeal nodes, jugulodigastric nodes, and deep posterior cervical nodes to other cervical nodal regions.

17.4.2.1 Retropharyngeal Lymph Nodes

RLN, especially those in the lateral group, provide one of the most important routes of spread in NPC. The incidence of RLN metastasis in NPC is

Table 17.6. Incidence of retropharyngeal lymph adenopathy in nasopharyngeal cancers (NPC)

Authors	Incidence of retropharyngeal lymph nodes (RLN) (percentage of total number of patients)		
	Overall	N− in Levels I-V	N+ in Levels I-V
Tang et al. (2009)[a]	679/924 (73.5)	195/333 (58.6)	484/591 (81.9)
Wang et al. (2009)[a]	392/618 (63.4)	35/110 (31.8)	357/508 (70.3)
Liu et al. (2006)[a]	175/275 (63.6)	40/100 (40)	135/175 (77.1)
Ng et al. (2004)[b]	73/101 (82)	4/16 (40)	69/85 (81.2)
Chua et al. (1997)[c]	106/364 (29)	21/134 (16)	85/230 (37)
Chong et al. (1995)[c]	Not stated	Not stated	59/91 (65)
McLaughlin et al. (1995)[c]	14/19 (74)	2/5 (40)	12/14 (86)

Numbers within parentheses are in percentage
[a]Lymph node of ≥5 mm or with central necrosis irrespective of size on MRI
[b]Lymph node of ≥5 mm or with central necrosis irrespective of size on MRI, or increased up FDG uptake on PET/CT
[c]Lymph node of ≥10 mm or with central necrosis irrespective of size on MRI and/or CT

approximately 70%, and the incidence of RLN metastasis in patients with N+ disease (include retropharyngeal nodes) approaches 86% (Tang 2009; Wang 2009; Ng 2006). Although the contribution of retropharyngeal lymph adenopathy in staging has not been determined, the results from a number of reports indicated that the prognoses of patients with unilateral or bilateral RLN involvement only (i.e., otherwise N0 neck) assimilated those with N1 disease (Tham et al. 2009b; Ma et al. 2007).

Among patients presented with cervical lymph adenopathy, approximately 25% have isolated metastasis in RLN without evidence of other cervical lymph node metastasis (Tang 2009; Wang 2009; Ng 2006). The incidence of metastatic RLN shows an orderly decrease from the level of C1 to C3 (Liu et al. 2006), and the majority of metastatic RLNs are located superior to the C2 vertebral level (Liu et al. 2006; Chong et al. 1995; King et al. 2000).

Table 17.6 provides the incidence or retropharyngeal lymph adenopathy in NPCs reported in literatures.

17.4.2.2
Level II Lymph Nodes

Level II is the most commonly involved nodal group among all cervical lymph nodes in NPC. In patients with clinically evident lymph adenopathy, 75%–95% has level II nodal involvement.

Although not included in the level II region according to the Consensus, the fatty space around the jugulocarotid vessels up to the jugular foramen, i.e., the retrostyloid space, is considered a high-risk region in patients with NPC because of its high propensity of level II and RLN metastasis. Retrograde lymph flow may carry cancer cells from level II nodes to the lymph nodes in the retrostyloid space (Fisch 1968). In addition, the retrostyloid space lies in close proximity of RLN, and direct extension of disease from an involved retropharyngeal node to the retropharyngeal space is not uncommon. In the delineation of CTV in nasopharyngeal IMRT, the retrostyloid space is usually encompassed by expansion of the RLN for set-up error. Therefore, it is reasonable to recommended to extend the upper border of level II

Table 17.7. Incidence and distribution of cervical lymph node metastasis in NPC (In MRI Era)

Clinical nodal metastases							
Authors	Patients with N+	Level Ib[a]	Level II	Level III	Level IV	Level V	Other
TANG et al. 2009	786 (85.1)	24 (3.1)	590 (75.1)	226 (28.8)	56 (7.1)	87 (11.1)	6[b] (0.8)
WANG et al. 2009	543 (87.8)	21 (3.9)	506 (93.2)	237 (43.7)	72 (13.3)	200 (36.8)	7[b] (1.3)
LIU et al. 2006	215 (78.2)	6 (2.8)	174 (80.9)	65 (30.2)	16 (7.4)	18 (8.4)	4[b] (1.9)
NG et al. 2004	89 (88.1)	2 (2.2)	85 (95.5)	54 (60.7)	31 (34.8)	24 (27)	13[c] (14.6)

Numbers within parentheses are in percentage
[a]Level Ia (submental) lymph adenopathy was not observed in any of these studies
[b]Including parotid lymph nodes
[c]Including parotid, level VI, mediastinal, and abdominal lymph nodes

to include the retrostyloid space up to the base of skull in NPC (GRÉGOIRE et al. 2006).

The incidence of RLN metastasis in patients with cervical lymph adenopathy is between 75% and 86.4%. And ~25% has isolated metastasis in RLN without level II nodes involvement, and ~15% of patients has isolated level II lymph adenopathy without ipsilateral RLN. Therefore, metastases to the retropharyngeal and level II lymph nodes are considered to be through two distinct pathways by many authors (NG et al. 2004; WAKISAKA et al. 2000; TANG 2009) (Table 17.7).

17.4.2.3
Level V Lymph Nodes

A distinct drainage may exist between the nasopharynx to the lymph nodes in the posterior triangle of the neck. Isolated metastasis to Level V lymph nodes occurs in about 10% of patients with NPC without any evidence of RLN and/or Level II lymph node metastases.

17.4.2.4
Level III and IV Lymph Nodes

Level III contains a highly variable number of lymph nodes and receives efferent lymphatics from levels II and V, and some efferent lymphatics from the retropharyngeal, pretracheal, and recurrent laryngeal nodes. Level IV contains a variable number of nodes and receives efferent lymphatics primarily from levels III and V, some efferent lymphatics from the retropharyngeal, pretracheal, and recurrent laryngeal nodes. The incidence of metastases to the Levels III and IV lymph nodes range between 30%–60% and 7%–35%, respectively; however, most patients with levels III and IV nodal involvement harbor disease in the retropharyngeal, level II, and/or level V lymph nodes, and isolated adenopathy at level III and/or level IV are relatively uncommon in NPC (NG et al. 2004; TANG et al. 2009).

17.4.2.5
Level I Lymph Nodes

Metastasis to Level Ia lymph nodes are exceedingly rare in NPC, and was not documented in most clinical reports in the MRI era. However, metastasis to Level Ib lymph nodes is of clinical significance. Although isolated metastases to level Ib nodes are uncommon, in patients with Level II lymph adenopathy, approximately 2%–4% of patients will harbor metastases in the submandibular lymph nodes (TANG et al. 2009; NG et al. 2004; WANG et al. 2008).

17.4.2.6
Supraclavicular Lymph Nodes

Supraclavicular region defined by GRÉGOIRE et al. (2006) includes the area bounded by the lower border of Level IV/Vb cranially, the sternoclavicular joint caudally, thyroid gland/trachea medially, lateral edge of the posterior scalenus muscle laterally, anterior edge of posterior scalenus muscle posteriorly, and sterno-clado-mastoid muscle, skin, or clavicle anteriorly (Table 17.3, Fig. 17.6). Lymph nodes in the supraclavicular region receives its drainage from levels III, IV, and V in most types of head and neck cancers including NPC. The probability of supraclavicular lymph node (as defined by Grégoire et al. in their 2006 supplement to the Consensus) and level I lymph node involvement is approximately 4% in NPC (Tang et al. 2009). And patients presented with metastatic supraclavicular lymph adenopathy usually harbor clinical evident disease in level IV or V lymph nodes, and isolated supraclavicular lymph node metastasis is exceedingly uncommon.

17.4.2.7
"Skip" Metastasis of Lymph Nodes

"Skip metastases" are metastases that bypass the orderly progression from one level to a contiguous level. As lymph node metastases from the nasopharynx usually initiate at retropharyngeal, level II, and less frequently level V nodes, isolated metastases to levels I, III, IV, and more distant lymph nodes can be considered as "skip metastases."

"Skip metastases" to cervical lymph nodes are not commonly observed in NPC. In a series reported by Sham et al., the incidence of skip lymph node metastases in the cervical lymph nodal regions was 3.9% (Sham et al. 1990). In a more recently reported series of 924 patients newly diagnosed with NPC, cervical lymph nodes were evaluated with MRI. Only two patients were found to have levels III and/or V metastases without evidence of lymph adenopathy in retropharyngeal and level II lymph nodes. In addition, two patients with lymph adenopathy in retropharyngeal or level II cervical nodes presented with level IV or supraclavicular nodal disease without involvement of level III or level V nodes. The incidence of "skip metastases" in the cervical lymph nodes was 0.6% in total (Tang et al. 2009). In a series of 89 patients with NPC reported by Ng and colleagues, the incidence of "skip metastases" including distant metastases to mediastinal and abdominal lymph nodes was 7.9% when both MRI and FDG-PET/CT were utilized (Ng et al. 2004). Nevertheless, the overall incidence of "skip metastases" in the cervical lymph node chain is less than 10%, thus whether elective irradiation of the lower neck in NPC patients with N0 disease or upper neck adenopathy is unknown.

17.4.2.8
Bilateral Cervical Node Involvement

Nasopharynx is a centrally located structure. In addition, submucosal extension of disease is not uncommon for disease initiated from an ipsilateral compartment. Therefore, bilateral lymph node metastases in the neck are common in NPC. Overall, 39.2%–50% of patients with cervical lymph adenopathy had bilateral diseases based on radiological diagnosis (Tang et al. 2009; Sham et al. 1990).

17.4.3
Selecting Clinical Target Volumes in the Neck

While the definition of the GTV is largely determined by the anatomical presentation of the disease and lymph adenopathy visualized on imaging studies such as CT, MRI, and FDG-PET/CT, the selection of the CTVs in the neck, i.e., in the lymph node draining area, of the NPC requires not only knowledge on the anatomical position of lymph nodes, but also the lymph drainage pattern in NPC.

Lymph node groups at higher risk for regional metastases in NPC included bilateral RNLs, Level II, and level V lymph nodes. Level III and level IV (lower neck) nodes are at high risk, especially when level II nodes are involved. In addition, level Ib in the submandibular region are at risk and should be included in the CTV if level II lymph nodes are clinically involved. Elective irradiation of neck lymph nodes, at least part of them, in patients with or without evidence of regional metastases is usually recommended. In a large retrospective study reported by Lee et al., (1989) the regional recurrence rate of patients treated with elective irradiation to cervical lymph nodes was 11%, when compared with 40% in those who only received irradiation to the primary diseases without elective neck irradiation.

The high-risk lymph node regions defined by the RTOG 0615 protocol include bilateral RLNs, upper deep jugular lymph nodes, and levels II–V lymph nodes. For patients with subdigastric lymph node involvement, extensive involvement of the hard palate, nasal cavity, or maxillary antrum, ipsilateral submandibular lymph nodes are also considered as high-risk, and should be included in the CTV. The outermost boundary of the CTV of the cervical lymph nodes should be at least 10 mm away from the involved lymph nodes and from the RLNs to ensure sufficient coverage of metastatic cervical nodes and RLNs by the high-dose region (Lee et al. 2006).

17.4.3.1 Clinical Target Volumes in N0 Disease

In the above-mentioned study reported by Lee et al., (1999) the regional recurrence rate of 40% in N0 patients who were devoid of elective neck irradiation was certainly unacceptable. However, as the entire cervical lymph node chain were omitted in the radiation portal, regional recurrence in the high-risk nodal regions such as level II and level III is foreseeable. And routine elective irradiation to upper neck lymph nodal regions including those in the posterior neck is necessary. In addition, the chance of level Ib, IV, and IVb nodes are at higher risk if the next node echelon, particularly levels II and III, are involved.

However, owing to the low risk of "skip metastasis" in NPC (Sham et al. 1990; Tang et al. 2009), it is reasonable to question the necessity of elective irradiation to the lower neck lymph nodes (such as levels IV and Vb) and supraclavicular nodes in patients with N0 disease.

Table 17.8. A proposed lymph node coverage scheme according to the nodal status in the treatment of NPC using intensity-modulated radiation therapy (IMRT)

Nodal classification (AJCC 1997)	Levels to be included in the CTV	
	Ipsilateral neck	Contralateral neck
N0	RP + II-III-Va	RP + II-III-Va
N1	RP + Ib-II-III-IV-V	RP + Ib[a]-II-III-IV-V
N2	RP + Ib-II-III-IV-V	RP + Ib-II-III-IV-V
N3	RP + Ib-II-III-IV-V ± adjacent structures based on clinical and radiological findings[b]	RP + Ib-II-III-IV-V

Specifics:
[a]The necessity of encompassing contralateral Ib nodes in patients with N1 NPC is not clear
CTV clinical target volume; *RP* retropharyngeal nodes
[b]Inclusion of supraclavicular nodes: in case of lymph node involvement in level IV and Vb, inclusion of supraclavicular nodes is suggested

In the above-mentioned study reported by Tang et al. (2009), 138 patients had N0 disease and were irradiated either to the superior border of the cricoid cartilage (37 patients) or the inferior border of the cricoid cartilage (101 patients). No patient experienced regional failure, although nine patients had distant failure. Furthermore, in a more recently reported series included 410 NPC patients with N0 disease by Gao et al. (2009), all patients were treated with conventional radiotherapy, but only lymph nodes in the upper neck nodes were electively irradiated. All nodal areas inferior to the inferior margin of the thyroid cartilage were spared from the radiation field. At 5-year follow-up, only one case (0.2%) of regional recurrence in the lower neck was observed. These results suggested that in patients diagnosed and staged with no cervical lymph adenopathy on physical examination and CT or MRI, spearing the lower neck nodes from radiation may be acceptable with a minimal risk of regional recurrence. However, further investigations are needed to confirm the above-mentioned optimal findings and before the limited neck field becomes the standard of CTV delineation in IMRT for NPC patients with N0 disease. Currently, most centers and research organizations advocate elective treatment of all lower level cervical lymph nodes including those in level IV, Vb, and supraclavicular lymph nodes in patients with N0 disease.

Table 17.8 summarized an evidence-based proposal for the lymph node coverage scheme in the treatment of NPC using IMRT.

17.4.3.2 Clinical Target Volumes in N+ Disease with Extracapsular Extension

In the node-positive neck, an important issue to consider is the probability of ECE and the extent of disease infiltration into the surrounding tissue, particularly muscle. As NPC is usually treated with radiation therapy, pathological evaluation of the probability of ECE and its implication to muscle invasion has not been performed. However, experience from other head and neck malignancies indicated that the risk of ECE is proportional to the size of the involved lymph node. For radiologically inevident but involved neck lymph nodes, extracapsular infiltration of cancer cells is usually found within 1 cm from the capsule (Apisarnthanarax et al. 2006). For lymph node smaller than 1 cm in diameter, the probability of ECE is approximately 25%, and for bulky lymph nodes of more than 3 cm in diameter, the probability increased to approximately 80% (Chao et al. 2002).

Therefore, for patients with lymph nodes with shortest diameter of more than 3 cm, clear evidence of ECE, it is important to consider the probability and extent of disease infiltration into the adjacent muscle during CTV delineation. And it is reasonable to encompass the adjacent muscle in the CTV, at least on the same CT slide of the lymph adenopathy to ensure sufficient coverage to subclinical disease. However, whether such volume is sufficient or excessive for disease control in the treatment of NPC is unknown.

17.5 Conclusions

The treatment of NPC is challenging. Accurate defining and delineation of tumor volumes in IMRT of NPC requires knowledge of the clinical diagnosis of the disease, patterns of disease spread and metastases, as well as a thorough understanding of radiological anatomy of the head and neck area. The current standard volume of IMRT for NPC usually encompasses regions of the primary disease and involved cervical lymph adenopathy, as well as lymph nodal drainage areas of nasopharynx for elective irradiation. Reduced-volume CTV in irradiation in the primary disease region seemed to provide acceptable outcome according to a large prospective series. In addition, omitting elective nodal irradiation in the lower neck seemed to be feasible, especially in patients with N0 disease. Further investigation is necessary to define the optimal clinical tumor volumes in the treatment of NPC using IMRT.

References

Adams S, Baum RP, Stuckensen T, et al (1998) Prospective comparison of 18F-FDG PET with conventional imaging modalities (CT, MRI, US) in lymph node staging of head and neck cancer. Eur J Nucl Med 25(9):1255–1260

Apisarnthanarax S, Elliott DD, El-Naggar AK, et al (2006) Determining optimal clinical target volume margins in head-and-neck cancer based on microscopic extracapsular extension of metastatic neck nodes. Int J Radiat Oncol Biol Phys 64(3):678–683

Chao KS, Wippold FJ, Ozyigit G, et al (2002) Determination and delineation of nodal target volumes for head-and-neck cancer based on patterns of failure in patients receiving definitive and postoperative IMRT. Int J Radiat Oncol Biol Phys 53(5):1174–1184

Chau RM, Teo PM, Choi PH, et al (2001) Three-dimensional dosimetric evaluation of a conventional radiotherapy technique for treatment of nasopharyngeal carcinoma. Radiother Oncol 58(2):143–153

Chau RM, Teo PM, Kam MK, et al (2007) Dosimetric comparison between 2-dimensional radiation therapy and intensity modulated radiation therapy in treatment of advanced T-classification nasopharyngeal carcinoma: to treat less or more in the planning organ-at-risk volume of the brainstem and spinal cord. Med Dosim 32(4):263–270

Chong VFH, Ong CK (2008) Nasopharyngeal carcinoma. Eur J Radiol 66:437–447

Chong VF, Fan YF, Khoo JB. Retropharyngeal lymphadenopathy in nasopharyngeal carcinoma. Eur J Radiol. 1995;21(2):100-5

Chua DT, Sham JS, Kwong DL, et al. Retropharyngeal lymphadenopathy in patients with nasopharyngeal carcinoma: a computed tomography-based study. Cancer. 1997;79(5):869–77

Emami B, Sethi A, Petruzzelli GJ (2003) Influence of MRI on target volume delineation and IMRT planning in nasopharyngeal carcinoma. Int J Radiat Oncol Biol Phys 57(2):481–488

Fisch U (1968) Lymphography of the cervical lymphatic system. WB Saunders, London

Gao Y, Zhu G, Lu JJ, et al (2009) Is prophylactic irradiation to the lower neck necessary for nasopharyngeal cancer patients with N0 disease? Int J Radiat Oncol Biol Phys

Grégoire V, Eisbruch A, Hamoir M, et al (2006) Proposal for the delineation of the nodal CTV in the node-positive and the post-operative neck. Radiother Oncol 79(1):15–20

Grégoire V, Levendag P, Ang KK, et al (2003) CT-based delineation of lymph node levels and related CTVs in the node-negative neck: DAHANCA, EORTC, GORTEC, NCIC,RTOG consensus guidelines. Radiother Oncol 69(3):227–236

Ho JHC (1978) Stage classification of nasopharyngeal carcinoma: a review. In: de The G, Ito Y (eds) Nasopharyngeal carcinoma: etiology and control, Vol 20. IARC Scientific Publications, Lyon, France, pp 99–113

Kam MK, Teo PM, Chau RM, et al (2004) Treatment of nasopharyngeal carcinoma with intensity-modulated radiotherapy: the Hong Kong experience. Int J Radiat Oncol Biol Phys 60(5):1440–1450

Kau RJ, Alexiou C, Laubenbacher C, et al (1999) Lymph node detection of head and neck squamous cell carcinomas by positron emission tomography with fluorodeoxyglucose F 18 in a routine clinical setting. Arch Otolaryngol Head Neck Surg 125(12):1322–1328

King AD, Ahuja AT, Leung SF, et al (2000) Neck node metastases from nasopharyngeal carcinoma: MR imaging of patterns of disease. Head Neck 22(3):275–281

King AD, Ma BB, et al (2008) The impact of 18F-FDG PET/CT on assessment of nasopharyngeal carcinoma at diagnosis. Br J Radiol 81(964):291–298

Kyzas PA, Evangelou E, Denaxa-Kyza D, et al 18F-fluorodeoxyglucose positron emission tomography to evaluate cervical node metastases in patients with head and neck squamous cell carcinoma: a meta-analysis. J Natl Cancer Inst. 2008;100(10):712–20

Lam WW, Chan YL, Leung SF, et al (1997) Retropharyngeal lymphadenopathy in nasopharyngeal carcinoma. Head Neck 19(3):176–181

Lee N, Pfister DG, Garden A, et al (2006) RTOG 0615, A phase II study of concurrent chemoradiotherapy using three-dimentional conformal radiotherapy (3D-CRT) or intensity-modulated radiation therapy (IMRT) + bevacizumab (BV) for locally or regionally advanced nasopharyngeal cancer.http://www.rtog.org/members/protocols/0615/0615.pdf Accessed on May 19

Lee N, Xia P, Quivey JM, et al (2002) Intensity-modulated radiotherapy in the treatment of nasopharyngeal carcinoma: an update of the UCSF experience. Int J Radiat Oncol Biol Phys 53(1):12–22

Lee AW, Sham JS, Poon YF, et al Treatment of stage I nasopharyngeal carcinoma: analysis of the patterns of relapse and the results of withholding elective neck irradiation. Int J Radiat Oncol Biol Phys. 1989;17(6):1183–90

Lin S, Pan J, Lu H, et al (2009) Nasopharyngeal carcinoma treated with reduced-volume intensity-modulated radiation therapy: report on the 3-year outcome of a prospective series. Int J Radiat Oncol Biol Phys. 2009 Apr 11. [Epub ahead of print]

Liu LZ, Zhang GY, Xie CM, et al (2006) Magnetic resonance imaging of retropharyngeal lymph node metastasis in nasopharyngeal carcinoma: patterns of spread. Int J Radiat Oncol Biol Phys 66(3):721–730

Ma J, Liu L, Tang L, et al (2007) Retropharyngeal lymphadenopathy in nasopharyngeal carcinoma: prognostic value and staging categories. Clin Cancer Res 13:1445–1452

McLaughlin MP, Mendenhall WM, Mancuso AA, et al Retropharyngeal adenopathy as a predictor of outcome in squamous cell carcinoma of the head and neck. Head Neck. 1995;17(3):190–8

Ng Sh, Chang TC, Ko SF, et al (1997) Nasopharyngeal carcinoma: MRI and CT assessment. Neuroradiology 39(10): 741–746

Ng SH, Chan SC, Yen TC, et al (2009) Staging of untreated nasopharyngeal carcinoma with PET/CT: comparison with conventional imaging work-up. Eur J Nucl Med Mol Imaging 36(1):12–22

Ng SH, Chang JT, Chan SC, et al Nodal metastases of nasopharyngeal carcinoma: patterns of disease on MRI and FDG PET. Eur J Nucl Med Mol Imaging. 2004;31(8):1073–80.

Ng WT, Lee AW, Kan WK, et al (2007) N-staging by magnetic resonance imaging for patients with nasopharyngeal carcinoma: pattern of nodal involvement by radiological levels. Radiother Oncol 82:70–75

Ogura I, Kaneda T, Kato M, et al (2004) MR study of lateral retropharyngeal lymph nodes at different ages. Oral Surg Oral Med Oral Pathol Oral Radiol Endod 98(3):355–358

Olmi P, Fallai C, Colagrande S, et al (1995) Staging and follow-up of nasopharyngeal carcinoma: magnetic resonance imaging versus computerized tomography. Int J Radiat Oncol Biol Phys 32(3):795–800

Robbins KT, Medina JE, Wolfe GT et al (1991) Standardizing neck dissection terminology. Official report of the Academy's Committee for Head and Neck Surgery and Oncology. Arch Otolaryngol Head Neck Surg 117: 601–605

Robbins KT, Clayman G, Levine PA, et al (2002) Neck dissection classification update: revisions proposed by the American Head and Neck Society and the American Academy of Otolaryngology-Head and Neck Surgery. Arch Otolaryngol Head Neck Surg 128(7):751–758

Robbins KT, Shaha AR, Medina JE, et al (2008) Consensus statement on the classification and terminology of neck dissection. Arch Otolaryngol Head Neck Surg 134(5): 536–538

Rouvière H. (Tobiar MT, Edwards JW, trans.) Anatomy of the Human Lymphatic System. Ann Arbor, MI, 1948

Sham JS, Choy D, Wei WI (1990) Nasopharyngeal carcinoma: orderly neck node spread. Int J Radiat Oncol Biol Phys 19(4):929–933

Som PM (1992) Detection of metastasis in cervical lymph nodes: CT and MR criteria and differential diagnosis. AJR Am J Roentgenol 158(5):961–969

Tang L, Mao Y, Liu L, et al The volume to be irradiated during selective neck irradiation in nasopharyngeal carcinoma: analysis of the spread patterns in lymph nodes by magnetic resonance imaging. Cancer. 2009;115(3):680–8

Tang L, Mao Y, Liu L, et al (2009) The volume to be irradiated during selective neck irradiation in nasopharyngeal carcinoma: analysis of the spread patterns in lymph nodes by magnetic resonance imaging. Cancer 115(3): 680–688

Tham IW, Hee SW, Yeo RM et al. (2009a) Treatment of Nasopharyngeal Carcinoma Using Intensity-Modulated Radiotherapy-The National Cancer Centre Singapore Experience. Int J Radiat Oncol Biol Phys. 2009 Apr 20. [Epub ahead of print]

Tham IW, Hee SW, Yap SP, et al (2009b) Retropharyngeal nodal metastasis related to higher rate of distant metastasis in patients with N0 and N1 nasopharyngeal cancer. Head and Neck 31(4):468–474

van den Brekel MW, Stel HV, Castelijns JA, et al (1990) Cervical lymph node metastasis: assessment of radiologic criteria. Radiology 177(2):379–384

Wakisaka M, Mori H, Fuwa N, et al (2000) MR analysis of nasopharyngeal carcinoma: correlation of the pattern of tumor extent at the primary site with the distribution of metastasized cervical lymph nodes. Preliminary results. Eur Radiol 10(6):970–977

Wang XS, Hu CS, Ying HM, et al (2009) Patterns of retropharyngeal node metastasis in nasopharyngeal carcinoma. Int J Radiat Oncol Biol Phys 73(1):194–201

Wang X, Li L, Hu C, et al. Patterns of level II node metastasis in nasopharyngeal carcinoma. Radiother Oncol. 2008;89(1):28-32

Wolden SL, Chen WC, Pfister DG, et al (2006) Intensity-modulated radiation therapy (IMRT) for nasopharynx cancer: update of the Memorial Sloan-Kettering experience. Int J Radiat Oncol Biol Phys 64(1):57–62

Post-treatment Follow-Up of Patients with Nasopharyngeal Cancer

Ivan W. K. Tham and Jiade J. Lu

CONTENTS

18.1 Introduction

Nasopharyngeal carcinoma (NPC) is one of the most radiosensitive malignancies, and radiation therapy is its mainstay modality for definitive treatment. With the advances of diagnostic and treatment technologies, as well as the utilization of concurrent chemoradiation therapy for locoregionally advanced disease, the majority of patients with non-metastatic NPC survive after definitive radiation therapy or combined chemoradiation therapy. Nevertheless, local, regional, and/or distant metastasis can occur despite aggressive treatment. Early detection of locoregional treatment failure is important in the management of NPC as limited locoregional recurrent foci can usually be effectively salvaged (Chua et al. 1998).

High-dose radiation inevitably induces acute and late toxicities to the normal organs within or adjacent to the irradiation field. Late toxicities from radiation or chemoradiation therapy can emerge months, even years after the completion of treatment. Assessment and prompt management of treatment-related toxicities are important for the long-term well-being of survivors. Furthermore, patients may continue to have psychosocial difficulties secondary to the disease or its therapy after successful treatment of the cancer (Ma 1996), especially in the first year following treatment. Even among those who had resumed normal or near-normal living, many patients may still note a subdued fear of disease recurrence (Lee et al. 2007).

All issues mentioned above make close follow-up crucial in the management of NPC and need to be addressed in the context of the long-term physician–patient relationship developed over the follow-up period. However, despite an evident necessity, the optimal follow-up schedule and regimen for patients treated for non-metastatic NPC have not been thoroughly addressed. A number of professional organizations have proposed guidelines for the management of NPC, and universally provided follow-up recommendations after treatment (Table 18.1). However, some of the recommendations were derived from those used for non-nasopharyngeal squamous cell carcinoma of head and neck (SCCHN) after radiation treatment. Furthermore, differences in treatment strategy and technique, at least in part, have caused substantial variations in those recommendations on follow-up management. As the biological behavior, treatment, and mode of recurrence of NPC differ substantially

Ivan W.K. Tham, MD
Jiade J. Lu, MD, MBA
Department of Radiation Oncology, National University Cancer Institute, National University Health System, National University of Singapore, 5 Lower Kent Ridge Road, Singapore 119074, Republic of Singapore

Table 18.1. Guidelines of follow-up management of nasopharyngeal cancer after definitive treatment

Summary of Guidelines by Professional Organizations			
	NCCN (2009)	ESMO (Chan et al. 2008)	AHNS (2009)
Modality			
Clinical	Physical examination Year 1: every 1–3 months Year 2: every 2–4 months Year 3–5: every 4–6 months >5 years: every 6–12 months Speech, hearing, swallowing evaluation, and rehabilitation when indicated	Periodic examination of the nasopharynx and neck, cranial nerve function, and systemic complaints	Periodic examinations (with optional use of endoscopy) as per NCCN schedule Clinical assessment for pituitary dysfunction Ophthalmic assessment if treatment portals included the orbit or optic nerves/chiasm
Laboratory	TSH every 6–12 months	Thyroid function EBV serology (might be useful)	TSH and free T4 in the first year, then repeat if clinically indicated. Liver enzymes, annually. EBV titers every 6 months for 5 years in those patients whose titers were elevated before therapy. (optional)
Imaging	Post-treatment baseline imaging, then repeat when clinically indicated Chest imaging when clinically indicated		MRI with suggested frequency Every 4 months: first year Every 6 months: second year Yearly: thereafter Annual chest X-ray
Others	Smoking cessation counseling Dental evaluation		Periodic examination by dentist

NCCN National Comprehensive Cancer Network; *ESMO* European Society for Medical Oncology; *AHNS* American Head and Neck Society; *TSH* thyroid-stimulating hormone; *T4* thyroxine; *EBV* Epstein–Barr virus; *MRI* magnetic resonance imaging

from SCCHN, adopting a common follow-up strategy may impede effective and efficient patient care, both medically and financially.

The purpose of this chapter is to discuss the value of the commonly utilized clinical studies including physical examination, laboratory and imaging tests, and their utilization in the follow-up of NPC after definitive radiation, and propose an evidence-based follow-up schedule and regimen.

18.2 Pattern of Pathological Response to Treatment

Although radiation-induced acute or subacute adverse effects can persist for weeks or months after the completion of therapy, and should be addressed during follow-up sessions, assessment of residual disease should only be initiated 10–12 weeks after the completion of radiation therapy. A number of clinical trials have addressed the pathological response of primary nasopharyngeal cancer to radiation therapy, and their results have indicated that primary tumor eradication could continue for weeks to months after the completion of treatment. In a prospective study reported by Sham et al. (1990), a series of biopsies performed twice a week were performed in patients with nonmetastatic NPC to study the pattern of tumor regression after radical radiotherapy. The results demonstrated that disease in the primary area may be persistent until 10 weeks after treatment, suggesting that residual disease could only be confirmed 10 weeks or more after the completion of the radiotherapy. The results reported by Kwong et al. (1999) confirmed the above-mentioned findings. In this larger series consisting of 803 patients with NPC, viable residual disease was observed in the postnasal space until 10 weeks after the completion of radiation.

In a study of 847 local recurrences out of 4,460 patients treated radically, Lee et al. (1999) reported that 52% of all local recurrences occurred within 2 years from commencement of primary radiotherapy, whereas 39% occurred between 2 and 5 years, and 9% more than 5 years after the radiotherapy. Since locoregional recurrence is more likely in the first 2–3 years after treatment, more intensive follow-up during this period may be justified to detect early locoregional recurrence. At the same time, follow-up should continue indefinitely because late local relapses can occur and may be associated with improved prognosis when compared with early local relapse (Lee et al. 1999). The National Comprehensive Cancer Network (NCCN) recommends monthly to 3-monthly reviews in the first year, 2–4 monthly reviews in the second year, and more infrequent visits thereafter.

18.3 Detection of Local, Regional, and Distant Treatment Failures and Recurrences

18.3.1 Clinical Examination and Endoscopy

In addition to a thorough history and physical examination during each follow-up, periodic nasopharyngoscopy (rigid or flexible) has been used to detect early mucosal recurrence. As nasopharyngoscopy provides direct visualization of the nasopharyngeal mucosa, it can facilitate in the early detection of exophytic or mucosal lesions. Ragab et al. (2008) showed that rigid endoscopy was useful in the follow-up assessment of NPC patients, demonstrating sensitivity, specificity, positive predictive and negative predictive values of 67%, 95%, 67%, and 95%, respectively. In contrast, Kwong et al. (2001) reported the sensitivity, specificity, positive predictive and negative predictive values of 29%, 86%, 35%, and 82%, respectively, using flexible endoscopy in the posttreatment setting, highlighting the difficulty in interpreting mucosal changes after irradiation due to edema, ulceration, and exudation from the radiation effect. In addition, recurrences occurring in the submucosa or deeper structures are usually not accessible by endoscopy. Ng et al. (1999) demonstrated that 28% of deep-seated recurrent NPC diagnosed by magnetic resonance imaging (MRI) were not detected on endoscopy. Therefore, clinical examination including endoscopic studies may not be sufficient for early detection of local recurrence in nasopharyngeal cancer after definitive radiation therapy.

18.3.2 Imaging for Locoregional Recurrence

Computed tomography (CT), MRI, and positron emission tomography (PET) are the most commonly used imaging modalities in the diagnosis and staging of NPC. Although imaging studies utilized for initial diagnosis and staging can be repeated to document the response to treatment, the value of post-radiation radiological studies in nasopharyngeal cancer has not been confirmed. In addition, guidelines from various professional bodies for nasopharyngeal cancer differ significantly regarding the diagnostic imaging studies to be recommended for detecting recurrence. For example, the American Head and Neck Society (AHNS) recommends using MRI during follow-up, whereas the NCCN and the European Society for Medical Oncology (ESMO) do not specify any particular technique.

CT scan of the head and neck area is a common diagnostic modality for follow-up after treatment of NPC. However, the clinical value of posttreatment CT scan on early detection of local or regional recurrence is unknown. Furthermore, the timing of CT scan is debatable. While pathological response to radiation completes within 16 weeks posttreatment, no correlation could be demonstrated between the pathological and radiological response on enhanced CT scan, according to a recently reported prospective study (Ma et al. 2006). "Persistent disease," including radiological evidence of disease progression, stable disease and partial response, was seen in close to 70% of patients on CT scans performed at 4 months after definitive radiation therapy. However, less than 5% had pathologically confirmed residual lesions. The sensitivity and specificity of posttreatment CT scans were 67% and 32%, respectively. These results suggested that CT scans might not provide sufficient value for differentiating persistent or recurrent disease vs. postradiation changes in the post nasal space.

MRI has been demonstrated to be superior to enhanced CT in distinguishing recurrent tumor from postradiation changes (Gong et al. 1991; Fujii and Kanzaki 1994; Chong and Fan 1997). The reported false-positive and false-negative rates of MRI were

17% and 14%, respectively, significantly lower than those of CT, which were 71% and 33%. MRI is also more sensitive than CT in detecting radiation-induced complications including soft tissue changes, masticator muscle fibrosis, arteriopathy, bone changes, central nervous system, and cranial nerve palsies (Ng et al. 1998). Nevertheless, it is limited in detecting early mucosal recurrence and to differentiate local recurrence from immature fibrosis, edema, granulation, and infection on the basis of MR signal intensity (Chong and Ong 2008).

The value of FDG-PET or FDG-PET/CT in detecting local, regional, and/or distant metastases has been a focus of study recently. A recently published systemic review (Liu et al. 2007) of 21 studies suggested that PET imaging was significantly more sensitive (95%) when compared with CT (76%) or MRI (78%) in detecting locally residual or recurrent tumor. A standard uptake values (SUV) cut-off of 4 at 3 months after completion of radiation therapy has been suggested as a diagnostic reference for recurrent or residual tumor (Yen et al. 2006). FDG-PET is especially valuable in patients presented with equivocal results in follow-up MRI after radiation treatment. In a study reported by Ng et al. (2004), 37 patients presented with questionable MRI findings in the primary site underwent FDG-PET. The results of the study demonstrated that the sensitivity of PET for detecting local, regional, and distant recurrences reached 91.6 %, 90 %, and 100%, respectively; furthermore, the specificities for those recurrences were 76%, 89%, and 90.6%, respectively. Despite the advantages of FDG-PET in detecting disease recurrence in NPC after definitive treatment, the high cost of the study at the present time prohibits many centers from using it routinely during follow-up. A cost–utility analysis in Taiwan (Yen et al. 2009) suggested that the use of PET only if an MRI showed an uncertain result provided the most cost-effective solution for early detection of locoregional NPC recurrence. Therefore, PET or PET/CT can be recommended as a complementary imaging modality to CT or MRI, rather than being relied on as the sole method of follow-up imaging in the head and neck region (Ng et al. 2002).

18.3.3 Imaging for Distant Metastases

The prevailing utilization of intensity-modulated radiation therapy (IMRT) and concurrent chemoradiation therapy for locoregionally advanced NPC has assured improved local and regional control of the disease. As such, distant recurrences have become a more predominant pattern of treatment failure for non-metastatic NPC at diagnosis (Lee et al. 2002). For patients with locally advanced disease receiving chemoradiation therapy, the rate of distant metastases may range between 13% and 21% (Kwong et al. 2004; Wee et al. 2005). In addition, it has been estimated that up to 54% of patients with local recurrence may harbor synchronous distant metastases (Lee et al. 1993).

Although the disease could spread to any organ or tissue in the body, the most common sites for distant metastatic NPC include bone, lung and liver (Al-Sarraf et al. 1998; Lee and Kong 2008). Detection of metastatic disease to these organs is largely through imaging studies. Metastatic foci in the lung can be detected by chest X-ray and/or CT of the thorax; liver metastases can be diagnosed by ultrasound and CT of the abdomen, and suspected bone metastases can be confirmed by bone scan and/or X-ray.

Recently published evidence suggests that PET scan or PET/CT is a sensitive modality for diagnosing recurrences and metastases in NPC after definitive therapy (Yen et al. 2005). The sensitivity, specificity, accuracy, positive and negative predictive value of FDG-PET images in the diagnosis of NPC recurrence or metastases and secondary primary cancers were 92%, 90%, 92%, 90%, and 91%, respectively, in patients with suspected disease recurrence. Furthermore, patients with FDG hypermetabolism had a poorer overall survival when compared with patients without increased FDG uptake. Similarly, a comparison of various methods to stage distant metastases showed that PET/CT was the most sensitive, specific, and accurate imaging modality when compared with conventional work-up consisting of chest X-ray, liver ultrasound, and skeletal scintigraphy, CT of the thorax, abdomen, and skeletal scintigraphy, and PET alone (Chua et al. 2009). The accuracy of FDG-PET or FDG-PET/CT for detecting distant metastases both exceed 90%, substantially higher than conventional work-up or CT with bone scan.

However, a number of important issues must be addressed before PET or PET/CT can be routinely considered in follow-up after definitive treatment of NPC. Firstly, although hematogenous spread is one of the most common modes of treatment failure in NPC, the prevalence of distant metastasis is relatively low, especially in patients without cervical lymph adenopathy after definitive treatment (Lin et al. 2009). Although distant metastasis has been observed in up to 20% of patients with locoregionally advanced NPC after chemoradiation therapy, a lower probability of detecting a metastatic focus in patients with no clinical indication such as bone pain, pathological fracture, hemoptysis, excessive cough, or impaired liver function is anticipated if all stages are included. Secondly, NPC with distant metastasis is usually considered an incurable condition. Although NPC is a chemo-sensitive disease and usually responds well to cisplatin-based chemotherapy, systemic treatment is hardly curative for NPC at its metastatic stage. Phase II studies using platinum-based chemotherapy have suggested a response rate of 50–90% in the metastatic setting, with median overall survival of 12–15 months (Loong et al. 2008). While long-term survival has been reported in a small subset of patients with metastatic disease (Fandi et al. 2000), particularly with isolated pulmonary metastasis after aggressive multimodality treatment (Cheng et al. 1996), it is unclear whether earlier detection and treatment of asymptomatic metastatic disease, whether isolated or multiple synchronous disease, would lead to improved survival, when compared with palliative treatment once active symptoms occur. In addition, the poor cost-effectiveness of PET/CT during routine follow-up of NPC patients after definitive treatment, in absence of clear clinical indication of disease recurrence, prevents the routine utilization of PET/CT in NPC follow-up.

Early detection of distant recurrence after definitive treatment of NPC is challenging, and the value of early detection and treatment on ultimate disease control, patients' overall survival, and quality of life is largely unknown. Currently, the AHNS recommends annual chest radiographs for follow-up, whereas NCCN and ESMO advocate imaging only when clinically indicated. Clearly, further investigation on the clinical value of early diagnosis and treatment of metastatic NPC is necessary. However, with the absence of clinical evidence supporting aggressive treatment to metastatic NPC, it may be reasonable to limit radiological investigations such as bone scan, liver ultrasound, CT of thorax or abdomen, or PET/CT to patients with clinical symptoms suggestive of metastases (NCCN 2009).

18.3.4
Plasma EBV DNA Measurement

Real-time quantitative polymerase chain reaction can be performed to quantify circulating tumor-derived EBV DNA in the follow-up management of patients with NPC. In a prospective study of 170 patients with locally advanced NPC, Chan et al. (2002) reported that plasma EBV DNA was a powerful prognostic marker with a relative risk for recurrence of 11.9 in patients with elevated levels after radiotherapy. This test also had positive and negative predictive values of 87 and 83%, respectively. Similarly, Lin et al. (2004) demonstrated that patients with detectable EBV DNA levels after radiotherapy had a poorer survival when compared with those with undetectable levels, and this was the most important prognostic factor for both overall and relapse-free survival in their study. However, plasma EBV DNA in itself is noted to be relatively insensitive in detecting local recurrence after RT (Loong et al. 2008).

18.3.5
EBV Serology Measurement

Serologic testing for immunoglobulin A (IgA) antibodies to viral capsid antigen (VCA) and EBV early antigen (EA) has been found to be useful as a marker for NPC in endemic areas (Gan et al. 1996). However, measurement of serum antibody titers of EBV VCA/IgA using the enzyme-linked immunoadsorbent assay method was shown to be less sensitive and specific when compared with measurement of plasma EBV DNA levels in the detection of recurrent disease (Shao et al. 2004). The same study suggested that change of the EBV titers after radiation therapy provided no significant association with outcome. Therefore, although measurement of EBV titers has been suggested by ESMO and AHNS, the justification for such a test requires further discussion.

18.4
Assessment of Treatment-Related Late Toxicities

The treatment of NPC with radiation therapy, with or without chemotherapy, has been associated with multiple late toxicities, including xerostomia, hormonal dysfunction, central nervous system abnormalities, and second malignancies. A detailed discussion on the mechanisms, prevalence, and treatment of radiation-induced long-term adverse effects is out of the scope of this discussion, and has been addressed in another chapter; however, accurate detection of these adverse effects is one of the crucial purposes of post-treatment follow-up for NPC. Effective preventative and treatment measures are lacking for some of the severe complications such as temporal lobe necrosis and brain stem/spinal cord damage once the complications occur. Nevertheless, other complications, such as pituitary and thyroid dysfunction, hearing impairment, poor dental hygiene, speech and swallowing dysfunction, and psychosocial stress can be effectively managed.

18.4.1 Endocrine Dysfunction

Radiation fields utilized in the definitive treatment for NPC usually encompass the pituitary and thyroid; thus radiation therapy is associated with both primary and secondary hypothyroidism (Tan and Kunaratnam 1966; Lam et al. 1991). The incidence of hypothyroidism can be more than 40% among patients receiving a radical radiotherapy dose to the low neck for head and neck cancer, with a median time to the development of hypothyroidism of between 1.4 and 2 years (Colevas et al. 2001; Mercado et al. 2001). Furthermore, patients receiving a high radiation dose to the hypothalamic–pituitary axis may suffer from hypopituitarism, especially if doses received exceed 40 Gy (Sklar and Constine 1995). The severity and frequency of the hormonal dysfunction correlates with the total radiation dose delivered, and the length of follow-up, with the somatotropic axis described as being the most vulnerable to radiation damage (Darzy and Shalet 2009).

Hypothyroidism can be effectively diagnosed with thyroid function screening tests, and thyroid hormone replacement treatment using thyroxine is an effective treatment of radiation-induced hypothyroidism. However, there is considerable variation among head and neck oncologists in the selection of tests, indication and timing of the laboratory assessment of hypothyroidism, as evidenced by a recent Dutch survey (Lo Galbo et al. 2009). In asymptomatic patients, testing the thyroid-stimulating hormone with free T4 as recommended by the AHNS, at an interval of 6–12 months as recommended by NCCN could be considered. Symptomatic patients would benefit from early directed laboratory tests and an endocrinology consultation if indicated.

18.4.2 Dental Care

Long-term follow-up with a dentist in a multidisciplinary setting is recommended, because close collaboration with the oncology team may minimize the rates of adverse dental events, e.g. osteoradionecrosis (Koga et al. 2008). Periodicity of appointments can be individualized.

18.4.3 Hearing

Sensorineural hearing loss can be expected in many patients after treatment, especially if platinum-based chemotherapy was added to radiation therapy (Low et al. 2006). Early detection and treatment may improve the patient's quality of life.

18.4.4 Speech and Swallowing

Continued follow-up with a speech therapist may be warranted, especially for patients at a high risk for late swallowing dysfunction following radiotherapy. Risk factors include bilateral neck irradiation, a large primary tumor (T3 or 4), weight loss >10%, addition of concurrent chemotherapy, or usage of accelerated radiotherapy (Langendijk et al. 2009).

18.4.5 Patient Support Groups

Many cancer centers have patient support groups for cancer survivors of various cancers, including NPC. These groups may provide a supportive environment for peer support, empower patients through knowledge, and provide counseling and psychosocial support if necessary. Common issues include problems related to disease relapse, late side effects such as xerostomia, and psychological issues including anxiety and depression. As many NPC survivors are in their 40s and 50s, employment and family issues are also significant concerns.

18.5 Summary

Assessment of residual disease should be done only about 10 weeks after the completion of radical radiotherapy or chemoradiotherapy. Locoregional recurrence commonly occurs within the first 2–3 years after treatment and follow-up should be more intense during this period. Clinical and radiological investigations

Table 18.2. A proposed recommendation for follow-up management of NPC patients after definitive treatment

Modality	Tests	Schedule
Clinical	Physical examination, including nasoendoscopy Speech, hearing, swallowing evaluation when indicated	Year 1: every 1–3 months Year 2: every 2–4 months Year 3–5: every 4–6 months >5 years: every 6–12 months
Laboratory	TSH, free T4 Other endocrine tests when clinically indicated EBV DNA monitoring (optional)	Every 6–12 months
Imaging	MRI of the head and neck Chest X-ray, CT of the thorax/abdomen, US liver, bone scan, PET/CT scan when clinically indicated	3 months after RT, then annually
Others	Smoking cessation counseling Dental evaluation Patient support group	

TSH thyroid-stimulating hormone; *EBV* Epstein–Barr virus; *MRI* magnetic resonance imaging; *RT* radiation therapy; *CT* computed tomography; *US* ultrasound; *PET* positron emission tomography

using MRI may detect early recurrences amenable to salvage treatment. Post-treatment measurement of plasma EBV DNA levels may be used to prognosticate patients. The role of routine body imaging to detect distant metastases on follow-up is poorly defined.

Hypothyroidism is common and should be screened with thyroid function tests regularly. The patient should continue follow-up with a dentist and other members of the multi-disciplinary team where indicated. Other investigations and interventions for late toxicity should be offered if necessary. The patient should also continue to be supported in the psychosocial domain. The proposed recommendations are summarized in Table 18.2.

References

Al-Sarraf M, LeBlanc M, Giri PGS, et al (1998) Chemoradiotherapy versus radiotherapy in patients with advanced nasopharyngeal cancer: phase III randomized intergroup study 0099. J Clin Oncol 16:1310–1317

American Head and Neck Society Practice Guidelines (2009) http://www.headandneckcancer.org/ clinicalresources/ docs/ nasopharynx.php. Accessed 23 Feb 2009

Chan AT, Felip E; ESMO Guidelines Working Group (2008) Nasopharyngeal cancer: ESMO clinical recommendations for diagnosis, treatment and follow-up. Ann Oncol 19(Suppl 2):ii81–ii82

Chan AT, Lo YM, Zee B, et al (2002) Plasma Epstein–Barr virus DNA and residual disease after radiotherapy for undifferentiated nasopharyngeal carcinoma. J Natl Cancer Inst 94(21):1614–1619

Cheng LC, Sham JS, Chiu CS, et al (1996) Surgical resection of pulmonary metastases from nasopharyngeal carcinoma. Aust N Z J Surg 66:71–73

Chong VFH, Fan YF (1997) Detection of recurrent nasopharyngeal carcinoma: MRI versus CT. Radiology 202: 463–470

Chong VFH, Ong CK (2008) Nasopharyngeal carcinoma. Eur J Radiol 66:437–447

Chua DT, Sham JS, Kwong DL, et al (1998) Locally recurrent nasopharyngeal carcinoma: treatment results for patients with computed tomography assessment. Int J Radiat Oncol Biol Phys 41(2):379–386

Chua ML, Ong SC, Wee JT, et al (2009) Comparison of 4 modalities for distant metastasis staging in endemic nasopharyngeal carcinoma. Head Neck 31(3):346–354

Colevas AD, Read R, Thornhill J, et al (2001) Hypothyroidism incidence after multimodality treatment for stage III and IV squamous cell carcinomas of the head and neck. Int J Radiat Oncol Biol Phys 51(3):599–604

Darzy KH, Shalet SM (2009) Hypopituitarism following radiotherapy revisited. Endocr Dev 15:1–24

Fandi A, Bachouchi M, Azli N, et al (2000) Long-term disease-free survivors in metastatic undifferentiated carcinoma of nasopharyngeal type. J Clin Oncol 18: 1324–1330

Fujii M, Kanzaki J (1994) The role of MRI for the diagnosis of recurrence of nasopharyngeal cancer. Auris Nasus Larynx 2(1):32–37

Gan YY, Fones-Tan A, Chan SH (1996) Molecular diagnosis of nasopharyngeal carcinoma: a review. Ann Acad Med Singapore 25(1):71–74

Gong QY Zheng GL Zhu HY (1991) MRI differentiation of recurrent nasopharyngeal carcinoma from postradiation fibrosis. Comput Med Imaging Graph 15:423–429

Koga DH, Salvajoli JV, Alves FA (2008) Dental extractions and radiotherapy in head and neck oncology: review of the literature. Oral Dis 14(1):40–44

Kwong DL, Nicholls J, Wei WI, et al (1999) The time course of histologic remission after treatment of patients with nasopharyngeal carcinoma. Cancer 85(7):1446–1453

Kwong DL, Nicholls J, Wei WI, et al (2001) Correlation of endoscopic and histologic findings before and after treatment for nasopharyngeal carcinoma. Head Neck 23(1):34–41

Kwong DL, Sham JS, Au GK, et al (2004) Concurrent and adjuvant chemotherapy for nasopharyngeal carcinoma: a factorial study. J Clin Oncol 22(13):2643–2653

Lam K, Tse V, Wang C, et al (1991) Effects of cranial irradiation on hypothalamic-pituitary function: a 5-year longitudinal study in patients with nasopharyngeal carcinoma. Q J Med 78:165–176

Langendijk JA, Doornaert P, Rietveld DH, et al (2009) A predictive model for swallowing dysfunction after curative radiotherapy in head and neck cancer. Radiother Oncol 90 (2):189–195

Lee AW, Foo W, Law SC, et al (1999) Recurrent nasopharyngeal carcinoma: the puzzles of long latency. Int J Radiat Oncol Biol Phys 44(1):149–156

Lee AW, Law SC, Foo W, et al (1993) Retrospective analysis of patients with nasopharyngeal carcinoma treated during 1976–1985: survival after local recurrence. Int J Radiat Oncol Biol Phys 26(5):773–782

Lee N, Kong L (2008)Nasopharyngeal cancer. In: Lu JJ, Brady LW (eds) Radiation oncology: an evidence-based approach. Springer, Berlin

Lee N, Xia P, Quivey JM, et al (2002) Intensity-modulated radiotherapy in the treatment of nasopharyngeal carcinoma: an update of the UCSF experience. Int J Radiat Oncol Biol Phys 53(1):12–22

Lee PW, Kwan TT, Kwong DL, et al (2007) A prospective study of the impact of nasopharyngeal cancer and radiotherapy on the psychosocial condition of Chinese patients. Cancer 109(7):1344–1354

Lin JC, Wang WY, Chen KY, et al (2004) Quantification of plasma Epstein–Barr virus DNA in patients with advanced nasopharyngeal carcinoma. N Engl J Med 350(24): 2461–2470

Lin S, Pan J, Lu H, et al (2009) Nasopharyngeal carcinoma treated with reduced-volume intensity-modulated radiation therapy: report on the 3-year outcome of a prospective series. Int J Radiat Oncol Biol Phys , article in press, published online 13 Apr 09

Liu T, Xu W, Yan WL, et al (2007) FDG-PET, CT, MRI for diagnosis of local residual or recurrent nasopharyngeal carcinoma, which one is the best? A systematic review. Radiother Oncol 85(3):327–335

Lo Galbo AM, de Bree R, Lips P, et al (2009) Detecting hypothyroidism after treatment for laryngeal or hypopharyngeal carcinomas: a nationwide survey in The Netherlands. Eur Arch Otorhinolaryngol 266(5):713–718

Loong HH, Ma BB, Chan AT (2008) Update on the management and therapeutic monitoring of advanced nasopharyngeal cancer. Hematol Oncol Clin North Am 22(6): 1267–1278

Low WK, Toh ST, Wee J, et al (2006) Sensorineural hearing loss after radiotherapy and chemoradiotherapy: a single, blinded, randomized study. J Clin Oncol 24(12): 1904–1909

Ma LC (1996) Psychosocial stresses and adjustment of nasopharyngeal carcinoma patients in Hong Kong: a panel study. Cancer Pract 4(5):258–266

Ma X, Lu JJ, Loh KS, et al (2006) Role of computed tomography imaging in predicting response of nasopharyngeal carcinoma to definitive radiation therapy. Laryngoscope 116(12):2162–2165

Mercado G, Adelstein DJ, Saxton JP, et al (2001) Hypothyroidism: a frequent event after radiotherapy and after radiotherapy with chemotherapy for patients with head and neck carcinoma. Cancer 92:2892–2897

National Comprehensive Cancer Center Clinical Practice Guidelines (2009) http://www.nccn.org/professionals/physician_gls/PDF/head-and-neck.pdf. Accessed 23 Feb 2009

Ng SH, Chang TC, Ko SF, et al (1999) MRI in recurrent nasopharyngeal carcinoma. Neuroradiology 41:862–885

Ng SH, Joseph CT, Chan SC, et al (2004) Clinical usefulness of 18F-FDG PET in nasopharyngeal carcinoma patients with questionable MRI findings for recurrence. J Nucl Med 45(10):1669–1676

Ng SH, Liu HM, Ko SF, et al (2002) Posttreatment imaging of the nasopharynx. Eur J Radiol 44(2):82–95

Ng SH, Wan YL, Ko SF, et al (1998) MRI of nasopharyngeal carcinoma with emphasis on relationship to radiotherapy. J Magn Reson Imaging 8:327–336

Ragab SM, Erfan FA, Khalifa MA, et al (2008) Detection of local failures after management of nasopharyngeal carcinoma: a prospective, controlled trial. J Laryngol Otol 122(11): 1230–1234

Sham JS, Wei WI, Kwan WH, et al (1990) Nasopharyngeal carcinoma. Pattern of tumor regression after radiotherapy. Cancer 65(2):216–220

Shao JY, Li YH, Gao HY, et al (2004) Comparison of plasma Epstein–Barr virus (EBV) DNA levels and serum EBV immunoglobulin A/virus capsid antigen antibody titers in patients with nasopharyngeal carcinoma. Cancer 100(6): 1162–1170

Sklar CA, Constine LS (1995) Chronic neuroendocrinological sequelae of radiation therapy. Int J Radiat Oncol Biol Phys 31(5):1113–1121

Tan BC, Kunaratnam M (1966) Hypopituitary dwarfism following radiotherapy for nasopharyngeal carcinoma. Clin Radiol 17:302–304

Wee J, Tan EH, Tai BC, et al (2005) Randomized trial of radiotherapy versus concurrent chemoradiotherapy followed by adjuvant chemotherapy in patients with American Joint Committee on Cancer/International Union against cancer stage III and IV nasopharyngeal cancer of the endemic variety. J Clin Oncol 23(27):6730–6738

Yen RF, Hong RL, Tzen KY, et al (2005) Whole-body 18F-FDG PET in recurrent or metastatic nasopharyngeal carcinoma. J Nucl Med 46(5):770–774

Yen RF, Yen MF, Hong RL, et al (2009) The cost-utility analysis of 18-fluoro-2-deoxyglucose positron emission tomography in the diagnosis of recurrent nasopharyngeal carcinoma. Acad Radiol 16(1):54–60

Yen TC, Lin CY, Wang HM, et al (2006) 18F-FDG-PET for evaluation of the response to concurrent chemoradiation therapy with intensity-modulated radiation technique for stage T4 nasopharyngeal carcinoma. Int J Radiat Oncol Biol Phys 65(5):1307–1314

Management of Patients with Failure Following Definitive Radiation Therapy: Reirradiation in Patients with Locally Recurrent Nasopharyngeal Carcinoma

19

Daniel Chua

CONTENTS

Daniel Chua, MD
Department of Clinical Oncology, Queen Mary Hospital, The University of Hong Kong, Rm PB-115, 1/F, Professorial Block, Queen Mary Hospital, Pok Fu Lam Road, Hong Kong SAR, P.R. China

19.1 Introduction

Although excellent control rates can be achieved after primary treatment for NPC, local relapse still represents a major cause of treatment failure, particularly in patients presented with advanced primary disease. In managing local failures of NPC, aggressive salvage treatment with curative intent should always be considered, since a significant proportion of these patients can still achieve long-term survival after successful retreatment. In a retrospective review of a large cohort of 275 patients with local failure of NPC, patients who received salvage treatment had a significantly better survival compared with those without receiving any salvage treatment (Yu et al. 2005). Although patients with less extensive recurrence and better performance were likely to be selected for salvage treatment, this large series still showed that only patients who underwent surgery or reirradiation had a chance of achieving long-term disease control and survival. Many salvage treatments are available, and the choice of method depends on several factors including extent of disease, site of disease, any synchronous nodal relapse, cumulative radiation dose already received by patient, patient's general condition and preference, and expertise available. In general, salvage treatments with curative intent can be classified into surgery and reirradiation. This chapter covers different approaches of reirradiation in salvaging local failures of NPC, which include brachytherapy using intracavitary intubation, mould application or gold grain implantation, stereotactic radiotherapy, and external beam radiation therapy.

19.2 Prognostic Factors

Important prognostic factors have been identified in patients receiving reirradiation of NPC. Table 19.1 lists these important prognostic factors. Most series reported T-classification, time of recurrence and reirradiation dose as significant prognostic factors for local control and/or survival. The most consistent prognostic factor being reported is recurrent T-classification, and patients treated for advanced recurrent disease in or adjacent to the nasopharynx had poor local control and survival after reirradiation. Patients with recurrent T4 disease had a particularly worse outcome, and successful salvage rate was low, and reirradiation often resulted in a high incidence of neurological complications. Another important prognostic factor commonly reported was the time interval from the completion of first radiotherapy to relapse. It is important to recognize a distinct group of patients with residual tumor that failed to regress within 6 months of completion of radiotherapy, commonly termed "persistent disease," as opposed to recurrent tumors diagnosed beyond 6 months, as the former group had a better outcome after salvage treatment using brachytherapy (Leung et al. 2000a, b; Kwong et al. 2001) or stereotactic radiotherapy (Chua et al. 2006; Wu et al. 2007). For patients with recurrent tumors, a longer time from primary radiotherapy was associated with a better outcome, and late isolated local relapse may actually represent second primary (Lee et al. 1999). There appears to be an important relationship between reirradiation dose and treatment outcome, with most series reporting poor tumor control with a dose below 60 Gy (Wang 1987; Lee et al. 1997; Öksüz et al. 2004). In one series that employed stereotactic radiotherapy as salvage treatment, the use of a dose equivalent to conventional fractionation of 55 Gy or above was associated with significantly better tumor control. Tumor volume smaller than 10 cm^3 was also reported to be associated with better local control after stereotactic radiotherapy using single or multiple fractions (Chua et al. 2006, Wu et al. 2007). Overexpression of epidermal growth factor receptor in recurrent tumor tissue was also associated with a poor outcome in patients treated by external beam reirradiation (Chua et al. 2008).

Table 19.1. Prognostic factors in nasopharyngeal carcinoma (NPC) patients receiving salvage reirradiation

Patient factors
Age
Performance score
Disease factors
Histology
Recurrent T classification
Persistent vs. recurrent tumor
Time interval from first course of radiation therapy
Tumor volume
Presence of synchronous nodal recurrence
Prior local failure
Epidermal growth factor receptor expression
Treatment factors
Reirradiation dose

19.3 Brachytherapy

19.3.1 Principle of Brachytherapy

The concept of application of brachytherapy is that with the application of the radiation source close to the tumor, the radiation dosage is the highest at the site of the radiation source and decreases rapidly as the distances increases from the radiation source towards the periphery. This enables a high dose of irradiation to be delivered to the residual or recurrent tumor in the nasopharynx, while the surrounding tissue only receives a much smaller dose at the same time. Brachytherapy radiation source also delivers radiation at a continuous low dose rate, which gives further radiobiological advantage over fractionated doses of external radiation. The procedural aspects of brachytherapy, especially those of interstitial brachytherapy, for the treatment of local recurrence of nasopharyngeal cancer is out of the scope of this chapter, and are detailed in Chap. 20.

19.3.2 Intracavitary Bracytherapy

Intracavitary brachytherapy has been used traditionally for NPC s (Wang et al. 1975). With this method,

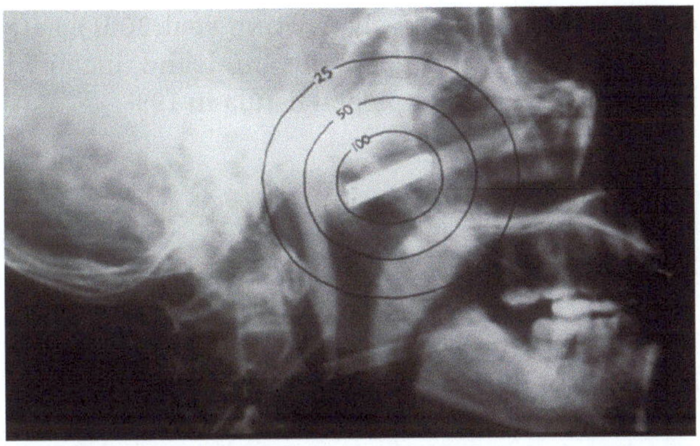

Fig. 19.1. Intracavitary bracytherapy for recurrent nasopharyngeal carcinoma (NPC). X-ray film showing position of intracavitary catheter inside nasopharynx and the isodose distribution

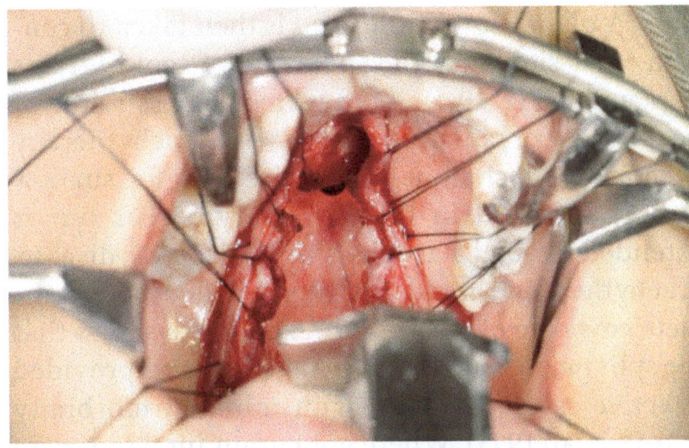

Fig. 19.2. Split palate approach for interstitial implantation of gold grain. The palate was split open to allow direct inspection of tumor and implantation of gold grain by clinician

the radiation source is placed either in a tube or a mould, and these devices are then inserted into the nasopharynx for therapy (Fig. 19.1). Intracavitary brachytherapy have also been reported to salvage local failure of NPC with success (Leung et al. 1996; Law et al. 2002), and considerable experience together with patient selection, are the key issues for a favorable outcome. Syed et al. (2000) analyzed 34 patients with persistent or recurrent disease managed with interstitial and intraluminal brachytherapy. Ten-year disease specific survival rate was 60%, and 10-year local control rate was 49%. Forty-five patients experienced some form of late complications. Using high-dose-rate intracavitary intubation, Leung et al. (2000a, b) reported an excellent 5-year local relapse-free survival rate of 85% in 87 NPC patients with persistent local disease after radiotherapy. The same group also reported a lower control rate when intracavitary brachytherapy alone was used in salvaging local recurrence in eight patients, with a 3-year local relapse-free survival rate of 42%. Intracavitary brachytherapy was also used as a boost treatment after external beam reirradiation for bulky disease. In the series by Lee et al. (1997), combined intracavitary brachytherapy and external beam radiotherapy yielded a superior 5-year local control rate of 45%, compared to 32% by external beam radiotherapy and 29% by brachytherapy.

19.3.3 Interstitial Implantation

In view of the irregular contour of the nasopharynx as well as the variation in dimension and location of tumor, it is usually difficult to position the radiation source accurately in the nasopharynx and in close proximity to the tumor to provide a tumoricidal dose by intracavitary brachytherapy. To circumvent this problem, radioactive interstitial implants have been used to treat small localized residual or recurrent tumor in the nasopharynx. At Queen Mary Hospital in Hong Kong, we frequently employed radioactive gold grains (^{198}Au) as the radiation source for this purpose. Gold grains can be implanted into the tumor either transnasally under endoscopic guidance (Harrison et al. 1987) or using the split-palate approach (Wei et al. 1990). The latter approach gives the surgeon a direct view of the tumor, its location and its extent in the nasopharynx. This enables the implant of the gold grains permanently into the tumor with great precision using the introducer. The procedure was carried out with the patient in supine position. A plastic plate with holes was placed behind his shoulder which allows the insertion of the ends of the rods to hold the mouth gag in position. A Dingman's mouth gag was inserted and the oral cavity rinsed with antiseptic solution. The soft palate was split in the midline to one side of the uvula and the mucoperiosteum over the hard palate was also lifted. The attachment of the soft palate to the posterior edge of the hard palate was detached from the hard palate and with retraction of the soft tissue; the tumor in the nasopharynx was exposed (Fig. 19.2). The surgeon inserted the endoscope into the nasopharynx, while the oncologist implanted the gold grains into the tumor under direct vision with the introducer (Fig. 19.3). The palatal wound was then closed in layers. During the closure, a thick lead shield was used to reduce the radiation dose to the body of the surgeon and his eyes were protected with a lead glass. A plain X-ray of the head is then taken to confirm the site and the number of gold grains implanted (Fig. 19.4). As the effectiveness range of the delivery of radiation energy with brachytherapy is short, the technique is effective only for shallow tumors localized in the nasopharynx. For tumor extended beyond nasopharynx and bulky disease, brachytherapy should not be used due to incomplete coverage of tumor. Our experience shows that the split palate implantation of gold grains provided effective salvage of NPC with minimal morbidity (Choy et al. 1993). Where gold grain implants were applied to treat persistent and recurrent tumors after radiotherapy, the 5-year local tumor control rates were 87% and 63% respectively, and the corresponding 5-year disease-free survival rates were 68% and 60% respectively (Kwong et al. 2001). Late complications were generally mild and included headache in 28% and palatal fistula in 19%.

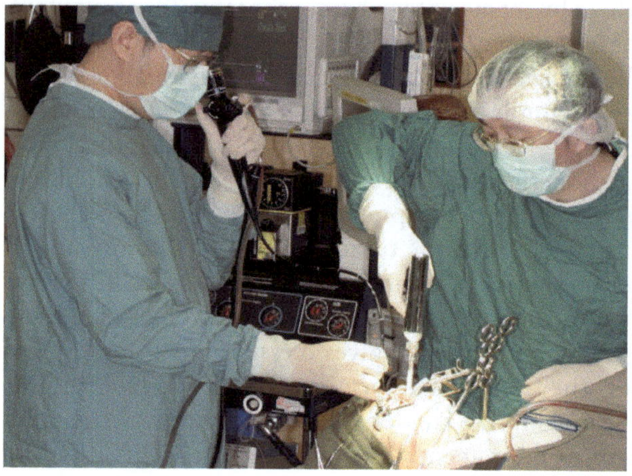

Fig. 19.3. Implantation of gold grain under direct vision into nasopharynx. Gold grains were implanted into the nasopharynx using a special gun and introducer to ensure even distribution of the radioactive source

19.4 Stereotactic Radiotherapy

19.4.1 Principle of Stereotactic Radiotherapy

Stereotactic radiosurgery is the technique in which a small target is stereotactically localized and irradiated by multiple convergent beams using a large single dose of radiation. The technique was originally developed for treatment of functional neurological disorder, but was later found to be useful for vascular malformations, benign intracranial/skull base neoplasm, and cerebral metastases. Stereotactic radiosurgery has also been used in NPC to deliver a boost dose after the second course of radiotherapy or as a salvage treatment of local recurrence. Unlike treating intracranial lesions, a wider margin is usually necessary during treatment planning, due to infiltrative nature of NPC (Fig. 19.5). With this technique, there is rapid dose fall-off beyond the target, thereby allowing sparing of adjacent tissues which is important in retreatment of NPC.

19.4.2 Stereotactic Radiosurgery

Most early reports of stereotactic radiotherapy employed single fraction treatment, or stereotactic radiosurgery, in salvaging local failure of NPC. The goal is to deliver an ablative dose of radiation to destroy the

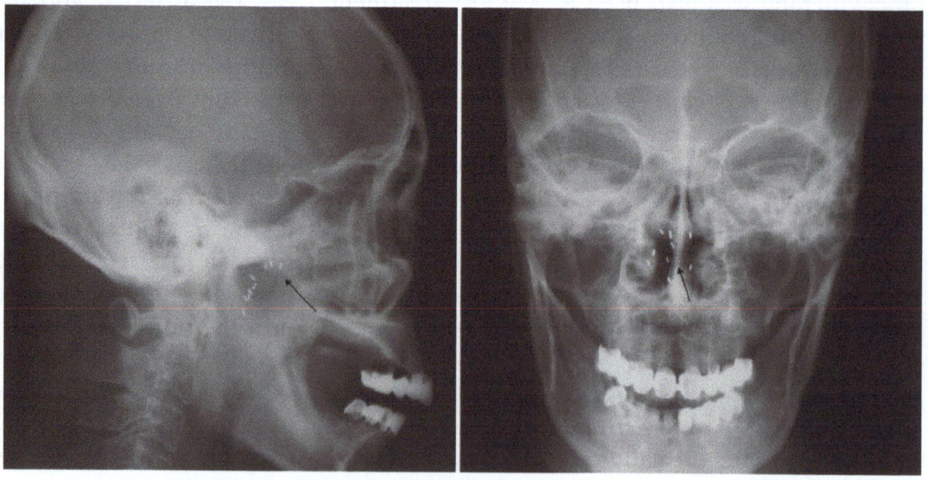

Fig. 19.4. Gold grain interstitial implantation. X-ray film showing the distribution of gold grains within the nasopharynx. *Right*: PA view. *Left*: lateral view

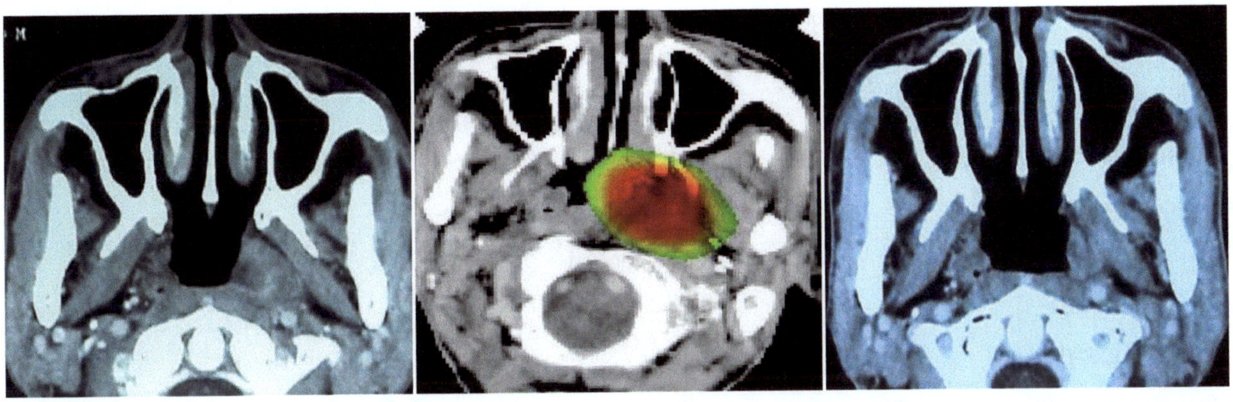

Fig. 19.5. Stereotactic radiosurgery for recurrent NPC. *Right*: pretreatment CT scan showing recurrent tumor in the left side of the nasopharynx extended to parapharyngeal space. *Middle*: target covered with single isocenter with a dose of 12.5 Gy delivered to 80% isodose line. *Left*: CT scan at 6 months after treatment showing complete resolution of tumor

Table 19.2. Results in literature on stereotactic radiosurgery for local failures of NPC

Study	No. of patients	rT stage	Dose (Gy)	Tumor control rate (%)	Any severe sequelae[a]
MILLER et al. (1997)	3	rT3–4	12–20	50 (1/2)	No
BUATTI et al. (1995)	3	rT2–4	12.5	50 (1/2)	Yes (50%, 1/2)
KOCHER et al. (1998)	5	rT3–4	15–24	67 (2/3)	Yes (60%, 3/5)
CMELAK et al. (1997)	9 (12 lesions)	rT3	15–20	58 (7/12)	Yes (11%, 1/9)
CHUA et al. (2006)	48	rT1–4	8–18	54 (26/48)	Yes (19%, 9/48)

[a]Severe sequelae includes brain necrosis, cranial neuropathy and massive hemorrhage

recurrent tumor. Table 19.2 summarizes the reported outcome using stereotactic radiosurgery for local failure of NPC. Using stereotactic radiosurgery alone to deliver a dose of 12–24 Gy to tumor periphery yielded a crude local control rate of 50%–67% for locally recurrent NPC (BUATTI et al. 1995; CMELAK et al. 1997; MILLER et al. 1997; KOCHER et al. 1998; CHUA et al. 2006). Although a wide range of dose was used in these early studies, our experience showed that tumor control rate was relatively good with a modest dose of 12.5 Gy for persistent disease and tumor confined to nasopharynx (CHUA et al. 2003, 2006). External beam radiotherapy and stereotactic radiosurgery have also been combined to retreat NPC, usually in the management of advanced recurrence. When stereotactic radiosurgery was administered as a boost dose after reirradiation, the 3-year control rate ranged from 52% to 58%. CHEN et al. (2001) reported the outcome of 11 patients with rT3–4 NPC after conformal radiotherapy and stereotactic radiosurgery. The radiosurgery dose ranged from 10 to 19 Gy with a median of 14 Gy. Significant regression of tumor was noted in five patients and limited regression in another three. Chang et al. (2000) reported 15 patients with locally recurrent NPC who received external reirradiation followed by radiosurgery using a dose ranged from 8 to 15 Gy, and noted a 3-year survival rate of 52%. PAI et al. (2000) reported 36 patients with recurrent NPC, also treated with external reirradiation followed by radiosurgery boost. The radiosurgery dose to target periphery ranged from 8 to 20 Gy with a median of 12 Gy. A 3-year local control rate of 58% was achieved.

19.4.3 Stereotactic Radiotherapy

The same technique may also be used to deliver multiple fractions of radiation and is termed stereotactic radiotherapy, and the control rates appeared to be similar to radiosurgery in the treatment of persistent disease (Table 19.3). For recurrent disease, stereotactic

Table 19.3. Results in literature on stereotactic radiotherapy for local failures of NPC

Study	No. of patients	rT stage	Dose (Gy)	Tumor control rate (%)	Any severe sequelae[a]
MITSUHASHI et al. (1999)	3	rT1	50–64	100 (3-year)	No
ORECCHIA et al. (1999)	13	rT1–4	24	31 (3-year)	No
AHN et al. (2000)	12	Not reported	45–65	92 (2-year)	No
XIAO et al. (2001)	49	rT1–4	14–35	47 (1-year)	Yes (16%)
YAU et al. (2004)	21	rT1–4	12–20	82 (3-year)	No
LEUNG et al. (2009)	30	rT1–4	32–57	57 (5-year)	Yes (36%)

[a]Severe sequelae includes brain necrosis, cranial neuropathy and massive hemorrhage

radiotherapy appears to be superior with a 3-year local control rate of 75% as reported in one large series, probably due to the higher dose delivered (WU et al. 2007). Based on these results, there is strong evidence indicating that stereotactic radiotherapy is an effective salvage treatment for local failures of NPC. Although most series reported a relatively low risk of late complications following stereotactic radiotherapy, massive hemorrhage resulting from carotid pseudoaneurysm represents one of the severe complications that frequently leads to fatal outcome (XIAO et al. 2001). Massive hemorrhage after radiosurgery was usually due to radiation damage to the carotid artery as a result of using large fraction dose and high cumulative dose. To minimize the risk of hemorrhage, use of multiple fractions with smaller dose is recommended in the presence of direct tumor encasement of carotid artery.

19.5 External Beam Reirradiation

Reirradiation of NPC with curative intent is often difficult due to the large numbers of important structures situated in the vicinity of the target that was already irradiated to a high dose during the primary course of radiotherapy. Whenever possible, brachytherapy or stereotactic radiotherapy should be considered as the first option for reirradiation of nasopharynx. Table 19.4 summarizes the treatment outcome using different techniques of external beam reirradiation for NPC, as reported in the literature. The reported 5-year survival rates after external beam reirradiation using conventional 2D planning and treatment delivery was poor and ranged from 8% to 36% (CHUA et al. 1998; CHANG et al. 2000; ÖKSÜZ et al. 2004). A high incidence of late complication, mostly neurological damage and soft tissue necrosis/fibrosis, was commonly seen after external beam reirradiation. The use of 3D conformal radiotherapy has improved the outcome of patients receiving reirradiation. In one study using 3D conformal radiotherapy for retreatment of NPC, 5-year local control rate was 71% but the actuarial incidence of major late toxicities was still high with 100% developing at least Grade 3 toxicity and 49% developing Grade 4 toxicity at 5 years (ZHENG et al. 2005).

In retreatment of NPC, intensity modulated radiotherapy (IMRT) can further improve the dosimetry and possibly the clinical outcome than 3D conformal radiotherapy. Hsiung et al. (2002) have demonstrated superior dose distribution and sparing of normal tissues with IMRT than 3D conformal radiotherapy for boost or salvage treatment of NPC. Several preliminary reports using IMRT for reirradiation of NPC reported good short-term control with a relatively low incidence of severe late toxicities. Using IMRT for high dose (68–70 Gy) reirradiation of NPC, Lu et al. (2004) reported 100% control rate in 49 patients without any severe late complications after a median follow-up of 9 months. Also using IMRT to deliver a median dose of 54 Gy for retreatment of NPC with or without induction chemotherapy and radiosurgery boost, we have initially reported 1-year loco-regional control rate of 56%, and the 1-year actuarial rate of Grade 3 late complications was 25% in 31 patients with disease not amenable to surgery or brachytherapy (CHUA et al. 2005a). These preliminary reports using IMRT for reirradiation of NPC suggests good short-term control, but longer follow-up is needed to assess long-term results and late complications. We updated the outcome of our cohort of 31 patients treated by IMRT recently and

Table 19.4. Results in literature on external beam reirradiation for local failure of carcinoma of the nasopharynx

Study	No. of patients	Radiation technique	Treatment outcome		Cumulative incidence of major late complications	
			5-year Local control (%)	5-year Survival (%)	Any (%)	Brain necrosis (%)
Teo et al. (1998)	123	2D RT	rT1: 43 rT2: 31 rT3–4: 16	rT1: 63 rT2: 48 rT3–4: 31	–	20
Lee et al. (1997)	654	2D RT	rT1: 35 rT2: 28 rT3–4: 11	16	26	3
Wang (1987)	51	2D RT	–	33	6	2
Pryzant et al. (1992)	53	2D RT	35	18	–	–
Yan et al. (1983)	219	2D RT	–	18	>29	>12
Chua et al. (1998)	97	2D RT	–	rT1–2: 57 rT3: 42 rT4: 17	–	16
Leung et al. (2000)	91	2D RT	38	30	57	27
Chang et al. (2000)	186	2D RT (81%) 3D CRT (19%)	–	rT1: 38.5(3-year) rT2: 23.7 rT3: 28.4 rT4: 3.7	2D RT: 23 3D CRT: 9	2D RT: 14 3D CRT: 0
Zheng et al. (2005)	86	3D CRT	rT1: 92 rT2: 81 rT3: 68 rT4: 41	rT1: 70 rT2: 52 rT3: 32 rT4: 10	44	16
Lu et al. (2004)	49	IMRT	100 (9-month)	–	–	–
Chua et al. (2005a)	31	IMRT	rT1–3: 100 rT4: 35 (1-year)	63	19	7

2D RT 2D treatment planning and radiation therapy; *3D CRT* 3D conformal radiation therapy; *IMRT*: Intensity-modulated radiation therapy

observed a 5-year local control rate of 43% for rT1–3 disease and 27% for rT4 disease. Late complications included cranial neuropathy in 32%, brain necrosis in 13%, soft tissue and osteoradionecrosis in 6%, and carotid pseudoaneurysm in 3%. These results suggest good long-term control with a relatively low risk of late complications compared with other series using conventional technique of reirradiation.

The challenging issue in external beam reirradiation is to retreat the target volume to a high dose (>54 Gy) while minimizing dose to adjacent critical tissues. Neurological tissues including optic apparatus, brain stem, temporal lobe and spinal cord usually represent the dose-limiting structures in treatment planning, and the dose constraint is usually set at 12%–20% of the prescription dose. In our experience, this is often difficult to achieve for advanced T stage recurrence and bulky tumor even with the use of IMRT, and induction chemotherapy is often used to improve target coverage and sparing of organs at risk. Newer techniques of radiotherapy allow better sparing of normal tissues and may further improve the outcome in locally recurrent NPC. Taheri-Kadkhoda et al. (2008) showed that three-field intensity modulated proton therapy was superior to nine-field IMRT using step and shoot technique, with respect to tumor coverage and reduction of the integral dose to organs at risk and nonspecific normal tissues. Lee et al. (2008) also showed that helical tomotherapy was superior to step and shoot IMRT with respect to target coverage and sparing of critical structures, with the mean and maximal dose of most organs at risk, except chaism, being significantly reduced with tomotherapy. Although these reports focused on the treatment of the newly diagnosed disease, the same advantage will be seen with perhaps a bigger impact in retreatment setting. The benefits of proton therapy and helical tomotherapy in retreatment of NPC deserve further exploration when these techniques become more widely available.

19.6 Combined Modality Approach

The application of chemotherapy and radiotherapy may also improve treatment outcome in locally recurrent NPC similar to the setting of newly diagnosed cases. One study employed induction chemotherapy with gemcitabine and cisplatin to shrink the tumor volume followed by reirradiation using IMRT, and reported 75% local control rate at 1-year (Chua et al. 2005b). Another study employed concurrent chemoradiotherapy with cisplatin followed by consolidation cisplatin and 5-FU, and reported 1-year progression-free rate of 42% (Poon et al. 2004). In patients with advanced local recurrence in which treatment planning for reirradiation is difficult, induction chemotherapy carries the advantage of shrinking the tumor, thereby facilitating subsequent radiotherapy planning and target coverage. This is of particular importance in the treatment of recurrent T4 disease with a significant component of intracranial extension. Induction chemotherapy may also be used to delay the course of external beam reirradiation in patients who relapse after a short time period following completion of first course of radiotherapy. Addition of molecular targeted agent may also improve the outcome in recurrent disease setting. In one study that employed induction chemotherapy with three cycles of gemcitabine and cisplatin followed by reirradiation using IMRT concurrent with weekly cetuximab in 16 patients with local failures of NPC, toxicity was manageable with 7% of patients developing grade 3 skin rash and 13% developing grade 3 mucositis. The 2-year local control rate was 47% and 2-year survival rate was 71% (Chua et al. 2009a). Based on these reports, the use of combined modality approach is likely to improve the outcome in local failures of NPC, although evidence from prospective phase III trial is lacking.

19.7 Patient Selection for Salvage Treatment

Currently, no prospective study that compares the relative efficacy and complication of different salvage treatments has ever been reported. Retrospective data, however, suggest that for local failure confined to nasopharynx, stereotactic radiotherapy appears to be comparable to brachytherapy using split palate gold grain (Chua et al. 2007). For recurrent disease and tumor extended beyond the nasopharynx, stereotactic radiotherapy using multiple fractions to deliver a higher total dose appears to be superior to single fraction treatment (Chua et al. 2009b). Stereotactic radiotherapy was also found to be superior to intracavitary brachytherapy for persistent NPC, with a 3-year local control rate of 82% for the former and 72% for the latter (Yau et al. 2004). For tumor localized to nasopharynx, surgery, bracytherapy and stereotactic radiotherapy are all effective salvage options and these treatments, rather than external beam reirradiation, should be used if it is technically feasible to retreat the tumor and with available expertise. For tumor extended beyond nasopharynx, the use of external beam reirradiation is often required, and the use of intensity-modulated radiotherapy, preferably in combination with chemotherapy, is recommended.

A multidisciplinary team comprising head and neck surgeon, medical oncologist, otorhinolaryngologist, radiation oncologist, and diagnostic radiologist should be always involved in joint assessment of patients with local failures and decision of salvage treatment. Table 19.5 summarizes the salvage treatments commonly employed at Queen Mary Hospital in Hong Kong and the treatment outcome. These results should not be compared directly due to different selection criteria; thus, patients treated by different salvage options had different disease characteristics. The results do suggest, however, that with good experience and careful patient selection, most salvage treatments can result in a long-term control rate of 50% or above. Since randomized trial comparing different salvage treatments are difficult to perform, one strategy to assist the clinician in selecting a salvage treatment is to define a model that predicts the outcome with a spe-

Table 19.5. Summary of Queen Mary Hospital's experience of using different salvage treatment for local failures of NPC

Salvage treatment	Time period	No. of patients	Tumor control rate (%)	Survival rate (%)
Nasopharyngectomy	1989–2008	236	67 (5-year)	52 (5-year)
Gold grain interstitial implantation	1986–1999	106	Persistent disease: 87 (5-year) Recurrent disease: 63 (5-year)	Persistent disease: 79 (5-year) Recurrent disease: 54 (5-year)
2D external beam radiotherapy	1984–1995	97	32 (5-year)	36 (5-year)
Stereotactic radiosurgery	1996–2005	48	52 (5-year)	47 (5-year)
Intensity modulated radiotherapy	2001–2004	31	rT1-3: 43 (5-year) rT4: 27 (5-year)	rT1-3: 38 (5-year) rT4: 14 (5-year)

cific type of treatment. Using five prognostic factors (age, recurrent T-classification category, time period from first radiotherapy, tumor volume, prior local failure), we have designed a prognostic scoring system for stereotactic radiosurgery, and the 5-year local control rates for good, intermediate and poor prognostic score were 100%, 43% and 10%, respectively (Chua et al. 2008). The scoring system was recently validated using published data in the literature (Chua et al. 2009c).

19.8 Future Directions

The technique of external beam radiation has evolved substantially over the past decade and the utilization of newer treatment techniques such as helical tomotherapy and proton therapy as salvage treatment of local failures of NPC may further improve the outcome. Improved target delineation using biological imaging is also important in salvage radiation due to the smaller margin that can be safely used. Integration of chemotherapy and molecular targeted agent may also play a role in the management of advanced recurrence, similar to the success observed in the treatment of newly diagnosed disease. Collaborative efforts in pooling data of salvage treatment from multiple centers should be encouraged, since it will allow the identification of important prognostic factors, and useful models may be developed to assist clinician in selecting the patient for a specific type of salvage treatment. This is of particular importance since prospective randomized trials comparing different salvage treatments are difficult to conduct.

References

Ahn YC, Lee KC, Kim DY, et al (2000) Fractionated stereotactic radiation therapy for extracranial head and neck tumors. Int J Radiat Oncol Biol Phys 48:501–505

Buatti JM, Friedman WA, Bova FJ, et al (1995) Linac radiosurgery for locally recurrent nasopharyngeal carcinoma: rationale and technique. Head Neck 17:14–19

Chang JT, See LC, Liao CT, et al (2000) Locally recurrent nasopharyngeal carcinoma. Radiother Oncol 54:135–142

Chen HJ, Leung SW, Su CY (2001) Linear accelerator based radiosurgery as a salvage treatment for skull base and intracranial invasion of recurrent nasopharyngeal carcinoma. Am J Clin Oncol 24:255–258

Choy D, Sham JS, Wei WI, et al (1993) Transpalatal insertion of radioactive gold grain for the treatment of persistent and recurrent nasopharyngeal carcinoma. Int J Radiat Oncol Biol Phys 25:505–512

Chua D (2009a) Phase II trial of induction chemotherapy followed by external beam re-irradiation and concurrent cetuximab for locoregionally recurrent nasopharyngeal carcinoma. Proceedings of 2nd International Conference on Innovative Approaches in Head and Neck Oncology, Abstract 56*

Chua DT, Hung KN, Lee V, et al (2009c) Validation of a prognostic scoring system for locally recurrent nasopharyngeal carcinoma treated by stereotactic radiosurgery. BMC Cancer 9: 131

Chua DT, Sham JS, Au GK (2005b) Induction chemotherapy with cisplatin and gemcitabine followed by reirradiation for locally recurrent nasopharyngeal carcinoma. Am J Clin Oncol 28:464–471

Chua DT, Sham JS, Hung KN, et al (2006) Predictive factors of tumor control and survival after radiosurgery of local failures of nasopharyngeal carcinoma. Int J Radiat Oncol Biol Phys 66:1415–1421

Chua DT, Sham JS, Kwong DL, et al (1998) Locally recurrent nasopharyngeal carcinoma: treatment results for patients with computed tomography assessment. Int J Radiat Oncol Biol Phys 41:379–386

Chua DT, Sham JS, Kwong PW, et al (2003) Linear accelerator-based stereotactic radiosurgery for limited, locally persistent, and recurrent nasopharyngeal carcinoma: efficacy and complications. Int J Radiat Oncol Biol Phys 56: 177–183

Chua DT, Sham JS, Leung LT, et al (2005a) Reirradiation of nasopharyngeal carcinoma with intensity-modulated radiotherapy. Radiother Oncol 77:290–294

Chua DT, Wei W, Sham JS, et al (2007) Stereotactic radiosurgery versus gold gain implantation in salvaging local failures of nasopharyngeal carcinoma. Int J Radiat Oncol Biol Phys 69:469–474

Chua DT, Wu SX, Lee V, et al (2009b) Comparison of single versus fractionated dose of stereotactic radiotherapy for salvaging local failures of nasopharyngeal carcinoma: a matched-cohort analysis. Head Neck Oncol 1:13

Chua D, Wong M, Wei W (2008) Epidermal growth factor receptor expression correlates with poor outcome in patients with locally recurrent nasopharyngeal carcinoma treated by external beam reirradiation. Proceedings of 50th Annual Meeting of American Society for Therapeutic Radiology and Oncology, Abstract 2479*

Cmelak AJ, Cox RS, Adler JR, et al (1997) Radiosurgery for skull base malignancies and nasopharyngeal carcinoma. Int J Radiat Oncol Biol Phys 37:997–1003

Harrison LB, Weissberg JB (1987) A technique for interstitial nasopharyngeal brachytherapy. Int J Radiat Oncol Biol Phys 13:451–453

Hsiung CY, Yorke ED, Chui CS, et al (2002) Intensity-modulated radiotherapy versus conventional three-dimensional conformal radiotherapy for boost or salvage treatment of nasopharyngeal carcinoma. Int J Radiat Oncol Biol Phys 53: 638–647

Kocher M, Voges J, Staar S, et al (1998) Linear accelerator radiosurgery for recurrent malignant tumors of the skull base. Am J Clin Oncol 21:18–22

Kwong DL, Wei WI, Cheng AC, et al (2001) Long term results of radioactive gold grain implantation for the treatment of persistent and recurrent nasopharyngeal carcinoma. Cancer 91:1105–1113

Law SC, Lam WK, Ng MF, et al (2002) Reirradiation of nasopharyngeal carcinoma with intracavitary mold brachytherapy: an effective means of local salvage. Int J Radiat Oncol Biol Phys 54:1095–1113

Lee AW, Foo W, Law SC, et al (1997) Reirradiation for recurrent nasopharyngeal carcinoma: factors affecting the therapeutic ratio and ways for improvement. Int J Radiat Oncol Biol Phys 38:43–52

Lee AW, Foo W, Law SC, et al (1999) Recurrent nasopharyngeal carcinoma: the puzzles of long lantency. Int J Radiat Oncol Biol Phys 44:149–156

Lee TF, Fang FM, Chao PJ, et al (2008) Dosimetric comparisons of helical tomotherapy and step-and-shoot intensity-modulated radiotherapy in nasopharyngeal carcinoma. Radiother Oncol 89:89–96

Leung TW, Tung SY, Sze WK, et al (2000a) Salvage brachytherapy for patients with locally persistent nasopharyngeal carcinoma. Int J Radiat Oncol Biol Phys 47:405–412

Leung TW, Tung SY, Sze WK, et al (2000b) Salvage radiation therapy for locally recurrent nasopharyngeal carcinoma. Int J Radiat Oncol Biol Phys 48:1331–1338

Leung TW, Tung SY, Wong VY, et al (1996) High dose rate intracavitary brachytherapy in the treatment of nasopharyngeal carcinoma. Acta Oncol 35:43–47

Leung TW, Wong VY, Tung SY (2009) Stereotactic radiotherapy for locally recurrent nasopharyngeal carcinoma. Int J Radiat Oncol Biol Phys [2009 Mar 25 (Epub)]

Lu TX, Mai WY, Teh BS, et al (2004) Initial experience using intensity-modulated radiotherapy for recurrent nasopharyngeal carcinoma. Int J Radiat Oncol Biol Phys 58: 682–687

Miller RC, Foote RL, Coffey RJ, et al (1997) The role of stereotactic radiosurgery in the treatment of malignant skull base tumors. Int J Radiat Oncol Biol Phys 39:977–981

Mitsuhashi N, Sakurai H, Katano S, et al (1999) Stereotactic radiotherapy for locally recurrent nasopharyngeal carcinoma. Laryngoscope 109:805–809

Öksüz DÇ, Meral G, Uzel Ö, et al (2004) Reirradiation for locally recurrent nasopharyngeal carcinoma: treatment results and prognostic factors. Int J Radiat Oncol Biol Phys 60: 388–394

Orecchia R, Redda MG, Regona R, et al (1999) Results of hypofractionated stereotactic re-irradiation on 13 locally recurrent nasopharyngeal carcinoma. Radiother Oncol 53:23–28

Pai P, Chuang C, Wei K, et al (2000) Stereotactic radiosurgery for locally recurrent nasopharyngeal carcinoma. Head Neck 24:748–753

Poon D, Yap SP, Wong ZW, et al (2004) Concurrent chemoradiotherapy in locoregionally recurrent nasopharyngeal carcinoma. Int J Radiat Oncol Biol Phys 59:1312–1318

Pryzant RM, Wendt CD, Delclos L, et al (1992) Re-treatment of nasopharyngeal carcinoma in 53 patients. Int J Radiat Oncol Biol Phys 22:941–947

Syed AM, Puthawala AA, Damore SJ, et al (2000) Brachytherapy for primary and recurrent nasopharyngeal carcinoma: 20 years' experience at long beach memorial. Int J Radiat Oncol Biol Phys 47:1311–1321

Taheri-Kadkhoda Z, Björk-Eriksson T, Nill S, et al (2008) Intensity-modulated radiotherapy of nasopharyngeal carcinoma: a comparative treatment planning study of photons and protons. Radiat Oncol 3:4

Teo PM, Kwan WH, Chan AT, et al (1998) How successful is high dose (≥60 Gy) reirradiation using mainly external beams in salvaging local failures of nasopharyngeal carcinoma? Int J Radiat Oncol Biol Phys 40:897–913

Wang CC (1987) Re-irradiation of recurrent nasopharyngeal carcinoma. Treatment techniques and results. Int J Radiat Oncol Biol Phys 13:953–956

Wang CC, Busse J, Gitterman M (1975) A simple afterloading applicator for intracavitary irradiation of carcinoma of the nasopharynx. Radiology 115:737–738

Wei WI, Sham JS, Choy D, et al (1990) Split-palate approach for gold grain implantation in nasopharyngeal carcinoma. Arch Otolaryngol Head Neck Surg 116:578–582

Wu SX, Chua DT, Deng ML, et al (2007) Outcome of fractionated stereotactic radiotherapy for 90 patients with locally persistent and recurrent nasopharyngeal carcinoma. Int J Radiat Oncol Biol Phys 69:761–769

Xiao JP, Xu GZ, Miao YJ (2001) Fractionated stereotactic radiosurgery for 50 patients with recurrent or residual nasopharyngeal carcinoma. Int J Radiat Oncol Biol Phys 51:164–170

Yan JH, Hu YH, Gu XZ (1983) Radiation therapy of recurrent nasopharyngeal carcinoma: report on 219 patients. Acta Radiol Oncol 22:23–28

Yau TK, Sze WM, Lee WM, et al (2004) Effectiveness of brachytherapy and fractionated stereotactic radiotherapy boost for persistent nasopharyngeal carcinoma. Head Neck 26:1024–1030

Yu KH, Leung SF, Tung SY, et al (2005) Survival outcome of patients with nasopharyngeal carcinoma with first local failure: a study by the Hong Kong Nasopharyngeal Carcinoma Study Group. Head Neck 27:397–405

Zheng XK, Ma J, Chen LH, et al (2005) Dosimetric and clinical results of three-dimensional conformal radiotherapy for locally recurrent nasopharyngeal carcinoma. Radiother Oncol 75:197–203

Surgery for Recurrent Nasopharyngeal Carcinoma

20

William Ignace Wei

CONTENTS

William Ignace Wei, MS FRCS, FRCSE, FRACS (Hon), FACS, FHKAM (Surg) (ORL)
Queen Mary Hospital, The University of Hong Kong, Pok Fu Lam Road, Hong Kong SAR, P.R. China

20.1 Introduction

The utilization of conformal radiation therapy and combined chemoradiation therapy has substantially improved the outcome of nasopharyngeal carcinoma (NPC) after treatment. However, local and/or regional recurrences remain a major concern of treatment failure. Therapeutic modalities are usually limited, and the outcome of nasopharyngeal cancer patients who experience local and/or regional recurrences is usually suboptimal.

Surgery plays a relatively limited role in the initial management of nasopharyngeal cancer; however, it is an important treatment option for patients who experience recurrence after definitive radiation therapy or chemoradiation therapy. Isolated recurrence in the cervical without evidence of distant metastasis or local recurrence in the nasopharynx can usually be successfully managed by surgery. For local recurrence in or around the nasopharynx, salvage treatment using reirradiation is a valid option. However, as most patients with recurrent NPC are previously treated with definitive dose of irradiation to the nasopharynx and its surrounding structures, high incidence of significant complications could result from the second course of irradiation. Alternative salvage measures have been introduced, in the treatment of recurrent disease in the nasopharynx this include the introduction of brachytherapy source into the tumor or surgical resection of the pathology. These treatment options are applicable especially when the residual or recurrent tumor is of limited size and is localized in the nasopharynx.

The aim of this chapter is to address the anatomical and pathological basis as well as the procedures of surgical management for the recurrent NPC in the neck or nasopharynx. As a thorough understanding of the surgical anatomy is crucial for the proper surgical management of recurrent NPC in the nasopharynx or the neck, the first section of the chapter is devoted to describe the anatomy of the nasopharynx and neck from a surgical perspective.

20.2 Surgical Anatomy

20.2.1 Surgical Anatomy of the Nasopharynx

The pharynx is separated arbitrarily into three parts and the upper one-third is defined as the nasopharynx. This is the region lying behind the nasal cavities and above the soft palate. The body of the sphenoid bone and the anterior wall of the sphenoid sinus form the slanting roof of the nasopharynx. The roof extends downward to merge with the posterior wall that is formed by the clivus, which in turn is connected by ligaments to the arch of the atlas and then the upper part of body of the axis vertebra. The anterior part of the floor of the nasopharynx is formed by the superior surface of the soft palate and the posterior part opens inferiorly into the oropharynx at the level of the soft palate (Fig. 20.1). The superior constrictor muscle with the opening of the Eustachian tube or the auditory tympanic tube forms the lateral wall. The medial portion of Eustachian tube is cartilaginous and situated between the skull base and upper edge of the superior constrictor muscle. The cartilage that surrounds the orifice of this tube is an incomplete ring, deficient in the inferolateral portion. The levator veli palatini muscle, attached to the lower edge of this cartilaginous ring, controls the patency of the aperture. The medial portion of the cartilage elevates the mucosa in the nasopharynx to form the medial crura. The slit-like recess located medial to the crura is the fossa of Rosenmüller, and its size and depth varies between individuals (Fig. 20.2); early nasopharyngeal carcinoma (NPC) is frequently found in this fossa. The anterior aspect of the nasopharynx is the posterior choanae that opens into the nasal cavity. The posterior part of the nasal septum is the vomer, which is attached to the anterior wall of the sphenoid and divides the nasopharynx incompletely into the right and left portions. Lying further laterally on the anterior aspect are the pterygoid plates with attachment of the pterygoid muscles, and in front of these is the maxillary sinus (Fig. 20.2).

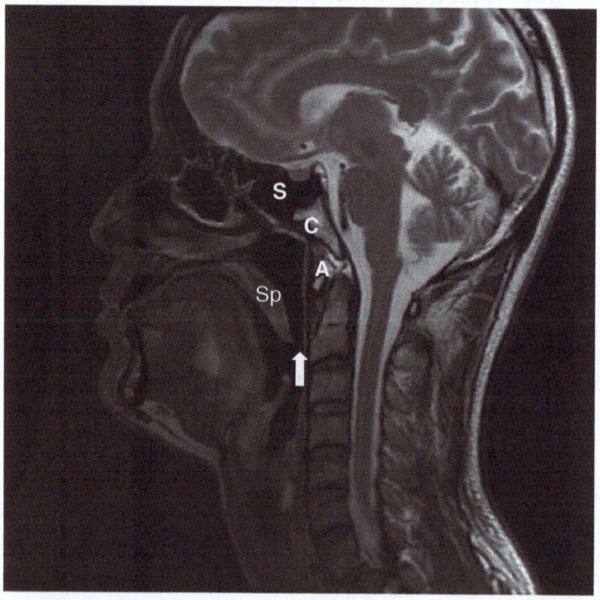

Fig. 20.1. MRI sagittal view of the nasopharynx showing the roof which is formed by the sphenoid sinus (S) and the clivus (C) with continues onto the Atlas vertebra (A) forming the posterior wall. The anterior part of the inferior wall is formed by the soft palate (Sp) and the posterior aspect continues into the oropharynx (*arrow*)

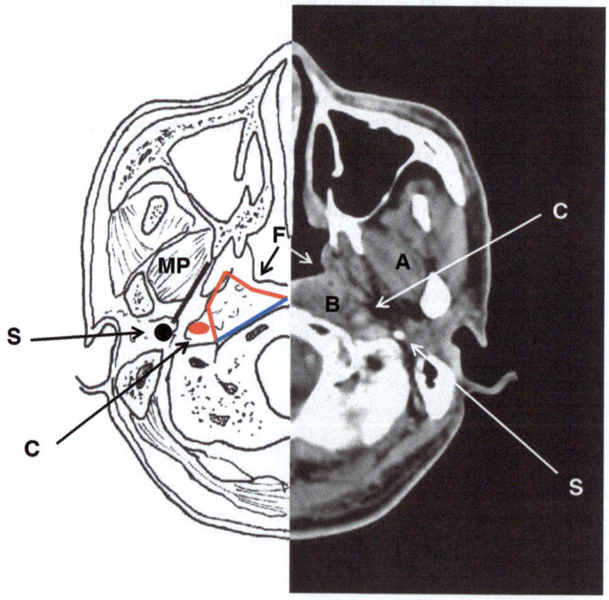

Fig. 20.2. Schematic CT showing the lateral boundaries of the nasopharynx. *C* internal carotid artery; *F* fossa of Rosenmuller; *MP* medial pterygoid muscle; *S* styloid process. The *black line* is the imaginary line joining the medial pterygoid plate to the styloid process. The space in front of the line is the prestyloid space (**A**) and behind the poststyloid space (**B**). The *Red line* is the pharyngobasilar fascia which joins with the fascia of the opposite side to form the median raphe. This fascia together with the prevertebral fascia (*Blue line*) encloses the retropharyngeal space

The mucosal lining of the nasopharynx varies; the posterior and superior wall is lined with stratified squamous cell while the pseudostratified ciliated epithelium is found in the region of the nasopharynx near the choana. The epithelium lies on a well-defined basement membrane and then on the lamina propria, which contains abundant lymphoid tissues. The superior constrictor forms the muscular layer of the nasopharynx and the auditory tympanic tubes pierce this muscular tube bilaterally at its superior portion. There is a thick fascia investing the superior constrictor muscle on the outside and this is the pharyngobasilar fascia. This fascia joins its counterpart from the opposite side to form the median raphe which extends from the skull base to the posterior pharyngeal wall at the hypopharynx level. The pharyngobasilar fascia together with the prevertebral fascia encloses the retropharyngeal space which harbors the node of Röuviere. This retropharyngeal space is part of the poststyloid space of the paranasopharyngeal space (Fig. 20.2). The last four cranial nerves, the carotid sheath, and the sympathetic trunk are located in this poststyloid space and they can be affected by direct tumor extension or involved by the enlarged retropharyngeal lymph node.

The lymphatic drainage channels of the nasopharynx are found mainly in the submucosal region, which subsequently drains into the retropharyngeal lymph nodes. Efferents from these nodes together with some lymphatics that come directly from the nasopharynx drain to the deep cervical lymph nodes.

20.2.2 Surgical Anatomy of the Neck

The patterns of lymph node distribution in the neck and lymphatic drainage in nasopharyngeal cancer have been detailed in Chap. 17. However, it is important to note that the radiological boundaries utilized in clinical tumor volume delineation are somewhat different from the boundaries described in surgery. The lymph node distribution pattern in the neck was originally described to be at five levels (Shah et al. 1981). The anatomical boundaries of these levels are as follows. Those lymphnodes situated in front of the anterior border of the sternomastoid muscle are in Level I and those lying behind the posterior edge of the muscle are in Level V. The nodes under the sternomastoid muscle are Level II, III, and IV lymph nodes. The position of the bifurcation of the carotid artery separates Level II from Level III and the lower edge of the thyroid cartilage or the omohyoid muscle marks the separation of Level III from Level IV nodes.

Surgery treatment of the neck nodes are the neck dissections. Different types of neck dissection have been defined following whether the nonlymphatic structures are removed and which levels of lymph nodes are resected (Robbins et al. 1991). When only the lymph nodes and lymphatic tissue are removed, they are the selective neck dissection. When all nodes, lymphatic structures and nonlymphatic structure are removed, it is the radical neck dissection. When some non lymphatic structures are preserved, they are the modified neck dissections. When the spinal accessory nerve is preserved, it is the Type I modified neck dissection, when both the spinal accessory nerve and the internal jugular vein (IJV) are preserved, it is Type II; when the nerve, the vein, and sternomastoid muscle are all preserved, it is Type III modified neck dissection.

The lymphatic drainage of the neck in general goes in an orderly fashion, from the high neck nodes to the lower ones, and this is also the pattern of metastasis of NPC in the cervical lymph nodes (Sham et al. 1990), going from the Levels I, II nodes and then to Levels III, IV, and V.

20.3 Management of Neck Recurrence in Nasopharyngeal Carcinoma

20.3.1 Recurrence in the Neck After Radiotherapy

One of the pathogenesis of nasopharyngeal cancer is its high propensity of metastasis to cervical lymph nodes. In a retrospective evaluation of the clinical features of over 4000 patients, enlarged lymph node were seen in 74.5% of patients (Lee et al. 1997). These metastasis in the cervical lymph nodes and their primary tumor are radiosensitive and in view of the high incidence of occult nodal metastasis, elective radiation of the neck is routinely carried out for all patients, even though no enlarged neck node is detected through clinical examination and imaging studies. This management strategy has shown to improve locoregional control of the disease (Lee et al. 1989).

The radiation dose for elective treatment of the neck is in the rage of 50–60 Gy. The control of disease for the N0 and N1 neck is 90%, but this dropped to 70% for N2 and N3 diseases (Chua et al. 2001). The application of concomitant chemoradiation, employing cisplatin and 5-fluorouracil in recent years, has improved locoregional disease control (Lee et al. 2005). The application of intensity-modulated radiotherapy also resolves the target-volume issue and dose uncertainty at the primary tumor and the upper lymph nodes in the neck. They can be treated with one single volume throughout, resulting in better tumor control (Kam et al. 2003).

Despite these measures, recurrent carcinoma in the neck node is still observed. In a report published 20 years ago on a large cohort of patients suffering from all stages of NPC, the incidence of recurrent disease in the neck following combined chemoradiation was less than 5% (Hung et al. 1985). Recently, with the application of IMRT, isolated recurrence in the neck was reported to be <1% (Lui et al. 2003). For patients with advanced nodal disease on presentation, the incidence of failure in the neck following concomitant chemoradiation could still be as high as 33% (Palazzi et al. 2004). The diagnosis of persistent or recurrent disease in the neck node is first suspected on clinical grounds. When the cervical lymph nodes fail to regress completely at 12 weeks after completion of treatment, either radiotherapy or concomitant chemoradiation, residual disease in the persistent node is likely to occur.

20.3.2 Diagnosis of Neck Recurrence

The presence of tumor in the node should also be suspected if the node reappears after its initial regression following treatment. The confirmation of the malignant nature of the lymph node is however not straightforward. In view of the increasing fibrosis in the neck nodes after radiation, fine needle aspiration cytology frequently yields equivocal results. Ultrasonography, computed tomography, or magnetic resonance imaging were able to show the presence of the lymph node, there are no special features to confirm the malignant nature of the node. When the imaging studies are carried out sequentially, then the progressive enlargement of the neck mass would suggest the presence of malignancy. Recently, positron emission tomography has been shown to be useful in the detection of this type of malignant disease in the neck (Yan et al. 2005), although the patient number is small. The tumor volume in the neck node is the critical factor that determines whether the various investigations are useful to reach the diagnosis.

20.3.3 Surgical Salvage Procedures

When the only site of malignant disease is in the neck following initial therapy, then further salvage therapy should be instituted to eradicate the disease. The efficacy of chemotherapy for the management of neck disease following previous treatment is expected to be low, and further radiotherapy has been reported to have a 5-year survival of 19.7% (Sham and Choy 1991). The second course of radiation is also associated with significant side effects. Surgical resection of the cervical lymph node recurrence then becomes the alternative choice. The most frequently performed surgical salvage procedure for persistent or recurrent disease in the neck node is radical neck dissection. The reported 5-year tumor control in the neck was 66% and 5-year actuarial survival for these patients was 37% (Wei et al. 1990a).

The radical neck dissection as a salvage procedure for the neck lymph nodes in these patients was carried out on irradiated tissue. To avoid complications of the surgery, the MacFee neck incision is advisable. These parallel neck incisions placed at least 7 cm apart would provide adequate circulation and prevent necrosis at the edge of the incisions. With this parallel incision, the neck skin flap has to be lifted for the radical neck dissection; the platysma should be left on the skin to ensure adequate perfusion of the skin (Wei 2004).

Patients with residual or recurrent neck disease after primary treatment usually present with one or two neck nodes clinically. When imaging studies were carried out for them, the number of cervical lymph node detected was usually limited, and frequently these lymph nodes were of small size. Thus, surgical salvage of the neck might focus only on these clinically obvious neck nodes. The extent of surgical resection might range from excision of the palpable lymph node to some form of neck dissection. The neck dissection might be a selective neck dissection, only removing the lymph nodes in Levels II, III, and upper part of V; or modified neck dissection, removing all the lymph nodes in the neck while preserving the nonlymphatic structures such as the spinal accessory nerve, the internal jugular vein, and the sternomastoid muscle; or radical neck dissection, removing all the lymph nodes in the neck together with all the nonlymphatic structures (Fig. 20.3). The extent of surgical resection depends on the pathological features of the carcinoma cells in these neck nodes. These include extent and pattern of lymph nodes

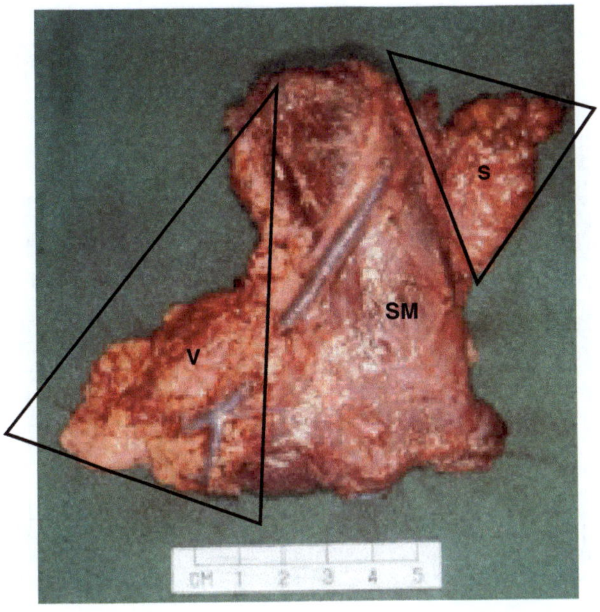

Fig. 20.3. Specimen of a right radical neck dissection showing the sternomastoid muscle covering the lymph nodes of levels II, III and IV. The submandibular gland and level I lymph nodes (S) and level V lymph nodes (V) are also shown

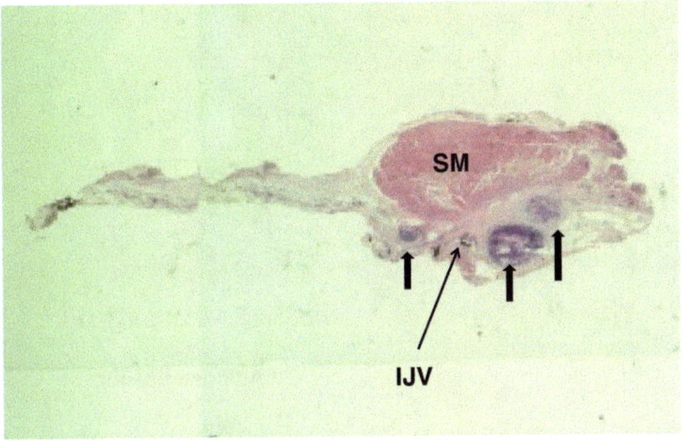

Fig. 20.4. Histological slide of a section of the neck dissection specimen showing multiple lymph nodes (*arrow*). The sternomastoid muscle (SM) and internal jugular vein (IJV) are also shown. (Haematoxylin and eosin × 40)

involved by the metastatic carcinoma cells, the potential and incidence of these malignant cells to exhibit extracapsular spread, and the tendency of these tumor cells to involve the nonlymphatic structures.

20.3.4 Pathological Basis of Surgical Salvage

These pathological behaviors were determined through a step serial sectioning of 43 specimens obtained following radical neck dissection carried out for residual or recurrent neck disease after initial radiation or chemoradiation (Wei et al. 1992). The study reported that in over 70% of the specimen studied, there were more lymph nodes harboring carcinoma cell than detected clinically or by imaging studies (Fig. 20.4). The distribution of the tumor-bearing lymph nodes was throughout the five levels in the neck, although most of them were located in Levels II and upper part of V. Among the lymph nodes that harbored malignant cells, in 60% of them there were extracapsular tumor extension. In many of the lymph nodes, the capsule had disintegrated (Fig. 20.5) and the tumor cells were infiltrating the surrounding tissue (Fig. 20.6). In 35% of the specimens, the carcinoma cells were infiltrating the nonlymphatic structures in the neck, such as the sternomastoid muscle (Fig. 20.7). In 28% of the specimens, malignant cells were seen infiltrating or lying close to the spinal accessory nerve (Fig. 20.8).

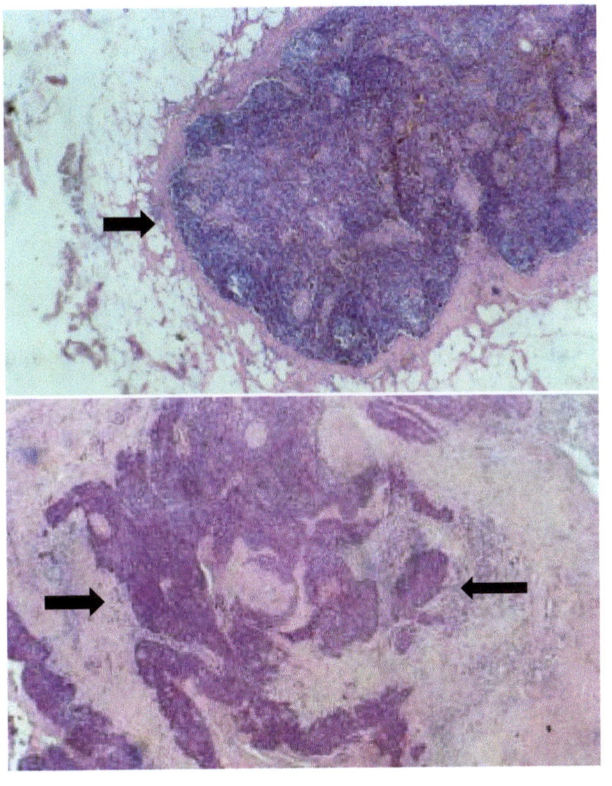

Fig. 20.5. Upper: Tumor seen within the capsule (*arrow*) of the lymph node. Lower: Capsule of the lymph node disintegrated (*arrow*) and tumor is in the surrounding soft tissue. (Haematoxylin and eosin × 150)

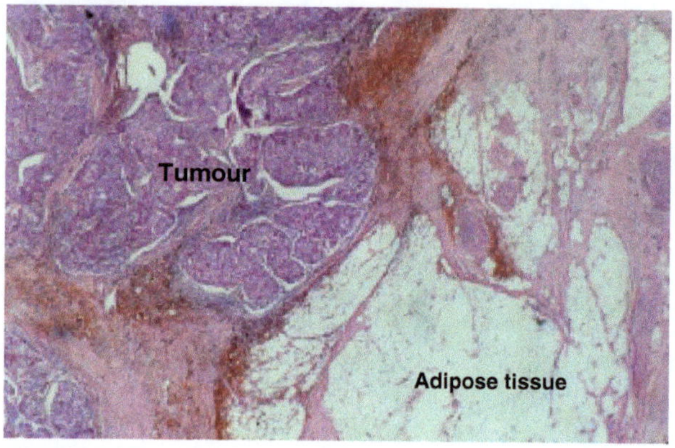

Fig. 20.6. Tumor infiltrating the soft tissue in the neck. (Haematoxylin and eosin × 150)

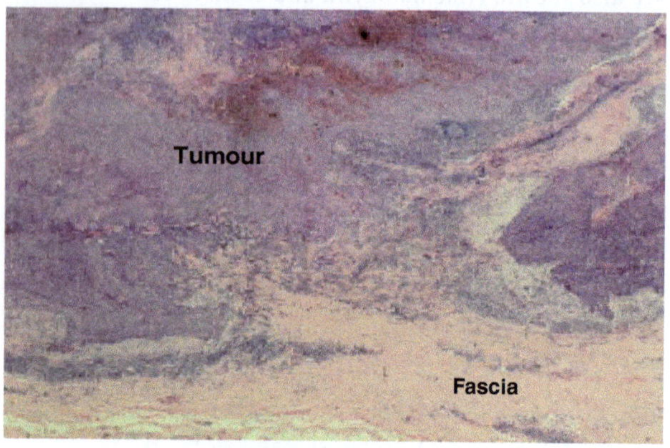

Fig. 20.7. Tumor infiltrating the fascia of the sternomastoid muscle. (Haematoxylin and eosin × 150)

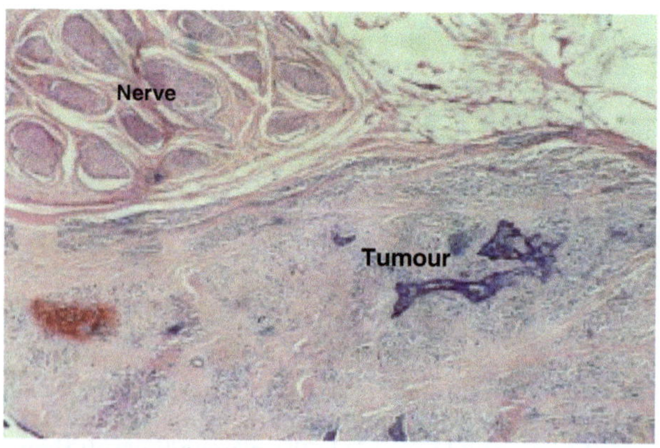

Fig. 20.8. Tumor lying close to the spinal accessory nerve. (Haematoxylin and eosin × 150)

In view of the extensive infiltrative nature of these recurrent or residual malignant cells in the cervical lymph nodes after radiation of chemoradiation, the surgical salvage procedure should be at least a radical

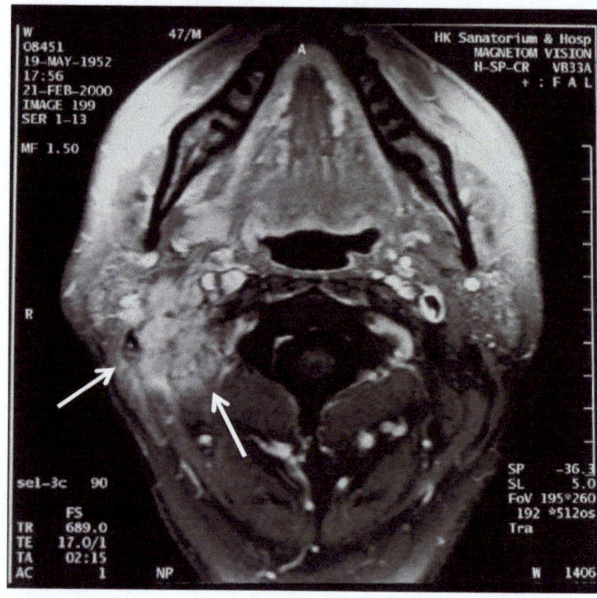

Fig. 20.9. MRI scan showing the multiple lymph nodes have infiltrated the overlying sternomastoid muscle and the muscle of the floor of the posterior triangle (*arrows*)

neck dissection. When a less-extensive salvage procedure is performed, then tumor cells might be left behind leading to failure of the salvage effort.

20.3.5 Salvage of Extensive Neck Recurrence

Sometimes the recurrent or residual disease might be extensive, lying close to or infiltrating the overlying skin or muscle of the floor of the posterior triangle (Fig. 20.9). Occasionally, during the radical neck dissection, the malignant lymph nodes could be macroscopically dissected off vital structures in the neck, such as the vagus nerve, internal carotid artery, or brachial plexus, the resection margins would be close. Further adjuvant therapeutic measures should be instituted to eradicate the possible microscopic malignant cells to ensure tumor clearance. As the neck of all these patients has been irradiated, further external radiation might lead to complications and would not be advisable.

After-loading brachytherapy to the surgical bed, however, could be considered when the clearance of the deep surgical margin is dubious. During the radical neck dissection, the area where microscopical tumor might be left behind is marked. Hollow nylon tubes are placed on this area; the tubes are placed at a regular distance from one another (Fig. 20.10). This distance depends on the radiation dosimeter of

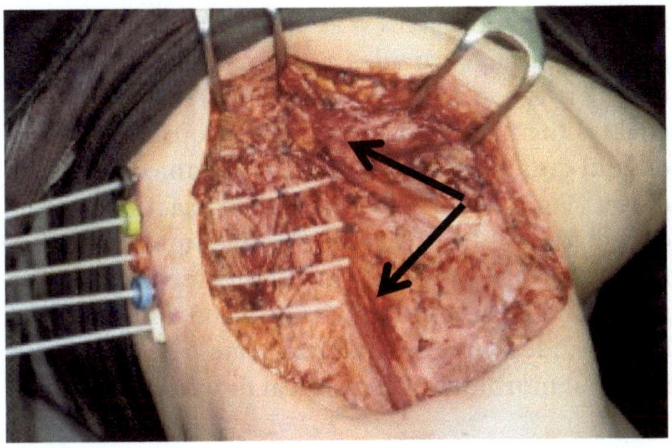

Fig. 20.10. Five empty nylon tubes are placed over the tumor bed (*arrows*) so that after-loading brachytherapy sources can be inserted

the brachytherapy source. The skin overlying the brachytherapy source is irradiated during the initial treatment, and might not be able to tolerate this additional brachytherapy. The area of neck skin lying on the brachytherapy source has to be removed with the specimen during radical neck dissection. The cutaneous defect should be reconstructed with nonirradiated skin from the chest wall, such as the deltopectoral flap or the pectoralis major myocutaneous flap (Fig. 20.11). Brachytherapy could start on seventh or eighth postoperative day, when the neck wound has healed and the nylon tubes could be removed after completion of brachytherapy.

When this adjuvant therapy was administered for patients with extensive recurrent or residual neck disease after radical neck dissection, a similar local tumor control rate could be achieved when compared to when the radical neck dissection was carried out for less-extensive neck disease (Wei et al. 2001).

20.4 Management of Recurrent Carcinoma in the Nasopharynx

20.4.1 Local Recurrence of Nasopharyngeal Carcinoma

As NPC is radiosensitive, the primary treatment of NPC is radiotherapy or concurrent chemoradiotherapy. Despite the fact that most of the tumor can be eradicated, in some patients the tumor might either persist or recur at the nasopharynx. It is still possible to manage the residual or recurrent tumor with a second course of external radiotherapy, usually at a greater dose than the initial course. A salvage rate of 32% together with a cumulative incidence of late postreirradiation sequelae of 24% and a treatment mortality of 1.8% has been reported (Lee et al. 1993). The problems associated with the second course of external radiotherapy affects significantly the quality of life of these patients.

To avoid this high incidence of significant complications resulting from the second course of irradiation, alternative salvage measures have been introduced. The surgical contributions in this aspect include the introduction of brachytherapy source into the tumor or surgical resection of the pathology. These treatment options are applicable when the residual or recurrent tumor is of limited size and is localized in the nasopharynx.

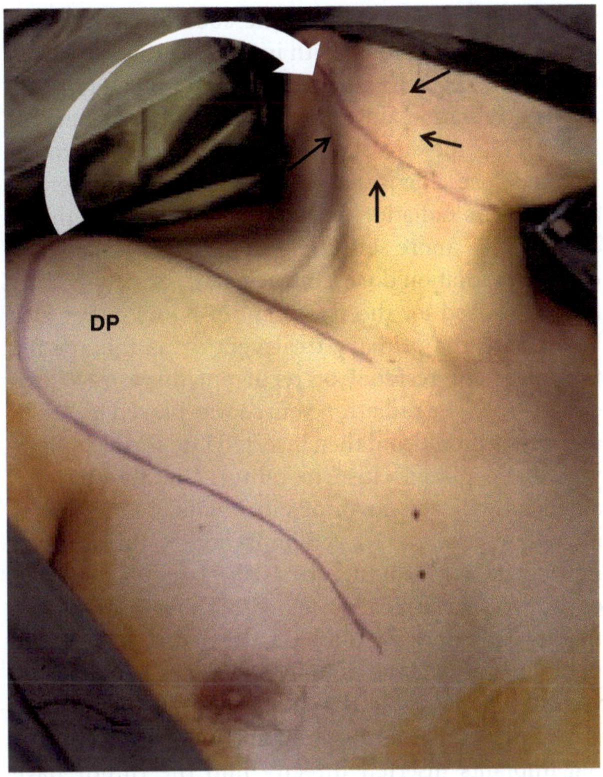

Fig. 20.11. Deltopectoral flap (DP) is planned to cover the cutaneous defect overlying the neck lymph node (*arrows*) after resection

20.4.2 Brachytherapy

Brachytherapy is most effective when the radiation source is inserted directly into the tumor. The radiation dose is highest at the source and declines gradually, proportional with increasing distance from the tumor. This thus allows the delivery of a high therapeutic radiation dose to the residual or recurrent NPC while the surrounding tissues receive a much smaller dose. The radiation source in brachytherapy also delivers radiation at a continuous rate and this is biologically more effective than the fractionated external radiation doses. Intracavitary brachytherapy has been used for the treatment of NPCs either as a boost with the primary treatment or as therapeutic treatment for residual or recurrent disease (Wang et al. 1975). The radiation source was placed either in a tube or a mould and then inserted into the nasopharynx to be placed close to tumor. Good result was achieved with this form of intracavitary brachytherapy (Law et al. 2002). The limitation of this form of intracavitary brachytherapy is the irregular contour of the primary tumor located within the nasopharynx that by itself does not have a uniform outline. It is difficult to apply the radiation source accurately into the vicinity of the whole tumor to obtain a tumoricidal dose. To circumvent this problem, radioactive interstitial implants inserted directly into the tumor have been used to treat small localized residual or recurrent tumor in the nasopharynx (Harrison and Weissber 1987).

One of the frequently used brachytherapy source is the radioactive gold grains (^{198}Au). These gold grains can be implanted directly into the tumor either transnasally with endoscopic guidance or using the split-palate approach (Wei et al. 1990b). The split-palate approach provides a direct view of the tumor for the surgeon and the oncologist (Fig. 20.12). This enables the implantation of the appropriate number of gold grains permanently into the tumor with precision (Fig. 20.13). This enables the exact dosimetry of radiation to be achieved in and around the tumor for the salvage purpose. For tumors localized in the nasopharynx, without bone invasion, this method has provided effective and high rate of salvage with minimal morbidity. The surgical procedure is simple

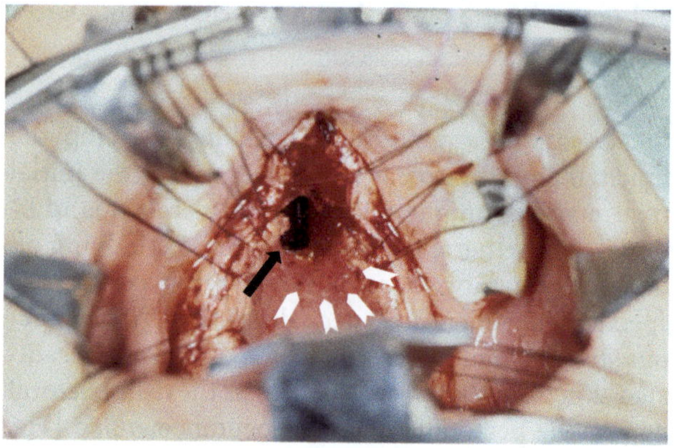

Fig. 20.12. The soft palate was split in the midline and together with the mucoperiosteum over the hard palate were retracted laterally. The black tip of a flexible endoscope (*arrow*) was inserted through the nose to provide better illumination. The edge of a shallow tumor could be seen (*arrow heads*)

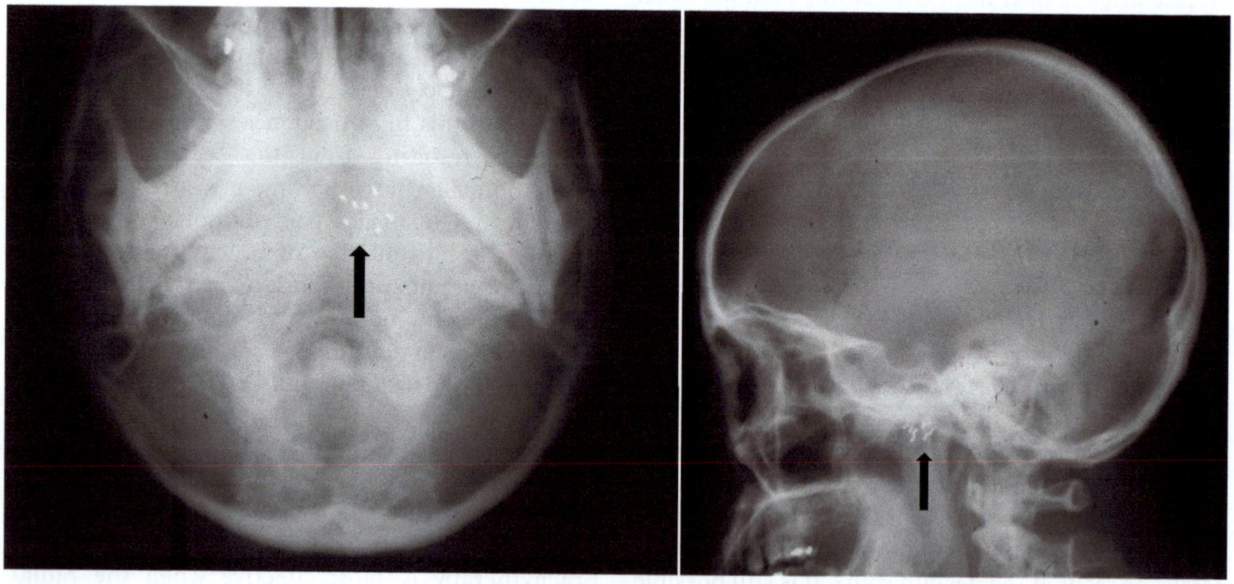

Fig. 20.13. Skull X-ray showing the inserted gold grains (*arrows*)

and in less than 10% of patients, they may develop a small palatal fistula and that can be managed with conservative measures, such as the wearing of a dental plate or can be repaired subsequently with a palatal flap (Choy et al. 1993). Lead shields however have to be used in the operating room during surgery to reduce the radiation hazards toward health-care workers. When gold grain implants were used to treat residual and recurrent tumors after the initial external radiotherapy, the 5-year local tumor control rates were reported to be 87% and 63%, respectively, and the corresponding 5-year disease-free survival rates were 68% and 60%, respectively, for these two groups of patients (Kwong et al. 2001).

20.4.3 Nasopharyngectomy

When the residual or recurrent tumor in the nasopharynx is of the size that the application of brachytherapy might not be useful, or if the tumor has extended to the paranasopharyngeal space (Fig. 20.14), then the next possible salvage option is surgery. Nasopharyngectomy, removing the tumor, the mucosa in the nasopharynx, and the Eustachian tube is effective in the eradication of localized disease in selected patients.

The nasopharynx is anatomically located in the center of the head; it is over 10 cm from the skin surface in all directions. It is difficult to expose the region adequately to allow an oncological resection to be

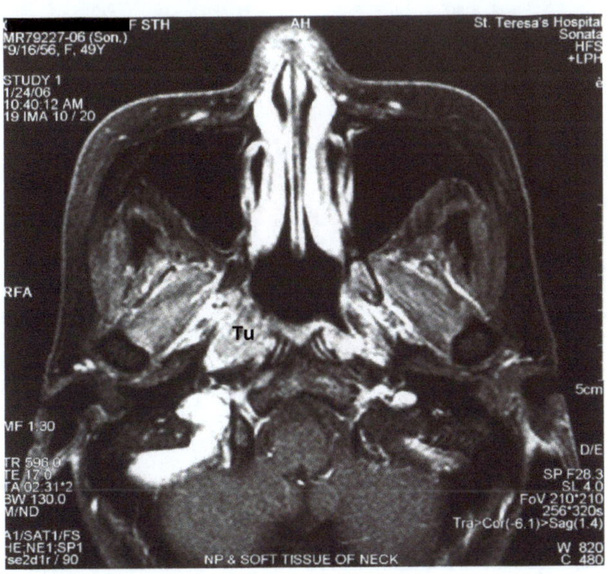

Fig. 20.14. MRI scan showing a large recurrent tumor in the right nasopharynx (Tu)

carried out, especially for a tumor in the nasopharynx which has extended to its vicinity. Resection of lesions in the nasal cavity and the nasopharynx under endoscopic guidance is frequently employed in recent years. Resection of residual or recurrent NPC with the endoscope is theoretically possible and this has been reported (Chen et al. 2007). This approach is applicable for small lesion localized in the central part of the posterior wall or superior wall, but not extending to the fossa of Rosenmüller. For small tumors in the location that can be removed with endoscopic approach, the same could also be adequately treated with brachytherapy. Most residual or recurrent NPC, however, involves the lateral wall of the nasopharynx, thus limiting the application of this minimal invasive surgical approach.

Over the years, a number of approaches have been used to expose the nasopharynx for a salvage nasopharyngectomy for more bulky tumors or those tumors that have extended to the paranasopharyngeal space. The brain and the spinal cord eliminated the superior and posterior routes. The transantral and midfacial deglove approaches can reach the nasopharynx from the front, but do not expose the lateral wall of the nasopharynx. These anterior approaches, even with the down fracture of the hard palate, only expose the central part of the nasopharynx including the superior and the posterior walls of the nasopharynx and not the posterolateral aspect of the paranasopharyngeal space. To approach the nasopharynx from the lateral aspect, through the infratemporal fossa, has been described over two decades ago (Fisch 1983). This route of entry started with a radical mastoidectomy and various structures have to be mobilized, these include the internal carotid artery, the cranial nerve, and the floor of the middle cranial fossa. The resultant morbidities are not negligible and with all these, it mainly exposes the lateral wall of the nasopharynx on the side of the surgery. It is hard to remove the lesion that has extended across the midline to the contralateral side. This procedure is also technically demanding, and it takes quite some time in dissection before the nasopharynx is exposed.

The nasopharynx can also be approached from the inferior aspect employing the transpalatal, transmaxillary, and transcervical approach (Fee et al. 1991; Morton et al. 1996). Again, this approach is useful for tumors located in the central part of the nasopharynx. For more extensive tumors, especially for those involving the lateral wall, the dissection of the paranasopharyngeal space is difficult from the inferior aspect. During the dissection, the internal carotid artery has to be protected, and it is not easy to control the superolateral margin of the tumor from below.

The anterolateral approach to the nasopharynx or the maxillary swing procedure has also been employed successfully for salvage nasopharyngectomy for nearly two decades since its first description in 1991 (Wei et al. 1991). Following osteotomies on the anterior wall of the maxilla, the hard palate, and between the maxillary tuberosity and the pterygoid plates, the maxilla antrum together with the hard palate attaches to the anterior cheek flap which can be swung laterally as one osteocutaneous complex (Figs. 20.15–17). This exposes the entire nasopharynx and the paranasopharyngeal space to allow an oncological surgical resection to be carried out adequately (Fig. 20.18). The entire nasopharynx together with the Eustachian tube on the side of the swing can be removed with the tumor en

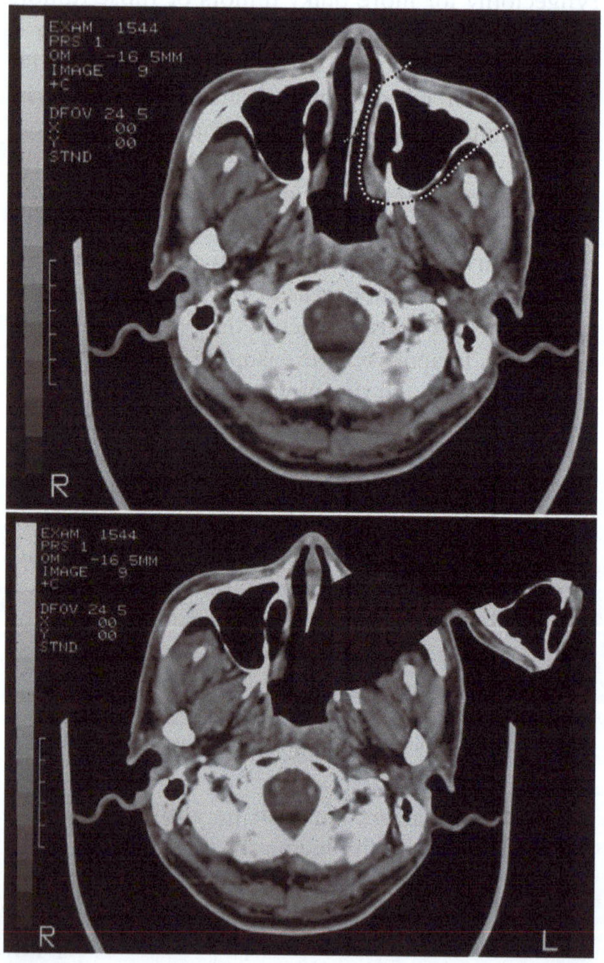

Fig. 20.15. Schematic computed tomography. *Upper*: the dotted lines mark the osteotomies. *Lower*: the maxilla is swung laterally to expose the nasopharynx, it is still attached to the anterior cheek flap

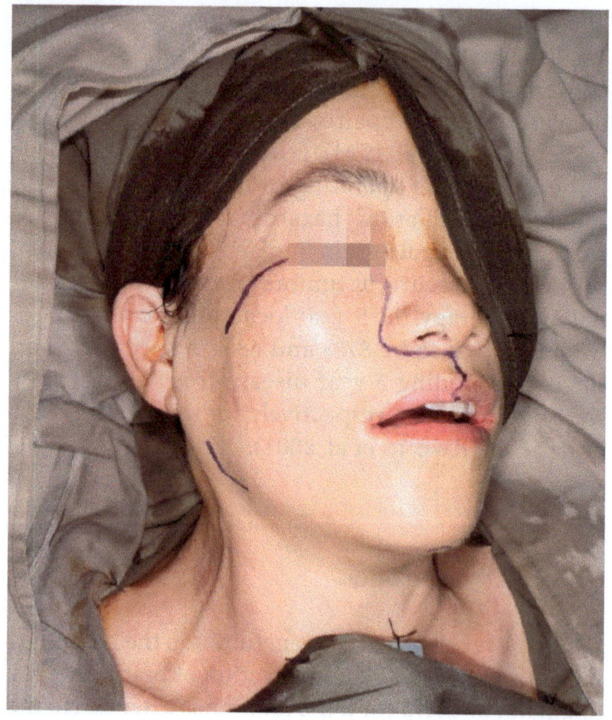

Fig. 20.16. Facial incision, in planning of right maxillary swing. The right angle of jaw is also marked

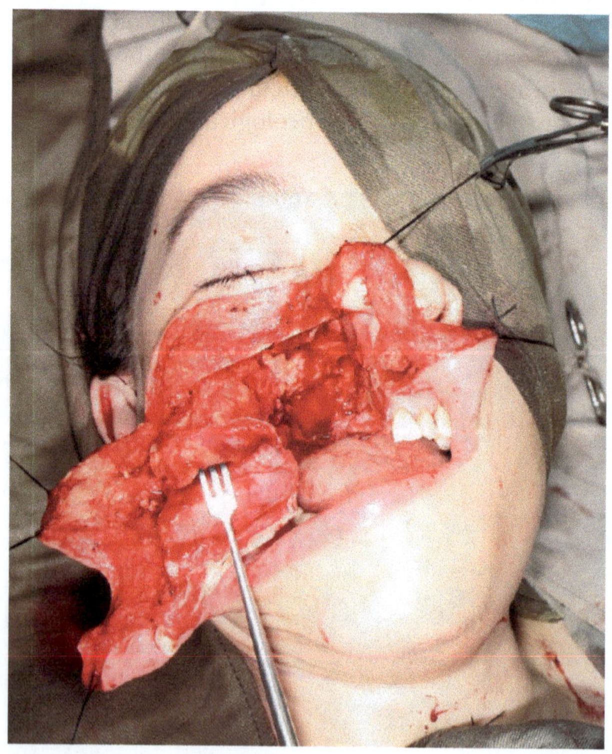

Fig. 20.17. Right maxilla swung laterally to expose the nasopharynx. The retractor is on the right inferior turbinate

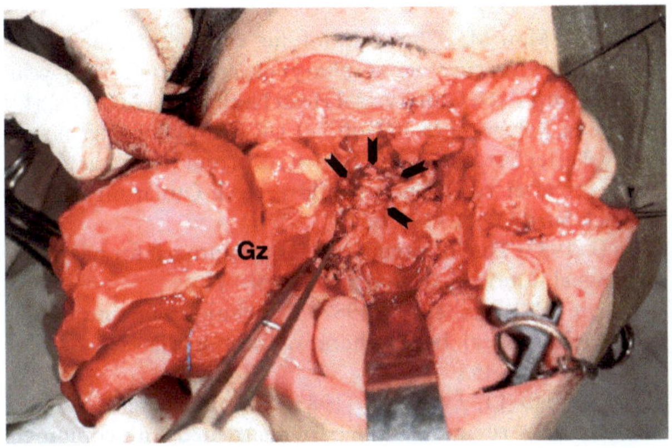

Fig. 20.18. The right maxilla is retracted laterally by a piece of gauz (Gz) to expose the tumor in the nasopharynx (*arrow heads*)

bloc (Fig. 20.19). With the resection of the posterior part of the nasal septum, tumor extended across the midline can also be adequately removed up to the edge of the opposite medial crura of the opening of the auditory tympanic tube. After the maxilla has been swung laterally, the dissection of the paranasopharyngeal LN can be done under direct vision. The internal carotid artery outside the pharyngobasilar fascia can be palpated and safe guarded during the dissection.

The mortalities associated with these salvage surgical procedures have been generally low and acceptable. As all these patients had previously undergone radical radiotherapy, complete wound healing might take some time. One of the initial complications associated with the maxillary swing approach was the development of a palatal fistula (Wei 2001). These patients have to wear a dental plate for swallowing and speech. Recently, the incision over the palate have been modified, the incision on the soft tissue and the osteotomy sites were designed to at different sites (Figs. 20.20 and 20.21) and this eliminated the formation of palatal fistula associated with this operation (Ng and Wei 2005). Many patients developed trismus after the nasopharyngectomy with the anterolateral approach, and this was related to the fibrosis of the pterygoid muscle following radiotherapy and surgery. This in general responded to passive stretching and did not affect significantly the quality of life of these patients who had undergone salvage nasopharyngectomy (Ng and Wei 2006). In general, as long as the persistent or recurrent tumor can be resected with a clear margin, the long-term results have been satisfactory. The 5-year actuarial control of tumors in the nasopharynx following salvage nasopharyngectomy has been reported to be around 65% and the 5-year disease-free survival rate is around 54% (Fee et al. 2002; Wei 2003).

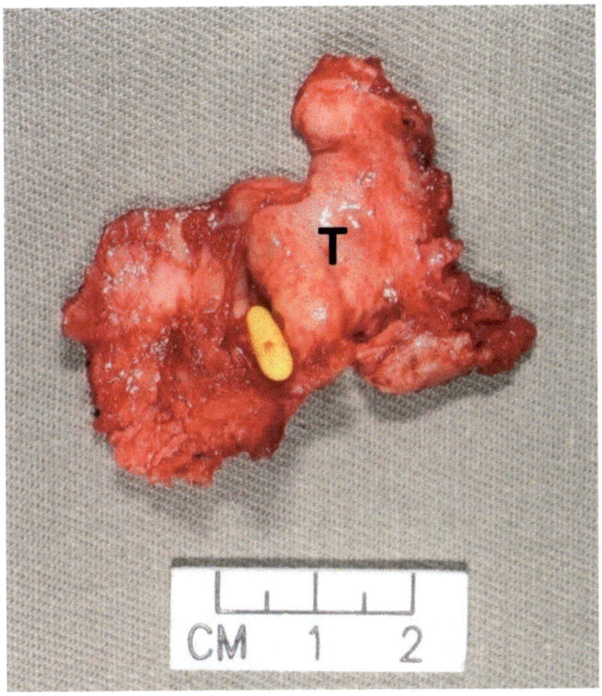

Fig. 20.19. The resected nasopharynx with the yellow tube marking the right Eustachian tube opening. The tumor (T) is resected with margin

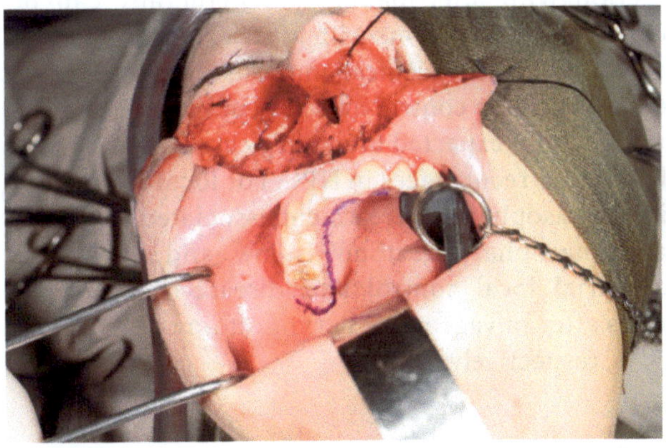

Fig. 20.20. The incision on the hard palate is modified to be a curved one, along the inner border of the upper alveolus

20.5 Summary

Local and/or regional recurrence after definitive treatment of NPC is a major concern of treatment failure. Although combined chemotherapy and reirradiation could be considered to treat the recurrent lesions in both neck and nasopharynx, a second

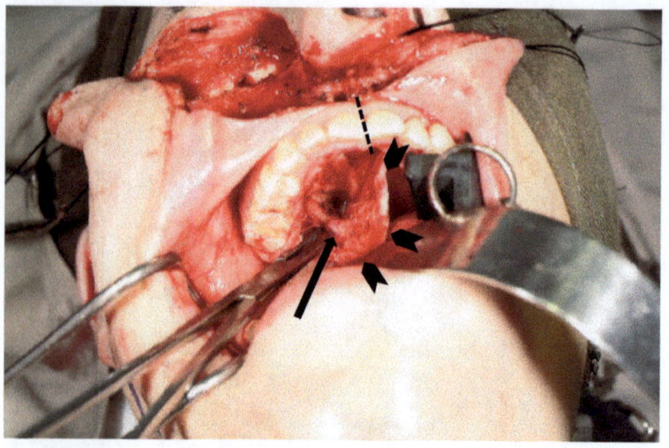

Fig. 20.21. The mucoperiosteum over the hard palate is lifted as a flap (*arrow heads*) after the division of the greater palatine vessel (*arrow*). Then the osteotomy between the two incisors (*dotted line*) will not be in the same plane as incision of the soft tissue

course of radiation therapy may be associated with significant treatment-induced complications.

Surgical salvage is a valid treatment option for nasopharyngeal cancer patients who experience local/regional recurrences. Radical neck dissection is a commonly utilized modality for patients with more limited neck recurrence, and radical neck dissection with after-loading brachytherapy can be considered for patients with more extensive disease, especially when surgical margins are dubious. A 66% of disease control and 37% of overall survival rates can be expected after surgical salvage for isolated neck recurrences in NPC. For local recurrence in the nasopharynx, treatment associated mortality after nasopharyngectomy is low, and the 5-year actuarial local control and disease-free survival rates after salvage nasopharyngectomy were 65 and 54%, respectively.

References

Chen MK, Lai JC, Chang CC, Liu MT (2007) Minimally invasive endoscopic nasopharyngectomy in the treatment of recurrent T1 - 2a nasopharyngeal carcinoma. Laryngoscope 117:894–896

Choy D, Sham JS, Wei WI, Ho CM, Wu PM (1993) Transpalatal insertion of radioactive gold grain for the treatment of persistent and recurrent nasopharyngeal carcinoma. Int J Radiat Oncol Biol Phys 25:505–512

Chua DT, Sham JS, Wei WI, et al (2001) The predictive value of the 1997 American Joint Committee on Cancer stage classification in determining failure patterns in nasopharyngeal carcinoma. Cancer 92:2854–2855

Fee WE Jr, Moir MS, Choi EC, Goffinet D (2002) Nasopharyngectomy for recurrent nasopharyngeal cancer: a 2- to 17-year follow-up. Arch Otolaryngol Head Neck Surg 128: 280–284

Fee WE Jr, Roberson JB Jr, Goffinet DR (1991) Long-term survival after surgical resection for recurrent nasopharyngeal cancer after radiotherapy failure. Arch Otolaryngol Head Neck Surg 117:1233–1236

Fisch U (1983) The infratemporal fossa approach for nasopharyngeal tumors. Laryngoscope 93:36–44

Harrison LB, Weissber JB (1987) A technique for interstitial nasopharyngeal brachytherapy. Int J Radiat Oncol Biol Phys 13:451–453

Hung SC, Lui LT, Lynn TC (1985) Nasopharyngeal cancer: study III. A review of 1206 patients treated with combined modalities. Int J Radiat Oncol Biol Phys 11:1789–1793

Kam MK, Chau RM, Suen J, et al (2003) Intensity-modulated radiotherapy in nasopharyngeal carcinoma: dosimetric advantage over conventional plane and feasibility of dose escalation. Int J Radiat Oncol Biol Phys 56:145–157

Kwong DL, Wei WI, Cheng AC, Choy DT, Lo AT, Wu PM, Sham JS (2001) Long term results of radioactive gold grain implantation for the treatment of persistent and recurrent nasopharyngeal carcinoma. Cancer 91:1105–1113

Lee AW, Foo W, Law SC, et al (1997) Nasopharyngeal carcinoma: presenting symptoms and duration before diagnosis. Hong Kong Med J 3:355–361

Lee AW, Lau WH, Tung SY, et al (2005) Preliminary results of a randomized study on therapeutic gain by concurrent chemotherapy for regionally-advanced nasopharyngeal carcinoma: NPC-9901 Trial by the Hong Kong Nasopharyngeal Cancer Study Group. J Clin Oncol 23:6966–6975

Lee AW, Law SC, Foo W, Poon YF, Cheung FK, Chan DK, Tung SY, Thaw M, Ho JH (1993) Retrospective analysis of patients with nasopharyngeal carcinoma treated during 1976–1985: survival after local recurrence. Int J Radiat Oncol Biol Phys 26:773–782

Lee AW, Sham JS, Poon YF, Ho JH (1989) Treatment of stage I nasopharyngeal carcinoma: analysis of the patterns of relapse and the results of withholding elective neck irradiation. Int J Radiat Oncol Biol Phys 17:1183–1190

Law SC, Lam WK, Ng MF, Au SK, Mak WT, Lau WH (2002) Reirradiation of nasopharyngeal carcinoma with intracavitary mold brachytherapy: an effective means of local salvage. Int J Radiat Oncol Biol Phys 54:1095–1113

Lui MT, Hsieh CY, Chang TH, et al (2003) Prognostic factors affecting the outcome of nasopharyngeal carcinoma. Jpn J Clin Oncol 33:501–508

Morton RP, Liavaag PG, McLean M, Freeman JL (1996) Transcervico-mandibulo-palatal approach for surgical salvage of recurrent nasopharyngeal cancer. Head Neck 18:352–358

Ng RW, Wei WI (2005) Elimination of palatal fistula after the maxillary swing procedure. Head Neck 27:608–612

Ng RW, Wei WI (2006) Quality of life of patients with recurrent nasopharyngeal carcinoma treated with nasopharyngectomy using the maxillary swing approach. Arch Otolaryngol Head Neck Surg 132:309–316

Palazzi M, Guzzo M, Bossi P, et al (2004) Regionally advanced nasopharyngeal carcinoma: long term outcome after sequential cheomtherpy and radiotherapy. Tumori 90:60–65

Robbins KT, Medina JE, Wolfe GT, Levine PA, Sessions RB, Pruet CW (1991) Standardizing neck dissection terminology: official report of the Academy's Committee for Head and Neck Surgery and Oncology. Arch Otolaryngol Head Neck Surg 117:601–605

Shah JP, Strong E, Spiro RH, Vikram B (1981) Surgical grand rounds: neck dissection: current status and future possibilities. Clin Bull 11:25–33

Sham JS, Choy D (1991) Nasopharyngeal carcinoma: treatment of neck node recurrence by radiotherapy. Australas Radiol 35:370–373

Sham JS, Choy D, Wei WI (1990) Nasopharyngeal carcinoma: orderly neck node spread. Int J Radiat Oncol Biol Phys 19:929–933

Wang CC, Busse J, Gitterman M (1975) A simple afterloading applicator for intracavitary irradiation of carcinoma of the nasopharynx. Radiology 115:737–738

Wei WI, Lam KH, Ho CM, et al (1990a) Efficacy of radical neck dissection for the control of cervical metastasis after radiotherapy for nasopharyngeal carcinoma. Am J Surg 160:439–442

Wei WI, Sham JS, Choy D, Ho CM, Lam KH (1990b) Split-palate approach for gold grain implantation in nasopharyngeal carcinoma. Arch Otolaryngol Head Neck Surg 116: 578–582

Wei WI, Lam KH, Sham JS (1991) New approach to the nasopharynx: the maxillary swing approach. Head Neck 13:200–207

Wei WI (2004) Salvage neck dissection after radiation and/or chemotherapy. Oper Tech Otolaryngol 15:269–272

Wei WI, Ho CM, Wong MP, Ng WF, Lau SK, Lam KH (1992) Pathological basis of surgery in the management of postradiotherapy cervical metastasis in nasopharyngeal carcinoma. Arch Otolaryngol Head Neck Surg 118:923–929

Wei WI (2001) Nasopharyngeal cancer: current status of management. Arch Otolaryngol Head Neck Surg 127:766–769

Wei WI, Ho WK, Cheng AC, Wu X, Li GK, Nicholls J, Yuen PW, Sham JS (2001) Management of extensive cervical nodal metastasis in nasopharyngeal carcinoma after radiotherapy: a clinicopathological study. Arch Otolaryngol Head Neck Surg 127:1457–1462

Wei WI (2003) Cancer of the nasopharynx: functional surgical salvage. World J Surg 27:844–848

Yan RF, Hong RL, Tzen KY, et al (2005) Whole body 18F-FDG PET in recurrent or metastatic nasopharyngeal carcinoma. J Nucl Med 46:770–774

Systemic Treatment for Incurable Recurrent and/or Metastatic Nasopharyngeal Carcinoma

21

Ye Guo and Bonnie S. Glisson

CONTENTS

Ye Guo, MD
Department of Medical Oncology, Fudan University Shanghai Cancer Center, 270 Dong An Road, Shanghai 200032, P.R. China
Bonnie S. Glisson, MD
Thoracic/Head & Neck Medical Oncology Department, Unit 432, UTMD Anderson Cancer Center, Houston, TX 77230-1402, USA

21.1 Introduction

Nasopharyngeal carcinoma (NPC) is poorly or undifferentiated in the vast majority of cases (70%–99% depending on geographic area). This characteristic histology combined with the abundant lymphatic network in its anatomic site of origin is most likely the major factors contributing to the higher rate of regional and distant metastasis when compared with squamous carcinoma arising in other mucosal sites of the head and neck (SCCHN).

Approximately, 20%–30% of patients with locoregional NPC will develop locoregional or distant recurrences, respectively, after definitive treatment using conventional radiation therapy (Lin et al. 2003; Lee et al. 2003). Risk of distant metastasis specifically is directly correlated with nodal stage and level. The incorporation of chemoradiation and, more recently, intensity-modulated radiation therapy (IMRT) in treatment have resulted in high locoregional control rates for locally advanced NPC, such that the major pattern of recurrence is now distant in nature (Kam et al. 2004; Wee et al. 2005).

The relatively unique chemosensitivity of NPC was first noted in the late-1970s when chemotherapy was first studied in patients with recurrent and/or metastatic SCCHN. Distinguished by higher rates of response, longer progression-free and overall survival, compared with tumors of other primary sites, the NPC data were initially subsumed in reports with mixed patient populations. Since then, patients with metastatic NPC have largely been segregated into separate trials or treated outside a study setting. However, no randomized trials have been reported in this particular setting and, thus, comparative effectiveness of various regimens and approaches is only estimated by comparing the results of single arm phase II trials. The data extant suggests that chemotherapy, while palliative in effect for the vast majority of patients, can result in long-term disease control in a small percentage of patients, with or without the incorporation of radiation to involved sites. Beyond conventional chemotherapy, molecularly targeted therapy and Epstein–Barr virus (EBV)-based immunotherapy approaches hold promise. However, published experience is minimal currently. Herein, we will review the currently available options for systemic treatment of incurable recurrent and/or metastatic NPC and identify potential avenues for future research.

21.2 Chemotherapy

On the basis of extrapolation from studies with neoadjuvant and concurrent regimens for NPC as well as data from studies in SCCHN of other primary sites, platin-based therapy has been most commonly investigated and utilized in practice for patients with incurable recurrent or metastatic NPC. While there have been no direct comparisons of various regimens, overall experience suggests that the single agent response rates of cisplatin (28%) and carboplatin (22%) (Chan et al. 2002) are augmented by a second active drug, but that no major incremental increase in response is obtained by adding a third or fourth drug. In addition, these latter regimens have been quite toxic and are not commonly utilized. The most commonly used regimens include a platin with 5-fluorouracil (5-FU) or a taxane.

21.2.1 Platin and Fluoropyrimidines

The preclinical and clinical evidence base for the efficacy of cisplatin and 5-FU (PF regimen) in the treatment of SCCHN and curative-intent treatment of locoregional NCP is substantial. Perhaps because it is commonly used during definitive therapy, its study in the setting of recurrent/metastatic NPC is not exhaustive. In a small phase II study conducted in Singapore (Au and Ang 1994), 24 chemotherapy-naïve patients were treated with cisplatin at 100 mg/m^2, and 5-FU 1,000 mg/m^2 daily by continuous infusion days 1–5, every 3 weeks. Responses were observed in 16/24 (66%); three patients responded completely. Median progression-free and overall survival times were 8 and 11 months, respectively. There was no treatment-related mortality, and the most common grade 3–4 toxicity was granulocytopenia, occurring in 10/24 (41%) patients. With the goal of reducing toxicity related to cisplatin, carboplatin was combined with 5-FU and studied in a larger trial of 42 patients (Yeo et al. 1996). Although the overall response rate was lower at 38%, the complete response rate of 17% and median survival of 12 months was similar to that obtained in the smaller trial with cisplatin. Notably, in a randomized trial of patients with newly diagnosed NPC, equivalent efficacy and reduced toxicity was observed with concurrent carboplatin and adjuvant carboplatin/5-FU, compared with cisplatin (Chitapanarux et al. 2007). Certainly, in a palliative-intent setting, it seems reasonable to consider use of carboplatin, especially in patients who have had substantial cisplatin exposure during curative-intent therapy and who may have persistent renal or neurologic toxicity, uncontrolled nausea/vomiting, or hearing loss.

The oral fluoropyrimidine, capecitabine was given as monotherapy in a phase II trial of 49 patients with recurrent/metastatic NPC with partial and complete response rates of 31% and 6%, respectively (Chua et al. 2008). Median progression-free and overall survival rates were 5 and 14 months, respectively. Hand-foot syndrome (HFS), seen in 86% of patients, was severe grade in 25%. This toxicity was especially severe at a dose of 1.25 g/m^2 bid for 14 days in the first 37 patients. A dose reduction to 1 g/m^2 given in the same schedule reduced the incidence and severity of HFS in the final 12 patients. Capecitabine and cisplatin were combined in a prospective trial of 48 patients with similar efficacy outcomes as PF in a recent phase II trial of patients with metastatic disease (Li et al. 2008). Li et al. reported an overall response rate of 62% (30/48) and median progression-free and overall survival rates of 7.7 and 13.3 months, respectively. Toxicity profile was similar to PF and judged manageable with neutropenia (15%), the only grade 3–4 effect observed in greater than 10% of patients. Severe grade HFS was seen in 4% of patients with capecitabine dose 1 gm/m^2 bid for 14 days. The convenience of oral administration and the avoidance of prolonged intravenous infusion make this an attractive option for patients who have a reasonable progression-free interval following prior fluoropyrimidine therapy.

21.2.2 Platin-Based Multidrug Regimens

Because NPC is chemosensitive, multiple active agents have been identified and studied further in platin-based regimens.

The addition of bleomycin, a drug devoid of hematologic toxicity, to PF was studied by a European and an Asian group with contrasting results (Boussen et al. 1991; Su et al. 1993). Boussen et al. observed an overall response rate of 79% (19% complete). However, both the overall and complete response rates were much lower in the trial by Su et al. at 40 and 3%, respectively. Further, despite a relatively low rate of grade 4 granulocytopenia (36%), 3/24 (12%) patients in the latter trial died due to sepsis. Toxic deaths were not observed in the European trial. Survival data were not reported in either study.

Anthracyclines, including doxorubin and epirubicin, and alkylating agents, such as cyclophosphamide and ifosfamide, have also been studied in NPC. Experience with an intense 5-drug regimen including cyclophosphamide, doxorubicin, cisplatin, methotrexate, and bleomycin (CAPABLE) in a phase I–II trial was reported by Siu et al. (1998). In the subset of patients with measurable persistent or recurrent locoregional disease, 7/17 (41%) responded; in the case of metastatic disease, responses were observed in 35/44 (80%). Despite promising survival rates of 16 and 14 months, respectively, in these two groups, the regimen has not been studied further due to excessive toxicity from myelosuppression, mucositis, and reactivation of hepatitis B, resulting in an 8% toxic death rate.

Similar results were obtained with the addition of epirubicin to either PF-bleomycin (Taamma et al. 1999) or PF-mitomycin (Hasbini et al. 1999) in trials of 26 and 44 patients, respectively, with incurable disease. Overall response rates of 78% and 52% were balanced by 6% and 9% toxic death rates. Although a percentage of patients in both trials had long-term disease control, these regimens were judged not feasible for common use.

21.2.3 Taxane-Based Regimens

The taxanes, including paclitaxel and docetaxel, are highly effective in the treatment of a number of solid tumors, including HNSCC where they are the most active single agents yet identified. They have both been studied in recurrent/metastatic NPC and the results of these investigations are detailed in Table 21.1. Only paclitaxel has been studied as monotherapy

Table 21.1. Studies using platin and taxane

Study	Schedule	ORR (%)	CR (%)	Median survival (months)
Yeo et al. (1998)	Paclitaxel 135 mg/m^2 day 1 Carboplatin AUC 6 day 1 Cycles repeated every 3 weeks	16/27 (59)	3/27 (11)	13.9
Tan et al. (1999)	Paclitaxel 175 mg/m^2 day 1 Carboplatin AUC 6 day 1 Cycles repeated every 3 weeks	24/32 (75)	1/32 (3)	12
Airoldi et al. (2002)	Paclitaxel 175 mg/m^2 day 1 Carboplatin AUC 5.5 day 1 Cycles repeated every 3 weeks	3/12 (25)	0/12 (0)	9.5
McCarthy et al. (2002)	Docetaxel 75 mg/m^2 day 1 Cisplatin 75 mg/m^2 day 1 Cycles repeated every 3 weeks	2/9 (22)	0/9 (0)	NR
Chua et al. (2005)	Docetaxel 60–75 mg/m^2 day 1 Cisplatin 60–75 mg/m^2 day 1 Cycles repeated every 3 weeks	12/19 (62)	1/19 (6)	12.4

NR not reported

resulting in responses in 5/24 (22%) patients and median response duration of 7.5 months (Au et al. 1998). Because of the problematic overlapping neurotoxicity with cisplatin, paclitaxel has been studied in combination with carboplatin in two trials in the front-line recurrent setting (Yeo et al. 1998; Tan et al. 1999). Rates of response and median survival were similar to that obtained with PF. Severe grade neutropenia observed in approximately 30% of patients was associated with a 28% incidence of neutropenic fever and one toxic death in the trial by Tan et al. (1999). This can be contrasted with a 3% rate of neutropenic fever observed by Yeo et al. (1998) with a lower dose of paclitaxel.

Activity in refractory patients was demonstrated in a small study performed by Airoldi et al. (2002). A response rate of 33% and median survival of 9.5 months were observed in 12 patients treated with paclitaxel and carboplatin in the third line setting.

For patients who have cisplatin-refractory disease, placlitaxel can be considered; the contribution of carboplatin to response is questionable in that setting.

Docetaxel is a semi-synthetic taxane that demonstrated more potent antineoplastic effect than paclitaxel in preclinical models. Its single agent activity in NPC is not documented to our knowledge. It was initially studied in patients with recurrent/metastatic NPC in combination with cisplatin by McCarthy et al. (2002). The trial was closed after accrual of nine patients when responses had been observed in only two patients. Grade 3–4 neutropenia was seen in all nine patients with three episodes of febrile neutropenia. Toxicity was stated to be manageable. Notably 8 of 9 patients were Asian. Similar myelosuppressive toxicity was observed with the same regimen in the study by Chua et al. in Chinese patients (Chua et al. 2005). In the initial 15 patients treated at 75 mg/m^2 for both drugs, febrile neutropenia occurred in 42% of patients and resulted in two toxic deaths. The second cohort of four patients was treated with dose reduction to 60 mg/m^2 with no instances of febrile neutropenia. Response rates and survival in this small trial were again reminiscent of rates with PF or paclitaxel and carboplatin. This experience with docetaxel in Asian patients with NPC is similar to experience with the drug in Asian patients with other solid tumors, such as non-small cell lung cancer, suggesting pharmacogenomic differences in drug disposition between Asians and the predominantly Caucasian population in the North America or Western Europe. In these groups, it is generally well tolerated at 75 mg/m^2 as monotherapy or in combination with a platin. This held true in a trial with docetaxel 75 mg/m^2 and carboplatin at an area under the curve (AUC) of 6 as neoadjuvant therapy for patients with advanced N stage NPC treated in North America (Johnson et al. 2004). In this trial, the incidence of febrile neutropenia was 22% and there were no toxic deaths.

These data in total suggest that a taxane/platin combination is a reasonable front-line therapy for incurable NPC. The regimen has definite advantages logistically when compared with P5FU, and is devoid of the mucosal toxicity and HFS of the fluoropyrimidines. Because many patients with recurrent disease will have had substantial exposure to cisplatin, carboplatin can be substituted and is preferred with pacliltaxel due to neurotoxicity. Docetaxel, which can be combined with either cisplatin or carboplatin, should be dosed at no greater than 60 mg/m^2 in Asian patients, especially if marrow growth factor support is not given. In view of roughly similar efficacy outcomes to platins combined with either a fluoropyrimidine or a taxane, it is unlikely that a randomized trial of these two approaches in the recurrent/metastatic setting will ever be undertaken.

21.2.4 Gemcitabine-Based Regimens

Gemcitabine is an antimetabolite with broad-spectrum antineoplastic activity. Although gemcitabine has not been intensively studied in SCCHN of other primary mucosal sites, it is an active drug in the treatment of NPC as reflected by the monotherapy trials in Table 21.2 (Foo et al. 2002; Ma et al. 2002; Zhang et al. 2008). The efficacy of gemcitabine/cisplatin is similar to the other platin-based doublets described above with a very reasonable safety profile (Ma et al. 2002; Ngan et al. 2002; Jiang et al. 2005). The majority of patients in all of these trials had been previously exposed to cisplatin with or without 5-FU, most commonly during definitive-intent treatment, and time to progression from prior chemotherapy and lines of prior treatment in the various trials is heterogeneous. In the trial reported by Wang, patients were required to have progressed while receiving cisplatin and thus the efficacy of gemcitabine/vinorelbine in that setting is notable (Wang et al. 2006).

The triplet regimen of gemcitabine, paclitaxel, and carboplatin followed by maintenance with 5-FU and leucovorin produced a high response rate and prolonged survival in patients who were either chemotherapy-naïve or had a minimum 6-month

Table 21.2. Studies with gemcitabine

Study	Schedule	ORR (%)	CR (%)	Median survival (MS)
Foo et al. (2002)	Gemcitabine 1,250 mg/m² days 1 and 8 q3 weeks	20/52 (38)	2/52 (4)	NR
Ma et al. (2002)	Gemcitabine1,000 mg/m² days 1,8,15 q3 weeks	6/18 (34)	1/18 (6)	NR (1 year 48%)
Zhang et al. (2008)	Gemcitabine 1,0000 mg/m² days 1, 8, 15 Cycles repeated every 4 weeks	4,414/32 (44)	0/32 (0)	16 (1 year 67%)
Ma et al. (2002)	Gemcitabine 1,000 mg/m² days 1,8,15 Cisplatin 70 mg/m² day 1 q3 weeks	9/14 (64)	2/14 (14)	NR (1 year 69%)
Ngan et al. (2002)	Gemcitabine 1,000 mg/m² days 1, 8, 15 Cisplatin 50 mg/m² days 1, 8 Cycles repeated every 4 weeks	32/44 (73)	9/44 (20)	NR (1 year 62%)
Jiang et al. (2005)	Gemcitabine 1,200 mg/m² days 1,8 Cisplatin 30 mg/m² days 1–3 q3 weeks	13/14 (93)	5/14 (21)	10.2 (1 year 47%)
Wang et al. (2006)	Gemcitabine 1,000 mg/m² days 1, 8 Vinorelbine 20 mg/m² days 1, 8 Cycles repeated every 3 weeks	14/39 (36)	1/39 (3)	11.9 (1 year 46%)
Leong et al. (2005)	Gemcitabine 1,250 mg/m² days 1, 8 Paclitaxel 70 mg/m² days 1, 8 Carboplatin AUC 5 Cycles repeated every 3 weeks (maximum 6) Maintenance 5-FU450 mg/m² and leucovorin 30 mg/m² weekly	24/28 (78)	3/28 (11)	22 (1 year 83%)

NR not reported

progression-free interval from chemotherapy given during curative-intent treatment (Leong et al. 2005) (Table 21.2). The toxicity of this triplet regimen was pronounced. Dose reduction and omissions were required in the majority of patients largely due to the high rate of grade 3/4 neutropenia (79%). Moreover, 42% of patients experienced grade 3/4 anemia and thrombocytopenia. Although the results are promising, clearly this was a highly selected group of patients. Further, the contribution of the maintenance therapy cannot be defined.

Gemcitabine clearly has activity in NPC; perhaps one of the greatest advantages over the taxanes and fluoropyrimidines is its therapeutic index. When combined with cisplatin, efficacy is similar to other platin-based doublets. Although the multidrug regimen studied by Leong et al. is of interest, its toxicity is reminiscent of the older multidrug regimens discussed above. The efficacy outcomes should be confirmed in additional studies.

21.2.5 Irinotecan

There is one published report on irinotecan for recurrent/metastatic NPC (Poon et al. 2005). Twenty-eight patients with metastatic disease that progressed within 3 months of platin or taxane-based therapy were treated with up to six cycles of irinotecan (100 mg/m² on days 1, 8, and 15, every 4 weeks). The response rate was 14% (4/28) with duration of response ranging from 5.6 to 12.2 months. Median follow-up was short at 7.5 months when the data were reported. Median progression-free survival of 3.9 months was observed. The median overall survival of

11.4 months is in question owing to short follow-up. Although response rate was low in this refractory population, responses were durable and irinotecan could be further studied in this setting.

21.2.6 Long-Term Survival

Chemotherapy confers short-term palliative benefit for the majority of patients with metastatic NPC. There is a very small subset of patients, however, who obtain long-term disease control greater than 3–5 years and apparent "cure," most commonly with multimodal treatment. In a series reported by Fandi et al. (2000), the most common site of metastatic disease in long-term survivors was bone followed by lung. Radiation to involved bony sites and surgery, in the case of pulmonary metastases, were frequently utilized in addition to chemotherapy. Radiation can also be applied to aid in control of mediastinal metastases. Teo et al. evaluated prognostic factors in a case series of 289 patients with recurrent/metastatic NPC (Teo et al. 1996). Survival greater than 5 years was observed in four patients, all of whom were <40 years of age and had isolated intrathoracic disease (Teo et al. 1996).

Locoregionally recurrent disease may be amenable to reirradiation with concurrent chemotherapy with prolonged disease control for a subset of patients as discussed elsewhere in this volume. In the series by Teo et al. (1996) mixed locoregional and distant recurrence predicted for poor outcome.

Given the variability in outcome for patients with recurrent/metastatic NPC, prognostic models have been derived. In a series of 172 patients, Toh et al. (2005) were able to validate a previously designed model and segregate patients into three prognostic categories based on independent variables including performance status, hemoglobin, disease-free interval, and metastasis at diagnosis. This model could ultimately prove useful in randomized trials in this setting.

21.3 Targeted Therapy for Recurrent/Metastatic NPC

NPC does commonly express EGFR although intensity of expression is generally lower than in squamous carcinomas of other mucosal sites in the head and neck. Its prognostic relevance has been inconsistent in two reports (Chua et al. 2004; Leong et al. 2004).

Cetuximab, a human–mouse chimeric monoclonal antibody (mAb), directed against the ligand-binding domain of EGFR was found to have single agent activity in vitro in 2/4 NPC cell lines. Both cisplatin and paclitaxel were additive to the antiproliferative effect only in the two sensitive cell lines (Sung et al. 2005).

Cetuximab and carboplatin were combined in 60 heavily pretreated platin-exposed patients (Chan et al. 2005). Cetuximab was administered at a loading dose of 400 mg/m^2 followed by weekly doses of 250 mg/m^2. Carboplatin AUC 5 was administered every 3 weeks up to a maximum of eight cycles. Although the treatment was well tolerated, the response rate was only 12%, most likely reflecting single-agent effects of cetixumab in this chemotherapy-refractory population. Moreover, the median progression-free and overall survival was disappointing at only 81 and 233 days. However, it is notable that the response rate in this trial is similar to that obtained with cetuximab in patients with refractory SCCHN and responses, though they occurred infrequently, were durable with median time to progression 5.8 months for responding patients. The EGFR tyrosine kinase inhibitor gefitinib had no activity in 19 patients with recurrent/metastatic NPC, ruling out a response rate of interest (Chua et al. 2008). There is no standard role as of now for EGFR inhibitors in the treatment of NPC.

21.4 Immunotherapy

EBV is uniformly detected in patients with undifferentiated and poorly-differentiated NPC and high-plasma viral DNA load after treatment has been associated with poor prognosis (Chan et al. 2002; Lin et al. 2004). There is strong evidence that cytotoxic T lymphocyte (CTL)-based immunotherapy is effective in post-transplant lymphoproliferative disorders, which is also EBV-associated. Therefore, EBV-based immunotherapy approaches are under active investigation, both in preclinical models and in clinical trials. Among these approaches, adoptive immunotherapy with autologous EBV-specific CTLs has been studied most and appears promising in limited experience. The experience with 20 patients enrolled in two pilot studies of adoptive immunotherapy have been reported (Straathof et al. 2005; Comoli et al. 2005). Both studies involved ex vivo expansion of EBV-specific CTLs through stimulation with EBV-transformed lymphoblastoid cell lines. Combining data from the two trials, infusion of CTLs resulted in two complete and three partial responses in a total of 16 patients with measureable disease, with response duration of 3–23 months. Moreover, two patients with stable disease were progression-free for 14 and 15 months. The only toxicity identified was grade 1–2 inflammatory reaction at tumor sites in three patients. Clearly, this approach is worthy of additional study and these are ongoing. Efficacy may be improved by cytoreducing with chemotherapy prior to CTL infusion and might be best applied to patients at high risk of progression following definitive therapy. Studies to define the optimal approach are also ongoing, selecting for dendritic cells, for example, and defining ways to enhance EBV-specific immunity. Other immunotherapy approaches are also under study (Lin et al. 2002).

21.5 Summary

Cytotoxic chemotherapy remains the treatment of choice for patients with recurrent or metastatic NPC. In the past 5–10 years taxanes and gemcitabine have demonstrated substantial efficacy and have been added to the armamentarium with platinating agents and fluoropyrimidines. At this time, platin-based doublets appear to be generally well tolerated and of palliative benefit. More aggressive multidrug regimens have been poorly tolerated and are not recommended outside of a trial setting. Monotherapy with a new class of agent can be considered as second- or third-line therapy in patients with retained performance status. Randomized clinical trials for patients with incurable NPC are needed and should stratify based on known prognostic factors, considering the heterogeneity in the population. Targeted therapy in NPC is to a great extent uncharted territory, and clinical trials, based on sound preclinical rationale, are clearly needed. Given the near universal association with EBV, viral-based adoptive immunotherapy is attractive and limited experience suggests promise and lack of significant toxicity. This approach is the subject of ongoing and planned investigation. However, current approaches are quite expensive and require a high level of technical expertise; this is prohibitive to broad clinical application or even large-scale clinical trials. Development of an international consortium at centers of excellence may help overcome these obstacles to progress.

References

Airoldi M, Pedani F, Marchionatti S, et al (2002) Carboplatin plus taxol is an effective third-line regimen in recurrent undifferentiated nasopharyngeal carcinoma. Tumori 88(4): 273–276

Au E, Ang PT (1994) hase II trial of 5-fluorouracil and cisplatinum in recurrent or metastatic nasopharyngeal carcinoma. Ann Oncol 5(1):87–89

Au E, Tan EH, Ang PT (1998) Activity of paclitaxel by three-hour infustion in Asian patients with metastatic undifferentiated nasopharyngeal cancer. Ann Oncol 9:327–329

Boussen H, Cvitkovic E, Wendling JL, et al (1991) Chemotherapy of metastatic and/or recurrent undifferentiated nasopharyngeal carcinoma with cisplatin, bleomycin, and fluorouracil. J Clin Oncol 9(9):1675–1681

Chan ATC, Teo PML, Johnson PJ (2002) Nasopharyngeal carcinoma. Ann Oncol 13(7):1007–1015

Chan AT, Hsu MM, Goh BC, et al (2005) Multicenter, phase II study of cetuximab in combination with carboplatin in patients with recurrent or metastatic nasopharyngeal carcinoma. J Clin Oncol 23(15):3568–3576

Chan AT, Lo YM, Zee B, et al (2002) Plasma Epstein–Barr virus DNA and residual disease after radiotherapy for undifferentiated nasopharyngeal carcinoma. J Natl Cancer Inst 94(21):1614–1619

Chitapanarux I, Lorvidhaya V, Kamnerdsupaphon P, et al (2007) Chemoradiation comparing cisplatin versus carboplatin in locally advanced nasopharyngeal cancer: randomized, non-inferiority, open trial. Eur J Cancer 43: 1399–1406

Chua DT, Nicholls JM, Sham JS, et al (2004) Prognostic value of epidermal growth factor receptor expression in patients with advanced stage nasopharyngeal carcinoma treated with induction chemotherapy and radiotherapy. Int J Radiat Oncol Biol Phys 59(1):11–20

Chua DT, Sham JS, Au GK (2005) A phase II study of docetaxel and cisplatin as first-line chemotherapy in patients with metastatic nasopharyngeal carcinoma. Oral Oncol 41: 589–595

Chua DT, Wei WI, Wong MP, et al (2008) Phase II study of gefitinib for the treatment of recurrent and metastatic nasopharyngeal carcinoma. Head Neck 30(7):863–867

Chua D, Wei WI, Sham JS, et al (2008) Capecitabine monotherapy for recurrent and metastatic nasopharyngeal cancer. Jpn J Clin Oncol 38(4):244–249

Comoli P, Pedrazzoli P, Maccario R, et al (2005) Cell therapy of stage IV nasopharyngeal carcinoma with autologous Epstein–Barr virus-targeted cytotoxic T lymphocytes. J Clin Oncol 23:8942–8949

Fandi A, bachouchi M, Azli N, et al (2000) Long-term disease-free survivors in metastatic undifferentiated carcinoma of nasopharyngeal type. J Clin Oncol 18:1324–1330

Foo KF, Tan EH, Leong SS, et al (2002) Gemcitabine in metastatic nasopharyngeal carcinoma of the undifferentiated type. Ann Oncol 13(1):150–156

Hasbini A, Mahjoubi R, Fandi A, et al (1999) Phase II trial combining mitomycin with 5-fluorouracil, epirubicin, and cisplatin in recurrent and metastatic undifferentiated carcinoma of nasopharyngeal type. Ann Oncol 10(4):421–425
Jiang Y, Wei WI, Luo F, et al (2005) Gemcitabine and cisplatin in advanced nasopharyngeal carcinoma: a pilot study. Cancer Invest 23(2):123–128
Johnson FM, Garden A, Palmer JL, et al (2004) A phase II study of docetaxel and carboplatin as neoadjuvant therapy for nasopharyngeal carcinoma with early T status and advanced N status.Cancer 100:991–998
Kam MK, Teo PM, Chau RM, et al (2004) Treatment of nasopharyngeal carcinoma with intensity-modulated radiotherapy: the Hong Kong experience. Int J Radiat Oncol Biol Phys 60(5):1440–1450
Lee AW, Foo W, Mang O, et al (2003) Changing epidemiology of nasopharyngeal carcinoma in Hong Kong over a 20-year period (1980–99): an encouraging reduction in both incidence and mortality. Int J Cancer 103(5):680–685
Leong JL, Lok KS, Putti TC, et al (2004) Epidermal growth factor receptor in undifferentiated carcinoma of the nasopharynx. Laryngoscope 114(1):153–157
Leong SS, Wee J, Tay MH, et al (2005) Paclitaxel, carboplatin, and gemcitabine in metastatic nasopharyngeal carcinoma: a phase II trial using a triplet combination. Cancer 103(3): 569–575
Li YH, Wang FH, Jiang WQ, et al (2008) Phase II study of capecitabine and cisplatin combination as first-line chemotherapy in Chinese patients with metastatic nasopharyngeal carcinoma. Cancer Chemother Pharmacol 62(3):539–544
Lin CL, Lo WF, Lee TH, et al (2002) Immunization with Epstein–Barr Virus peptide-pulsed dendritic cells induces functional CD8 + T-cell immunity and may lead to tumor regression in patients with EBV-positive nasopharyngeal carcinoma. Cancer Res 62(23):6952–6958
Lin JC, Jan JS, Hsu CY, et al (2003) Phase III study of concurrent chemoradiotherapy versus radiotherapy alone for advanced nasopharyngeal carcinoma: positive effect on overall and progression-free survival. J Clin Oncol 21(4): 631–637
Lin JC, Wang WY, Chen KY, et al (2004) Quantification of plasma Epstein–Barr virus DNA in patients with advanced nasopharyngeal carcinoma. N Engl J Med 350(24):2461–2470
Ma BB, Tannock IF, Pond GR, et al (2002) Chemotherapy with gemcitabine-containing regimens for locally recurrent or metastatic nasopharyngeal carcinoma. Cancer 95(12):2516–2523
McCarthy J, Tannock I, Degendorfer P, et al (2002) A Phase II trial of docetaxel and cisplatin in patients with recurrent or metastatic nasopharyngeal carcinoma. Oral Oncol 38(7):686
Ngan RK, Yiu HH, Lau WH, et al (2002) Combination gemcitabine and cisplatin chemotherapy for metastatic or recurrent nasopharyngeal carcinoma: report of a phase II study. Ann Oncol 13(8):1252–1258
Poon D, Chowbay B, Cheung YB, et al (2005) Phase II study of irinotecan (CPT-11) as salvage therapy for advanced nasopharyngeal carcinoma. Cancer 10(3):576–581
Siu LL, Czaykowski PM, Tannock IF (1998) Phase I/II study of the CAPABLE regimen for patients with poorly differentiated carcinoma of the nasopharynx. J Clin Oncol 16(7):2514–2521
Straathof KC, Bollard CM, Popat U, et al (2005) Treatment of nasopharyngeal carcinoma with Epstein–Barr virus-specific T lymphocytes. Blood 105:1898–1904
Sung FL, Poon TC, Hui EP, et al (2005) Antitumor effect and enhancement of cytotoxic drug activity by cetuximab in nasopharyngeal carcinoma cells. In Vivo 19:237–245
Su WC, Chen TY, Kao RH, et al (1993) Chemotherapy with cisplatin and continuous infusion of 5-fluorouracil and bleomycin for recurrent and metastatic nasopharyngeal carcinoma in Taiwan. Oncology 50(4):205–208
Taamma A, Fandi A, Azli N, Wibault P, et al (1999) Phase II trial of chemotherapy with 5-fluorouracil, bleomycin, epirubicin, and cisplatin for patients with locally advanced, metastatic, or recurrent undifferentiated carcinoma of the nasopharyngeal type. Cancer 86(7):1101–1108
Tan EH, Khoo KS, Wee J, et al (1999) Phase II trial of a paclitaxel and carboplatin combination in Asian patients with metastatic nasopharyngeal carcinoma. Ann Oncol 10(2):235–237
Teo PM, Kwan WH, Lee WY, et al (1996) Prognosticators determining survival subsequent to distant metastasis from nasopharyngeal carcinoma. Cancer 77:2423–2431
Toh CK, Heng D, Ong YK, et al (2005) Validation of a new prognostic index score for disseminated nasopharyngeal carcinoma. Br J Cancer 92(8):1382–1387
Wang CC, Liu TW, Lin CY, et al (2006) Phase II study of gemcitabine plus vinorelbine in the treatment of cisplatin-resistant nasopharyngeal carcinoma. Head Neck 28(1):74–80
Wee J, Tan EH, Tai BC, et al (2005) Randomized trial of radiotherapy versus concurrent chemoradiotherapy followed by adjuvant chemotherapy in patients with American Joint Committee on Cancer/International Union against cancer stage III and IV nasopharyngeal cancer of the endemic variety. J Clin Oncol 23(27):6730–6738
Yeo W, Leung TW, Chan AT, et al (1998) A Phase II study of combination paclitaxel and carboplatin in advanced nasopharyngeal carcinoma. Eur J Cancer 34:2027–2031
Yeo W, Leung TW, Leung SF, et al (1996) Phase II study of the combination of carboplatin and 5-fluorouracil in metastatic nasopharyngeal carcinoma. Cancer Chemother Pharmacol 38(5):466–470
Zhang L, Zhang Y, Huang PY, et al (2008) Phase II clinical study of gemcitabine in the treatment of patients with advanced nasopharyngeal carcinoma after the failure of platinum-based chemotherapy. Cancer Chemother Pharmacol 61:33–38

Long-Term Complications in the Treatment of Nasopharyngeal Carcinoma

22

Simon S. Lo, Jiade J. Lu, and Lin Kong

CONTENTS

Simon S. Lo, MD
Department of Radiation Medicine, Arthur G. James Cancer Hospital, Ohio State University Medical Center, 300 West 10th Avenue, Ste 088A, Columbus, OH 43210, USA
Jiade J. Lu., MD, MBA
Department of Radiation Oncology, National University Cancer Institute, National University Health System, National University of Singapore, 5 Lower Kent Ridge Road, Singapore 119074, Republic of Singapore
Lin Kong, MD
Department of Radiation Oncology, Fudan University, Shanghai Cancer Center, 270 Dong An Road, Shanghai 200032, P.R. China

22.1 Introduction

Radiation therapy is the mainstay therapeutic modality for nasopharyngeal carcinoma (NPC). In the last two decades, advances in the diagnostic and treatment techniques in cancer management have significantly improved prognosis of NPC, including the long-term local and regional disease control as well as patients' overall survival. With definitive radiation therapy for early stage disease and combined chemoradiotherapy for locoregionally advanced disease, the overall survival of NPC patients exceed 80% at 5 years (Wee et al. 2005; Cheng et al. 2000).

However, the advances in the management of NPC and the improved outcome are not without consequences. Although we celebrate the progresses in cancer management, better understanding of treatment-related, long-term complications is imperative. Among all treatment-induced side effects in the management of NPC, late complications including xerostomia, hearing deficit, and soft-tissue fibrosis are commonly observed. Other late complications such as radiation-induced spinal cord myelopathy, brain stem and temporal lobe necrosis, and second primary tumor (SPT), although rare, are usually devastating to patients and are associated with severe impairment of quality of life. Clearly, treatment-induced late complication is an important entity in the management of NPC. This chapter aims to discuss the pathogenesis, diagnosis, prevention, and management of the long-term complications secondary to the treatment of NPC.

22.2 Xerostomia

Saliva is produced by the major and minor salivary glands. The average daily production of saliva of a healthy individual is approximately 1,000–1,500 ml. The three major glands including the parotid, submandibular, and submental glands are responsible for 90% of the total saliva production. The parotid glands account for approximately 80% of the total saliva from major glands. As radiation therapy is the main treatment modality for nasopharyngeal cancer and parotid glands are positioned close to the nasopharynx, dysfunction of the parotid gland is one of the major concerns in NPC treatment.

22.2.1 Pathogenesis of Radiation-Induced Salivary Hypofunction

The serous acinar cells of the parotid glands are very sensitive to ionizing radiation (Stephens et al. 1986), and is affected earlier in the course of radiation therapy when compared with mucous cells (Parsons 1994). Radiation damage of acinar cells in the forms of apoptosis can be observed at low dose of irradiation. Clinically, xerostomia has been reported after merely 2 or 3 fractions of irradiation at conventional dose. Within 1–2 weeks of radiation therapy and a dose of merely 20 Gy or less encompassing the major salivary glands, the salivary output declines by up to 60% (Wescott et al. 1978), thereby making saliva more viscous. However, the mechanism of the high sensitivity of salivary glands in the early phase of radiotherapy with relatively low dose of radiation is not fully understood.

The probability and severity of long-term salivary hypofunction and xerostomia are directly related to the volume and dose of parotid gland irradiated (Liu et al. 1990). Once the mean dose to the parotid glands exceeds 26 Gy, recovery of salivary function is uncommon (Eisbruch et al. 2001). Conventional radiotherapy for NPC usually causes high-dose irradiation to the bilateral parotid glands. With a dose approaching curative dose for NPC, degenerative changes, fibrosis, and/or atrophy of the parotid and/or submandibular glands are nearly universal.

The use of chemotherapy in the treatment of NPC may also cause an increased risk for xerostomia. Certain medications such as 5-FU may have synergistic effect with ionizing irradiation for xerostomia (Kies et al. 2001). However, whether the most commonly used chemotherapy drug in NPC, i.e., cisplatin is significantly associated with xerostomia is largely unknown.

The reduction of saliva reduces the wetting medium for the function of chemoreceptors on the tongue and palate. This hypofunction, together with radiation-induced damage to the taste buds, diminish the stimuli from foods for salivation, and induce a vicious cycle for salivary dysfunction in radiotherapy for head and neck cancer including NPC.

22.2.2 Clinical Manifestations and Diagnosis

As both parotid glands are usually irradiated in conventional radiation therapy for NPC, salivary hypofunction with resultant xerostomia is one of the most common acute and late side effects in the management. Although radiation-induced xerostomia is usually discussed as a late complication, reduction of saliva production usually begins soon after the initiation of radiotherapy, as mentioned above. Approximately 95% of patients treated with conventional radiation therapy for their head and neck malignancies experience xerostomia. Furthermore, more than 70% of the symptoms were reported as moderate or severe (Eisbruch et al. 2001). Xerostomia may result in dry and burning sensation of the tongue, oral mucosa, and throat. Some other commonly observed long-term complications such as infection (particularly oral candidiasis), dental decay,

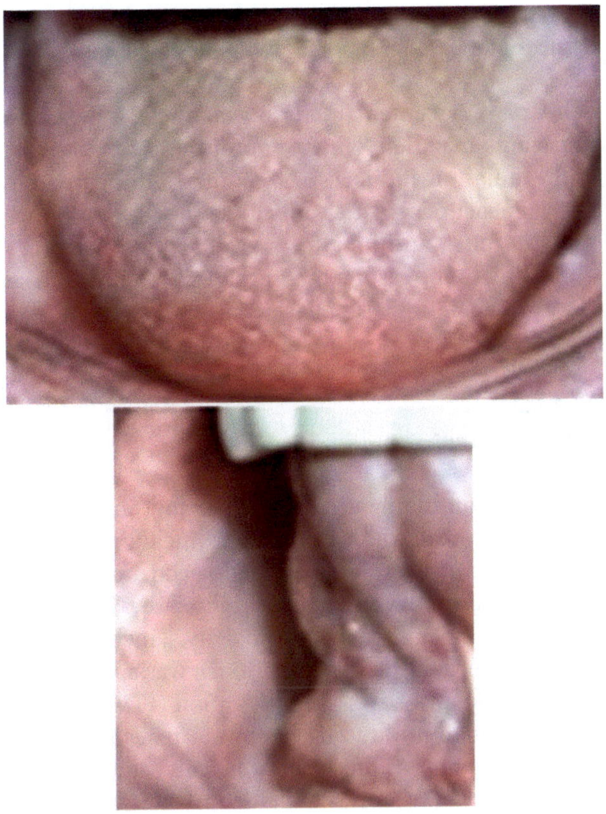

Fig. 22.1. Radiation-induced xerostomia. (Courtesy of Michael Kahn, DDS)

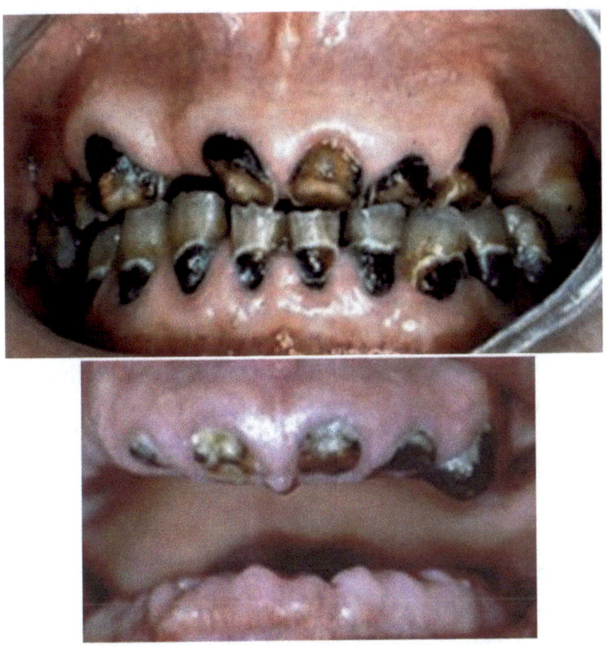

Fig. 22.2. Dental caries secondary to radiation therapy. (Courtesy of Michael Kahn, DDS) (Permission to use picture granted by Dr. Michael Kahn, DDS)

reduction of taste acuity, dysphagia, poor denture fitting, and dysfunction of phonation are also associated, at least in part, with xerostomia (Figs. 22.1 and 22.2).

NPC is a highly curative malignancy, especially in its early stages by radiation therapy and the majority of NPC patients become long-term cancer survivors. The occurrence of moderate to severe xerostomia is nearly universal after convention radiation therapy for NPC (Lee et al. 1992, 2009). As in any other types of squamous cell carcinoma (SCC) of the head and neck treated by radiation therapy, the chronic adverse-effects secondary to radiotherapy affect patients' quality-of-life (Spielman 1990; Harrison et al. 1997; Epstein et al. 1999).

With significant xerostomia and other complications such as mucositis, substantial loss of appetite will lead to reduction in dietary intake. Treatment-induced weight loss in NPC certainly affects patients' quality of life during treatment. In addition, substantial weight loss may cause body contour change that is significant enough to alter the radiation dose distribution, thus adversely affecting the treatment outcome (Wang et al. 2009).

The diagnosis of radiation-induced xerostomia is usually subjective, and the assessment of severity of the symptoms can be achieved by using self-report instruments and visual analog scales. Objective assessment of the severity of xerostomia utilizes parameters such as stimulated and unstimulated salivary flow rates. The scoring criteria for both acute and late salivary gland toxicity advocated by the Radiation Therapy Oncology Group and the European Organization for Research and Treatment of Cancer (RTOG/EORTC) largely depend on subjective measure of xerostomia (Table 22.1 and 22.2) (Cox et al. 1995). The Common Terminology Criteria for Adverse Events v3.0 (CTCAE v3.0) that are used for both acute and late effects of

Table 22.1. RTOG scoring for acute radiation-induced salivary gland morbidity (Nicolatou-Galitis et al. 2003)

Grade	Criteria
0	No change over baseline
1	Mid dryness, slightly thickened saliva, and slightly altered or metallic taste
2	Moderate to complete dryness, thick sticky saliva, and markedly altered taste
3	Not defined for acute xerostomia
4	Acute salivary gland necrosis

Table 22.2. Detal caries secondary to radiation therapy RTOG-EORTC scoring criteria for late radiation-induced salivary gland morbidity (Nicolatou-Galitis et al. 2003)

Grade	Criteria
0	None
1	Slight dryness of mouth with good response to stimulation
2	Moderate dryness of mouth with poor response to stimulation
3	Complete dryness of mouth with no response to stimulation
4	Fibrosis

Table 22.3. CTCAE v3.0 scoring criteria for xerostomia (Koukourakis 2002; Eisbruch et al. 1999)

Grade	Criteria
0	None
1	Symptomatic (dry or thick saliva) without significant dietary alteration; unstimulated saliva flow >0.2 ml/min
2	Symptomatic and significant oral intake alteration (e.g., copious water, other lubricants, diet limited to purees and/or soft, moist foods); unstimulated saliva 0.1–0.2 ml/min
3	Symptoms leading to inability to adequately aliment orally; IV fluids, tube feedings, or TPN indicated; unstimulated saliva <0.1 ml/min

xerostomia combines both subjective and objective findings (Table 22.3) (Trotti et al. 2003).

22.2.3 Management of Radiation-Induced Xerostomia

The substantial adverse effects of treatment-induced xerostomia on the long-term quality of life of NPC patients make its effective management important. A number of therapeutic measures can be used for treating xerostomia. However, as in many other diseases and conditions, the most effective treatment of radiotherapy- associated salivary dysfunction is prevention. In the case of NPC radiation therapy, prevention of salivary damage can be achieved by cytoprotectants and salivary-sparing radiation therapy using more advanced treatment technology.

22.2.3.1 Symptomatic Relief Using Salivary Replacements

Salivary replacement including artificial saliva and lubricants may help with symptom relief in patients with radiation-induced xerostomia. Unfortunately, such a measure provides only ultra short-term symptomatic relief, and its effects are hardly satisfactory according to the results of a randomized clinical trial (Levine et al. 1987; Jellema et al. 2001).

22.2.3.2 Cytoprotectant

The most commonly used cytoprotectant in radiation therapy for head and neck cancers including NPC is amifostine. Amifostine is a broad-spectrum cytoprotectant against adverse effects caused by ionization radiation including nephrotoxicity, myelotoxicity, mucositis, and salivary dysfunction. It was approved by the US Food and Drug Administration (FDA) for preventing radiation-induced xerostomia in head and neck cancer patients. Amifostine is usually administered intravenously (IV) or subcutaneously (SQ) prior to each fraction of radiation. Results from clinical trials have demonstrated that 200 mg/m^2 given IV or 500 mg/m^2 subcutaneously 30–60 min before radiation provide significant improvement in xerostomia in long-term follow-up (Anne et al. 2007; Buntzel et al. 1998; Vacha et al. 2003; Koukourakis et al. 2000). Furthermore, conditions associated with radiation-induced xerostomia such as oral infection and dental caries could also be improved with the use of amifostine (Rudat et al. 2000; Nicolatou-Galitis et al. 2003).

The use of amifostine could be limited by its side effects, which include hypotension, nausea, and vomiting. Hypotension caused by amifostine delivered intravenously could be severe, thus pretreatment hydration is usually required before its use on daily basis (Koukourakis 2002). Amifostine delivered subcutaneously provides similar therapeutic effect but is associated with reduced adverse effects (Anne et al. 2007; Koukourakis et al. 2000).

22.2.3.3 Salivary-Sparing Radiotherapy

The fields used in the conventional radiation therapy for NPC technique usually encompass both parotid and submandibular glands bilaterally. As a result of high-dose irradiation, grade 3 or 4 xerostomia is one of the most commonly observed long-term complications in conventional radiation for NPC (Lee et al. 1992; Lee et al. 2009). The utilization of intensity-modulated radiation therapy (IMRT) allows effective differentiation of dose coverage to the gross, clinical, and planning target volumes vs. organs at risk (OARs). As indicated above, recovery of parotid function is highly unlikely after a mean dose of 26 Gy (Eisbruch et al. 1999).

Experience from United States and Asia unanimously demonstrated that limiting irradiation to the parotid glands could effectively preserve the salivary function, if the mean dose to parotid glands is restricted to 26 Gy or lower. In one of the largest series reported by Lin et al. (2009), grade 3 and 4 xerostomia was not observed during long-term follow-up in their series of more than 300 NPC patients treated using IMRT. In addition, parotid sparing IMRT was not associated with a compromised disease control, and no significant increase of marginal local recurrence was observed. These results paralleled those reported by Lee et al. (2002).

The long-term xerostomia associated quality of life of patients treated using parotid-sparing radiation such as IMRT has also been addressed using a validated quality of life (QoL) instrument. Subjective differences regarding xerostomia-associated symptoms were reported between patients treated using parotid-sparing radiation when compared with those treated with convention radiotherapy for head and neck cancers (Eisbruch et al. 2001, 2003; Malouf et al. 2003; Henson et al. 2001).

22.2.3.4
Medical Treatment of Xerostomia

Effective treatment options for radiation-induced xerostomia is relatively limited. Radiation damage of the exocrine tissue of salivary glands is not reversible once occurred. Therefore, the purpose of medical treatment for xerostomia after NPC radiation therapy is to enhance the function of the remaining salivary function.

Pilocarpine is a US FDA approved muscarinic agonist for treatment of xerostomia in head and neck cancer patients treated with radiation therapy. When indicated, pilocarpine is recommended after the completion of radiation therapy for symptomatic relief. A titrated dosage between 5 and 10 mg administrated orally 3–4 times a day with a maximum daily dose of 30 mg have been shown effective for increasing salivary output and symptomatic reduction (Johnson et al. 1993; LeVeque et al. 1993; Rieke et al. 1995; Hamlar et al. 1996). The use of pilocarpine after IMRT for managing mild to moderate xerostomia has not been thoroughly investigated. However, for those whose dose to parotid glands exceeds the tolerance, and who have developed xerostomia, medical treatment should be considered.

The use of pilocarpine treatment may cause substantial side effects including excessive perspiration, bowel and bladder irritation, and hot sensation. Furthermore, the use of pilocarpine during radiotherapy with an intention to reduce the probability and severity of xerostomia has not been proven effective, thus is not routinely recommended (Jacobs and van der Pas 1996; Warde et al. 2002; Fisher et al. 2003).

22.2.3.5
Management of Infection and Dental Caries

As mentioned above, oral candidiasis is a commonly observed complication of xerostomia during radiation therapy for head and neck cancer. However, the frequency of candidiasis in long-term follow-up after the completion of radiation is not as frequent. In addition, long-term use of antifungal agents is usually not necessary. Once occurred, oral rinse using Nystatin is recommended, and systemic antifungal therapy such as ketaconazole is usually not indicated unless refractory candidiasis is observed. Frequent dental examination and preventative treatment scheduled every 3–6 months and maintenance of oral hygiene are important in management of infection and preventing dental caries. In addition, smoking cessation, low sugar diet, avoiding caffeinated drinks, frequent teeth brushing using soft bristle toothbrush, and antiseptic mouth wash can reduce the risk of infection and dental caries.

22.3
Hearing Deficit

A high dose of radiation is needed to eradicate NPC. However, the proximity of the nasopharynx to the auditory organ subjects NPC patients who receive radiation therapy to risks of conductive and/or sensorineural hearing loss. Patients with NPC may present with unilateral hearing loss from serous otitis media as a result of the blockage of one of the

Eustachian tubes by tumor. Sensorineural hearing loss may be induced by cisplatin-based chemotherapy, which is commonly used as a radiosensitizer.

The reported incidence of hearing deficits after radiotherapy for NPC is variable. In a large series from Hong Kong, the rate of hearing deficit was 19.2% and patients who received accelerated fractionated radiotherapy had a higher rate of hearing deficit (Lee et al. 2009). Other series reported rates of hearing loss exceeding 50% (Yeh et al. 2005; Chan et al. 2009; Chen et al. 2006). The sensorineural hearing loss is typically in the high frequency range and is related to the mean radiation dose exposure to the cochlea and the concurrent cisplatin dose (Chan et al. 2009).

22.3.1 Pathogenesis

Radiation can cause late toxicities in the external ear including skin atrophy, skin ulceration, external canal stenosis, and external otitis (Jereczek-Fossa et al. 2003). Decreased wax secretion can occur as a result of epithelial damage and destruction of sebaceous and apocrine glands. Those changes can potentially lead to some degree of conductive hearing deficit (Jereczek-Fossa et al. 2003).

During head and neck radiation therapy, especially in patients with NPC, the components of the middle ear including the ossicles, the Eustachian tubes, and the middle ear cavity frequently receive a significant radiation dose, sometimes close to tumor dose, especially when conventional radiotherapy techniques are used. Otitis media can occur as a result of tumefaction of the mucosa and blockage within the cartilaginous part or at the pharyngeal orifice of the Eustachian tubes (Jereczek-Fossa et al. 2003). Gas resorption by the middle ear mucosa coupled with compromised mechanism of pressure equilibration during swallowing or yawning can result in reduction of pressure in the middle ear cavity, retraction of the tympanic membrane, and increased tension in the ossicles leading to impairment of sound conduction. If this condition persists, transudation of fluid from engorged capillaries will lead to chronic effusion inside the middle ear cavity (Jereczek-Fossa et al. 2003). This will cause metaplasia of the normal epithelium into mucus-secreting pseudostratified, columnar, ciliated epithelium. A tenacious deposit will then accumulate and this may cause formation of fibrovascular granulation tissue or inflammatory polyps, which will lead to tympanic drum performation. If atrophic otitis or necrosis of the ossicles occur, the conductive hearing loss will become permanent (Jereczek-Fossa et al. 2003).

Sensorineural hearing loss typically occurs several months after completion of radiotherapy and is usually chronic, progressive, and irreversible. Radiation-induced vascular insufficiency has been implicated in the mechanism of sensorineural hearing loss (Jereczek-Fossa et al. 2003). The process can lead to progressive degeneration and atrophy of the inner ear sensory structures, fibrosis, and possibly ossification of the inner ear fluid spaces. Histologic examination of irradiated temporal bone showed hemorrhage in inner ear spaces and edema of membranous labyrinth, loss of cells in the organ of Corti, atrophy of stria vascularis, atrophy of spiral ganglion cells and cochlear nerve, reduced number of capillaries, and degeneration of endothelium in vessels (Chan et al. 2009; Jereczek-Fossa et al. 2003; Gamble et al. 1968).

22.3.2 Clinical Manifestation and Diagnosis

Otologic deficits caused by both tumor and radiation effects are common in patients with NPC. A significant proportion of patients may present with some conductive hearing loss as a result of otitis media with effusion. Otologic evaluation is usually prompted by persistent or new onset of progressive hearing loss. In patients with serous otitis media caused by radiotherapy, they usually start to have some conductive hearing loss during treatment and the deficit does not improve. Cisplatin-induced sensorineural hearing loss usually occurs acutely, with effects apparent within a few days after drug administration (Chen et al. 2006). The deficit is more severe in higher frequency range and is proportional to the cumulative cisplatin dose. On the contrary, in patients with radiation-induced sensorineural hearing loss, there is usually a latent period of 6–12 months. Similar to cisplatin-induced sensorineural hearing loss, the deficit is also more severe in higher frequency range. Such patterns of hearing deficit will manifest as difficulty in hearing in a noisy environment and increased susceptibility to masking by low-frequency background noise (Chan et al. 2009).

A complete baseline otologic evaluation including microscopic otoscopy and functional tests such as pure tone audiometry, tympanometry, and stapedial reflexes is necessary to evaluate patients with otologic complications caused by radiation therapy or prior to treatment (Jereczek-Fossa et al. 2003). Microscopic otoscopy allows for evaluation of different forms of external and middle ear inflammation. Air and bone conduction pure tone audiometry, which is usually performed at frequencies of the speech range, evaluates subjective hearing thresholds and detects and defines the nature of hearing loss. Tympanometry measures acoustic impedance of the middle ear and evaluates aeration of the middle ear, the mobility of the ossicles, and the function of Eustachian tube. The testing of stapedial reflexes provides information on the integrity of the neural reflex loop (Jereczek-Fossa et al. 2003). If any of the above tests is abnormal, a more extensive otologic examination is necessary. Radiation-induced injury to the auditory pathway such as labyrinthitis, neuronitis, inner ear space hemorrhage, and white matter changes are readily detectable on magnetic resonance imaging (MRI) (Jereczek-Fossa et al. 2003).

22.3.3 Management

The best strategy is to avoid the occurrence of hearing deficit by limiting the radiation dose to the auditory system, particularly the inner ear. With advances in radiation therapy treatment planning, it is possible to achieve this goal. With the use of intensity-modulated radiation therapy technique, it is possible to steer the radiation dose away from the cochlea while still adequately covering the target volume. Data in the literature shows that when the mean dose to the cochlea exceeds 48 Gy, there is an increased risk of sensorineural deficit (Chen et al. 2006). With the use of intensity-modulated radiation therapy, the dose to bilateral cochlea can be limited to below the tolerance level. In patients receiving concurrent cisplatin, the dose constraint of the cochlea should be further lowered because it has been shown that the threshold cochlear dose for hearing loss is as low as 10 Gy when concurrent cisplatin is given (Hitchcock et al. 2009).

Some investigators recommended the insertion of ventilation tubes prophylactically to decrease the risk of conductive hearing loss. In a study from Hong Kong, 115 patients with NPC were randomized to undergoing insertion of ventilation tubes or no intervention after radiotherapy for NPC. There was an improvement in hearing, with a reduction of averaged air-bone gap among patients with ventilation tubes (Chowdhury et al. 1988). However, other studies did not show similar benefits of using ventilation tubes (Skinner et al. 1988; Lau et al. 1992).

There is no standard therapy for sensorineural hearing loss. Steroid therapy has been used to treat edema and inflammation of the inner ear caused by radiation (Jereczek-Fossa et al. 2003). However, it is not consistently effective. Hyperbaric oxygen has also been used with variable success. Classical conduction hearing aid may be used to improve hearing in patients with sensorineural hearing loss. Successful cochlear implants have been reported in a patient who developed bilateral deafness as a result of radiation-induced acoustic neuritis and labyrinthitis (Formanek et al. 1998).

22.4 Soft Tissue Fibrosis

A high dose of radiation is required to control NPC and as a result, the head and neck region including the skull base are typically treated to a high dose. Radiation-induced fibrosis can manifest as neck soft tissue fibrosis, cranial nerve entrapment (discussed in Sect. 20.5), trismus, or dysphagia. Cancer centers with anecdotal experience with the use of hypofractionated regimens have observed a higher incidence of symptomatic radiation-induced fibrosis of the soft tissue (Lee et al. 1992). In modern series where typically a more conventional fractionation (≤2 Gy) was used, the reported rates of radiation fibrosis were much lower (Lee et al. 2002, 2009, 2005; Sultanem et al. 2000; Kam et al. 2004). In a study by Lee et al., major late toxicities after conformal radiotherapy for NPC in 422 patients were analyzed. The rate of grade 2 or higher soft tissue damage ranged from 0 to 4.3%. The rate of grade 3 or higher trismus ranged from 0 to 1% (Lee et al. 2009).

22.4.1 Pathogenesis

Traditional teaching attributed late radiation injury to vascular/microvascular damage that led to tissue hypoxia and nutritional depletion (O'Sullivan and Levin 2003). Subsequently, it was believed that the linear-quadratic equation could predict the normal tissue response, which was determined by the radiosensitivity of parenchymal cells. Most recently, molecular pathways are implicated in the development of radiation-induced fibrosis. Irradiation of soft tissue causes tissue injury, which leads to activation of monocytes, macrophages, and platelets, which in turn causes release cytokine and growth factors (O'Sullivan and Levin 2003). This results in recruitment and proliferation of fibroblasts, increased synthesis of extracellular matrix, and decreased degradation of extracellular matrix and all these events contribute to eventual fibrosis.

22.4.2 Clinical Manifestation and Diagnosis

For neck soft tissue fibrosis, the earliest feature is the loss of tissue elasticity and mild induration (O'Sullivan and Levin 2003). More severe degree of fibrosis will result in rigidity of surface layers of tissue and loss of normal surface contours. Other associated changes any include hyperpigmentation, skin dryness, epilation, loss of vascularity, and changes in the epidermis. In the most severe case, necrosis or ulceration may occur. Trismus is result of fibrosis of the temporomandibular joints and the muscles of mastication. The dental gap may be narrowed to an extent such that feeding becomes difficult (Lee 1999). Dysphagia can be a result of swallowing dysfunction caused by radiation fibrosis. However, damage to the IX and X nerves from radiotherapy and/or late lymphedema may also contribute to dysphagia (Murphy and Gilbert 2009).

The diagnosis of radiation-induced fibrosis is mainly clinical. A combination of a history of radiotherapy for NPC and one or more of the above symptoms and signs substantiates the diagnosis. For patients with dysphagia, the physician should have a high index of suspicion for potential aspiration if there are symptoms like coughing or clearing of the throat prior to, during, and after eating (Murphy and Gilbert 2009). An official swallowing assessment should be performed by certified speech-language pathologists. The most common tests used include modified barium swallow study (MBSS) and flexible endoscopic evaluation of swallowing safety (FEES). MBSS allows for evaluation of oral and pharyngeal function whereas FEES allows for direct visualization of the upper aerodigestive tract and evaluation of vital functions including management of secretions, sensory function, and muscular function of the pharyngeal muscles. It also allows for direct visualization of the larynx and evaluation of any dysfunction of the larynx.

22.4.3 Management

There are several strategies that have been used for the treatment of radiation fibrosis. Several pharmacologic agents have been used. Pentoxifylline has been used alone or together with vitamin E with fair results (O'Sullivan and Levin 2003). In a study by Chua et al., 16 NPC patients who developed severe radiation-induced trismus that resulted in a dental gap of 25 mm or less. Pentoxifylline 400 mg 2–3 times a day was given for 8 weeks. Ten (62.5%) patients had measured increase in dental gap ranging from 2 to 25 mm and six (37.5%) had an increase of dental gap of 5 mm or more (Chua et al. 2001). In a study by Delanian et al., where 40 patients with radiation-induced fibrosis were treated with pentoxifylline and vitamin D, 24 (60%) patients showed at least 50% regression and the mean surface area regression was 53% (Delanian et al. 1999). Liposomal Cu/Zn superoxide dismutase has also been used for the treatment of radiation-induced fibrosis with impressive results. Among the 34 patients treated with twice weekly intramuscular injections of 5 mg for a total dose of 30 mg, all showed some clinical regression of fibrosis after 3 weeks with maximal effect observed after 2 months (Delanian et al. 1994). However, this agent is not available as an approved treatment. The role of corticosteroid in the management of radiation-induced fibrosis is uncertain.

Apart from pharmacologic measures, hyperbaric oxygen, physical therapy, and microcurrent therapy have also been used (O'Sullivan and Levin 2003). Hyperbaric oxygen works by increasing oxygen diffusibility, collagen synthesis, and neo-angiogenesis, thus allowing healing of damaged soft tissue. However, there has not been conclusive evidence that hyperbaric oxygen can significantly affect the degree of fibrosis (O'Sullivan and Levin 2003). Physical therapy, namely jaw exercise, may be useful in decreasing the degree of trismus when it is done during and after radiotherapy. Microcurrent therapy has been demonstrated to improve range of motion of the neck in 81%–92% of 26 patients with established radiation fibrosis of the neck in a study and the effect was sustained for more than 3 months (Lennox et al. 2002). However, no other confirmatory studies are available.

In patients with radiation-induced dysphagia, the goals of swallowing therapy are avoiding aspiration, improving swallowing function over time, and modifications in diet to render safe oral intake possible. The techniques used in swallowing therapy include postural techniques, sensory techniques, motor exercise, swallowing maneuvers, and change in diet (Murphy and Gilbert 2009).

With modern radiotherapy technology such as IMRT, it is possible to decrease the risk of radiation fibrosis. The temporomandibular joints can be contoured as avoidance structures and they can potentially be spared using IMRT. Since there is a dose–response relationship between dysphagia and the radiation dose delivered to the superior and middle pharyngeal constrictors, if those structures can be spared using IMRT without risking a geographic miss of disease, the risk of dysphagia can be reduced (Murphy and Gilbert 2009).

22.5 Cranial Neuropathy

Among all long-term complications, radiation-induced cranial neuropathy (CNP) is one of the least studied and understood entities. Although the biologic basis of radiation-induced nerve damage is not well understood, there is a notion that peripheral nerve is relatively resistant to radiation damage (Janzen and Warren 1942). However, once occurred, peripheral nerve damage can be debilitating and even life-threatening. The low incidence of cranial neuropathy after the completion of radiation, as well as the long latent of the onset of the condition, make prospective studies of the topic not possible.

22.5.1 Pathogenesis

Cranial nerves are a special group of the peripheral nerves in the cranium. It is generally accepted that peripheral nerve is highly resistant to radiation damage (Janzen and Warren 1942). However, the mechanisms of radiation-induced neuropathy are not well studied and understood. Like other types of peripheral nerves, cranial nerve trunks are composed of numerous nerve fascicles. The nerve fascicle contains individual nerve fibers. The cranial nerve trunks are surrounded by a fibrous connective tissue epineurium; the nerve fascicles are surrounded by a fibrous perineurium; and the nerve fibers are embedded in fibrous endoneurium. Each nerve fiber consists of an axon, which is surrounded by a myelin sheath or unmyelinated depending on its size. The cell bodies of the axon may be in the brainstem or peripheral ganglia. The epineurium carries major blood supply to the nerve trunk, and the arteries become arterioles in the perineurium; the arterioles then become capillaries in the endoneurium.

When damage to a peripheral nerve occurs, the death of an axonal cell body will cause the death of the nerve fiber. However, if only a portion of axon was damaged, it may form sprouts and regenerate. Schwann cells, the composing cells of the myelin sheath, can regenerate after damage including radiation-induced damage.

The knowledge of anatomy of the peripheral nerves is important in the understanding of radiation-induced damage. Peripheral neuropathy induced by high-dose irradiation may occur in two phases. Radiation may have early and direct effect on nerve fibers that may cause changes in electrophysiology and histochemistry. However, the later phase of radiation damage to the nerve may be caused by the changes in the surrounding fibrotic structures and its embedded blood supply to nerve fibers (Mendes et al. 1991).

Radiation-induced fibrosis of neck muscle may be a secondary cause of cranial neuropathy. Lin et al. (2002) reported 19 cases of radiation-induced cranial nerve palsy and found that the most frequently involved nerves were the hypoglossal nerve, the vagus nerve, and the recurrent laryngeal nerve. All three cranial nerves pass through the high-dose irradiated neck regions. Results of other retrospective series also supported that muscle fibrosis after irradiation might be the cause of cranial nerve palsy (Huang and Chu 1981; Saunders and Hodgson 1979; Marks et al. 1982; Mesic et al. 1981). In a more recently completed cross-sectional study, Kong and Lu et al. (2009 , unpublished data) studied 98 NPC patients who experienced cranial nerve palsy after definitive radiation therapy, and discovered that the probability of involvement of lower group of cranial nerves (i.e., CN IX–XII) was significantly higher than that of the anterior group. In addition, muscle fibrosis was a significant predictive factor for cranial nerve palsy.

Radiation-induced fibrosis of skeletal muscle may cause nerve entrapment with secondary demyelination. Furthermore, the fibrotic process of muscle, epineurium, perineurium, and endoneurium may also induce damage of the vasculature of the nerve (Mendes et al. 1991; Stryker et al. 1990). The significantly higher probability of neuropathy in the posterior group of cranial nerves suggests that the radiation-induced changes particularly fibrosis in the surrounding tissue may be a more significant cause of cranial neuropathy in the management of NPC, when compared to direct nerve damage caused by radiation.

Interestingly, the adjacent anatomic structures significantly influence the probability of radiation-induced neuropathy: severe (grade 3 or 4) muscle fibrosis is significantly related to the onset of cranial nerve deficits, thus significantly more patients developed posterior than anterior cranial nerve palsy. The above findings could also account for the manifestation of the peripheral neuropathy in terms of their function: it seems that motor nerves are more sensitive to fibrosis of the surrounding soft tissues, and sensory/motor nerves are more sensitive to direct radiation damage.

The probability and severity of cranial nerve neuropathy are associated with total radiation dose and large daily fraction. The incidence of cranial neuropathy has been addressed in two studies. In an analysis of 4527 NPC patients from Hong Kong, the incidence of CNP was reportedly 5% (Lee et al. 1992). However, the experience with 1032 patients from Taiwan showed that the incidence was only 1% after definitive radiation therapy (Huang and Chu 1981). The reason for this substantial discrepancy was not fully understood. However, all patients in the Hong Kong series were treated with 2.5 Gy or 4.2 Gy per daily fraction, whereas all patients in the Taiwan series were treated with conventional fractions. The discrepancy in the occurrence of CNP after radiation may indicate that dose fractionation plays a major role in the development of radiation-induced cranial neuropathy. In the above-mentioned cross-sectional study, total dose of radiation and radiation scheme are both predictive of neuropathy in the anterior cranial nerve, which are not embedded in skeletal muscle (Kong and Lu et al. 2009, unpublished data). The studies of radiation- induced peripheral neuropathy in brachial plexus after adjuvant radiation for breast cancer also supported that both higher total dose and hypofractionation were associated with higher incidence of brachial plexopathy (Rubin et al. 2001; Gillette et al. 1995).

The threshold dose of radiation for cranial neuropathy has not been clearly defined. The TD5/5 of radiation-induced peripheral neuropathy is 60 Gy (Emami et al. 1991). CNP is uncommon when a total radiation dose is less than 60 Gy delivered using conventional fractionation (Gillette et al. 1995). Furthermore, the probability of radiation-induced CNP is significantly related to the total radiation dose delivered to the postnasal space, and total radiation dose is an independent predictive factor for CNP (Kong and Lu et al. 2009, unpublished data).

Currently, the standard treatment modality for locoregionally advanced NPC is concurrent chemoradiation therapy. The addition of concurrent chemotherapy may sensitize cranial nerves to radiation injury. Although no literature has addressed the synergistic effect of chemotherapy on cranial neuropathy in the management of NPC, one needs to recognize that cisplatin-based chemotherapy induces peripheral neuropathy.

22.5.2 Clinical Manifestations

Clinical manifestations of cranial neuropathy secondary to radiation therapy depend on the cranial nerve involved and the nature of the damage. Cranial neuropathy is a descriptive term that does not indicate the underlying etiology and mechanism of damage.

Cranial nerves III, IV, and VI dysfunction results in limited extraocular muscle movement leading to diplopia. Dysfunction of the CN VIII results in sensorineural hearing deficit. However, differentiation between sensorineural hearing loss caused by irradiation and that from other etiology such as aging, or conductive hearing loss is difficult. As such, many clinical studies on cranial nerve damage excluded hearing dysfunction as a reliable indicator for CN VIII palsy. Damage to other cranial nerves is diagnosed by dysfunction of the particular nerve. For example, vagus nerve palsy is featured by simultaneous vocal cord paralysis and loss of motor function of the uvula. And tongue deviation to one side with atrophy is indicative of hypoglossal nerve palsy.

The diagnosis of radiation-induced cranial neuropathy is usually by exclusion, and injury of the nerve(s) by recurrent or progressive tumor must be excluded by radiological studies such as CT or MRI. Once occurred, a 3–6 months observation is recommended to exclude disease recurrence as the cause of nerve palsy (Lin et al. 2002; Konga and Lu et al. 2009).

Diagnosis of peripheral neuropathy after radiation therapy by imaging studies has not been well reported. MRI of patients with plexopathy may reveal subtle changes in adjacent tissues, but the nerve itself may appear normal (Hoeller et al. 2004). In a historical report on the pathologic finding of radiation-induced peripheral neuropathy, Stoll et al. (1966) demonstrated loss of myelin, fibrosis, thickening of the neurolemma sheath, and hyalinization and obliteration of the vasonervorum to the brachial plexus after radiation. All findings indicated focal compression of the nerve by fibrosis or chronic nerve ischemia as the causes of neuropathy (Stoll et al. 1966).

25.5.2.1 Latent Period of CNP

It was reported that the median interval between completion of radiotherapy and occurrence of neurologic symptoms was 1–4 years (Stoll et al. 1966; Powell et al. 1990), although the symptoms of neuropathy could be progressive after many years post-treatment (Johansson et al. 2000, 2002).

The results of the above-mentioned cross-sectional study revealed that the median time to occurrence of CNP was 8 years, and the incidence of the onset of cranial neuropathy within 5 years, between 5 to 10 years, 10–15 years, and 15–20 years postradiation varied between 10% and 14%, without substantial differences (Kong and Lu et al. 2009, unpublished data). Therefore, late onset of radiation-induced peripheral neuropathy after 15 years is not uncommon, and the probability remains constant for a considerable portion of the patients' life after the completion of radiation. This is of special relevance when the overall treatment outcome for cancer patients improves, and the long-term survival becomes prevailing.

Once developed, peripheral neuropathy may steadily progress or stabilize, and only few patients experience improvement (Kong and Lu et al. 2009, Pierce et al. 1992; Harper et al. 1989; Salner et al. 1981).

22.5.3 Management

Understanding of the cause of peripheral neuropathy is important for the proper treatment of cranial nerve palsy induced by high-dose irradiation. Radiation-induced posterior cranial neuropathy and brachial plexopathy are proven to be associated with muscle fibrosis of the neck after radiation. Thus, symptomatic alleviation of muscle fibrosis by surgical intervention for releasing cranial nerve from entrapment could be therapeutic (Lin et al. 2002; Hoeller et al. 2004; Bowen et al. 1996; Fathers et al. 2002). Surgical intervention for posterior cranial neuropathy caused by cervical muscle fibrosis should be postponed for at least 6–12 months after the onset of cranial nerve palsy to allow the stabilization of the symptoms.

Although neurolysis or neurolysis with omental grafting aimed to relief fibrosis of epi- and perineurium has been reported to be effective in some patients with brachial plexopathy (LeQuang 1989; Killer and Hess 1990), such a procedure is usually not feasible in the case of nasopharyngeal cancer due to the critical location of most cranial nerves.

Radiation-induced neuropathy in the anterior group of cranial nerves is more likely to be caused by direct damage from radiotherapy. Unfortunately, no proven effective treatment for radiation-induced nerve damage is available. Limited data supported the use of hyperbaric oxygen (HBO) and steroids for symptomatic control in the acute phase of radiation-induced cranial neuropathy; however, no effective long-term control has been demonstrated with any type of therapeutic efforts (Mihalcea and Arnold 2008; Boschetti et al. 2006; Levy and Miller 2006).

As no effective treatment is available for radiation-induced peripheral nerve damage, efforts should be directed at preventative measures. Reduction in radiation field size and fraction size has been demonstrated to reduce late complication severity (Stinson et al. 1991). The utilization of IMRT in the treatment of NPC requires delineation of a number of neurological OARs including optic nerve, optical chiasm, and cochlea. Limiting dose to nerves may help in reducing the probability of cranial neuropathy. However, for patients with locally advanced NPC, especially T4 lesions, irradiating the cranial nerves involved or in proximity to the primary tumor are usually unavoidable.

22.6 Brainstem and Spinal Cord Injury (Encephalomyelopathy)

Because of the pattern of tumor invasion, the clivus frequently receives a high dose of radiation during radiotherapy for nasopharyngeal cancer. Given the proximity of the clivus to the brainstem and upper cervical spinal cord, those two structures are at risk of radiation-induced injury. In cases of extensive posterior skull base involvement, the risk of injury to the brain stem and cervical spinal cord is further elevated. Brainstem and spinal cord injury is the most devastating complication from head and neck radiotherapy. Injury to the brainstem and/or spinal cord can result in spastic paraparesis or quadraparesis and more than half of those patients progress rapidly to a debilitated state with a significant proportion eventually dying of the complication (LEE et al. 1992). Fortunately, this complication mainly occurred in the old radiotherapy era where two-dimensional techniques were used, in which shielding was based on bony landmarks without the actual structures volumetrically contoured. Furthermore, without the advantage of three-dimensional computer planning, the radiation doses delivered to the brainstem and cervical spinal cord might be underestimated. In cases where matching fields were used, suboptimal treatment set-up accuracy might result in overdosing of the spinal cord. In a study from Hong Kong, all the patients who developed brainstem and/or spinal cord injury were patients treated before 1983 (LEE et al. 1992). With the utilization of more sophisticated radiation therapy technology, it is possible to accurately estimate the radiation doses delivered to the brainstem and spinal cord and to protect those structures without compromising target coverage. In most modern series, the occurrence of brainstem and spinal cord injury is extremely rare (LEE et al. 2009, 2002, 2005; SULTANEM et al. 2000; KAM et al. 2004).

22.6.1 Pathogenesis

The mechanisms of injury to the brainstem and spinal cord are likely similar. According to Schultheiss et al., the main morphologic features of radiation-induced myelopathy are demyelination and necrosis of the spinal cord, although they are not pathognomomic of radiation injury. Vasculopathies and glial reaction can also be seen in radiation-induced myelopathy (SCHULTHEISS et al. 1995). Damage to the microvasculature has been implicated as one of the mechanisms of radiation-induced myelopathy. Cytokine network in the central nervous system may also have a role on the development of radiation myelopathy (SCHULTHEISS et al. 1995).

22.6.2 Clinical Manifestation and Diagnosis

Patients may present with slowly progressive spastic paraparesis or quadraparesis and in patients with brainstem injury, multiple cranial nerve deficits may coexist (LEE 1999). Since the posterior parts of the brainstem and cervical spinal cord are farther away from the target volume, when injury occurs in the brainstem or the cervical spinal cord, the anteriorly located corticospinal tracts are at the highest risk. As a result, on clinical examination, the predominant deficits are motor with mild or absent associated sensory deficits. The majority of patients will progress and develop severe motor debilitation. In one series from Hong Kong, 59% of patients with encephalomyelopathy became debilitated and 34% eventually succumbed to the complication (LEE et al. 1992).

To make a definite diagnosis of radiation-induced brainstem and spinal cord injury (encephalomyelopathy), it is crucial that certain criteria are fulfilled. First of all, the localization of the neurologic findings must match the anatomic region of the brainstem or spinal cord treated with radiation therapy. It is important to rule out other causes of encephalomyelopathy such as tumor progression as well. In addition, the latent period between the occurrence of the neurologic deficits and the completion of radiotherapy has to be considered. In the classical radiation oncology teaching, a latency period of less than 6 months is rare. In a study by Lee et al. from Hong Kong, the median latent period was 3 years (LEE et al. 1992). On MRI, the regions affected typically show increased signal intensity on T2-weighted images and decreased signal intensity on T1-weighted images. Brainstem auditory evoked potentials may reveal brainstem dysfunction (LEE 1999).

22.6.3 Management

No effective treatment is currently available for radiation-induced brainstem and/or spinal cord injury. Corticosteroid therapy has been used and may be able to temporarily delay progression of the injuries and symptomatic progression (ST CLAIR et al. 2003). Clinical and radiographic improvement of radiation-induced myelopathy has been reported after treatment with heparin and coumadin (GLANTZ et al. 1994). Hyperbaric oxygen has also been used without substantial success although clinical improvement has been reported in a case report where a patient with radiation myelopathy who was not responding to steroid therapy was treated with 20 dives of hyperbaric oxygen (CALABRO and JINKINS 2000).

Because of the lack of effective treatment for brainstem injury and myelopathy, the best strategy of prevention cannot be overemphasized. With the prevailing utilization of modern treatment techniques such as three-dimensional conformal and IMRT, it is possible to avoid overdosing the brainstem and spinal cord. With the use of IMRT, a highly concave isodose distribution can be achieved. Whenever possible, it is important to keep the maximum brainstem and spinal cord doses to 50–54 Gy and 45 Gy, respectively (Emami et al. 1991).

22.7 Temporal Lobe Necrosis

Given the proximity of the temporal lobes to the sphenoid sinus, which is typically included in the radiation field or clinical target volume in NPC, they are at risk for radiation-induced injury including necrosis. Temporal lobe necrosis is one of the most feared complications in the management of NPC because it accounts for 65% of deaths from radiation-induced complications (Lee et al. 1992). Fortunately, the reported rates of temporal lobe necrosis are relatively low in most series and they ranged from 0% to 6% (Lee et al. 1992, 2009, 2002, 2005; Yeh et al. 2005; Kam et al. 2004).

The incidence of temporal lobe necrosis depends on a number of factors including the fractional dose, total dose, and the volume of brain irradiated (Lee 1999; Lee et al. 2002 1998, 1999; Jen et al. 2001). When altered fractionation is used, the interfraction time interval impacts on the rate of temporal lobe necrosis. Clinical evidence suggested that an interfraction interval of 6 h may not be adequate for complete repair of radiation damage (Lee et al. 1999). In a study by Lee et al., the incidence of temporal lobe necrosis was 0% for patients who received 66 Gy in 33 fractions (2 Gy per fraction, five times a week), 24% for those who received 59.5 Gy in 17 fractions (3.5 Gy per fraction, three times a week), and 33% for those who received 71.2 Gy in 40 fractions over 35 days (Lee et al. 2002).

22.7.1 Pathogenesis

In radiation-induced necrosis of brain parenchyma, the histopathologic changes are typically limited to the white matter but can occasionally extend to the gray matter. The pathologic changes seen under the microscope include focal coagulative and fibrinoid necrosis and demyelination (Schultheiss et al. 1995; Sloan et al. 2003). Recognizable cells and structures are completely lost. The areas of necrosis are positive in fibrin stains but older lesions may lose the intense staining for fibrin stain. At the margins of the necrosis, gliosis are present. Occasionally, stromal edema and microvascular proliferation are seen. Dystrophic calcium deposits may be present in the necrotic focus.

22.7.2 Clinical Manifestation and Diagnosis

Patients with temporal lobe necrosis can present with very subtle symptoms that may be missed if the physician does not have a high index of suspicion. In the series by Lee et al., 16% of the 102 patients with temporal lobe necrosis were asymptomatic and 39% presented with vague symptoms such as mild dizziness, memory impairment, or personality change. Only 31% of patients with temporal lobe necrosis presented with classical temporal lobe epilepsy and 14% with nonspecific neurologic findings such as headache, mental confusion, or general seizures (Lee et al. 1988). On physical examination, only a small percentage of patients showed signs of raised intracranial pressure such as papilledema (4%) or 6th nerve palsy (14%) (Lee 1999). The median latent period was 5 years (range, 1.5–13 years). Neurocognitive deficit can occur in patients with temporal lobe necrosis. The general intelligence is usually intact (Cheung et al. 2000). The degree of neurocognitive deficit is dependent on the volume and site of necrosis in the temporal lobe (Cheung et al. 2003).

The diagnosis of temporal lobe necrosis is usually confirmed using imaging studies. Computerized tomography (CT) of the brain usually demonstrates a small necrotic foci at the inferomedial aspect of each of the temporal lobes associated with edema. Irregular "finger-like" hypodense areas in the white matter are seen (Lee 1999). In a minority of cases, well-defined lesions with central liquefaction may be obvious. However, in some cases, patients with temporal lobe necrosis may have a negative brain CT. In such cases, MRI of the brain will be useful. MRI is superior to CT in terms of sensitivity and can demonstrate a small area of necrotic focus in the brain. On T1-weighted images, temporal lobe necrosis shows up as very low intensity areas; on T2-weighted spin echo sequence images, it shows up as high signal intensity areas (Lee 1999). Liquefaction within edematous brain parenchyma is ready demonstrated as a roundish area of hypointensity on proton-density sequence.

22.7.3 Management

Increased capillary permeability and brain edema occur as a result of vascular injury from radiation therapy before the development of brain parenchymal necrosis (Sloan et al. 2003). Corticosteroids are frequently used for temporal lobe necrosis. In a report by Lee et al., 72 patients with temporal lobe necrosis were treated with tapering doses of corticosteroids and 35% of them achieved a durable response (Lee et al. 1988). Steroid therapy is found to be most effective when it is used in the early stage of temporal lobe necrosis where there is significant reactive edema (Lee 1999). It provides a delaying or retarding effect on the progressive pathologic process during the early phase of temporal lobe necrosis. Some patients may even show radiographic improvement with steroid therapy. However, long-term use of steroid may put patients at risk for severe and sometimes fatal infection (Lee et al. 1988). When temporal lobe necrosis reaches a later stage where there is cystic liquefaction, it is very unlikely that steroid therapy will have any significant effect (Lee 1999). In the study by Lee et al., none of the patients with cystic necrosis responded to steroid therapy (Lee et al. 1988). Therefore, once cystic liquefaction develops, the only definitive treatment is surgical resection. However, bilateral temporal lobectomy can be problematic because of the risk of Kluver–Bucy syndrome and should be avoided as much as possible (Kluver and Bucy 1997; Lee et al. 1993). Lee et al. reported a case where a patient with temporal lobe necrosis underwent sequential bilateral temporal lobectomy and subsequently had dramatic response with no significant neurologic deficits (Lee 1999). At Queen Elizabeth Hospital of Hong Kong, among six patients who underwent bilateral temporal lobectomy for bilateral temporal lobe necrosis, none had developed Kluver–Bucy syndrome as of 2006 (Lee et al. 2008). Unilateral temporal lobectomy may produce short-term relief but recurrence of contralateral temporal necrosis are common (Lee 1999). The effect of aspiration of the cystic necrosis is usually very short-lived. Seizures caused by temporal lobe necrosis is treated with anticonvulsants.

Given the difficulty with the management of temporal lobe necrosis, prevention is the best strategy of management. As mentioned above, the most important factors predicting the risk of development of temporal lobe necrosis are fractional dose, total dose, and total brain volume irradiated. With the prevailing utilization of modern radiation therapy technology especially with IMRT, it is possible to limit the amount of temporal lobe brain parenchyma irradiated. When three-dimensional conformal radiation therapy or IMRT planning is used, the temporal lobes should be contoured as organs at risk, so they can be blocked or spared appropriately. Data from the literature on altered fractionation for NPC show increased risk of development of temporal lobe necrosis (Lee et al. 2002, 1998, 1999; Jen et al. 2001). Given the significantly increased risk of temporal lobe necrosis and the lack of significant benefits in terms of disease control and survival, the use of altered fractionation should be avoided.

22.8 Neuroendocrine Deficits

The sphenoid sinus is typically included in the radiation treatment field in NPC; therefore, radiation dose delivered to the hypothalamic–pituitary axis can be substantial, especially when the NPC is locally advanced. However, the incidence of symptomatic neuroendocrine disturbance is low overall. In a study by Lee et al., the reported rate of symptomatic neuroendocrine disturbance was 9.7% (Lee et al. 2009). The latency period is reported to be 5 years although when a detailed endocrine evaluation is performed, biochemical changes can be detected in as early as 1 year after the completion of radiotherapy (Lee et al. 1992; Lam et al. 1987).

22.8.1 Pathogenesis

The hypothalamus–pituitary axis is considered an integrated endocrine organ that controls the peripheral endocrine function. Deficiencies of releasing or inhibitory factors are observed in NPC patients after radiotherapy suggesting that the predominant damage occurs in the hypothalamus (Lam et al. 1987, 1986). Growth hormone production by the hypothalamus–pituitary axis is most prone to radiation injury. Secretion of gonadotropin is more resistant to damage by radiation. Secretion of corticotrophin and thyrotropin is even more resistant to damage by radiation (Fajardo and Anderson 2001). Microscopic changes such as cell degeneration, early and late necrosis, epithelial cell atrophy, and extensive fibrosis in the anterior pituitary have been described after particle beam therapy but the radiation doses given were significantly higher than the level of radiation exposure from radiotherapy for NPC.

22.8.2 Clinical Manifestation and Diagnosis

As mentioned above, the overall incidence of symptomatic hypothalamus–pituitary axis deficiency is relatively low. However, when detailed endocrine evaluation is performed, the 5-year incidence can be as high as 62% (Lam et al. 1991). The most commonly diagnosed endocrine deficiency is growth hormone deficiency, followed by gonadotropin, corticotrophin, and thyrotropin deficiencies.

The diagnosis of hormonal deficiency is based on clinical and biochemical findings. A strong clinical suspicion can lead to early diagnosis asymptomatic neuroendocrine deficiencies. A full endocrine panel, including growth hormone, insulin-like growth factor-1, prolactin, corticotrophin, free cortisol, thyroid-stimulating hormone, free T3 and T4, follicle-stimulating hormone, and luteinizing hormone, should be performed. The evaluation is best performed by an endocrinologist.

In adult patients with growth hormone deficiency, reduction of muscular and adipose tissue of the body is observed. Gonadotropin deficiency may present as secondary amenorrhea and sexual dysfunction. Symptoms of hypoadrenalism and hypothyroidism may occur in patients with deficiencies of corticotrophin and thyrotropin, respectively. Since the whole neck is typically irradiated in NPC patients treated with conventional radiation therapy, radiation-induced damage to the thyroid may also contribute to hypothyroidism. Female patients may develop amenorrhea and/or galactorrhea as a result of hyperprolactinemia (Lee et al. 2008).

22.8.3 Management

The most effective management of radiation-induced neuroendocrine deficits is by prevention. With a combination of modern imaging modalities such as positron emission tomography/CT (PET/CT) and MRI, accurate delineation of the tumor extent in skull base is possible. In early stage nasopharyngeal cancer, shielding or sparing (when IMRT is used) of the hypothalamic–pituitary axis can be safely achieved without risking a geographic miss (Sham et al. 1994).

It is advisable that prior to the initiation of treatment, a complete baseline endocrine profile is obtained. After the completion of radiation therapy, continued follow-up of endocrine profile is necessary. When endocrine deficits are detected, hormonal replacement therapy should be considered.

22.9 Second Primary Tumor

Second primary tumor (SPT) is probably the most devastating complication a cancer patients may face after the successful treatment of their first malignancy. Although the incidence of SPT is relatively low, it is a true clinical entity in cancer management. The understanding and study of SPT after treatment of nasopharyngeal cancer are very limited when compared with other types of upper aerodigestive track cancer, especially squamous cell carcinoma. Therefore, much of the knowledge on this topic for NPC is derived from that of other head and neck cancers.

22.9.1 Pathogenesis

SPTs in patients with squamous cell carcinoma of the head and neck (SCCHN) area are not uncommon after definitive treatment, with a cumulative incidence of 10%–20%. The mechanism of SPT in SCCHN is not completely understood. Two mechanisms of the occurrence of SPT after treatment of the primary disease have been proposed: The "condemned mucosa syndrome" and "field cancerization" theories.

"Condemned mucosa syndrome" theory was based on a hypothesis that synchronous transformation of multiple cells is rare and that SPTs are caused by widespread migration of cancer cells to other tissues or organs in the aerodigestive tract (Bedi et al. 1996). In contrast, in the "field cancerization" theory proposed by Slaughter et al. states that the mucosa accumulates genetic alterations that result in the induction of multiple and independent, malignant lesions after repeated carcinogenic exposure. This theory is widely accepted now and is supported by research results in molecular biology (Slaughter et al. 1953; Ronchetti et al. 2005; Homann et al. 2001; van Oijen et al. 2000).

Radiation is a known weak carcinogen, and it belongs to the common carcinogen group that may be responsible for "field cancerization." However, our understanding of the mechanisms of radiation-induced malignancy is limited. In a population-based study of 20,074 patients with laryngeal cancer, Gao et al. (2003) reported an incidence of 17.6% for SPTs, and radiotherapy was associated with a 68% excess risk of developing a second head and neck cancer in patients who survived 5 years or longer. However, more than 60% of the SPTs occurred were of upper aerodigestive tract primary and are of squamous cell nature (Dikshit et al. 2005; Yamamoto et al. 2002; Leon et al. 1999). It is not easy to differentiate primary malignancies from radiation-induced malignancies of same pathology with current technology. The high incidence of SPT after radiation therapy for laryngeal cancer could be a manifestation of a suboptimal management of the primary disease.

The identified carcinogens such as EBV infection in NPC are not clearly associated with most types of malignancy diagnosed in the upper aerodigestive tract. In addition, the most commonly diagnosed pathology in NPC, i.e., undifferentiated carcinoma is relatively unique for nasopharynx. In the largest series on SPT in NPC patients after definitive radiotherapy, Kong et al. (2006) intended to study the incidence of SPT in NPC after radiotherapy and any significant risk factors responsible for the increase of the incidence of SPT. Although the cumulative incidence of SPT in NPC after definitive treatment exceeded 5% at 5 years, the incidence for those occurred within the radiation portal (mostly in the upper aerodigestive tract) was 1.2%. Furthermore, except for an advanced age of >50 years, no other factors was identified to be associated with an increased of SPT incidence. The cumulative incidence of SPT at 5-years after treatment in NPC was much less than that of SCCHN of other primary. The diagnosed SPT in the radiation therapy portal including SCCs of the squamous epithelium, adenoid cystic carcinoma of the parotid, epidermoid carcinoma of the hard palate, and pleomorphic sarcoma in the neck. And whether "field cancerization" from common etiologies (including radiotherapy) can be used to explain the etiology of SPT in NPC is largely unknown.

22.9.2 Clinical Manifestations and Diagnosis

Not all SPT diagnosed after radiation therapy are treatment-induced. Three diagnostic criteria need to be met before a diagnosis of a radiation-induced SPT can be made: the tumor should be of different pathology from the initial diagnosis, should occurs within the radiation portal, and should be diagnosed after 5 years from the completion of radiation therapy (Kong and Lu 2009). Such criteria made the diagnosis of an SPT in NPC after definitive treatment straightforward. The majority cases of NPC are of poorly- or un-differentiated nonkeratinizing SCC, and similar pathology in the upper aerodigestive track are relatively uncommon. Therefore, a poorly- or un-differentiated carcinoma in the head and neck area (including the radiation portal) is usually considered as a recurrence from NPC. Whereas in patients with keratinizing SCC of the upper aerodigestive system, a true second primary SCC with similar etiology such as cigarette smoking and/or excessive alcohol use or due to field cancerization is not uncommon.

22.9.3 Management

The treatment of SPT after radiation therapy for any malignancy depends on the pathology of the disease, patient's performance status and preference, and previous treatment utilized for the primary disease. As radiation therapy is the mainstay treatment modality for NPC, and definitive treatment of nonmetastatic NPC usually requires a total dose of 66–70 Gy to the head and neck areas, the use of high-dose re-irradiation is usually limited. Surgical resection is usually considered as the primary treatment modality for nonmetastatic disease. If surgical resection is not feasible, combined chemotherapy (if indicated) and radiation therapy of advanced technology such as IMRT or stereotactic radiosurgery can be considered.

22.10 Summary

Treatment-induced late adverse effects are clinically important and could be dose-limiting for radiation therapy. Commonly observed late effects include xerostomia, hearing deficit, and soft-tissue fibrosis. Rare complications such as SPT, temporal lobe necrosis, and cranial nerve palsy could be life threatening. Most conditions can substantially affect quality of life physiologically or psychologically. The pathogenesis of treatment-induced, mostly radiation-induced, late complications are complex and not well understood. Currently, no effective management is available for most types of radiation-induced late complications except for symptomatic palliation. Advanced treatment technology and utilization of radioprotectant such as amifostine could reduce the probability of the occurrences of certain late complications.

References

Anne PR, Machtay M, Rosenthal DI, et al (2007) A phase II trial of subcutaneous amifostine and radiation therapy in patients with head-and-neck cancer. Int J Radiat Oncol Biol Phys 67(2):445–452

Bedi GC, Westra WH, Gabrielson E, Koch W, Sidransky D (1996) Multiple head and neck tumors: evidence for a common clonal origin. Cancer Res 56(11):2484–2487

Boschetti M, De Lucchi M, Giusti M, et al (2006) Partial visual recovery from radiation-induced optic neuropathy after hyperbaric oxygen therapy in a patient with Cushing disease. Eur J Endocrinol 154(6):813–818

Bowen BC, Verma A, Brandon AH, Fiedler JA (1996) Radiation-induced brachial plexopathy: MR and clinical findings. AJNR Am J Neuroradiol 17(10):1932–1936

Buntzel J, Kuttner K, Frohlich D, Glatzel M (1998) Selective cytoprotection with amifostine in concurrent radiochemotherapy for head and neck cancer. Ann Oncol 9(5):505–509

Calabro F, Jinkins JR (2000) MRI of radiation myelitis: a report of a case treated with hyperbaric oxygen. Eur Radiol 10(7): 1079–1084

Chan SH, Ng WT, Kam KL, et al (2009) Sensorineural hearing loss after treatment of nasopharyngeal carcinoma: a longitudinal analysis. Int J Radiat Oncol Biol Phys 73(5):1335–1342

Cheng SH, Jian JJ, Tsai SY, et al (2000) Long-term survival of nasopharyngeal carcinoma following concomitant radiotherapy and chemotherapy. Int J Radiat Oncol Biol Phys 48(5):1323–1330

Chen WC, Jackson A, Budnick AS, et al (2006) Sensorineural hearing loss in combined modality treatment of nasopharyngeal carcinoma. Cancer 106(4):820–829

Cheung MC, Chan AS, Law SC, Chan JH, Tse VK (2003) Impact of radionecrosis on cognitive dysfunction in patients after radiotherapy for nasopharyngeal carcinoma. Cancer 97(8): 2019–2026

Cheung M, Chan AS, Law SC, Chan JH, Tse VK (2000) Cognitive function of patients with nasopharyngeal carcinoma with and without temporal lobe radionecrosis. Arch Neurol 57(9):1347–1352

Chowdhury CR, Ho JH, Wright A, Tsao SY, Au GK, Tung Y (1988). Prospective study of the effects of ventilation tubes on hearing after radiotherapy for carcinoma of nasopharynx. Ann Otol Rhinol Laryngol 97(2 Pt 1):142–145

Chua DT, Lo C, Yuen J, Foo YC (2001) A pilot study of pentoxifylline in the treatment of radiation-induced trismus. Am J Clin Oncol 24(4):366–369

Cox JD, Stetz J, Pajak TF (1995) Toxicity criteria of the Radiation Therapy Oncology Group (RTOG) and the European Organization for Research and Treatment of Cancer (EORTC). Int J Radiat Oncol Biol Phys 31(5):1341–1346

Delanian S, Baillet F, Huart J, Lefaix JL, Maulard C, Housset M (1994) Successful treatment of radiation-induced fibrosis using liposomal Cu/Zn superoxide dismutase: clinical trial. Radiother Oncol 32(1):12–20

Delanian S, Balla-Mekias S, Lefaix JL (1999) Striking regression of chronic radiotherapy damage in a clinical trial of combined pentoxifylline and tocopherol. J Clin Oncol 17 (10):3283–3290

Dikshit RP, Boffetta P, Bouchardy C, et al (2005) Risk factors for the development of second primary tumors among men after laryngeal and hypopharyngeal carcinoma. Cancer 103(11):2326–2333

Eisbruch A, Kim HM, Terrell JE, Marsh LH, Dawson LA, Ship JA (2001) Xerostomia and its predictors following parotid-sparing irradiation of head-and-neck cancer. Int J Radiat Oncol Biol Phys 50(3):695–704

Eisbruch A, Ship JA, Dawson LA, et al (2003) Salivary gland sparing and improved target irradiation by conformal and intensity modulated irradiation of head and neck cancer. World J Surg 27(7):832–837

Eisbruch A, Ten Haken RK, Kim HM, Marsh LH, Ship JA (1999) Dose, volume, and function relationships in parotid salivary glands following conformal and intensity-modulated irradiation of head and neck cancer. Int J Radiat Oncol Biol Phys 45(3):577–587

Emami B, Lyman J, Brown A, et al (1991) Tolerance of normal tissue to therapeutic irradiation. Int J Radiat Oncol Biol Phys 21(1):109–122

Epstein JB, Emerton S, Kolbinson DA, et al (1999) Quality of life and oral function following radiotherapy for head and neck cancer. Head Neck 21(1):1–11

Fajardo L-G LF, Berthrong M, Anderson RE (eds) (2001) Endocrine glands: hypothalamic-hypophyseal axis. In: Radiation pathology. Oxford University Press, New York, pp 331–336

Fathers E, Thrush D, Huson SM, Norman A (2002) Radiation-induced brachial plexopathy in women treated for carcinoma of the breast. Clin Rehabil 16(2):160–165

Fisher J, Scott C, Scarantino CW, et al (2003) Phase III quality-of-life study results: impact on patients' quality of life to reducing xerostomia after radiotherapy for head-and-neck cancer – RTOG 97-09. Int J Radiat Oncol Biol Phys 56(3): 832–836

Formanek M, Czerny C, Gstoettner W, Kornfehl J (1998) Cochlear implantation as a successful rehabilitation for radiation-induced deafness. Eur Arch Otorhinolaryngol 255(4): 175–178

Gamble JE, Peterson EA, Chandler JR (1968) Radiation effects on the inner ear. Arch. Otolaryngol. 88:64–69

Gao X, Fisher SG, Mohideen N, Emami B (2003) Second primary cancers in patients with laryngeal cancer: a population-based study. Int J Radiat Oncol Biol Phys 56(2):427–435

Gillette EL, Mahler PA, Powers BE, Gillette SM, Vujaskovic Z (1995) Late radiation injury to muscle and peripheral nerves. Int J Radiat Oncol Biol Phys 31(5):1309–1318

Glantz MJ, Burger PC, Friedman AH, Radtke RA, Massey EW, Schold SC Jr (1994) Treatment of radiation-induced nervous system injury with heparin and warfarin. Neurology 44(11): 2020–2027

Hamlar DD, Schuller DE, Gahbauer RA, et al (1996) Determination of the efficacy of topical oral pilocarpine for postirradiation

xerostomia in patients with head and neck carcinoma. Laryngoscope 106(8):972–976
Harper CM Jr, Thomas JE, Cascino TL, Litchy WJ (1989) Distinction between neoplastic and radiation-induced brachial plexopathy, with emphasis on the role of EMG. Neurology 39(4):502–506
Harrison LB, Zelefsky MJ, Pfister DG, et al (1997) Detailed quality of life assessment in patients treated with primary radiotherapy for squamous cell cancer of the base of the tongue. Head Neck 19(3):169–175
Henson BS, Inglehart MR, Eisbruch A, Ship JA (2001) Preserved salivary output and xerostomia-related quality of life in head and neck cancer patients receiving parotid-sparing radiotherapy. Oral Oncol 37(1):84–93
Hitchcock YJ, Tward JD, Szabo A, Bentz BG, Shrieve DC (2009) Relative contributions of radiation and cisplatin-based chemotherapy to sensorineural hearing loss in head-and-neck cancer patients. Int J Radiat Oncol Biol Phys 73(3):779–788
Hoeller U, Bonacker M, Bajrovic A, Alberti W, Adam G (2004) Radiation-induced plexopathy and fibrosis. Is magnetic resonance imaging the adequate diagnostic tool? Strahlenther Onkol 180(10):650–654
Homann N, Nees M, Conradt C, et al (2001) Overexpression of p53 in tumor-distant epithelia of head and neck cancer patients is associated with an increased incidence of second primary carcinoma. Clin Cancer Res 7(2):290–296
Huang S, Chu G (1981) Nasopharyngeal cancer: study II. Int J Radiat Oncol Biol Phys 7(6):713–716
Jacobs CD, van der Pas M (1996) A multicenter maintenance study of oral pilocarpine tablets for radiation-induced xerostomia. Oncology (Williston Park) 10(3 Suppl):16–20
Janzen AH, Warren S (1942) Effect of roentgen rays on the peripheral nerve of the rat. Radiology 38:333–337
Jellema AP, Langendijk H, Bergenhenegouwen L, et al (2001) The efficacy of Xialine in patients with xerostomia resulting from radiotherapy for head and neck cancer: a pilot-study. Radiother Oncol 59(2):157–160
Jen YM, Hsu WL, Chen CY, et al (2001) Different risks of symptomatic brain necrosis in NPC patients treated with different altered fractionated radiotherapy techniques. Int J Radiat Oncol Biol Phys 51(2):344–348
Jereczek-Fossa BA, Zarowski A, Milani F, Orecchia R (2003) Radiotherapy-induced ear toxicity. Cancer Treat Rev 29(5): 417–430
Johansson S, Svensson H, Denekamp J (2000) Timescale of evolution of late radiation injury after postoperative radiotherapy of breast cancer patients. Int J Radiat Oncol Biol Phys 48(3):745–750
Johansson S, Svensson H, Denekamp J (2002) Dose response and latency for radiation-induced fibrosis, edema, and neuropathy in breast cancer patients. Int J Radiat Oncol Biol Phys 52(5):1207–1219
Johnson JT, Ferretti GA, Nethery WJ, et al (1993) Oral pilocarpine for post-irradiation xerostomia in patients with head and neck cancer. N Engl J Med 329(6):390–395
Kam MK, Teo PM, Chau RM, et al (2004) Treatment of nasopharyngeal carcinoma with intensity-modulated radiotherapy: the Hong Kong experience. Int J Radiat Oncol Biol Phys 60(5):1440–1450
Kies MS, Haraf DJ, Rosen F, et al (2001) Concomitant infusional paclitaxel and fluorouracil, oral hydroxyurea, and hyperfractionated radiation for locally advanced squamous head and neck cancer. J Clin Oncol 19(7):1961–1969
Killer HE, Hess K (1990) Natural history of radiation-induced brachial plexopathy compared with surgically treated patients. J Neurol 237(4):247–250
Kluver H, Bucy PC (1997) Preliminary analysis of functions of the temporal lobes in monkeys. J Neuropsychiatry Clin Neurosci Fall;9(4):606–620
Kong L, Lu JJ (2009) Second primary tumor. In: Schwab M (ed) Encyclopedia of cancer. Springer, Berlin
Kong L, Lu JJ, Hu C, Guo X, Wu Y, Zhang Y (2006) The risk of second primary tumors in patients with nasopharyngeal carcinoma after definitive radiotherapy. Cancer 107(6): 1287–1293
Koukourakis MI (2002) Amifostine in clinical oncology: current use and future applications. Anticancer Drugs 13(3): 181–209
Koukourakis MI, Kyrias G, Kakolyris S, et al (2000) Subcutaneous administration of amifostine during fractionated radiotherapy: a randomized phase II study. J Clin Oncol 18(11): 2226–2233
Lam KS, Ho JH, Lee AW, et al (1987) Symptomatic hypothalamic-pituitary dysfunction in nasopharyngeal carcinoma patients following radiation therapy: a retrospective study. Int J Radiat Oncol Biol Phys 13(9):1343–1350
Lam KS, Tse VK, Wang C, Yeung RT, Ho JH (1991) Effects of cranial irradiation on hypothalamic-pituitary function – a 5-year longitudinal study in patients with nasopharyngeal carcinoma. Q J Med 78(286):165–176
Lam KS, Tse VK, Wang C, Yeung RT, Ma JT, Ho JH (1987) Early effects of cranial irradiation on hypothalamic-pituitary function. J Clin Endocrinol Metab 64(3):418–424
Lam KS, Wang C, Yeung RT, et al (1986) Hypothalamic hypopituitarism following cranial irradiation for nasopharyngeal carcinoma. Clin Endocrinol (Oxf) 24(6):643–651
Lau SK, Wei WI, Sham J, Hui Y, Choy D (1992) Effect of irradiation on middle ear effusion due to nasopharyngeal carcinoma. Clin Otolaryngol Allied Sci 17(3):246–250
Lee A (1999) Complications of radiation therapy. In: Van Hasselt CA, Gibb AG (eds) Nasopharyngeal carcinoma. 2nd ed. The Chinese University of Hong Kong Press & Greenwich Medical Media, Hong Kong, pp 255–275
Lee AW, Foo W, Chappell R, et al (1998) Effect of time, dose, and fractionation on temporal lobe necrosis following radiotherapy for nasopharyngeal carcinoma. Int J Radiat Oncol Biol Phys 40(1):35–42
Lee AW, Kwong DL, Leung SF, et al (2002) Factors affecting risk of symptomatic temporal lobe necrosis: significance of fractional dose and treatment time. Int J Radiat Oncol Biol Phys 53(1):75–85
Lee AW, Lau WH, Tung SY, et al (2005) Preliminary results of a randomized study on therapeutic gain by concurrent chemotherapy for regionally-advanced nasopharyngeal carcinoma: NPC-9901 Trial by the Hong Kong Nasopharyngeal Cancer Study Group. J Clin Oncol 23(28): 6966–6975
Lee AW, Law SC, Ng SH, et al (1992) Retrospective analysis of nasopharyngeal carcinoma treated during 1976–1985: late complications following megavoltage irradiation. Br J Radiol 65(778):918–928
Lee AWMPC, Law SCK, Chua DTT, Wei WI, Chong V (2008) Nasopharynx. In: Halperin EC, Perez C, Brady LW (eds)

Perez and Brady's principles and practice of radiation oncology. 5th ed. Lippincott, Philadelphia, pp 820–857
Lee AW, Ng SH, Ho JH, et al (1988) Clinical diagnosis of late temporal lobe necrosis following radiation therapy for nasopharyngeal carcinoma. Cancer 61(8):1535–1542
Lee AW, Ng SH, Tse VK, Chiu HM, Thaw M (1993) Bilateral temporal lobectomy for necrosis induced by radiotherapy for nasopharyngeal carcinoma. Acta Oncol 32(3):343–344
Lee AW, Ng WT, Hung WM, et al (2009) Major late toxicities after conformal radiotherapy for nasopharyngeal carcinoma-patient- and treatment-related risk factors. Int J Radiat Oncol Biol Phys 73(4):1121–1128
Lee AW, Sze WM, Fowler JF, Chappell R, Leung SF, Teo P (1999) Caution on the use of altered fractionation for nasopharyngeal carcinoma. Radiother Oncol 52(3):207–211
Lee N, Harris J, Garden AS (2009) Intensity-modulated radiation therapy with or without chemotherapy for nasopharyngeal carcinoma: Radiation Therapy Oncology Group Phase II Trial 0225. J Clin Oncol
Lee N, Xia P, Quivey JM, et al (2002) Intensity-modulated radiotherapy in the treatment of nasopharyngeal carcinoma: an update of the UCSF experience. Int J Radiat Oncol Biol Phys 53(1):12–22
Lennox AJ, Shafer JP, Hatcher M, Beil J, Funder SJ (2002) Pilot study of impedance-controlled microcurrent therapy for managing radiation-induced fibrosis in head-and-neck cancer patients. Int J Radiat Oncol Biol Phys 54(1):23–34
Leon X, Quer M, Diez S, Orus C, Lopez-Pousa A, Burgues J (1999) Second neoplasm in patients with head and neck cancer. Head Neck 21(3):204–210
LeQuang C (1989) Postirradiation lesions of the brachial plexus. Results of surgical treatment. Hand Clin 5(1):23–32
LeVeque FG, Montgomery M, Potter D, et al (1993) A multicenter, randomized, double-blind, placebo-controlled, dose-titration study of oral pilocarpine for treatment of radiation-induced xerostomia in head and neck cancer patients. J Clin Oncol 11(6):1124–1131
Levine MJ, Aguirre A, Hatton MN, Tabak LA (1987) Artificial salivas: present and future. J Dent Res 66:Spec No 693–698
Levy RL, Miller NR (2006) Hyperbaric oxygen therapy for radiation-induced optic neuropathy. Ann Acad Med Singapore 35(3):151–157
Lin S, Pan J, Han L, Zhang X, Liao X, Lu JJ (2009) Nasopharyngeal carcinoma treated with reduced-volume intensity-modulated radiation therapy: report on the 3-year outcome of a prospective series. Int J Radiat Oncol Biol Phys Apr 11. [Epub ahead of print]
Lin YS, Jen YM, Lin JC (2002) Radiation-related cranial nerve palsy in patients with nasopharyngeal carcinoma. Cancer 95(2):404–409
Liu RP, Fleming TJ, Toth BB, Keene HJ (1990) Salivary flow rates in patients with head and neck cancer 0.5 to 25 years after radiotherapy. Oral Surg Oral Med Oral Pathol 70(6):724–729
Malouf JG, Aragon C, Henson BS, Eisbruch A, Ship JA (2003) Influence of parotid-sparing radiotherapy on xerostomia in head and neck cancer patients. Cancer Detect Prev 27(4): 305–310
Marks JE, Bedwinek JM, Lee F, Purdy JA, Perez CA (1982) Dose-response analysis for nasopharyngeal carcinoma: an historical perspective. Cancer 50(6):1042–1050
Mendes DG, Nawalkar RR, Eldar S (1991) Post-irradiation femoral neuropathy. A case report. J Bone Joint Surg Am 73(1):137–140
Mesic JB, Fletcher GH, Goepfert H (1981) Megavoltage irradiation of epithelial tumors of the nasopharynx. Int J Radiat Oncol Biol Phys 7(4):447–453
Mihalcea O, Arnold AC (2008) Side effect of head and neck radiotherapy: optic neuropathy. Oftalmologia 52(1):36–40
Murphy BA, Gilbert J (2009) Dysphagia in head and neck cancer patients treated with radiation: assessment, sequelae, and rehabilitation. Semin Radiat Oncol 19(1):35–42
Nicolatou-Galitis O, Sotiropoulou-Lontou A, Velegraki A, et al (2003) Oral candidiasis in head and neck cancer patients receiving radiotherapy with amifostine cytoprotection. Oral Oncol 39(4):397–401
O'Sullivan B, Levin W (2003) Late radiation-related fibrosis: pathogenesis, manifestations, and current management. Semin Radiat Oncol 13(3):274–289
Parsons J (1994)Time-dose-volume relations in radiation therapy. In: Million RR CN (ed) Management of head and neck cancer a multidisciplinary approach, 2nd edn. Lippincott, Philadelphia, PA, pp 204–244
Pierce SM, Recht A, Lingos TI, et al (1992) Long-term radiation complications following conservative surgery (CS) and radiation therapy (RT) in patients with early stage breast cancer. Int J Radiat Oncol Biol Phys 23(5):915–923
Powell S, Cooke J, Parsons C (1990) Radiation-induced brachial plexus injury: follow-up of two different fractionation schedules. Radiother Oncol 18(3):213–220
Rieke JW, Hafermann MD, Johnson JT, et al (1995) Oral pilocarpine for radiation-induced xerostomia: integrated efficacy and safety results from two prospective randomized clinical trials. Int J Radiat Oncol Biol Phys 31(3): 661–669
Ronchetti D, Arisi E, Neri A, et al (2005) Microsatellite analyses of recurrence or second primary tumor in head and neck cancer. Anticancer Res 25(4):2771–2775
Rubin DI, Schomberg PJ, Shepherd RF, Panneton JM (2001) Arteritis and brachial plexus neuropathy as delayed complications of radiation therapy. Mayo Clin Proc 76(8):849–852
Rudat V, Meyer J, Momm F, et al (2000) Protective effect of amifostine on dental health after radiotherapy of the head and neck. Int J Radiat Oncol Biol Phys 48(5):1339–1343
Salner AL, Botnick LE, Herzog AG, et al (1981) Reversible brachial plexopathy following primary radiation therapy for breast cancer. Cancer Treat Rep 65(9–10):797–802
Saunders WH, Hodgson SE (1979) Bilateral hypoglossal nerve paralysis after irradiation therapy. Ann Otol Rhinol Laryngol 88(4 Pt 1):515–517
Schultheiss TE, Kun LE, Ang KK, Stephens LC (1995). Radiation response of the central nervous system. Int J Radiat Oncol Biol Phys 31(5):1093–1112
Sham J, Choy D, Kwong PW, et al (1994) Radiotherapy for nasopharyngeal carcinoma: shielding the pituitary may improve therapeutic ratio. Int J Radiat Oncol Biol Phys 29(4):699–704
Skinner DW, Lesser TH, Richards SH (1988) A 15 year follow-up of a controlled trial of the use of grommets in glue ear. Clin Otolaryngol Allied Sci 13(5):341–346
Slaughter DP, Southwick HW, Smejkal W (1953) Field cancerization in oral stratified squamous epithelium; clinical implications of multicentric origin. Cancer 6(5):963–968
Sloan AE, Arnold SM, St Clair WH, Regine WF (2003) Brain injury: current management and investigations. Semin Radiat Oncol 13(3):309–321
Spielman AI (1990) Interaction of saliva and taste. J Dent Res 69(3):838–843

St Clair WH, Arnold SM, Sloan AE, et al (2003) Spinal cord and peripheral nerve injury: current management and investigations. Semin Radiat Oncol 13(3):322–332

Stephens LC, King GK, Peters LJ, Ang KK, Schultheiss TE, Jardine JH (1986) Unique radiosensitivity of serous cells in rhesus monkey submandibular glands. Am J Pathol 124(3):479–487

Stinson SF, DeLaney TF, Greenberg J, et al (1991) Acute and long-term effects on limb function of combined modality limb sparing therapy for extremity soft tissue sarcoma. Int J Radiat Oncol Biol Phys 21(6):1493–1499

Stoll BA, Andrews JT (1966) Radiation-induced peripheral neuropathy. Br Med J 1:834–837

Stryker JA, Sommerville K, Perez R, Velkley DE (1990) Sacral plexus injury after radiotherapy for carcinoma of cervix. Cancer 66(7):1488–1492

Sultanem K, Shu HK, Xia P, et al (2000) Three-dimensional intensity-modulated radiotherapy in the treatment of nasopharyngeal carcinoma: the University of California-San Francisco experience. Int J Radiat Oncol Biol Phys 48(3):711–722

Trotti A, Colevas AD, Setser A, et al (2003) CTCAE v3.0: development of a comprehensive grading system for the adverse effects of cancer treatment. Semin Radiat Oncol 13(3): 176–181

Vacha P, Fehlauer F, Mahlmann B, et al (2003) Randomized phase III trial of postoperative radiochemotherapy +/- amifostine in head and neck cancer. Is there evidence for radioprotection? Strahlenther Onkol 179(6):385–389

van Oijen MG, Leppers Vd Straat FG, Tilanus MG, Slootweg PJ (2000) The origins of multiple squamous cell carcinomas in the aerodigestive tract. Cancer 88(4):884–893

Wang X, Lu JJ, Xiong X, et al (2009) Anatomic and dosimetric changes during the treatment course of intensity-modulated radiotherapy for locally advanced nasopharyngeal carcinoma? Med Dosim

Warde P, O'Sullivan B, Aslanidis J, et al (2002) A Phase III placebo-controlled trial of oral pilocarpine in patients undergoing radiotherapy for head-and-neck cancer. Int J Radiat Oncol Biol Phys 54(1):9–13

Wee J, Tan EH, Tai BC, et al (2005) Randomized trial of radiotherapy versus concurrent chemoradiotherapy followed by adjuvant chemotherapy in patients with American Joint Committee on Cancer/International Union against cancer stage III and IV nasopharyngeal cancer of the endemic variety. J Clin Oncol 23(27):6730–6738

Wescott WB, Mira JG, Starcke EN, Shannon IL, Thornby JI (1978) Alterations in whole saliva flow rate induced by fractionated radiotherapy. AJR Am J Roentgenol 130(1): 145–149

Yamamoto E, Shibuya H, Yoshimura R (2002) Miura M. Site specific dependency of second primary cancer in early stage head and neck squamous cell carcinoma. Cancer 94(7):2007–2014

Yeh SA, Tang Y, Lui CC, Huang YJ, Huang EY (2005) Treatment outcomes and late complications of 849 patients with nasopharyngeal carcinoma treated with radiotherapy alone. Int J Radiat Oncol Biol Phys 62(3):672–679

Nasopharyngeal Cancer in Pediatric and Adolescent Patients

23

Enis Ozyar and Inci Ayan

CONTENTS

Enis Ozyar, MD
Professor of Radiation Oncology, Acibadem Maslak Hospital Acibadem University,Department of Radiation Oncology Maslak, 34457, Turkey
Inci Ayan MD
Professor of Pediatric Oncology, Acibadem Maslak Hospital Acibadem University, Department of Pediatrics, Maslak, 34457, Turkey

23.1 Introduction

Nasopharyngeal carcinoma (NPC) is a rare disease in children with distinct epidemiological and etiological features, histopathological characteristics, and clinical presentation. The incidence of pediatric NPC varies widely around the world, and both genetic and environmental factors contribute to the development of the disease. Children with NPC almost always have the undifferentiated variant of the disease, which is associated with advanced locoregional spread and distant metastases. Currently, cisplatin-based induction chemotherapy followed by high-dose radiotherapy is the treatment of choice. Although multimodality treatment has increased the 5-year survival to 70%–90%, late morbidity is a major concern. Immune-modulation with interferon has resulted in excellent outcome, and studies have been extended to investigate the impact of immunotherapy on survival, in combination with less toxic chemoradiotherapy.

The aim of this chapter is to address the current management strategy of pediatric NPC, as well as discuss the future direction of research for improved treatment of the disease.

23.2 Etiological and Epidemiological Features

NPC is one of the few malignancies in childhood that emerge from the epithelium, and constitutes 1%–5% of all pediatric cancers and 20%–50% of all primary nasopharyngeal malignant tumors in children (Ayan et al. 2003). Several studies indicated the distinct clinical features of pediatric NPC when compared with its adult counterpart (Ayan and Altun 1996). Young patients have a higher rate of lymph node metastasis, fewer WHO Type 1 (keratinizing) tumors, and a better prognosis when compared with adults (Huang 1982).

NPC is a malignant tumor with a variable range of incidence depending on age, ethnicity, and geographic localization (Wei and Sham 2005). In Southeast Asia, where the incidence is the highest in the world, the incidence of NPC demonstrates a single peak at about the age of 50 years (Huang 1982). However, NPC shows a bimodal age distribution in nonendemic countries and the first peak is seen in the second decade in addition to the second peak at more advanced age (Selek et al. 2005) While the rate of pediatric patients accounts for 6%–18% of all NPC patients in nonendemic countries like Argentina, Turkey, India, Israel, Morocco, Tunisia, Algeria, and Uganda, the rate is reported to be less than 1% of all NPCs in the endemic countries (Zubizarretta et al. 2000; Berberoglu et al. 2001; Laskar et al. 2004; Bar-Sela et al. 2005; Cammoun et al. 1974; Ayan I et al 2003; Sahraoui et al. 1999; Schmauz et al. 1972). Although NPC has the highest incidence worldwide, in Southeast China, first peak does not exist (Sham et al. 1990). The number of patients less than 15 years of age is reported to be 53 (0.1%) among 54,304 NPC patients treated between 1964 and 1983 in Guangdong Province of China, where NPC has the highest incidence (Huang et al. 1990). However, the rate of pediatric cases is reported to be 5% in Liaoning Province, one of the areas with lowest risk for NPC in China, from where a retrospective analysis of 117 Chinese pediatric or adolescent NPC patients was reported recently (Cao et al. 2006).

Although the incidence of NPC is less frequent in Mediterranean basin countries than in Southeast China, there is an additional minor peak between the ages of 10 and 20 years besides the second peak at the fifth decade. There is a significant number of reports in the literature which reported the treatment results of pediatric and adolescent NPC patients from the Maghrep countries, Egypt, Israel, and Turkey (Serin et al. 1998; Har-Kedar et al. 1974). A few studies reported a substantial number of pediatric NPC in France; however, more than two-thirds of accrued patients were originally from Maghrep countries (Habrand et al. 2004). However, data from Portugal, Italy, and Greece suggested that the incidence of pediatric NPC is not as high as in southern and eastern Mediterranean countries (Polychronopoulou et al. 2004).

Southern and eastern Mediterranean countries with high incidence of pediatric NPC share two important characteristics. They are all developing and are Muslim countries, except Israel, although approximately 30% of Israel's population consists of Muslim Arabs. A case-control study was carried out to assess the genetic and environmental risk factors in Maghreb countries (Northern Africa countries bordering the Mediterranean) by the International Agency for Research of Cancer (Feng et al. 2007). This study postulated that consanguinity (15%–30% of marriages) might have increased the level of genetic homozygozity which may have caused a recessive susceptibility. We may partly explain the higher proportion of young cases observed in the Mediterranean basin countries, especially Muslim countries of this region like Turkey, Morocco, Egypt, Tunisia, and Algeria, when compared with the Southeastern Asian countries where consanguinity is socio-culturally rare. However, results of this study have shown no significant difference between the proportion of cases and controls reporting consanguinity in parents (18.3% vs. 19.8%, p = 0.48) (Feng et al. 2007).

In the United States, only 3% of NPC occurs in patients younger than 19 years of age according to Surveillance, Epidemiology and End Results (SEER) data (Marks et al. 1998), and pediatric NPC is more prevelant among African-Americans and its geographic distribution favours southern states (Greene et al. 1977). Furthermore, approximately and 38% of the cases in NPC patients younger than 20 years or between 20 and 40 years were undifferentiated subtype, respectively, whereas patients older than 40 years were often diagnosed with keratinizing squamous cell carcinoma. The randomized study conducted by the Pediatric Oncology Group (POG) enrolled 18 patients from 59 institutions to the POG 9486 study, and majority of patients from the United States were from Southeastern or Southern–Midwestern institutions. Among all the accrued patients, 65% were reportedly of African-American origin (Rodriguez-Galindo et al. 2005).

Most of the reports on pediatric NPC have demonstrated a male predominance (Uzel et al. 2001). The largest series in the literature published by the Rare Cancer Network (RCN) have shown a male to female preponderance of 2:1 in 165 patients (Ozyar et al. 2006).

The differences between endemic and nonendemic NPC suggests underlying etiologic variations between children and adults. It is postulated that distinct oncogenic mechanisms exists for the pediatric form of NPC in the literature (Khabir et al. 2003). Major risk factors for NPC include diet, Epstein–Barr virus (EBV) reactivation, and genetic susceptibility (Jeannel et al. 1999). Common risk factors among

Catonese, Arabs, and Inuits for NPC include high consumption of preserved foods and dried meats in childhood, when compared with the controls in an earlier study (Hubert and De-The 1982). In the intermediate- to high-risk Chinese populations such as those from the Southern provinces, consumption of salted fish, especially during weaning in childhood, has been found to be associated with increased risk of NPC (Yuan et al. 2000).

Earlier reports and favorable treatment outcomes have demonstrated that pediatric form of NPC has features reminiscent of lymphomas. Recently, a few researchers pointed to the role of EBV in the pathogenesis of various neoplasms including Hodgkin's disease and NPC, and indicated that both malignancies have the same type II EBV latency and show bimodal age distribution (Barista et al. 2007).

Specific human leukocyte antigens (HLA) and alleles have been associated with adult NPC in several populations including Asian and North African populations (Goldsmith et al. 2002; Dardari et al. 2001). A similar study was presented recently on young Turkish patients with an age of less than 30 years (Daglikoca et al. 2007). In this study, four of the genes (BLU, RASSF1, p16-INK4a, and UBAP1), previously implied on adult NPC cases, were chosen and analyzed, with the hypothesis that these genes may cause liability to childhood NPC in a recessive manner. The homozygosity frequency of the patient group was found to be twice as high as the frequency of the control group, and the authors concluded that their result provides strong evidence to support the hypothesis that p16-INK4a causes liability to NPC, but it is not sufficient to support the hypothesis that it causes liability to childhood-specific NPC.

Distinct clinical features of pediatric NPC led the investigators to search for biological characteristics, which may explain this clinical difference between the pediatric and adult NPCs (Ayan and Altun 2003). Expression of p53, Bcl-2 family, Ki67, c-Kit, cyclooxygenase-2, epidermal growth factor receptor, and EBV latent membrane protein (EBV LMP1) was evaluated in a cohort of pediatric NPC patients, and prediction of survival, recurrence, lymph node metastasis was found in some (Khabir et al. 2000; Fang et al. 2007).

Khabir et al. (2000) previously demonstrated that p53 accumulation is much less frequent in younger patients. The same group of researchers investigated Bcl-2 and Bcl-X expression by immunohistochemistry in patients below 30 years of age or those aged over 30 years. The average Bcl-2 score was found to be much lower for patients below 30 years of age, and concluded that this finding strengthened their hypothesis that oncologic mechanisms may be different for pediatric and adult patients. Their comparison of clinical data revealed a major difference between patients below 30 years of age or older in terms of frequency of lymph node involvement also. While all patients below 30 years of age had clinical lymph node invasion, the figure was 66% for patients older than 30 years of age. The same observation was made previously by Maalej et al. (1995), and they found that almost all the patients in their series with T4N0 disease were over 30 years of age.

23.3 Treatment Strategy

The optimal treatment modality for pediatric NPC has not been established; however, any potential reduction in radiation field and doses is desirable due to the significant chronic morbidity among long-term survivors. While the concomitant chemotherapy and radiation, with or without adjuvant chemotherapy, is the current standard for adult patients with NPC, neoadjuvant chemotherapy with radiotherapy has gained popularity parallel to other paediatric treatment protocols in various solid tumors (Al-Sarraf et al. 1998; Ayan et al. 2000).

23.4 Radiation Therapy

Radiation therapy (RT) has been the mainstay of the treatment in both adult and pediatric NPC (Wei and Sham 2005; Ozyar et al. 1999). Owing to the rarity of pediatric NPC, most of the published series are relatively heterogeneous in terms of patient, tumor, and treatment characteristics. Moreover, radiotherapy dose for disease control in paediatric NPC has reportedly ranged from 50 to 70 Gy in the literature (Fernandez et al. 1976; Gasparini et al. 1988).

Literature on RT for pediatric NPC can be classified into the following three groups: historical retrospective series published in the late 1970s and early 1980s, more recent retrospective series, and prospective series. Reports in the first group of literature typically included few patients, with inadequate staging, and with suboptimal treatment strategies such as radiotherapy using orthovoltage or Co-60 techniques and noncisplatin-based chemotherapy regimens (Lombardi et al. 1982; Deutsch et al. 1978; Jenkin et al. 1981; Jereb et al. 1980; Berry et al. 1980). Results of these reports generally proposed the use of total tumor radiation doses in the range of 35–86 Gy and pointed out the need for effective systemic treatment in addition to radiotherapy.

The second group of papers were published in the 1990s, with improved local and systemic staging of the disease and improved treatment parameters (mostly linear accelerator external-beam radiation therapy (EBRT), including reports with CT treatment planning and cisplatin-based chemotherapy) (Pao et al. 1989; Ingersoll et al. 1990; Martin et al. 1994; Ghim et al. 1998; Wolden et al. 2000; Daoud et al. 2003; Kupeli et al. 2005). The majority of these retrospective studies found the optimum dose to the primary tumor to be between 50 and 70 Gy, with the suggestion of higher efficacy with doses greater than 60–66 Gy in some reports (Laskar et al. 2004; Ozyar et al. 2006). Superior results were reported with the use of cisplatin-based chemotherapy and neoadjuvant chemotherapy when compared with the regimens without cisplatin and adjuvant chemotherapy schedules (Ayan et al. 2000; Kupeli et al. 2005).

The RCN study is the largest retrospective analysis in the literature aimed to analyze the results in terms of local control, survival, and the possible prognostic factors in 165 paediatric NPC patients collected worldwide (Ozyar et al. 2006). The patient's age at diagnosis ranged from 7 to 17 years. There was a predominance of males (66.1%). Histopathological classification revealed 23 (13.9%) patients with WHO type II and 142 (86.1%) patients with WHO type III. All patients were treated with fractionated EBRT to a median dose of 66 Gy. While 13% of the patients were treated with radiotherapy alone, 87% of the patients received chemotherapy in addition to radiotherapy. The actuarial overall 5-year survival (OS) was 78%, whereas the actuarial 5-year local relapse-free survival (LRFS), loco-regional relapse free survival (LRRFS), distant metastasis-free survival (DMFS), and disease-free survival (DFS) rates were 88%, 82%, 81.5%, and 69%, respectively. In multivariate analysis, statistically significant unfavorable factors were age older than 14 years for LRC; male gender for DMFS; T3, T4 disease for LRFS; N3 disease for DFS and OS; total nasopharyngeal EBRT dose of less than 66 Gy for LRFS and LRRFS; and patients treated with radiotherapy alone for LRFS, LRRFS, and DFS. The nodal tumor bulk seems to be the major parameter affecting survival, and nasopharyngeal dose of ≥66 Gy turned out to be still important in achieving local control according to this retrospective review. As this study is a retrospective comparison between experiences at multiple institutions, one may argue that patient-selection bias may have impacted the results. Although a randomized study is always preferable, the results of this retrospective review would still provide valuable contribution to understanding the basic behavior of pediatric NPC, regarding the outcome and treatment approach.

Recently, retrospective analysis of 74 pediatric NPC patients treated between 1978 and 2004 at the Gustave Roussy Institute (IGR) was reported in 2004 as an abstract (Habrand et al. 2004). Almost 75% of the patients were originally from Maghreb countries and treated with different cisplatin-based chemotherapy multiregimens. Either low-dose radiotherapy (50 Gy) was administered to good responders to neoadjuvant chemotherapy (54% of the patients) or high-dose radiotherapy (65–70 Gy). Despite a similar locoregional recurrence rate in the two groups, event-free survival (EFS) and OS rates were better in the low-dose radiotherapy group. In addition, late toxicity was improved in the low-dose group as well. Thus, the authors concluded that response-adapted dose reduction seems to be possible in selected pediatric NPC patients.

Recent data supporting response-adapted dose-reduced radiotherapy have been published by Institut Curie, from France (Orbach et al. 2008). Thirty-four children were treated for 27 years and 20 out of 34 were reported to be of North African origin. The cervical nodal irradiation dose was reduced to less than 50 Gy in the case of a good response to chemotherapy. All but one child received neoadjuvant chemotherapy with various regimens, and the overall chemotherapy response rate was reported to be 78%. Fifteen patients had dose-reduced cervical nodal irradiation (range: 45–50 Gy). The primary tumor dose ranged between 45 and 66 Gy. Local and distant failure rates were 10% and 18%, respectively. The 5-year OS was 73% and the EFS was 75%. The authors concluded that cervical nodal failure rate was low despite radiotherapy dose reduction in the case of a good response to neoadjuvant chemotherapy, and they proposed a dose reduction for primary disease less than 50 Gy in the case of good response to initial chemotherapy.

There are only two reported prospective studies in the literature on the management of pediatric NPC, and these constitute the third group of publications in the literature (Mertens et al. 1997, 2005; Rodriguez-Galindo et al. 2005). A prospective German trial, conducted in the early 1990s, treated patients with neoadjuvant chemotherapy with adjuvant recombinant IFN-β (MERTENS et al. 1997). A total dose of 59.4 Gy was given to all patients, independent of their T-status, with a response rate of 91%. Definitive results of this study were reported recently for 59 patients treated between 1992 and 2003, with a median follow-up time of 48 months (MERTENS et al. 2005). In their study, 58 of 59 patients responded to three courses of chemotherapy and only one patient progressed during chemotherapy. Based on the potentially strong role of EBV infection in the pathogenesis of the disease, all the patients received adjuvant recombinant IFN-β. Using this approach, an excellent outcome was reported with only distant relapse in three and local recurrence in one patient. A new treatment protocol was initiated by the same group by changing several treatment parameters with the primary aim to further improve the outcome in this patient group. The major changes were as follows: methotrexate was omitted from combined schedule due to the severe mucositis with this agent, chemoradiation therapy introduced based on adult studies that showed enhanced survival, and a total radiotherapy dose reduction to 54 Gy, instead of 59 Gy, was made in patients with complete response (CR) after three courses of chemotherapy, with the intent of reducing late-term fibrosis and bone necrosis.

The second prospective study was reported recently by the Pediatric Oncology Group (POG 9486) (RODRIGUEZ-GALINDO et al. 2005). This study included 18 patients less than 22 years of age treated from 1990 to 1994. All the patients were enrolled from south eastern or midwestern United States. About 65% of the patients were African-Americans. Stage I–II patients were treated with radiotherapy alone and stage III–IV patients were treated with four courses of preradiation chemotherapy. The primary tumor and involved lymphatics were treated to a total tumor dose of 61.2 Gy with a shrinking-field technique volume. The target volume was the prechemotherapy volume as defined by any combination of CT/MRI scans or nasopharyngeal examination. The overall response rate to induction chemotherapy was 93.7% with 4-year EFS and OS rates of 77% and 75%, respectively. The investigators initiated the new ARAR 0331 study, in which they explored the use of induction chemotherapy with cisplatin and 5-FU, followed by concurrent chemotherapy similar to the German protocol.

Both the studies revealed that the total primary radiotherapy dose reduction to 60 Gy is feasible. However, the OS and disease-free survival rates were superior in the German study when compared with the U. S. study, despite the fact that the POG-study patients received one chemotherapy cycle more and a slightly higher total dose of radiation. The results of RCN study, by some means, conflict with the abovementioned prospective studies opposing dose reduction; however, both the patients and neoadjuvant chemotherapy schedules in these centers were not homogeneous. Therefore, this divergence might indicate that higher doses still play an important role in the absence of effective chemotherapy regimens and response-directed radiotherapy schedules.

At this time, the standard treatment of pediatric NPC consists of high-dose radiotherapy and chemotherapy. The primary disease, the structures surrounding nasopharynx and the entire neck should be included in the high-dose radiation portal. Although pediatric NPC patients usually have an excellent acute tolerability to the treatment, long-term radiation-induced toxicities such as dental caries, trismus, xerostomia, hearing impairment, growth retardation of the facial bones, and soft-tissue fibrosis are major concerns.

Pediatric NPC is one of the pediatric malignancies where significant reduction in radiation dose have not yet been proven, although the results of the two prospective studies and retrospective IGR analysis suggest such measure may be possible. Therefore, every effort should be made to prevent these patients from severe late sequelae without jeopardizing the good disease control. These efforts may include the use of high-tech treatments like intensity-modulated radiotherapy (IMRT), use of radioprotectors (e.g., amifostine) during radiotherapy, response-based total radiotherapy dose reduction, radiotherapy field reductions (e.g., omitting supraclavicular fields, except in patients with N3b disease), use of brachytherapy, use of new chemotherapeutic agents or modifiying their administration sequence when managing pediatric NPCs (CHUA et al. 2005; SELEK et al. 2005).

Intracavitary brachytherapy was used to reduce EBRT after 50–55 Gy by several centers in the literature (OZYAR et al. 2002; NAKAMURA et al. 2005). Although early T-disease can be treated adequately by brachytherapy boost, patients with locally-advanced diseases are not good candidates for brachytherapy because of the nonhomogenous dose distribution. A large cohort of pediatric NPC patients treated with brachytherapy boost dose was recently reported from a center at Brazil (NAKAMURA et al. 2005). A total of 16 patients received neoadjuvant chemotherapy, EBRT, and high dose-rate brachytherapy boost and adjuvant chemotherapy. The total dose of 10 Gy was given in two fractions under local anesthesia using metallic applicators. At the median follow-up time of 54 months, the local control was achieved in 15 out of 16 patients. However, one should be cautious when evaluating these results as other series had high rates of local control with similar external radiotherapy doses.

It was shown that IMRT provides superior target coverage and normal tissue sparing when compared with conventional radiotherapy (CRT) in adult patients with NPC (Kam et al. 2004). However, when compared with CRT, a twofold increase in the integral dose has been theoretically estimated with the use of IMRT due to the larger treatment volumes. In the pediatric setting, the risk could be significant due to a higher inherent susceptibility of tissues. However, as the risk of secondary cancers related with IMRT was estimated to be 2% when compared with 1% for CRT, it seems logical to utilize IMRT in pediatric NPC to decrease the significant late effects. The efficacy of IMRT in reducing the acute and late toxicity in children with NPC was recently reported by two centers (Louis et al. 2007; Laskar et al. 2008). A single institution experience with five pediatric NPC patients who were treated with chemotherapy and IMRT was reported (Louis et al. 2007). With a median follow-up of 6.3 years, all the patients experienced ≥3 of acute and late toxicities. The most common toxicities were reported to be hypothyroidism, xerostomia, hearing loss, and dental disease. The authors concluded that they did not observe a significant decrease in the long-term toxicities with IMRT plus chemotherapy in their small cohort of pediatric NPC patients. The second study was reported from the Tata Memorial Center in India (Laskar et al. 2008). A total of 36 children were included in this retrospective study. All the patients had undifferentiated carcinoma and were treated with a combination of chemotherapy and radiation therapy. Of the 36 patients, 19 underwent IMRT and 17 underwent CRT. The average mean dose to the first and second planning target volume was 71.8 and 62.5 Gy with IMRT, when compared with 66.3 and 64.4 Gy with CRT, respectively. After a median follow-up of 27 months, the 2-year locoregional control, DFS, and OS rate was 76.5%, 60.6%, and 71.3%, respectively. A significant reduction in acute Grade 3 toxicities of the skin, mucous membrane, and pharynx was noted with the use of IMRT. The median time to the development of Grade 2 toxicity was delayed with IMRT (skin, 35 vs. 25 days; mucous-membrane, 39 vs. 27 days; and larynx, 50 vs. 28 days). They concluded that IMRT could significantly reduce and delay the onset of acute toxicity, resulting in improved tolerance and treatment compliance for children with NPC. However, the number of studies with IMRT in pediatric NPC was very limited and other centers' experiences are required.

Integration of new chemotherapeutic agents or modifiying their administration sequence when managing pediatric NPCs is another way to improve results. In a randomized phase III study, it was demonstrated that patients with squamous-cell carcinoma of the head and neck who received docetaxel plus cisplatin and fluorouracil induction chemotherapy plus chemoradiotherapy had a significantly longer survival than those who received cisplatin and fluorouracilinductionchemotherapypluschemoradiotherapy (Posner et al. 2007). This study led the investigators to explore the role of docetaxel in pediatric NPC. An international randomized study recently compared two- vs. three-drug regimen including docetaxel in 72 pediatric NPC. The results of this study are expected for the optimal chemotherapy regimen for neoadjuvant use.

Another recent major modification of treatment algorithm is to use concomitant chemoradiotherapy after the induction chemotherapy in pediatric NPC. This modification was introduced based on adult studies that revealed improved survival and is currently evaluated by the German and U. S. groups within randomized studies. However, one should be cautious on the synergistic effect of cisplatin on hearing apparatus when used concurrent with radiotherapy, until the mature results of these studies are available.

The investigations should be encouraged to determine the optimal radiotherapy dose and field reductions in selected patients, while investigating the optimal chemotherapy schedule and timing. Regional or international collaboration would facilitate to clarify and refine the etiology, pathogenesis, and treatment of this rare malignancy.

23.5 Systemic Treatments

Owing to the rarity of NPC in children and adolescents, the majority of published studies on chemotherapy for the disease are of retrospective nature with long-term experiences. This type of literature is usually complicated with high heterogeneous patient population and disease characteristics, staging methods, and treatment modalities. Therefore, it is usually difficult to interpret the historical and more recent results within the same study or to compare them with other studies.

During the past three decades, studies on the treatment of adults and children with NPC have identified several factors that can explain the rationale underlying chemotherapy in the management of childhood and young adolescence NPC:

1. Undifferantiated histopathology associated with advanced locoregional disease at presentation.
2. Propensity to systemic metastasis.
3. ltough highly sensitive to high dose radiotherapy initially, high rate of distant and locoregional recurrences might be observed.
4. Radiation volume and doses adopted from adults have serious acute and late effects including second malignancies in young patients.
5. Undifferantiated NPC is highly chemosensitive.
6. Preradiation chemotherapy minimizes the risk of distant recurrence through eradication of micrometastases.
7. Complete response or marked and rapid reduction in tumor volume can be achieved by preradiation chemotherapy resulting in improvement in locoregional disease control.
8. Preradiation chemotherapy may render to reduce radiation dose and volume in children by decreasing the tumor volume.
9. Concurrent administration of chemotherapy with radiation as a radiosensitizer may have a role in improving DMFS, perhaps through better loco-regional control.
10. Better OS and DFS by the integration of chemotherapy.

As with other malignancies, attempts on chemotherapy in NPC started in the mid-1960s. Single agents (mostly cyclophosphamide) or different chemotherapeutic combinations of noncisplatin agents adopted from the adult NPC trails have been employed as an adjuvant treatment, following 35–83 Gy radiotherapy, in patients with advanced diseases. The results of these early studies suggested that combined modality treatment may be of value (Deutsch et al. 1978; Jenkin et al. 1981). By the 1990s, several long-term and heterogeneous data from single or multiinstitutional series have provided valuable information and contributed to our understanding of childhood and adolescence NPC regarding biological and clinical characteristics, as well as the utilization of chemotherapy following radiotherapy. Various combinations of cyclophosphamide, vincristin, doxorubicin, actinomycin-D, 5-FU, methotrexate, and bleomycin have been used in postradiation setting, and 5-year OS rates of 30%–58% have been reported in these studies (Table 23.1).

Unfortunately, the postradiation chemotherapy studies did not provide a standard chemotherapy regimen in terms of drug combination, doses, and treatment duration. Furthermore, these studies did not result in an improved outcome when compared with the trials used for radiotherapy alone in children with NPC. It was suggested that the unsatisfactory results might be due to inadequate drug-dose intensity, ineffective chemotherapy combinations, insufficient courses of treatment, delay in systemic disease control in the setting of postradiation, and/or the lack of randomized studies because of small sample sizes.

One of the early studies on preradiation chemotherapy reported by Lobo-Sanahuja et al. (1986) demonstrated a 100% (12/12) clinical response rate to 6-week trail of preradiation cyclophosphamide alternated with adriamycine. The same chemotherapy regimen was continued following reduced doses (45–60 Gy) of radiotherapy for 30 more weeks, resulting in a 67% OS rate at 5 years. This limited experience indicated that pre and postradiation chemotherapy was effective in prolonging DFS and may allow a decrease in the radiation dose. Another improved result in pediatric NPC patients were reported by Gasparini et al. (1988), who, in a small series of children, demonstrated a 2-year relapse-free survival of 75% with preradiation VAC followed by radiation therapy. Several retrospective studies have been published thereafter. In most of these series, cisplatin-based preradiation chemotherapy combinations were used, and OS rates of 45%–91% have been reported (Table 23.1). Some of the chemotherapy regimens used in these studies are provided in Table 23.2.

Excellent overall response rates were achieved with these induction regimens. A single-institution experience from Argentina demonstrated a 100% overall response rate in 11 children, 5 (45%) of whom had CR with three courses of bleomycin, cisplatin, and 5-FU (Zubizarreta et al. 2000). In another single-institution study from Turkey, we have reported 100% overall response rate (22% CR, 39% very good partial response (VGPR), and 39% partial response (PR)) following three cycles of bleomycin, epirubicin, and cisplatin in

Table 23.1. Pre and/or postradiation chemotherapy studies in children and adolescents with advance stage nasopharyngeal carcinoma (NPC)

Patient Number (age)	Chemotherapy	Radiotherapy (Gy; tm/nod)	Locoregioal control (%)	Survival (%)	Study-years/Author (Reference)
11	Post-RT	45/77	–	45	1965–1980 LOMBARDI et al. (1982)
10	Post-RT	50/60	–	40	1970–1983 LOBO-SANAHUJA et al. (1986)
12	Pre and post-RT	45–60/50	–	67	
(<13 year)				$p < 0.05$	
13	None	66/50	65	36	1971–1998 WOLDEN et al. (2000)
20	Pre and post-RT or concurrent and post-RT	66/50	84	76	
(<20 year)			$p = 0.25$	$p < 0.05$	
19	Post-RT	50/70	–	30.9	1972–2002 KUPELI et al. (2005)
65	Pre-RT	50/70	–	63.4	
(<17 year)	Without platin			80	
	With platin			$p = 0.001$	
23	None	62/50	52	46	1976–1993 AYAN and ALTUN (1996)
13	Post-RT	62/50	71	58	
12	Pre-RT	62/50	89	76	
(<16 year)				$p > 0.05$	
21	None	66	65	62	1978–2003 OZYAR et al. (2002)
144	Pre-RT ± concurrent and/or post-RT	66	85	80	
(<18 year)			$p = 0.02$	$p = 0.1$	
20	None	70/40–54	74.7	75	1978–1998 UZEL et al. (2001)
12	Pre-RT		100	73.3	
(<16 year)			$p = 0.1$	$p = 0.6$	
32	None	66/66	61	42	1979–1996 SERIN et al. (1998)
24	Pre ± post-RT or concurrent	66/66	63	58	
(<20 year)					
30	None	60–70/60–65	–	38	1980–1993 SAHRAOUI et al. (1999)
22	Pre-RT	60–70/60–65		52	
(<15 year)				$p < 0.001$	
11 (<14 year)	Pre-RT	55/45	–	91	1988–1997 ZUBIZARRETA et al. (2000)
4	None	50–72/45–50	88	63	1989–1999 BERBEROGLU et al. (2001)
29 (<17 year)	Pre and/or post-RT	50–72/45–50			
10 (<16)	Pre-RT	56/66	–	75	GASPARINI et al. (1988)
7	None	55–70	–	36	1990–2000 LASKAR et al. (2004, 2008)
57	Pre-RT			67	
(<18 year)				$p = 0.296$	
36 (7–16 year)	Pre-RT	55–72	–	86.5	1990–2004 ALTUN et al. (2008)
37 (17–25 year)	Pre-RT	62–75	–	71.5	
12	None	58–74	96–100	83.3	1994–2001 SELEK et al. (2005)
47 (<30 year)	Pre ± post-RT ± concurrent	± brakiterapi		65 (<16 year 90.5)	
				$p = 0.34$	

Table 23.2. Chemotherapy combinations for children and adolescents with NPC[a]

MPF	Methotrexate: 120 mg/m² IV on day 1
	Cisplatin: 100 mg/m²/6 h. IV infusion on day 2
	5FU: 1,000 mg/m²/24 h. IV infusion on days 1–3 or 5
PF	Cisplatin: 100 mg/m²/4 h. IV infusion on day 1
	Or 20 mg/m²/1 h. IV infusion on days 1–5
	5-FU: 1,000 mg/m²/24 h. IV infusion on days 1–5
BEC	Bleomycin: 15 mg/m² IV bolus dose on day 1, and
	12 mg/m²/24 h. IV infusion on days 1–5
	Epirubicin: 70 mg/m²/1 h. IV infusion on day 1
	Cisplatin: 100 mg/m²/4 h. IV infusion on day 5
Or BEC	Variants with reduced doses
PMB	Cisplatin: 20 mg/m²/1 h. IV infusion on days 1–5
	Methotrexate: 50 mg/m² IV on days 1, 8, 15
	Bleomycin: 20U/m² IV on days 1, 8, 15

[a]Chemotherapy combinations are given with 3-weekly intervals for two to four courses before radiation

18 children (Ayan et al. 2000). An updated and combined 36 children and 37 adolescents data revealed rapid and high response rates both in the primary tumor and the involved neck nods with the same three cycles combination of bleomycin, epirubicin, and cisplatin. The treatment outcome was relatively high both for children and adolescents, with 5- and 10-years OS rates of 86.5% and 71.5% respectively (Altun et al. 2008). The same combination with reduced doses of all the three drugs was used in 22 children (Sahraoui et al. 1999). Although the response rates to preradiaton chemotherapy was not indicated in the study, the 5-year OS rate of patients who received chemotherapy was 52% and was significantly better than the 38% OS rate of radiation-only patient population ($p < 0.001$). Laskar et al. reported 42% CR and 44% PR rates following two cycles of preradiation bleomycin, 5-FU, and cisplatin combination in 57 patients of age less than 18 years. Further analyses on prognosis revealed that patients with CR had signifi cantly better OS (86% vs. 61% vs. 16%, p 0.0001) and DFS (69% vs. 36% vs. 25%, p 0.0001) than those with PR and no response (NR) (Laskar et al. 2004).

A similar result regarding the prognostic significance of induction response was reported by Kupeli et al. In this retrospective series, 65 of 84 patients less than 17 years of age were given preradiation chemotherapy. According to the time period, noncisplatin and cisplatin-based combinations were used. The assessment following induction revealed 48.8% CR and 33.3% PR for the entire group; the OS rates (68% vs. 0%, $p = 0.0003$) were significantly better in complete responders when compared with NR patients. Although the induction combinations were heterogeneous in this pediatric series, it was demonstrated that the cisplatin-based combinations resulted in a significantly better OS (80% vs. 63.4% vs. 30.9%, $p = 0.001$) than noncisplatin regimens and post-RT cyclophasphamide monotherapy, respectively (Kupeli et al. 2005).

In the GPOH Study NPC-91, where three cycles of preradiation methotrexate, cisplatin, and 5-FU have been used, 56 of 58 high-risk patients had good clinical tumor response (14% CR, 86% PR) (Mertens et al. 2005). In POG study 9486, 16 patients received four courses of methotrexate, 5-FU, and cisplatin. An overall response rate of 93.75% with 5 CR (31.25%) and 10 PR (62.5%) were achieved before radiation (Rodriquez-Galindo et al. 2005). Recently, the efficacy of preradiation docetaxel and cisplatin combination was investigated in newly diagnosed pediatric and young adult NPC patients. Ten patients received four cycles of cisplatin of 100 mg/m² and docetaxel of 75 mg/m² on day 1 with 3 weekly intervals, followed by 59.4 Gy median dose of radiotherapy. The induction chemotherapy combination yielded 1 CR, 5 PR, 3 stable, and 1 progressive disease. No major chemotherapy toxicity was reported, and the 2-year OS and EFS was 90% and 70%, respectively. It was concluded that cisplatin and docetaxel combination is safe and efficacious for NPC (Varan et al. 2009). A RCN study evaluated 165 nonmetastatic NPC patients <18 years of age from 16 institutions, retrospectively. In this RCN study, 144 (87.3%) patients were treated with preradiation (132 patients) ± concurrent chemoradiotherapy (19 patients/12 treated with concurrent chemoradiotherapy alone) and/or postradiation chemotherapy (52 patients). The majority (72.2%) of the chemotherapy combinations included cisplatin.

and 127 (96.3%) out of 132 patients treated with preradiation chemotherapy responded either completely or partially to 2–4 cycles of various combinations of chemotherapy. The univariate and multivariate analysis demonstrated statistically significant differences for LRFS (92% vs. 65%), LRRFS (85% vs. 65%), and DFS (72% vs. 51%), but not for OS rates, between patients who were treated with combined chemoradiation therapy to radiation therapy and who were treated with radiation alone (Ozyar et al. 2006).

Although some retrospective studies demonstrated the superiority of preradiation chemotherapy on survival, such conclusion has not been confirmed. Results on local and locoregional control are very heterogenous and there is no consensus on the response evaluation. Nevertheless, improved local or locoregional control rates with combined modality treatments have been achieved in most retrospective series demonstrated in Table 23.1. The RCN study has collected the largest data of pediatric NPC. The data revealed the benefit of chemotherapy on LRFS, LRRS, and DFS, but the conclusive data on the impact of chemotherapy on survival, drug doses, combinations, and scheduling with RT has to be collected from prospective cooperative group studies.

As mentioned earlier, only two published prospective multiinstitutional studies are available on the management of pediatric NPC. In GPOH Study NPC-91 from Germany, 58 high-risk patients less than 25 years of age were treated with three cycles of preradiation chemotherapy combination of methotrexate, cisplatin, and 5-FU followed by radiation therapy. After irradiation, all the patients were treated with recombinant IFN-β for 6 months. The rationale for postradiation immunotherapy was: suppressed immunological response in patients with NPC at diagnosis, the strong role of EBV infection in the pathogenesis of disease, antiangiogenic effect of interferon, and a 10%–15% response to IFN-β as a single agent in patients with recurrent NPC. Excellent results have been achieved from this study with 91% DFS and 95% OS rates. Among 58 high-risk patients, one patient showed tumor progression during chemotherapy, and another patient had only one cycle of treatment because of acute cardiotoxicity. Distant and local recurrences were reported in three and one patients, respectively. It was concluded that the combination of preradiation chemotherapy, relatively low cumulative radiotherapy dose (59.4 Gy to primary site, 45 Gy for neck area), and postradiation interferon improved the outcome of children and adolescents with high-risk NPC. The study group has launched out a new treatment protocol with the intent to investigate the role of concurrent chemoradiotherapy with cisplatin followed by 6 months treatment of interferon after three cycles of preradiation cisplatin and 5-FU.

The second prospective multiinstitutional study (i.e., POG 9486) from the U.S., where 16 high-risk patients less than 22 years of age were treated with four cycles of preradiation chemotherapy consisted of methotrexate, cisplatin, and 5-FU followed by radiotherapy. Only one patient had progression during preradiation chemotherapy and the overall response rate to four cycles of induction chemotherapy was 93.7%. The overall 4-year EFS and OS rates were 77% and 75%, respectively. All treatment failures occurred in systemic sites in spite of the four cycles of preradiation chemotherapy. It was reported that the severity of mucositis and the need for nutritional support was greater than expected, and it was mainly related to methotrexate. In their new protocol, the same study group will explore the use of less toxic preradiation chemotherapy with cisplatin and 5-FU, followed by concurrent chemoradiotherapy. The circulating EBV-DNA levels will also be measured to evaluate the prognostic significance in an attempt to create risk-adapted, less toxic but effective therapies.

The results from these two trials indicated that incorporation of chemotherapy improved the outcome and allowed radiation dose reduction to 60 Gy in chemo-responsive patients, thus, approving the previous suggestions. The other important result was that the OS and the DFS rates of patients in GPOH study was superior to that of POG study, although patients in the POG study had one more cycle of similar chemotherapy and a slightly higher dose of radiotherapy. The difference may be explained by the incorporation of immunotherapy with interferon in GPOH study and/or the severe toxicity of four cycles of preradiation chemotherapy used in POG study, which might have reduced the dose intensity and/or caused delay of radiotherapy.

In view of the results of these retrospective and prospective nonrandomized studies, early induction with chemotherapy improved the outcome of childhood and adolescence NPC by increasing the locoregional control and to some extent, the systemic control. Induction chemotherapy has allowed radiation dose reduction to 60 Gy. Further reductions may be possible in good responders to chemotherapy, as it was demonstrated that these patients have superior survival and that initial response to induction chemotherapy is a strong predictor of the outcome.

The combination of cisplatin and 5-FU as an induction regimen gained popularity due to excellent results of prospective studies, and possibly continue to act as a standard regimen until less toxic combinations take their place.

It is still unclear if an extended preradiation chemotherapy or the addition of postradiation and/or concurrent chemoradiotherapy may improve survival without jeopardizing the organ functions with toxicity. Immunotherapy with interferon seemed to yield excellent results when combined with chemoradiotherapy.

23.6 Treatment-Induced Adverse Effects

23.6.1 Acute Toxicities

Reports on adverse effects of chemotherapy are mainly related to acute toxicities, and depend on the type and doses of the chemotherapy agents used. Major side effects include nausea and vomiting, myelosuppression, mucositis, infection due to neutropenia, electrolyte imbalances, and organ toxicities. In their study, Mertens et al. (2005) who used three cycles of cisplatin, methotrexate, and 5-FU with leucovorin rescue followed by radiotherapy, nausea and vomiting was reported in all except one patient. Furthermore, leucopenia was reported in 52 out of 57 patients, mucositis in all the patients, septicemia in 5, renal toxicity in 5, cardiotoxicity in 2, ototoxicity in 7, xerostomia in 42, and trismus in 5 patients. No second malignancy was observed in this study within the median follow-up time of 47.6 months. Serin et al. (1998) reported two nephrotoxicities following cisplatin-based chemotherapy which resulted in death (Serin et al. 1998). To maintain high quality of life, efforts have to be made to prevent or minimize the adverse effects of both treatment modalities in children and young adults, without jeopardizing the improved outcome. Radioprotectants like amifostine, imaging-based radiotherapy techniques, immunotherapy with interferon, and vaccination for EBV infections may promise future effort in the prevention and treatment of NPC in children and adolescents.

Acute toxicity of radiotherapy include mild to severe xerostomia, odynophagia, pharyngitis, mucositis, anorexia, moderate to severe weight loss which may necessitate tube feeding or parenteral nutrition, and a high rate of actinic dermatitis.

23.6.2 Late Toxicities

Knowledge on the treatment-induced adverse effects in childhood and adolescence NPC are limited and mainly concentrated on late effects of radiotherapy. Late endocrine effects, soft-tissue fibrosis, bone and dental problems, and second primary malignancies have been reported as a consequence of high-dose radiotherapy with or without chemotherapy. Reports on long-term experiences demonstrated that up to 70% of irradiated children developed hypothyroidism and needed hormone supplementation. Less-frequently encountered endocrine effects included the hypothalamo-pituitary dysfunction, late onset of puberty, secondary amenorrhea, and stunted growth (Sahraoui et al. 1999; Uzel et al. 2001).

Mild and moderate neck fibrosis is another common late adverse effect, and occured in about 30%–60% of the cases reported in literature. Neck fibrosis strongly related to the radiation dose, technique, and the age of patients during the treatment (Zubizarreta et al. 2000; Selek et al. 2005). Uzel et al. (2001) reported skeletal growth retardation as a consequence of facial, cervical, and clavicular bone damage in 5 of 23 patients alive after treatment, who were followed-up with a median of 107 months. Moderate to severe dental damage occurred from 2 to 17 years in seven patients, and two resulted in total dental prosthesis in the same report. Serin et al. reported dental caries in 23 children among 41 patients available for toxicity assessment (Serin et al. 1998). These findings were supported by two additional reports. Severe teeth damage were observed in 30%–50% of patients after combined chemoradiation therapy (Zubizarretta et al. 2000; Sahraoui et al. 1999).

Mild to moderate xerostomia and chronic sinusitis are common side effects of head and neck irradiation, and are reported in high frequencies in pediatric NPC series. It is reported that medication for xerostomia may relieve the dryness of the mouth and the symptom may subside as the years pass. Hearing deficit due to irradiation occurs as a result of eustachian tube dysfunction and influence the low frequencies (<4,000 Hz). This pattern of hearing loss is different from cisplatin toxicity and can be treated by ventilation tube insertions. Trismus and myelitis are the other reported adverse effects of radiotherapy.

One of the serious late effects of high-dose radiotherapy is the second malignancies. We have reported 3 second malignant tumors in 48 treated children, after a median of 77 months. Two of the second malignancies

(Hodgkin's disease and chondrosarcoma) occurred within the radiation field, while the other one (gastric carcinoma) was outside the field (ALTUN et al. 2008). Ingersol et al. reported the occurrence of second malignancies in three patients (two in field, one outside the field) out of 57 children with NPC, 6–11 years following treatment (INGERSOLL et al. 1990).

In the RCN study, two infield secondary cancers have been reported. One was fibrosarcoma and the other was basal cell carcinoma (OZYAR et al. 2006). KÜPELI et al. (2005) reported second malignancies (one dysgerminoma, one renal cell carcinoma), both of which occurred outside the treatment field. Combined modality treatments may increase the frequency of second malignancies, thus long-term follow up of patients have to be considered.

23.7 Summary

NPC is a rare disease in children with distinct epidemiological and etiological features, histopathological characteristics, and clinical presentation. Children with NPC almost always have the undifferentiated variant of the disease, which is associated with advanced locoregional spread and distant metastases. While the concomitant chemotherapy and radiation, with or without adjuvant chemotherapy, is the current standard for adult patients with NPC, neoadjuvant chemotherapy with radiotherapy has gained popularity parallel to other paediatric treatment protocols in various solid tumors. Although multimodality treatment has increased the 5-year OS to 70%–90%, late morbidity is a major concern. Any potential reduction in radiation field and doses is desirable due to the significant chronic morbidity among the long-term survivors.

References

Al-Sarraf M, LeBlanc M, Giri PG, et al (1998) Chemoradiotherapy versus radiotherapy in patients with advanced nasopharyngeal cancer: phase III randomized Intergroup study 0099. J Clin Oncol 16:1310–1317

Altun M, Ayan I, Dizdar Y, et al (2008) Nasopharyngeal carcinoma of children, adolescents and young adults. 40th Congress of the International Society of Pediatric Oncology. (2–6 Oct) SIOP Abstract Book 2008; 142, D118 (abstract) Berlin, Germany

Ayan I, Altun M (1996) Nasopharyngeal carcinoma in children: retrospective review of 50 patients. Int J Radiat Oncol Biol Phys 35:485–492

Ayan I, Kaytan E, Ayan N (2003) Childhood nasopharyngeal carcinoma: from biology to treatment. Lancet Oncol 4:13–21

Ayan I, Meral R, Kebudi R, et al (2000) Efficacy of cisplatinum based preradiation chemotherapy in childhood nasopharyngeal carcinoma. Med Pediatr Oncol 35:277

Barista I, Varan A, Ozyar E (2007) Bimodal age distribution in Hodgkin's disease and nasopharyngeal carcinoma. Med Hypotheses 68(6):1421

Bar-Sela G, Ben Arush MW, Sabo E, et al (2005) Nasopharyngeal carcinoma: better prognosis and increased c-Kit expression as compared to adults. Pediatr Blood Cancer 45:291–297

Berberoglu S, Ilhan I, Cetindag F, et al (2001) Nasopharyngeal carcinoma in Turkish children: review of 33 cases. Pediatr Hematol Oncol 18:309–315

Berry MP, Smith CR, Brown TC, et al (1980) Nasopharyngeal carcinoma in the young. Int J Radiat Oncol Biol Phys 6:415–421

Cammoun M, Hoerner V, Mourali N (1974) Tumors of the nasopharynx in Tunisia. An anatomic and clinical study based on 143 cases. Cancer 33:184–192

Cao KJ, Li Y, Xie GF, et al (2006) Prognostic factors in nasopharyngeal carcinoma in childhood and adolescence. Zhonghua Zhong Liu Za Zhi 28:134–137

Chua DT, Sham JS, Au GK (2005) A phase II study of docetaxel and cisplatin as first-line chemotherapy in patients with metastatic nasopharyngeal carcinoma. Oral Oncol 41: 589–595

Daglikoca ED, Ozyar E, Atay Ç, et al (2007) Determination of tumor suppressor genes in childhood nasopharyngeal carcinoma: Genetic linkage data of Turkish population. Second Regional Congress of Cancer and Blood Diseases of Childhood, Nasopharyngeal Carcinoma Symposium. (Sep 6–8) Amman, Jordan

Daoud J, Toumi N, Bouaziz M, et al (2003) Nasopharyngeal carcinoma in childhood and adolescence: analysis of a series of 32 patients treated with combined chemotherapy and radiotherapy. Eur J Cancer 39:2349–2354

Dardari R., Khyatti M, Jouhadi H, et al (2001) Study of human leukocyte antigen class I phenotypes in Moroccan patients with nasopharyngeal carcinoma. Int J Cancer 92:294–297

Deutsch M, Mercado R Jr, Parsons JA (1978) Cancer of the nasopharynx in children. Cancer 41:1128–1133

Fang FM, Li CF, Chien CY, et al (2007) Immunohistochemical expression of epidermal growth factor receptor and cyclooxygenase-2 in pediatric nasopharyngeal carcinomas: no significant correlations with clinicopathological variables and treatment outcomes. Int J Pediatr Otorhinolaryngol 71(3):447–455

Feng BJ, Jalbout M, Ayoub WB, et al (2007) Dietary risk factors for nasopharyngeal carcinoma in Maghrebian countries. Int J Cancer 121:1550–1555

Fernandez CH, Cangir A, Samaan NA, et al (1976) Nasopharyngeal carcinoma in children. Cancer 37:2787–2791

Gasparini M, Lombardi F, Rottoli L, et al (1988) Combined radiotherapy and chemotherapy in stage T3 and T4 nasopharyngeal carcinoma in children. J Clin Oncol 6: 491–494

Ghim TT, Briones M, Mason P, et al (1998) Effective adjuvant chemotherapy for advanced nasopharyngeal carcinoma in children: a final update of a long-term prospective study in a single institution. J Pediatr Hematol Oncol 20:131–135

Goldsmith DB, Morton TM, West R (2002) HLA associations with nasopharyngeal carcinoma in Southern Chinese: a meta analysis. Clin Otolaryngol 27:61–67

Greene MH, Fraumeni JF, Hoover R (1977) Nasopharyngeal cancer among young people in the United States:racial variations by cell type. J Natl Cancer Inst 58:1267–1270

Habrand J, Valls DG, Petras S, et al (2004) Carcinoma of the nasopharynx in children and adolescents treated with initial chemotherapy followed by adapted doses of radiotherapy. Proceedings of 46th Annual ASTRO Meeting. Int J Radiat Oncol Biol Phys S247:191

Har-Kedar I, Chaitchik S, Hercberg A (1974) Nasopharyngeal carcinoma at the Tel-Hashomer Government Hospital, Israel. A 20 year survey (1951–1970). Clin Radiol 25:403–407

Huang TB (1982) Multiple primary malignant tumors. Clinicopathologic study of 188 cases. Zhonghua Zhong Liu Za Zhi 4(4):290–293

Huang TB (1990) Cancer of the nasopharynx in childhood. Cancer 66:968–971

Hubert A, De-The G (1982) Dietary behavior, way of life, and nasopharyngeal cancer. Bull Cancer 69:476–482

Ingersoll L, Woo SY, Donaldson S, et al (1990) Nasopharyngeal carcinoma in the young: a combined M.D. Anderson and Stanford experience. Int J Radiat Oncol Biol Phys 19:881–887

Jeannel D, Bouvier G, Hubbert A (1999) Nasopharyngeal carcinoma: an epidemiological approach to carcinogenesis. Cancer Surv 33:125–155

Jenkin RD, Anderson JR, Jereb B, et al (1981) Nasopharyngeal carcinoma–a retrospective review of patients less than thirty years of age: a report of Children's Cancer Study Group. Cancer 47:360–366

Jereb B, Huvos AG, Steinherz P, et al (1980) Nasopharyngeal carcinoma in children review of 16 cases. Int J Radiat Oncol Biol Phys 6:487–491

Kam MK, Teo PM, Chau RM, et al (2004) Treatment of nasopharyngeal carcinoma with intensity-modulated radiotherapy: the Hong Kong experience. Int J Radiat Oncol Biol Phys 60:1440–1450

Khabir A, Ghorbel A, Daoud J, et al (2003) Similar BCL-X but different BCL-2 levels in the two age groups of north African nasopharyngeal carcinomas. Cancer Detect Prev 27:250–255

Khabir A, Sellami A, Sakka M, et al (2000) Contrasted frequencies of p53 accmulation in the two age groups of North African nasopharyngeal carcinomas. Clin Cancer Res 6:3932–3936

Kupeli S, Varan A, Ozyar E, et al (2005) Treatment results of 84 patients with nasopharyngeal carcinoma in childhood. Pediatr Blood Cancer 46(4):454–458

Laskar S, Bahl G, Muckaden M, et al (2008) Nasopharyngeal carcinoma in children:comparison of conventional and intensity-modulated radiotherapy. Int J Radiat Oncol Biol Phys 72(3):728–736

Laskar S, Sanghavi V, Muckaden MA, et al (2004) Nasopharyngeal carcinoma in children: ten years' experience at the Tata Memorial Hospital, Mumbai. Int J Radiat Oncol Biol Phys 58:189–195

Lobo-Sanahuja F, Garcia I, Carranza A, et al (1986) Treatment and outcome of undifferentiated carcinoma of the nasofarenx in children: a 13-year experience. Med Pediatr Oncol 14:6–11

Lombardi F, Gasparini M, Gianni C, et al (1982) Nasopharyngeal carcinoma in childhood. Med Pediatr Oncol 10:243–250

Louis CU, Paulino AC, Gottschalk S, et al (2007) A single institution experience with pediatric nasopharyngeal carcinoma: high incidence of toxicity associated with platinum-based chemotherapy plus IMRT. J Pediatr Hematol Oncol 29: 500–505

Maalej M, Daoud J, Bouaouina N, et al (1995) Clinical and evaluative aspects of nasopharyngeal T4N0 neoplasms. Bull Cancer 82:728–731

Marks JE, Phillips JL, Menck HR (1998) The National Cancer Data Base report on the relationship of race and national origin to the histology of nasopharyngeal carcinoma. Cancer 83:582–588

Martin WD, Shah KJ (1994) Carcinoma of the nasopharynx in young patients. Int J Radiat Oncol Biol Phys 28:991–999

Mertens R, Granzen B, Lassay L, et al (1997) Nasopharyngeal carcinoma in childhood and adolescence: concept and preliminary results of the cooperative GPOH study NPC-91. Gesellschaft fur Padiatrische Onkologie und Hamatologie. Cancer 80:951–959

Mertens R, Granzen B, Lassay L, et al (2005) Treatment of nasopharyngeal carcinoma in children and adolescence: definitive results of a multicenter study (NPC-91-GPOH). Cancer 104:1083–1089

Nakamura RA, Novaes PERS, Antoneli CBG, et al (2005) High-dose-rate brachytherapy as part of a multidisciplinary treatment of nasopharyngeal lymphoepithelioma in childhood.Cancer 104:535–531

Orbach D, Brisse H, Helfre S, et al (2008) Radiation and chemotherapy combination for nasopharyngeal carcinoma in children: Radiotherapy dose adaptation after chemotherapy response to minimize late effects. Pediatr Blood Cancer 50:849–853

Ozyar E, Selek U, Laskar S, et al (2006) Treatment results of 165 pediatric patients with non-metastatic nasopharyngeal carcinoma: a Rare Cancer Network study. Radiother Oncol 81:39–46

Ozyar E, Yildiz F, Akyol FH, et al (1999) 1988 and 1997 classifications for nasopharyngeal carcinoma. American joint committee on cancer. Int J Radiat Oncol Biol Phys 44: 1079–1087

Ozyar E, Yildz F, Akyol FH, et al (2002) Adjuvant high-dose-rate brachytherapy after external beam radiotherapy in nasopharyngeal carcinoma.Int J Radiat Oncol Biol Phys 52(1):101–108

Pao WJ, Hustu HO, Douglass EC, et al (1989) Pediatric nasopharyngeal carcinoma: long term follow-up of 29 patients. Int J Radiat Oncol Biol Phys 17:299–305

Polychronopoulou S, Kostaridou S, Panagiotou JP, et al (2004) Nasopharyngeal carcinoma in childhood and adolescence: a single institution's experience with treatment modalities during the last 15 years. Pediatr Hematol Oncol 21: 393–402

Posner MR, Hershock DM, Blajman CR, et al; TAX 324 Study Group (2007) Cisplatin and fluorouracil alone or with docetaxel in head and neck cancer. N Engl J Med 357: 1705–1715

Rodriguez-Galindo C, Wofford M, Castleberry RP, et al (2005) Preradiation chemotherapy with methotrexate, cisplatin, 5-Fluorouracil, and Leucovorin for pediatric nasopharyngeal carcinoma. Results of Pediatric Oncology Group (Now

Children's Oncology Group) Study 9486. Cancer 103: 850–857
Sahraoui S, Acharki A, Benider A, et al (1999) Nasopharyngeal carcinoma in children under 15 years of age: a retrospective review of 65 patients. Ann Oncol 10:1499–1502
Schmauz R, Templeton AC (1972) Nasopharyngeal carcinoma in Uganda. Cancer 29:610–621
Selek U, Ozyar E, Ozyigit G Varan A, et al (2005) Treatment results of 59 young patients with nasopharyngeal carcinoma. Int J Pediatr Otorhinolaryngol 69:201–207
Serin M, Erkal H, Elhan AH, et al (1998) Nasopharyngeal carcinoma in childhood and adolescence. Med Pediatr Oncol 31:498–505
Sham JS, Poon YF, Wei WI, et al (1990) Nasopharyngeal carcinoma in young patients. Cancer 65:2606–2610
Uzel O, Yoruk SO, Sahinler I, et al (2001) Nasopharyngeal carcinoma in childhood: long-term results of 32 patients. Radiother Oncol 58:137–141
Varan A, Ozyar E, Corapçioğlu F, Köksal Y, Aydin B, Yazici N, Akyüz C, Büyükpamukçu M (2009) Pediatric and young adult nasopharyngeal carcinoma patients treated with preradiation Cisplatin and docetaxel chemotherapy. Int J Radiat Oncol Biol Phys 73(4):1116–20
Wei W, Sham JST (2005) Nasopharyngeal carcinoma. Lancet 365:2041–2054
Wolden SL, Steinherz PG, Kraus DH, et al (2000) Improved long-term survival with combined modality therapy for pediatric nasopharynx cancer. Int J Radiat Oncol Biol Phys 46:859–864
Yuan JM, Wang XL, Xiang YB, et al (2000) Preserved foods in relation to risk of nasopharyngeal carcinoma in Shanghai, China Int J Cancer 85:358–363
Zubizarreta PA, D'Antonio G, Raslawski E, et al (2000) Nasopharyngeal carcinoma in childhood and adolescence: a single-institution experience with combined therapy. Cancer 89:690–695

Staging of Nasopharyngeal Carcinoma

24

Brian O'Sullivan and Eugene Yu

CONTENTS

Brian O'Sullivan, MD, FRCPC
Department of Radiation Oncology, Princess Margaret Hospital, University of Toronto, 610 University Avenue, Toronto, ON M5G, 2M9, Canada
Eugene Yu, MD, FRCPC
Department of Medical Imaging, Princess Margaret Hospital, University of Toronto, 610 University Avenue, Toronto, ON, M5G 2M9, Canada

24.1 Introduction

In oncology, "to stage" a patient implies two intentions. The first uses clinical examination and investigations to describe the extent of disease to permit a rational treatment strategy to be formulated. The second employs an agreed classification system to categorize extent of disease within risk hierarchies that predict outcome following conventional treatment strategies. For the latter, the foremost priority is given to the risk of death and is provided by the joint TNM classification of the International Union Against Cancer (UICC) and the American Joint Committee on Cancer (AJCC), a discussion about which will comprise the majority of this chapter. In the creation of the TNM, a strong emphasis is paid to ensure that the classification is both useful for clinicians and researchers, while also being applicable in regions of the world where nasopharyngeal carcinoma (NPC) has its highest incidence. These goals may engender conflict between the latest scientific discoveries and practical application in jurisdictions, where such advances are difficult to implement. This is particularly relevant to NPC and often some compromise is needed to permit all stakeholders to embrace an international classification.

In the sections that follow, the accepted guidelines for staging investigations for NPC are outlined briefly. In addition, attention will be paid to the recent evolution in stage classifications for NPC and the rationale for their design. This will include discussion of the most recent version of TNM for its forthcoming 7th edition. We will also discuss additional descriptions of anatomic extension of disease, or molecular or volumetric measures that may be considered for inclusion in TNM or may modify the classification in the future.

24.2 Investigation of Individual Patients

24.2.1 The Anatomic Spread of NPC

The location of the nasopharynx, in the sanctuary of the skull base, provides great opportunity for tumor extension to regions of relative inaccessibility. Distinct issues present themselves early in the natural history of NPC (Dubrulle et al. 2007). For example, the parapharyngeal space (PPS) separates the wall of the nasopharynx from more extreme degrees of lateral extension to the masticator space (also variously termed the *infratemporal fossa* as discussed later in Sect. 24.5.1). Invasion of the PPS is found in approximately 70% of cases (Liao et al. 2008) and may lead to invasion of the masticator muscles or the mandibular nerve (Fig. 24.1). In turn, this may result in tumor extension through the foramen ovale intracranially without bone destruction, as manifested on magnetic resonance imaging (MRI), yet may be non-visible on computerized tomography (CT). The PPS is also important because of its particular location with respect to the local vulnerable anatomy that must be protected from the full prescribed radiotherapy dose. The consequence with previous radiotherapy techniques was potential tumor underdosage in this region as the PPS is juxtaposed to the spine and brain stem.

Cervical adenopathy is very common in NPC (seen in 75%) (Heng et al. 1999). Typically, both the anterior deep cervical lymph nodes (levels II, III, and IV), and level V are at risk. In NPC, low neck disease is traditionally described with respect to the supraclavicular zone or fossa (SCF) originally described by Ho (1978a), but recent evidence suggests that it may also be reasonable to depart from this convention in favor of the more usual topographic convention used for other head and neck sites (see discussion in Sect. 24.5.2). The retropharyngeal lymph nodes are the primary echelon but are bypassed in about 35% of cases. A rich avalvular and well-organized lymph capillary network exists in the mucous membrane. Two major lymph collecting pathways converge in the PPS laterally and posteriorly and enter multiple first-tier lymph nodes (Pan et al. 2009). Distant metastasis may be seen at presentation in approximately 8% of patients (Chua et al. 2009), and in M0 patients also, it is a discouragingly frequent subsequent event evident in approximately 20% of patients in some series (Chan et al. 2009).

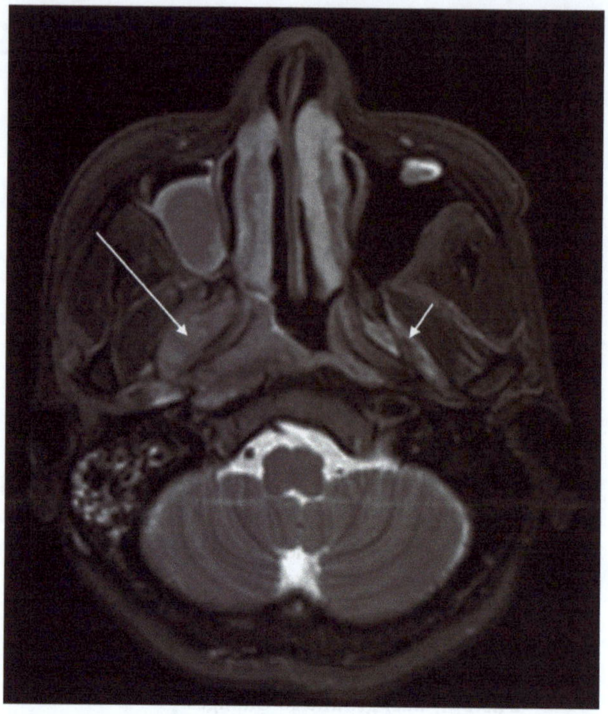

Fig. 24.1. Axial T2 weighted magnetic resonance scan with fat saturation. The *solid short arrow* points to the left normal third division of the trigeminal (V3) nerve. The V3 nerve is a good radiographic landmark for the masticator space. The tumor mass on the right side (*long solid arrow*) is seen to be invading laterally such as to envelope and obscure the V3 nerve. This is masticator space involvement by virtue of V3 disease

24.2.2 Staging to Evaluate Disease Extent

Among the published guidelines, those of the National Comprehensive Cancer Network (NCCN) are most helpful, because they are frequently updated through evidence review and judgment by multidisciplinary panels from its member institutions. The NCCN guidelines recommend that every NPC patient should undergo physical examination that includes nasopharyngeal inspection and biopsy as well as chest imaging to exclude distant metastases (NCCN 2009). For imaging of the nasopharynx and base of skull, MRI with gadolinium is normally recommended and would usually include the regional lymph node regions down to the level of clavicles. Alternatively, positron emission tomography–computerized tomography (PET/CT) and CT with contrast may be performed. Imaging for distant metastases is essential, especially for nonkeratinizing lesions and in patients with N2 and N3 disease. Evaluation of at risk patients should include bone scan and CT of the chest and liver. Alternatively, PET/CT may be preferred to exclude distant disease (NCCN 2009). In general, evidence suggests that MRI is superior to PET/CT for the assessment of locoregional invasion and retropharyngeal nodal metastasis (Liao et al. 2008). PET/CT seems more accurate than MRI in determining cervical lymph node metastasis, and its sensitivity, specificity, and accuracy suggest that PET/CT can replace conventional work-up in the detection of distant metastasis (Chua et al. 2009). Therefore, a combination of PET/CT and head-and-neck MRI has been suggested for the initial staging of NPC patients (Ng et al. 2009).

24.3 A Milestone in the TNM Classification

24.3.1 The 5th edition TNM

Since anatomic features are so important in NPC, a relevant and reproducible system of stage classification has always been a priority. The absence of an international consensus had previously resulted in the proliferation of stage classifications (Lee et al. 1996b). The majority were derived from the anatomic extent of disease, but one also used nonanatomic factors (Neel and Taylor 1989). Mounting enthusiasm for the revision of UICC/AJCC TNM commenced in the early 1990s, in preparation for the publication of the 5th edition TNM in 1997. This initiative arose from a recognition that the staging system in frequent use in southeast Asia was that of Ho and that this and other classifications were superior to the UICC and AJCC TNM (Teo et al. 1991a; Teo et al. 1991b; Lee et al. 1996a). The consequence was a complete revision of the earlier UICC/AJCC 4th edition classification (Fleming et al. 1997; Sobin and Wittekind 1997), establishing a milestone for the classification that was developed jointly, and by consultation involving an international task force comprised mainly of radiation oncologists in south-east Asia and elsewhere, in collaboration with the UICC and the AJCC.

24.3.2 Background to Changes in the 5th Edition TNM

24.3.2.1 Modification of the Ho T-Classification

The Ho classification had never separated different subsites of involvement within the nasopharynx, which the UICC and AJCC had classified as T1 and T2 categories, a subdivision that lacked validity (Sham et al. 1992). The absence of attention to PPS involvement in the TNM was considered a weakness, although its true place in the stage classification was problematic even then (Sham and Choy 1991; Chua et al. 1996; Teo et al. 1996a). This was, in part, because of the changing ability to identify PPS disease with contemporary imaging (thereby introducing "stage creep" effect), the influence of treatment modifications to account for it in many centers (thereby potentially modifying its effect), and the problem of definitions (thereby rendering the data difficult to interpret). However, the view at the time of the 5th edition revision was that PPS should be included in an intermediate T-category (e.g., within categories T2 or T3 of a four category T system, and identified separately).

Complicating the discussions were the different ways of subdividing the involvement of the PPS. One system involved classification based on lateral extension by NPC across the PPS (Sham and Choy 1991), another separated the pre vs. poststyloid components of the PPS (Min et al. 1994), while another subdivided the PPS into paranasopharynx vs. paraoropharynx at the C1/C2 interspace (Tsao 1993).

For the TNM 5th edition revision, much reliance was given at the time to unpublished data concerning PPS involvement from the Queen Elizabeth Hospital (QEH) in Hong Kong for Ho T2 disease (tumor extension to adjacent soft tissue). Although cancer specific survival was worse in the presence of PPS involvement, this was largely explained on multivariate analysis by the fact that PPS extension was associated with higher neck stage (William Foo, personal communication). Nevertheless, the need for a consistent classification overshadowed the problem of discordant beliefs about the importance of PPS invasion or how it should be weighted or described. It was incorporated in the TNM classification as a subcategory within T2 (T2b rather than as T3). The rationale for this decision is discussed elsewhere (LEE et al. 1999).

The T4 category was also amended to include extreme lateral extension to soft tissue described as the infratemporal fossa (or what is probably most usually termed the masticator space today) or hypopharynx in addition to gross intracranial extension and/or cranial nerve involvement. Bone involvement alone was also relegated to the T3 category in the 5th edition.

24.3.2.2 Modification of the Ho N-Classification

Traditionally, in the Ho classification, the N-categories were distinguished by the position of palpable lymph nodes as they related to topographic landmarks in the neck, which create three echelons of levels and takes no account of lymph node size (HO 1978b; HO 1978a). N3 also included skin involvement together with disease, wholly or partially in the supraclavicular fossa.

Different results have been reported about lymph node descriptions and whether nodal size was independently significant (SHAM et al. 1990; LEE et al. 1996b; TEO et al. 1996b) in NPC. To resolve this, a detailed analysis from Hong Kong on almost 5,000 cases without distant metastasis formed the basis for the task force recommendations (LEE et al. 1996b). Lymph node size (greatest diameter ≤6 vs. >6 cm), level (upper-mid vs. supraclavicular), and laterality (unilateral vs. bilateral) constituted the criteria for N-categorization in the 5th edition TNM (LEE et al. 1996b). Multiplicity and fixation were not included due to combination of factors, including varied statistical significance, absence of definition, or interrelationship with other parameters of lymph node description (JOHNS et al. 1984; LEE et al. 1999).

24.3.3 Validation of the 5th and 6th Edition TNM

A very extensive literature has now emerged on the value of the 5th edition (and the virtually unchanged 6th edition) TNM and include evidence that it is valid in both endemic regions as well as in the regions where the disease is less common including North America, Australia and Europe (COOPER et al. 1998; HENG et al. 1999; LEE et al. 1999; OZYAR et al. 1999; SAKATA et al. 1999; HONG et al. 2000; CHUA et al. 2001; MA et al. 2001; AU et al. 2003; CORRY et al. 2004; KALOGERA-FOUNTZILA et al. 2006), and in pediatric patients (CASANOVA et al. 2001). The consistent view from these studies is that the 5th and 6th editions were a significant improvement over the 4th edition, carrying superior distribution of cases across groups, and better discrimination between prognostic groups. The acceptance of the classification is further underlined by the fact that the 5th edition TNM remained essentially unchanged in the 2002 6th edition, but for some minor rewording for clarification.

24.4 The Upcoming 7th Edition TNM

The AJCC and UICC are currently reviewing the overall TNM classification for all diseases in preparation for the 7th edition that is anticipated for the coming year. An important element in this process is the need to maintain relevance with current management approaches and to respond to the availability of new data that may be considered in the revisions to the classifications. This process involves collaboration between both organizations that is accomplished by a series of disease specific task forces. In the area of head and neck, this process is led in a joint collaboration chaired by Dr Jatin Shah for the AJCC, and Dr Brian O'Sullivan, the original chair of the international task force that developed the 5th edition NPC TNM, for the UICC. A number of resources are available to the task forces and include, especially, a structured process for introducing changes to the TNM classification. The elements of the TNM process include the development of unambiguous criteria for the information and documentation required to consider changes in the classification, establishment of a well-defined process for the annual review of relevant literature, formation of site-specific expert panels, and the participation of experts from all over the world in the TNM review process (GOSPODAROWICZ et al. 2004). In considering the forthcoming 7th edition, a number of areas have been considered by the head and neck task forces for modification of the NPC TNM classification and are summarized below.

24.4.1 The Significance of Parapharyngeal Space Involvement Today

Over the period since the 5th edition, management has changed and perhaps most especially in the area of radiotherapy delivery with enhanced spatial targeting, principally related to computerized planning and delivery systems such as intensity modulated radiotherapy, as well as in more universal use of MRI to evaluate the local region of invasion by the tumor. As noted earlier, the PPS has held a special place in the staging of NPC. But evidence appears to suggest that the spatial importance of parapharyngeal extension is diminishing due to the ability to encompass this postero-lateral extension with modern radiotherapy technique (Ng et al. 2008). At the same time, parapharyngeal extension seems also to be associated with a unique predisposition for risk of distant metastases (approximately 11%) potentially mediated by the passage of tumor through the parapharyngeal venous plexus and seems to be associated with risk as great or greater than regional lymph node involvement (Cheng et al. 2005). Differences in identifying this risk may also relate to differences in the imaging techniques used by different investigators (i.e., CT vs. MRI) or to differences in the definition of the regional anatomy (King et al. 2000; Liao et al. 2008).

24.4.2 Adjustment in T1, T2a, and T2b Categories

In considering potential modifications to TNM, several groups in Asia have reminded us of the contribution and importance of the 5th and 6th edition TNM, but have also identified areas for improvement (Lee et al. 2004; Low et al. 2004; Liu et al. 2008). This extends to definitions of some of the elements: for example within the spectrum of the existing T2a subcategory, different interpretations of nasal fossa involvement seem to have prevailed with different incidences of this subcategory between series (Au et al. 2003; Low et al. 2004; Liu et al. 2008). Multivariate analysis quantifying different hazards of failure and death have shown discrepancies in the stage classification, though some of these may relate to small number of patients in some groups and the consequence this may have on subset analysis and the decision to modify the classification. Nonetheless, a relatively consistent finding has been the absence of a difference in outcome between T1 and T2a tumors, other than potentially for very extensive nasal involvement (Low et al. 2004), leading to a recommendation for reclassification of patients with soft tissue disease involvement of the oropharynx and nasal fossa to the T1 category (Lee et al. 2004; Liu et al. 2008) This will be included in the forthcoming classification (Table 24.1).

As well, in the substantial series from Hong Kong that influenced the preceding recommendation concerning the T2a category, 1,006 patients had T2b disease (those with parapharyngeal extension). Analysis of this subset indicated that they remain as a distinct group with unfavorable prognosis compared to the proposed T1 category, exhibiting a significantly higher hazard of local and distant failure, with consequent significant impact on cancer-specific death (Table 24.2). This effect was even more apparent when restricted to patients without lymph node involvement (Lee et al. 2004). An additional large series from mainland China that included 309 patients with T2b disease confirmed these findings, therefore justifying that this sub-category continue independently as a T2 category within the TNM (Liu et al. 2008). The latter series and that of Lee et al. from Hong Kong both demonstrated a more even rise in the hazard ratio for adverse events with the redistributed new T-categories contained in the upcoming 7th edition TNM (i.e., T2a is reassigned to T1, and T2b remains as a T2 category) (Table 24.2).

24.4.3 Regional Lymph Nodes (Especially Retropharyngeal Nodes)

Retropharyngeal nodes have an iconic presence in NPC but have not been classified uniformly. For example, heterogeneous approaches among centers have considered them as N1 if unilateral, N2 if bilateral, N1 irrespective of laterality, N1 if discrete, or T2b if abutting adjacent soft tissue tissues, or unclassified (Lee et al. 2004). Some of these approaches reflect historic inadequacies in imaging prior to the era of cross-sectional imaging, especially MRI, and consistent principles have not been identified in TNM. Recent series have assessed the prognostic importance of retropharyngeal nodes including the method by which they should be classified. In general, it seems compelling that MRI is superior to CT and resulted in the identification of abnormal retropharyngeal nodes in an excess of 70% of patients in a large series from Guangzhou, China (Tang et al. 2008), compared to approximately 50% in a series from Singapore, where CT was the predominant imaging modality (Tham et al. 2009). Evidence from

Table 24.1. UICC Nasopharynx TNM Classification (7th edition, in preparation)

T-primary tumor			
T1	Tumor confined to nasopharynx, or tumor extends to soft tissue of oropharynx and/or nasal fossa without parapharyngeal extension		
T2	Tumor with parapharyngeal extension		
T3	Tumor invades bony structures and/or paranasal sinuses		
T4	Tumor with intracranial extension and/or involvement of cranial nerves, infratemporal fossa, hypopharynx, orbit, or masticator space		
N-regional lymph nodes			
N0	No regional lymph node metastasis		
N1	Unilateral metastasis in lymph node(s), 6 cm or less in greatest dimension, above the supraclavicular fossa and/or unilateral or bilateral, retropharyngeal lymph nodes 6 cm or less in greatest dimension		
N2	Bilateral metastasis in lymph node(s), 6 cm or less in greatest dimension, above the supraclavicular fossa		
N3	Metastasis in lymph node(s) greater than 6 cm in dimension or in the supraclavicular fossa		
N3a	Greater than 6 cm in dimension		
N3b	In the supraclavicular fossa		
Stage I	T1	N0	M0
Stage II	T1	N1	M0
	T2	N0, N1	M0
Stage III	T1	N2	M0
	T2	N2	M0
	T3	N0, N1, N2	M0
Stage IVA	T4	N0, N1, N2	M0
Stage IVB	Any T	N3	M0
Stage IVC	Any T	Any N	M1

UICC TNM Prognostic Factors Committee, Geneva, 2009 (UICC 7th edition, in preparation). Format and wording may differ from the AJCC version, in preparation

both studies shows that patients with retropharyngeal nodes alone have a risk of distant metastasis that it similar to N1 disease (Tang et al. 2008; Tham et al. 2009). In addition, the proposal that they should be correspondingly classified as N1 disease, and that this should be independent of laterality (Tham et al. 2009) forms the basis for revision of this element in the 7th edition of TNM (Table 24.1).

Within the more advanced N-categories, potential areas for improvement may also exist. Thus while N3 disease is associated with the least favorable prognosis, this appears to be confined to the circumstance where regional nodes extend to the supraclavicular fossa (N3b disease). N3a disease, a subcategory representing less than 5% of cases, appears not to have adverse impact beyond N2 (Lee et al. 2004; Low et al. 2004; Liu et al. 2008), but this has not been modified for the 7th edition, in part due to the statistical issues associated with the small number of cases.

24.5 Anatomic Issues Relevant to Contemporary Imaging

24.5.1 Lateral Tumor Extension

As discussed above, in the forthcoming TNM classification, T2 disease will refer to instances of parapharyngeal extension, defined as "posterolateral infiltration of tumor", as it was in the 5th and 6th editions. However with contemporary imaging, this definition is unduly vague. This is especially true since many of the main components of the pre and poststyloid

Table 24.2. Significance of original and modified T-categories by multivariate analysis

T-category	Hazard ratio (95% confidence interval)		
	Local recurrence	Distant failure	Cancer-specific death
Original 5th and 6th edition TNM			
T1	1	1	1
T2a	1.24 (0.75–2.06)	0.70 (0.44–1.12)	0.96 (0.59–1.55)
T2b	1.80 (1.20–2.69)	0.33 (0.97–1.84)	1.42 (0.996–2.03)
T3	2.51 (1.62–3.87)	1.42 (0.99–2.05)	1.83 (1.24–2.71)
T4	3.17 (2.08–4.83)	2.17 (1.55–3.05)	3.01 (2.09–4.32)
Modified TNM with T2a considered to be T1, and T2b considered to be T2			
T1	1	1	1
T2	1.62 (1.18–2.22)	1.54 (1.17–2.03)	1.45 (1.08–1.94)
T3	2.26 (1.59–3.22)	1.63 (1.18–2.25)	1.86 (1.33–2.60)
T4	2.86 (2.04–4.01)	2.50 (1.86–3.36)	3.05 (2.26–4.13)

Adapted from Lee et al. (2004)

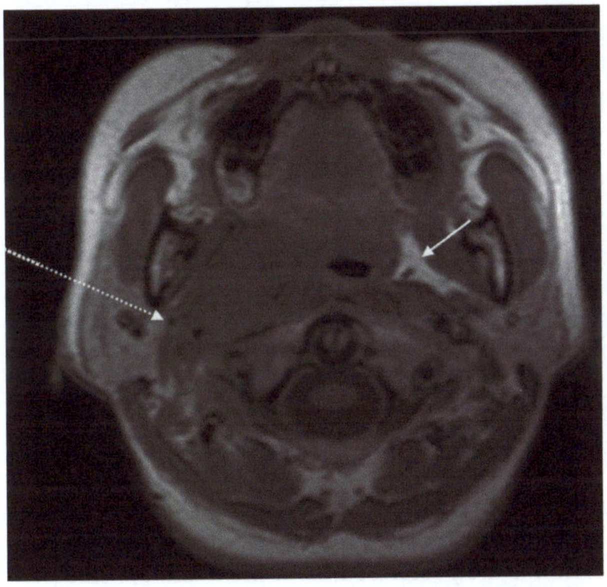

Fig. 24.2. Axial T1 magnetic resonance weighted image shows tumor extending to involve the right poststyloid parapharyngeal space (PPS) (*dashed arrow*). The two dark rounded structures are the carotid and jugular vessels which are encased by tumor. The normal PPS fat is seen on the left side as a wedge-shaped area of bright T1 signal (*solid arrow*)

compartments of the PPS are radiographically visible on MRI. For example, infiltration of the fatty component of the PPS is often visible on T1-weighted imaging (Fig. 24.2). This appears as intermediate signal tumor and invades into the bright fat of the PPS. Also, it is often possible to delineate the pharyngobasilar fascia (PBF), the tensor veli palatini and levator palatini muscles which are key components in the delineation of the PPS. Violation of the PBF (Fig. 24.3), infiltration of the tensor veli palatini, and breach of the pharyngeal portion of the levator veli palatini muscle are radiographically consistent with PPS involvement.

The traditional AJCC TNM classification criterion for defining infratemporal fossa extension is the presence of disease beyond the anterior surface of the lateral pterygoid muscle, or lateral extension beyond the postero-lateral wall of maxillary antrum or pterygomaxillary fissure (Fleming et al. 1997). The UICC on the other hand did not specify a definition and some centers may use an alternative definition, for example employing a line drawn from the free edge of the medial pterygoid plate to the lateral surface of the carotid artery for demarcation (Lee et al. 2004). The term *masticator space* was added as one of the criteria for T4 in the UICC/AJCC 6th edition, and considered as synonymous with infratemporal fossa and has used the same definition (Greene et al. 2002). Both terms are currently used to both acknowledge the traditional method described by Ho (Ho 1978b) and to allow the more favored contemporary approach used by radiologists. In reality, most head and neck radiologists would prefer to exclusively use the term masticator space. As discussed below, it is clear is that they are not synonymous, and resolution of this controversy is probably needed to avoid

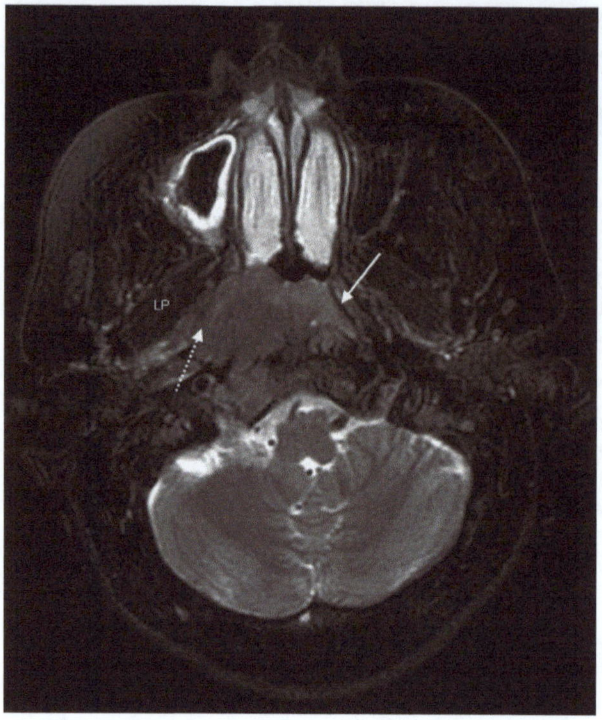

Fig. 24.3. Axial T2 magnetic resonance weighted image in the superior nasopharynx shows the normal left pharyngobasilar fascia (PBF, *solid arrow*). The tumor mass on the right is extending to breach the PBF, which is no longer visible (*dashed arrow*). The masticator space is spared since the lateral pterygoid muscle (LP) remains intact. Please note that the medial pterygoid muscles lie inferior to this plane and is also not invaded by tumor

unnecessary confusion, since it is also likely that less significant degrees of lateral tumor extension also may not be associated with the significant adverse outcome found with very bulky disease invading deeply into the full masticator space (Lee et al. 2004).

24.5.1.1 Definition of the Parapharyngeal Space

The PPS is also known as the pharyngomaxillary or lateral pharyngeal space. It refers to a fascially defined space lateral to the pharyngeal mucosal space and medial to the masticator space. It extends from the skull base lateral to the site of attachment of the PBF but medial to the foramen ovale down to the level of the angle of the mandible. In fact, inferiorly it has been variously described in the literature as extending to the styloglossus muscle, the hyoid bone and posterior belly of the digastric muscle. The anterior boundary is generally considered to be the peterygomandibular raphe, which forms the interface between the buccopharyngeal fascia and the interpterygoid fascia (Som and Curtin 2003). The lateral boundary is the medial fascial boundary of the masticator space and the fascia of the deep lobe of the parotid. Posteriorly, the boundary is the prevertebral fascia, and the medial border is the PBF and buccopharyngeal fascia that contain the pharynx.

The posterior boundary is the most controversial because variation exists as to whether the carotid sheath belongs to the PPS, or whether it should be termed the carotid space (Som and Curtin 2003). A fascial layer known as the tensor-vascular-styloid fascia (TVSF) subdivides the PPS into a prestyloid and retrostyloid component (poststyloid or carotid space) (Fig. 24.4). The TVSF incorporates fibers from the tensor veli palatini muscle and extends from the medial pterygoid plate to the styloid process. The resulting prestyloid compartment predominantly contains fatty tissue. The deep parotid tissue also extends into this area. The poststyloid compartment consists of fatty tissue and the carotid sheath structures.

24.5.1.2 Definition of the Infratemporal Fossa

There is considerable variation in the exact definition of the intratemporal fossa (ITF), partly because it lacks fascial containment. It is generally considered as an irregular space behind the maxilla and lateral to the nasopharynx and pterygomaxillary fissure and peterygomaxillary fossa. The borders of the ITF can be considered as follows: the greater wing of the sphenoid superiorly with the alveolar border of the maxilla inferiorly; the anterior demarcation is the posterior wall of the maxilla, while posteriorly, it is the articular tubercle of the temporalis bone and spine of the sphenoid; the ramus of the mandible forms the lateral boundary, while the pterygoid plates form the medial limit. Laterally, it communicates with the deeper aspect of the buccal space just anterior to the masticator space. Harnsberger has described the ITF as the nasopharyngeal portion of the masticator space (Harnsberger 1995). Mafee has indicated that the ITF contains the masticator muscles, the internal maxillary vessels, and the mandibular and auriculo-temporal nerves. The foramen ovale and foramen spinosum open through the roof of the fossa (Mafee 2005). While some of

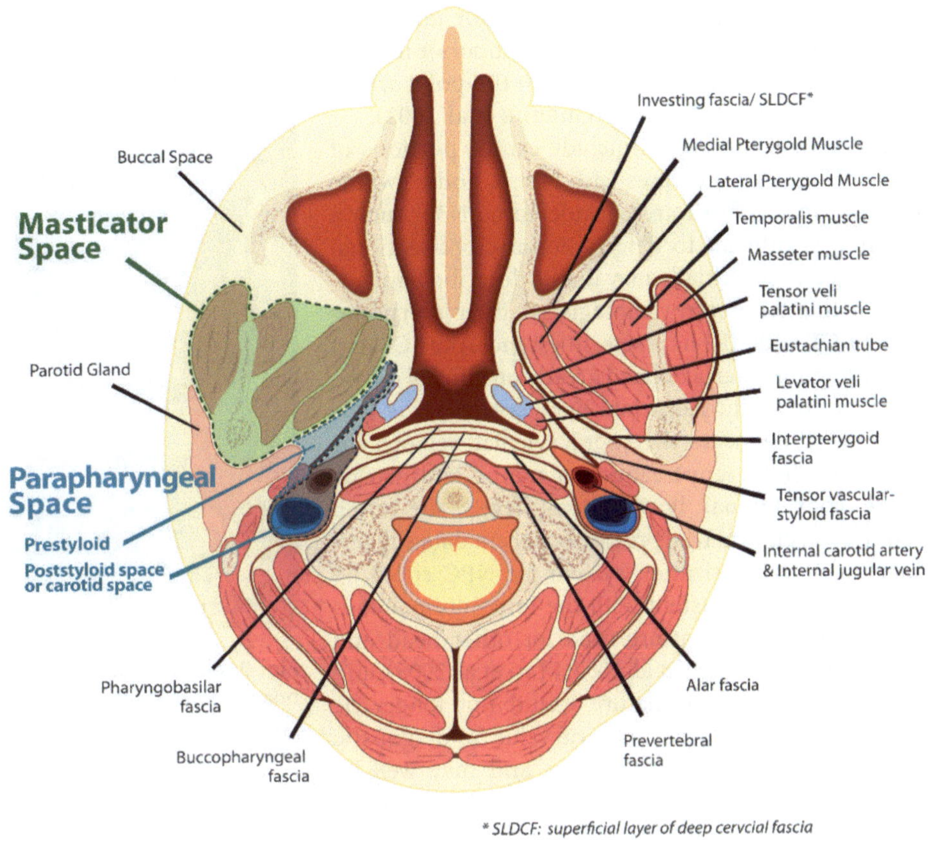

Fig. 24.4. Schematic axial view with color overlays on left side at the level of the nasopharynx demonstrating the fascial boundaries of the masticator (*green overlay*) and PPS (*blue overlay*). Note that the tensor-vascular-styloid fascia subdivides the PPS into a prestyloid and poststyloid (carotid space) (see text for additional details)

the definitions overlap with the masticator space, it lacks the definitional precision of the latter and is less frequently used in radiologic practice to describe nasopharyngeal disease extension.

24.5.1.3 Definition of the Masticator Space

The masticator space (MS) also describes the anatomic region below the middle cranial fossa. This term is generally preferred in the radiology community and has the advantage that there are clear anatomic boundaries defined by fascial planes defining it. The main fascial boundary is related to the superficial layer of the deep cervical fascia (SLDCF). This is also known as the investing fascia. The investing fascia is formed when the SLDCF splits at the lower margin of the body of the mandible and rises to enclose the muscles of mastication. Medially, the fascia combines with another fascia, the interpterygoid fascia, and then rises up to the skull base (Som and Curtin 2003) (Fig. 24.4). Laterally, the fascia rises up above the level of the zygomatic arch and covers the temporalis muscle. The zygomatic arch is used to subdivide the MS into a suprazygomatic MS (portion above the zygomatic arch) and the nasopharyngeal MS (portion below the level of the zygomatic arch). The contents of the MS include the mandibular divison of the fifth cranial nerve, the muscles of mastication, sections of the internal maxillary artery, the pterygoid plexus, and the ramus and coronoid of the mandible.

24.5.2 Description of Lymph Node Neck Levels

The distribution and the prognostic impact of regional lymph node spread from nasopharynx cancer differ from other head and neck mucosal cancers and have involved the use of a different N classification scheme as introduced in the 5th edition. In this context, the SCF is based primarily on clinical landmarks and has been described as the triangular region originally described by Ho (Ho 1978a). It is defined by three points: (1) the superior margin of the sternal end of the clavicle, (2) the superior margin of the lateral end of the clavicle, (3) the point where the neck meets the shoulder (Greene et al. 2002).

As defined this would include caudal portions of levels IV and VB. All cases with lymph nodes (whole or part) in the fossa are considered as N3b. Such a division is difficult to determine on cross-sectional imaging and potentially may not be described universally in this manner by radiologists in their interpretation of CT and MRI data sets. In essence, the SCF and the N staging criteria depend greatly on clinical examination, especially palpation. Furthermore, it is also difficult to delineate the supracavicular regions for modern radiotherapy treatment planning, and instead, more conventional lymph node levels are often required in clinical trial protocols. Recent data suggest that the N categorization system for NPC could be adapted to be consistent with the international consensus guidelines that are used for other head and neck disease sites (Ng et al. 2007; Mao et al. 2008), and the traditional nomenclature would not longer be needed. This would have practical value for diagnostic reporting, radiotherapy planning, and may well be more consistent (Mao et al. 2008). While the actual terms used to describe low lying neck disease would change if the international consensus guidelines for topographic lymph node description were adopted, it would neither change the NPC TNM neck classification itself nor would it affect the stage grouping.

24.5.3 Base of Skull and Intracranial Invasion

Skull base invasion is apparent in about one-third of patients with NPC (Roh et al. 2004) and cranial nerve dysfunction has been reported in approximately 10% of patients (Liu et al. 2009). However, invasion of the base of skull is a heterogeneous condition with a range of potential diagnostic settings. These include minimal asymptomatic disease detected with high quality MRI, frank gross intracranial disease with a presentation spectrum ranging from a subtle bony erosion of the skull base to extensive intracranial invasion that may rarely include brain invasion. Subtle paralysis of cranial nerves, especially the abducens nerve, may accompany minimal disease but gross paralysis of multiple cranial nerves in NPC usually indicates significant direct erosion of the skull base, especially in patients with intracranial extension. Frequently, this may result from the involvement of the cavernous sinus directly by the primary disease, but perineural disease extension may also occur, especially along the third division of the trigeminal nerve (Fig. 24.5). There is evidence that minimal invasion of the skull base or minimal cranial nerve involvement is by no means as prognostically detrimental as very gross intracranial extension (Nishioka et al. 2000), further emphasizing the rationale for why the AJCC has emphasized the importance of clinical evaluation of cranial nerves in staging assessments (Greene et al. 2002). NPC patients with cranial nerve palsy and intracranial extension are both still classified as T4 by the current TNM, and there is no sufficient data available yet to create a subclassification of T4 (e.g., T4a vs T4b) such as that introduced in the 6th edition TNM for other head and neck cancers (Greene et al. 2002; Sobin and Wittekind 2002). Future explorations of TNM will likely consider this issue, and investigators should attempt to assemble larger and more robust data sets to permit base of skull and intracranial disease to be better characterized. By this means, this generally ominous but heterogeneous situation may be classified more optimally in the future.

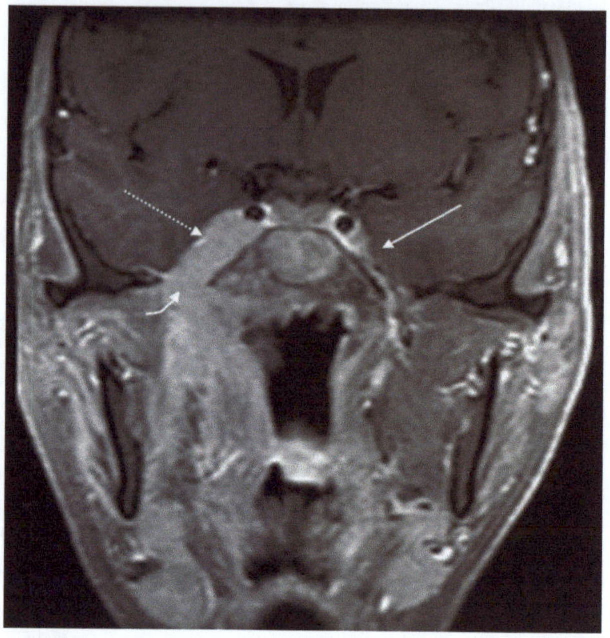

Fig. 24.5. Coronal contrast enhanced magnetic resonance image shows abnormal thickening and enhancement of the right cavernous sinus due to intracranial disease extension (*dashed arrow*). There is also perineural tumor tracking along V3 across the widened right foramen ovale (*curved arrow*). The *solid arrow* shows the normal appearing left cavernous sinus

24.5.4 Prevertebral Space Invasion

Prevertebral space invasion in NPC suffers from similar problems as base of skull invasion. Thus again the entity is heterogeneous and prone to the problems of "stage creep" resulting from the use of high quality MRI and there may be judgment identifying this phenomenon in patients with gross prevertebral longus muscle invasion (Fig. 24.6). Obviously, these investigations have significant potential to improve the quality of radiotherapy targeting for affected patients. The alternative consequence is that they make interpretation of the available data problematic from a prognostic standpoint, and interseries comparisons may be challenging. Lee et al. (2008) from Taiwan most recently proposed that prevertebral space involvement should at least be considered together with the TNM classification to predict prognosis and potentially to influence treatment strategies. In a modest retrospective series where all patients underwent magnetic imaging of the prevertebral space (n = 106), these investigators reported that 43 patients had baseline prevertebral space involvement and experienced statistically significant worse overall and metastasis-free survival compared to the 63 patients without this attribute. In a larger series, also from Taiwan, Feng et al. reported the experience of 181 of 521 patients deemed to have prevertebral muscle involvement. This finding was associated with a statistically significant detriment in loco-regional and distant recurrence, and a borderline significant risk in terms of overall survival (Feng et al. 2006). To what degree the regional anatomy affects these outcomes needs to be considered in future studies, and in particular, the significance, if any, of prevertebral muscle vs. space invasion, as well as the local hematogenous and lymphatic drainage that may influence the risk of distant metastasis (Feng et al. 2006; Lee et al. 2008). In the same manner as discussed for base of skull and intracranial disease, the community would benefit from additional work in this area to determine if it should be considered for inclusion in the future editions of the stage classification.

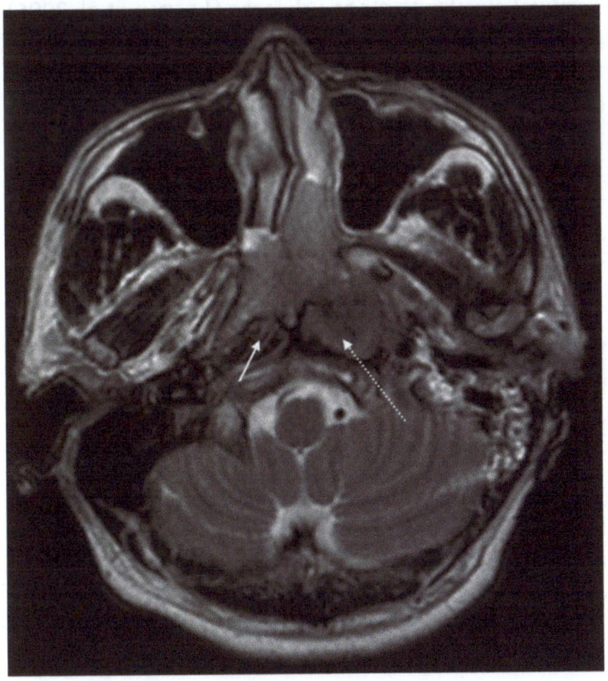

Fig. 24.6. Axial T2 weighted magnetic resonance image shows abnormal expansion and signal change in the left longus musculature (*dashed arrow*). The contralateral longus muscle shows a normal slender shape and internal striations (*solid arrow*)

24.6 Surrogates of Disease Burden

24.6.1 Tumor Volume Assessment

Since the publication of the 5th edition, classification based on tumor volume instead of strict anatomic extent alone has been reported as a significant prognostic factor in the treatment of NPC. In turn, this has prompted investigators to suggest the incorporation of tumor volume into the TNM staging system. Indeed, an extensive literature has now emerged that addresses this topic, but will not be discussed exhaustively. Nonetheless, if tumor volume is to be used as an independent prognostic factor, the methods for volume measurement need to be standardized (Chong and Ong 2008). Unfortunately, the technical challenges to implement this in the clinical setting routinely need to be resolved if it is to be used to classify patients using a TNM system. Not only is the measurement of tumor volume a tedious process requiring the tumor to be outlined digitally on cross-sectional imaging, but the results are prone to difficulties created by both intra and interobserver discrepancy. To overcome this problem, several investigators have developed semi-automated systems to reduce interoperator as well as intraoperator variability (Chong and Ong 2008). To overcome the technical

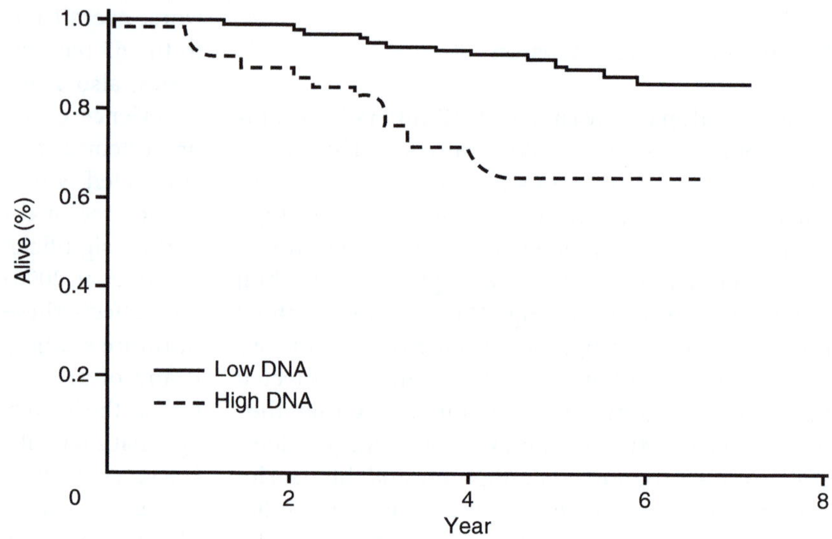

No. of patients at risk:

Low DNA 108	106	94	48
High DNA 47	42	31	6

Fig. 24.7. Actuarial survival curve for early stage (I and II) nasopharyngeal carcinoma segregated according to high vs. low Epstein–Barr virus (EBV) DNA titer prior to treatment. Low DNA denotes low EBV DNA levels of less than 4,000 copies/mL, and high DNA denotes high EBV DNA levels equal or greater than 4,000 copies/mL. The subgroup with high titers have outcome that appears inferior to Stage III disease in the remainder of the study. Reproduced with permission from reference (Leung et al. 2006)

and manpower considerations, alternative more simple methods have also been suggested, including standard bidimensional measurements (King et al. 2007; Lee et al. 2009). While there seems to be no doubt that tumor volume provides a robust predictor of outcome in NPC, the manpower issues and other problems have not yet been resolved, including the determination of agreed potential cut-points that might be used to create a classification that meets the needs of clinicians and scientists throughout the regions where NPC is prevalent.

24.6.2 Assessment of EB Viral Copy Number

Among mucosal head and neck cancers, NPC has additional uniqueness in possessing a robust circulating tumor marker that can be expected to be employed clinically. One of the uses is the correlation of circulating EBV DNA with disease staging, using quantitative real-time polymerase chain reaction (PCR) technology (Lo 2001). By means of its production by NPC cells, EBV DNA level has been shown to be more powerful than existing staging system in predicting outcomes by providing an index of disease burden in the individual patient and has been investigated now by numerous authors (Chan and Lo 2002). In particular, Leung et al. showed that pretherapy circulation of EBV DNA load is an independent prognostic factor for overall survival in NPC. Thus patients with early stage disease can be segregated by EBV DNA levels into a poor-risk subgroup with survival similar to that of stage III disease and a good-risk subgroup with survival similar to stage I disease (Leung et al. 2006) (Fig. 24.7). While this provides a very attractive and undeniable concept, it also faces challenges in whether it can be applied universally at this time, especially in regions where the disease is most prevalent and resources are not as plentiful as in the developed world. A possibility may be to use it presently as an additional tool within clinical trials to augment prognostic assessment and disease monitoring.

24.7 Summary

The dominant theme of prognosis in NPC continues to be the complex anatomic issues that occur in this disease and in particular, the proximity of disease to critical adjacent anatomy which may be injured by high dose radiotherapy. For this reason, the development of a relevant world-wide anatomic staging system was an important step forward in the 5th edition of TNM. The classification remained stable for the 6th edition but changes are to be included it the 7th edition, largely related to the ability to spatially target regions that were previously less accessible to radiotherapy and their prognostic importance has diminished. Additional factors also need clarification, and there is opportunity to improve and agree on definitions for some anatomic structures that should facilitate modification of future revisions to the stage classification. The complexity and expense of assessment and management continue to provide challenges for the introduction of improvements in staging in all jurisdictions where this disease is diagnosed. However, it is hoped that the future will bring the promise of a better understanding of treatment and prognosis, including additional discoveries of molecular alterations in this rare disease that can also be used to complement the anatomic TNM classification.

References

Au JS, Law CK, Foo W, et al (2003) In-depth evaluation of the AJCC/UICC 1997 staging system of nasopharyngeal carcinoma: prognostic homogeneity and proposed refinements. Int J Radiat Oncol Biol Phys 56:413–426

Casanova M, Ferrari A, Gandola L, et al (2001) Undifferentiated nasopharyngeal carcinoma in children and adolescents: comparison between staging systems. Ann Oncol 12: 1157–1162

Chan KC, Lo YM (2002) Circulating EBV DNA as a tumor marker for nasopharyngeal carcinoma. Semin Cancer Biol 12:489–496

Chan SC, Chang JT, Wang HM, et al (2009) Prediction for distant failure in patients with stage M0 nasopharyngeal carcinoma: the role of standardized uptake value. Oral Oncol 45:52–58

Cheng SH, Tsai SY, Yen KL, et al (2005) Prognostic significance of parapharyngeal space venous plexus and marrow involvement: potential landmarks of dissemination for stage I–III nasopharyngeal carcinoma. Int J Radiat Oncol Biol Phys 61:456–465

Chong VF, Ong CK (2008) Nasopharyngeal carcinoma. Eur J Radiol 66:437–447

Chua DT, Sham JS, Kwong DL, et al (1996) Prognostic value of paranasopharyngeal extension of nasopharyngeal carcinoma. A significant factor in local control and distant metastasis. Cancer 78:202–210

Chua DT, Sham JS, Wei WI, et al (2001) The predictive value of the 1997 American Joint Committee on Cancer stage classification in determining failure patterns in nasopharyngeal carcinoma. Cancer 92:2845–2855

Chua ML, Ong SC, Wee JT, et al (2009) Comparison of 4 modalities for distant metastasis staging in endemic nasopharyngeal carcinoma. Head Neck 31:346–354

Cooper JS, Cohen R, Stevens RE (1998) A comparison of staging systems for nasopharyngeal carcinoma. Cancer 83: 213–219

Corry J, Fisher R, Rischin D, et al (2004) Clinical verification of the superiority of the current International Union Against Cancer staging criteria in an Australian population of patients with nasopharyngeal carcinoma. Australas Radiol 48:509–515

Dubrulle F, Souillard R, Hermans R (2007) Extension patterns of nasopharyngeal carcinoma. Eur Radiol 17:2622–2630

Feng AC, Wu MC, Tsai SY, et al (2006) Prevertebral muscle involvement in nasopharyngeal carcinoma. Int J Radiat Oncol Biol Phys 65:1026–1035

Fleming I, Cooper J, Henson D, Hutter R, Kennedy B, Murphy G, O'Sullivan B, Yarbo J, Sobin L (eds) (1997) AJCC cancer staging manual, 5th edn. Lippincott-Raven, Philadelphia

Gospodarowicz MK, Miller D, Groome PA, et al (2004) The process for continuous improvement of the TNM classification. Cancer 100:1–5

Greene FL, Page D, Norrow M, Balch C, Haller D, Fritz A, Fleming ID (eds) (2002) AJCC cancer staging manual, 6th edn. Springer, New York

Harnsberger HR (1995) The masticator space. In: Harnsberger HR (ed) Handbook of head and neck imaging, 2nd edn. Mosby, St. Louis, pp 46–59

Heng DM, Wee J, Fong KW, et al (1999) Prognostic factors in 677 patients in Singapore with nondisseminated nasopharyngeal carcinoma. Cancer 86:1912–1920

Ho J (1978a) An epidemiologic and clinical study of nasopharyngeal carcinoma. Int J Radiat Oncol Biol Phys 4:183–198

Ho J (1978b) Stage classification of nasopharyngeal carcinoma: a review in nasopharyngeal carcinoma, etiology and control. IARC Sci Publ 20:99–113

Hong MH, Mai HQ, Min HQ, et al (2000) A comparison of the Chinese 1992 and fifth-edition International Union Against Cancer staging systems for staging nasopharyngeal carcinoma. Cancer 89:242–247

Johns M, Neal D, Cantrell R (1984) Staging of cervical lymph node metastasis: comparison of two systems. Ann Otol Rhinol Laryngol 93:330–332

Kalogera-Fountzila A, Karanikolas D, Katodritis N, et al (2006) Prognostic factors and significance of the revised 6th edition of the AJCC classification in patients with locally advanced nasopharyngeal carcinoma. Strahlenther Onkol 182:458–466

King AD, Teo P, Lam WW, et al (2000) Paranasopharyngeal space involvement in nasopharyngeal cancer: detection by CT and MRI. Clin Oncol (R Coll Radiol) 12:397–402

King AD, Zee B, Yuen EH, et al (2007) Nasopharyngeal cancers: which method should be used to measure these irregularly shaped tumors on cross-sectional imaging? Int J Radiat Oncol Biol Phys 69:148–154

Lee AW, Au JS, Teo PM, et al (2004) Staging of nasopharyngeal carcinoma: suggestions for improving the current UICC/AJCC Staging System. Clin Oncol (R Coll Radiol) 16: 269–276

Lee AW, Foo W, Law CK, et al (1996a) N-staging of nasopharyngeal carcinoma: discrepancy between UICC/AJCC and Ho systems. Clin Oncol (R Coll Radiol) 8:155–159

Lee AW, Foo W, Law SC, et al (1999) Staging of nasopharyngeal carcinoma: from Ho's to the new UICC system. Int J Cancer 84:179–187

Lee AW, Foo W, Poon YF, et al (1996b) Staging of nasopharyngeal carcinoma: evaluation of N-staging by Ho and UICC/AJCC systems. Clin Oncol (R Coll Radiol) 8:146–154

Lee CC, Chu ST, Chou P, et al (2008) The prognostic influence of prevertebral space involvement in nasopharyngeal carcinoma. Clin Otolaryngol 33:442–449

Lee CC, Ho HC, Su YC, et al (2009) Bidimensional measurement of nasopharyngeal carcinoma: a simple method to predict outcomes. Clin Otolaryngol 34:26–33

Leung SF, Zee B, Ma BB, et al (2006) Plasma Epstein–Barr viral deoxyribonucleic acid quantitation complements tumor-node-metastasis staging prognostication in nasopharyngeal carcinoma. J Clin Oncol 24:5414–5418

Liao XB, Mao YP, Liu LZ, et al (2008) How does magnetic resonance imaging influence staging according to AJCC staging system for nasopharyngeal carcinoma compared with computed tomography? Int J Radiat Oncol Biol Phys 72:1368–1377

Liu L, Liang S, Li L, et al (2009) Prognostic impact of magnetic resonance imaging-detected cranial nerve involvement in nasopharyngeal carcinoma. Cancer 115:1995–2003

Liu MZ, Tang LL, Zong JF, et al (2008) Evaluation of sixth edition of AJCC staging system for nasopharyngeal carcinoma and proposed improvement. Int J Radiat Oncol Biol Phys 70:1115–1123

Lo YM (2001) Prognostic implication of pretreatment plasma/serum concentration of Epstein-Barr virus DNA in nasopharyngeal carcinoma. Biomed Pharmacother 55: 362–365

Low JS, Heng DM, Wee JT (2004) The question of T2a and N3a in the UICC/AJCC (1997) staging system for nasopharyngeal carcinoma. Clin Oncol (R Coll Radiol) 16:581–583

Ma J, Mai HQ, Hong MH, et al (2001) Is the 1997 AJCC staging system for nasopharyngeal carcinoma prognostically useful for Chinese patient populations? Int J Radiat Oncol Biol Phys 50:1181–1189

Mafee MF (2005) Nasopharynx. In: Mafee MF, Valvassori GE, Becker M (eds) Imaging of the head and neck, 2nd edn. Thieme, Stuttgart, pp 555–578

Mao YP, Liang SB, Liu LZ, et al (2008) The N staging system in nasopharyngeal carcinoma with radiation therapy oncology group guidelines for lymph node levels based on magnetic resonance imaging. Clin Cancer Res 14:7497–7503

Min H, Hong M, Ma J, et al (1994) A new staging system for nasopharyngeal carcinoma in China. Int J Radiat Oncol Biol Phys 30:1037–1042

NCCN (2009) National comprehensive cancer network – head and neck. http://www.nccn.org/professionals/physician_gls/PDF/head-and-neck.pdf. Accessed 1 Jun 2009

Neel HB, Taylor WF (1989) New staging system for nasopharyngeal carcinoma. Long-term outcome. Arch Otolaryngol Head Neck Surg 115:1293–1303

Ng SH, Chan SC, Yen TC, et al (2009) Staging of untreated nasopharyngeal carcinoma with PET/CT: comparison with conventional imaging work-up. Eur J Nucl Med Mol Imaging 36:12–22

Ng WT, Chan SH, Lee AW, et al (2008) Parapharyngeal extension of nasopharyngeal carcinoma: still a significant factor in era of modern radiotherapy? Int J Radiat Oncol Biol Phys 72:1082–1089

Ng WT, Lee AW, Kan WK, et al (2007) N-staging by magnetic resonance imaging for patients with nasopharyngeal carcinoma: pattern of nodal involvement by radiological levels. Radiother Oncol 82:70–75

Nishioka T, Shirato H, Kagei K, et al (2000) Skull-base invasion of nasopharyngeal carcinoma: magnetic resonance imaging findings and therapeutic implications. Int J Radiat Oncol Biol Phys 47:395–400

Ozyar E, Yildiz F, Akyol FH, et al (1999) Comparison of AJCC 1988 and 1997 classifications for nasopharyngeal carcinoma. American Joint Committee on Cancer. Int J Radiat Oncol Biol Phys 44:1079–1087

Pan WR, Suami H, Corlett RJ, et al (2009) Lymphatic drainage of the nasal fossae and nasopharynx: preliminary anatomical and radiological study with clinical implications. Head Neck 31:52–57

Roh JL, Sung MW, Kim KH, et al (2004) Nasopharyngeal carcinoma with skull base invasion: a necessity of staging subdivision. Am J Otolaryngol 25:26–32

Sakata K, Hareyama M, Tamakawa M, et al (1999) Prognostic factors of nasopharynx tumors investigated by MR imaging and the value of MR imaging in the newly published TNM staging. Int J Radiat Oncol Biol Phys 43:273–278

Sham JS, Choy D (1991) Prognostic value of paranasopharyngeal extension of nasopharyngeal carcinoma on local control and short-term survival. Head Neck 13:298–310

Sham JS, Choy D, Choi PH (1990) Nasopharyngeal carcinoma: the significance of neck node involvement in relation to the pattern of distant failure. Br J Radiol 63:108–113

Sham JS, Wei WI, Nicholls J, et al (1992) Extent of nasopharyngeal carcinoma involvement inside the nasopharynx. Lack of prognostic value on local control. Cancer 69:854–859

Sobin LH, Wittekind C (eds) (1997) TNM classification of malignant tumors, 5th edn. Wiley, New York

Sobin LH, Wittekind C (eds) (2002) TNM classification of malignant tumors, 6th edn. Wiley, New York

Som PM, Curtin HD (2003) Fascia and spaces of the neck. In: Som PM, Curtin HD (eds) Head and neck imaging, 4th edn. Mosby, St Louis, pp 1805–1827

Tang L, Li L, Mao Y, et al (2008) Retropharyngeal lymph node metastasis in nasopharyngeal carcinoma detected by magnetic resonance imaging: prognostic value and staging categories. Cancer 113:347–354

Teo P, Lee WY, Yu P (1996a) The prognostic significance of parapharyngeal tumour involvement in nasopharyngeal carcinoma. Radiother Oncol 39:209–221

Teo P, Leung SF, Yu P, et al (1991a) A retrospective comparison between different stage classifications for nasopharyngeal carcinoma. Br J Radiol 64:901–908

Teo P, Yu P, Lee WY, et al (1996b) Significant prognosticators after primary radiotherapy in 903 nondisseminated nasopharyngeal carcinoma evaluated by computer tomography. Int J Radiat Oncol Biol Phys 36:291–304

Teo PM, Leung SF, Yu P, et al (1991b) A comparison of Ho's, International Union Against Cancer, and American Joint Committee stage classifications for nasopharyngeal carcinoma. Cancer 67:434–439

Tham IW, Hee SW, Yap SP, et al (2009) Retropharyngeal nodal metastasis related to higher rate of distant metastasis in patients with N0 and N1 nasopharyngeal cancer. Head Neck 31:468–474

Tsao S (1993) A new working staging system for nasopharyngeal carcinoma (NPC). In: Tursz T, Pagano J, Ablashi D, de The G, Lenoir G, Pearson G (eds) The Epstein–Barr virus and associated diseases, vol 225. John Libby Eurotext, Paris, pp 727–734

Subject Index

A

B

C

D

E

F

G

H

I

O

P

Q

R

S

T

U

V

W

X

Z

List of Contributors

RON R. ALLISON, MD
Department of Radiation Oncology
The Brody School of Medicine at ECU
600 Moye Blvd.
Greenville, NC 27834
USA

Email: allisonr@ecu.edu

INCI AYAN, MD
Department of Pediatrics
Acibadem Maslak Hospital
Acibadem University
Maslak, 34457
Turkey

Email: inci.ayan@acibadem.edu.tr

KONG BING TAN, MD
Department of Pathology
National University Health System
National University of Singapore
5 Lower Kent Ridge Road
Singapore 119074
Republic of Singapore

Email: pattankb@nus.edu.sg

SUMEI CAO, MD
DEPARTMENT OF RADIATION ONCOLOGY
CANCER CENTER OF SUN YAT-SEN UNIVERSITY
651 EAST DONGFENG ROAD
GUANGZHOU, GUANGDONG 510060
P.R. CHINA

Email: caosumei@mail.sysu.edu.cn

ANTHONY CHAN, MD
Department of Clinical Oncology at the Sir YK Pao Centre for Cancer
State Key Laboratory in Oncology in South China
The Chinese University of Hong Kong
Shatin, NT
Hong Kong SAR
P. R. China

Email: anthony@clo.cuhk.edu.hk

CHIEN-JEN CHEN, ScD
Genomics Research Center
Academia Sinica
Academia Road Section 2
Nankang, Taipei 115
Taiwan
ROC

Email: chencj@gate.sinica.edu.tw

Graduate Institute of Epidemiology
College of Public Health
National Taiwan University
Taipei 100
Taiwan
ROC

YIN-CHU CHIEN, PhD
Genomics Research Center
Academia Sinica
Academia Road Section 2
Nankang, Taipei 115
Taiwan
ROC

Email: ycchien219@ntu.edu.tw

VINCENT FOOK HIN CHONG, MBBA, MBA, FRCR
Department of Diagnostic Radiology
National University Health System
National University of Singapore
5 Lower Ket Ridge Road
Singapore 119074
Republic of Singapore

Email: dnrcfhv@nus.edu.sg

DANIEL T. CHUA, MD
Department of Clinical Oncology
Queen Mary Hospital
The University of Hong Kong
Rm PB-115, 1/F, Professorial Block
Pok Fu Lam Road
Hong Kong SAR
P.R. China

Email: dttchua@hku.hk

Jay S. Cooper, MD, FACR, FACRO, FASTRO
Department of Radiation Oncology
Maimonides Cancer Center
6300 Eighth Avenue
Brooklyn, NY 11220
USA
Email: jcooper@maimonidesmed.org

Bonnie S. Glisson, MD
Thoracic/Head and Neck Medical Oncology Department
Unit 432
UTMD Anderson Cancer Center
Houston, TX 77230-1402
USA
Faculty Center Building
1400 Holcombe Blvd.
Room FC9.3065
Houston, TX 77030-4008
USA
Email: bglisson@mdanderson.org

Boon Cher Goh, MD
Department of Medical Oncology
National University Cancer Institute
National University Health System
National University of Singapore
5 Lower Kent Ridge Road
Singapore 119074
Republic of Singapore
Email: Goh_Boon_Cher@nuh.com.sg

Vincent Grégoire, MD, PhD
Radiation Oncology Department and Center of Molecular Imaging, and Experimental Radiothearpy
Université Catholique de Louvain
St-Luc Univesity Hospital
10 Avenue Hippocrate
1200 Bruxelles
Belgium
Email: vincent.gregoire@uclouvain.be

Ye Guo, MD
Department of Medical Oncology
Fudan University Shanghai Cancer Center
270 Dong An Road
Shanghai, 200032
P.R. China
Email: pattrick_guo@msn.com

Wan-Lun Hsu, MD
Genomics Research Center
Academia Sinica
Academia Road Section 2
Nankang, Taipei 115, Taiwan
ROC
Email: lun0112@ms26.hinet.net

Lin Kong, MD
Department of Radiation Oncology
Fudan University Shanghai Cancer Center
270 Dong An Road
Shanghaia 200032
P.R. China
Email: konglinj@gmail.com

Quynh-Thu Le, MD
Department of Radiation Oncology
Stanford University
875 Blake Wilbur Dr, MC 5847
Stanford, CA 94350-5847
USA
Email: qle@stanford.edu

Anne W.M. Lee, MD
Department of Clinical Oncology
Pamela Youde Nethersole Eastern Hospital
3 Lok Man Road
Chai Wan, Hong Kong SAR
P. R. China
Email: awmlee@ha.org.hk

Nancy Lee, MD
Department of Radation Oncology
Memorial Sloan Kettering Cancer Center
1275 York Avenue, Box 22
New York, NY 10021
USA
Email: leen2@mskcc.org

Jin-Ching Lin, MD, PhD
Department of Radiation Oncology
Taichung Veterans General Hospital
No. 160, Sec. 3, Taichung-Kang Road
Taichung City 407, Taiwan
ROC
Email: jclin@vghtc.gov.tw

Shaojun Lin, MD
Department of Radiation Oncology
Cancer Hospital of Fujian Medical University
91, Fumalu Maluding Road
Fuzhou, Fujian 350014
P.R. China

Simon S. Lo, MD
Department of Radiation Medicine
Arthur G. James Cancer Hospital
Ohio State University Medical Center
300 West 10th Avenue, Ste 088A
Columbus, OH 43210
USA

Email: simon.lo@osumc.edu

Pei-Jen Lou, MD, PhD
Department of Otolaryngology,
College of Medicine,
National Taiwan University,
Taipei 100, Taiwan
ROC

Email: pjlou@ha.mc.ntu.edu.tw

Jiade J. Lu, MD, MBA
Department of Radiation Oncology
National University Cancer Institute
National University Health System
National University of Singapore
5 Lower Kent Ridge Road
Singapore 119074
Republic of Singapore

Email: jiade.lu.2005@anderson.ucla.edu

Brigette B.Y. Ma, MD
Department of Clinical Oncology at the Sir YK Pao Centre for Cancer,
State Key Laboratory in Oncology in South China,
The Chinese University of Hong Kong,
Shatin, NT,
Hong Kong SAR
P.R. China

Email: brigette@clo.cuhk.edu.hk

Jun Ma, MD
Department of Radiation Oncology
Cancer Center of Sun Yat-sen University
651 East Dongfeng Road
Guangzhou, Guangdong 510060
P.R. China

Email: drjunma@hotmail.com

Cheng Kang Ong, MBBS (Hons), MRCS (Eng), FRCR
Department of Diagnostic Radiology
National University Health System
National University of Singapore
5 Lower Kent Ridge Road
Singapore 119074
Republic of Singapore

Email: ongck22@hotmail.com

Brian O'Sullivan, MD, FRCPC
Department if Radiation Oncology
Princess Margaret Hospital
610 University Avenue
Toronto, ON M5G 2M9
Canada

Email: brian.osullivan@rmp.uhn.on.ca

Roger Ove, MD, PhD
Department of Radiation Oncology
Leo Jenkins Cancer Center
The Brody School of Medicine at ECU
600 Moye Blvd.
Greenville, NC 27834
USA

Email: OVER@ecu.edu

Enis Ozyar, MD
Department of Radiation Oncology
Acibadem Maslak Hospital
Acibadem University
Maslak, 34457
Turkey

Email: enis.ozyar@acibadem.edu.tr

Thomas C. Putti, MD
Department of Pathology
National University Health System
National University of Singapore
5 Lower Kent Ridge Road
Singapore 119074
Republic of Singapore

Email: pattcp@nus.edu.sg

Kwok Seng Loh, MD, FRCS
Department of Otolaryngology Head and Neck Surgery
National University Health System
National University of Singapore
5 Lower Kent Ridge Road
Singapore 119074
Republic of Singapore

Email: entv5@nus.edu.sg

Ivan W.K. Tham, MD
Department of Radiation Oncology
National University Cancer Institute
National University Health System
National University of Singapore
5 Lower Kent Ridge Road
Singapore 119074
Republic of Singapore

Joseph Wee, MD, FRCR
Duke-NUS Graduate Medical School
8 College Road
Singapore 169857
Republic of Singapore.
Department of Radiation Oncology
Division of Clinical Trials and Epidemiological Sciences
The Humphrey Oei Institute of Cancer Research
National Cancer Center
11 Hospital Drive
Singapore 169610
Republic of Singapore

Email: trdwts@nccs.com.sg

William I. Wei, MS FRCS, FRCSE, FRACS(Hon), FACS, FHKAM(Surg)(ORL)
The University of Hong Kong,
Queen Mary Hospital
The University of Hong Kong
Pok Fu Lam Road
Hong Kong SAR
P.R. China

Email: hrmswwi@hkucc.hku.hk

Eugene Yu, MD, FRCPC
Department if Medical Imaging
Princess Margaret Hospital
610 University Avenue
Toronto, ON M5G 2M9
Canada

Email: Eugene.yu@.uhn.on.ca

Mu-Sheng Zeng, PhD, MD
State Key Laboratory of Oncology in Southern China
Cancer Center of Sun Yat-sen University
651 East Dongfeng Road
Guangzhou, Guangdong 510060
P.R. China

Email: zengmsh@mail.sysu.edu.cn

Yi-Xin Zeng, MD
Cancer Center of Sun Yat-sen University
651 East Dongfeng Road
Guangzhou, Guangdong 510060
P.R. China

Email: zengyix@mail.sysu.edu.cn

Medical Radiology Diagnostic Imaging and Radiation Oncology

Titles in the series already published

Diagnostic Imaging

Radiological Imaging of Sports Injuries
Edited by C. Masciocchi

Modern Imaging of the Alimentary Tube
Edited by A. R. Margulis

Diagnosis and Therapy of Spinal Tumors
Edited by P. R. Algra, J. Valk and J. J. Heimans

Interventional Magnetic Resonance Imaging
Edited by J. F. Debatin and G. Adam

Abdominal and Pelvic MRI
Edited by A. Heuck and M. Reiser

Orthopedic Imaging
Techniques and Applications
Edited by A. M. Davies and H. Pettersson

Radiology of the Female Pelvic Organs
Edited by E. K. Lang

Magnetic Resonance of the Heart and Great Vessels
Clinical Applications
Edited by J. Bogaert, A. J. Duerinckx, and F. E. Rademakers

Modern Head and Neck Imaging
Edited by S. K. Mukherji and J. A. Castelijns

Radiological Imaging of Endocrine Diseases
Edited by J. N. Bruneton in collaboration with B. Padovani and M.-Y. Mourou

Radiology of the Pancreas
2nd Revised Edition
Edited by A. L. Baert. Co-edited by G. Delorme and L. Van Hoe

Trends in Contrast Media
Edited by H. S. Thomsen, R. N. Muller, and R. F. Mattrey

Functional MRI
Edited by C. T. W. Moonen and P. A. Bandettini

Emergency Pediatric Radiology
Edited by H. Carty

Liver Malignancies
Diagnostic and Interventional Radiology
Edited by C. Bartolozzi and R. Lencioni

Spiral CT of the Abdomen
Edited by F. Terrier, M. Grossholz, and C. D. Becker

Medical Imaging of the Spleen
Edited by A. M. De Schepper and F. Vanhoenacker

Radiology of Peripheral Vascular Diseases
Edited by E. Zeitler

Radiology of Blunt Trauma of the Chest
P. Schnyder and M. Wintermark

Portal Hypertension
Diagnostic Imaging and Imaging-Guided Therapy
Edited by P. Rossi.
Co-edited by P. Ricci and L. Broglia

Virtual Endoscopy and Related 3D Techniques
Edited by P. Rogalla, J. Terwisscha van Scheltinga and B. Hamm

Recent Advances in Diagnostic Neuroradiology
Edited by Ph. Demaerel

Transfontanellar Doppler Imaging in Neonates
A. Couture, C. Veyrac

Radiology of AIDS
A Practical Approach
Edited by J. W. A. J. Reeders and P. C. Goodman

CT of the Peritoneum
A. Rossi, G. Rossi

Magnetic Resonance Angiography
2nd Revised Edition
Edited by I. P. Arlart, G. M. Bongartz, and G. Marchal

Applications of Sonography in Head and Neck Pathology
Edited by J. N. Bruneton in collaboration with C. Raffaelli, O. Dassonville

3D Image Processing
Techniques and Clinical Applications
Edited by D. Caramella and C. Bartolozzi

Imaging of the Larynx
Edited by R. Hermans

Pediatric ENT Radiology
Edited by S. J. King and A. E. Boothroyd

Imaging of Orbital and Visual Pathway Pathology
Edited by W. S. Müller-Forell

Radiological Imaging of the Small Intestine
Edited by N. C. Gourtsoyiannis

Imaging of the Knee
Techniques and Applications
Edited by A. M. Davies and V. N. Cassar-Pullicino

Perinatal Imaging
From Ultrasound to MR Imaging
Edited by F. E. Avni

Diagnostic and Interventional Radiology in Liver Transplantation
Edited by E. Bücheler, V. Nicolas, C. E. Broelsch, X. Rogiers and G. Krupski

Imaging of the Pancreas
Cystic and Rare Tumors
Edited by C. Procacci and A. J. Megibow

Imaging of the Foot & Ankle
Techniques and Applications
Edited by A. M. Davies, R. W. Whitehouse and J. P. R. Jenkins

Radiological Imaging of the Ureter
Edited by F. Joffre, Ph. Otal and M. Soulie

Radiology of the Petrous Bone
Edited by M. Lemmerling and S. S. Kollias

Imaging of the Shoulder
Techniques and Applications
Edited by A. M. Davies and J. Hodler

Interventional Radiology in Cancer
Edited by A. Adam, R. F. Dondelinger, and P. R. Mueller

Imaging and Intervention in Abdominal Trauma
Edited by R. F. Dondelinger

Radiology of the Pharynx and the Esophagus
Edited by O. Ekberg

Radiological Imaging in Hematological Malignancies
Edited by A. Guermazi

Functional Imaging of the Chest
Edited by H.-U. Kauczor

Duplex and Color Doppler Imaging of the Venous System
Edited by G. H. Mostbeck

Multidetector-Row CT of the Thorax
Edited by U. J. Schoepf

Radiology and Imaging of the Colon
Edited by A. H. Chapman

Multidetector-Row CT Angiography
Edited by C. Catalano and R. Passariello

Focal Liver Lesions
Detection, Characterization, Ablation
Edited by R. Lencioni, D. Cioni, and C. Bartolozzi

Imaging in Treatment Planning for Sinonasal Diseases
Edited by R. Maroldi and P. Nicolai

Clinical Cardiac MRI
With Interactive CD-ROM
Edited by J. Bogaert, S. Dymarkowski, and A. M. Taylor

Dynamic Contrast-Enhanced Magnetic Resonance Imaging in Oncology
Edited by A. Jackson, D. L. Buckley, and G. J. M. Parker

Contrast Media in Ultrasonography
Basic Principles and Clinical Applications
Edited by E. Quaia

Paediatric Musculoskeletal Disease
With an Emphasis on Ultrasound
Edited by D. Wilson

MR Imaging in White Matter Diseases of the Brain and Spinal Cord
Edited by M. Filippi, N. De Stefano, V. Dousset, and J. C. McGowan

Imaging of the Hip & Bony Pelvis
Techniques and Applications
Edited by A. M. Davies, K. Johnson, and R. W. Whitehouse

Imaging of Kidney Cancer
Edited by A. Guermazi

Magnetic Resonance Imaging in Ischemic Stroke
Edited by R. von Kummer and T. Back

Diagnostic Nuclear Medicine
2nd Revised Edition
Edited by C. Schiepers

Imaging of Occupational and Environmental Disorders of the Chest
Edited by P. A. Gevenois and P. De Vuyst

Virtual Colonoscopy
A Practical Guide
Edited by P. Lefere and S. Gryspeerdt

Contrast Media
Safety Issues and ESUR Guidelines
Edited by H. S. Thomsen

Head and Neck Cancer Imaging
Edited by R. Hermans

Vascular Embolotherapy
A Comprehensive Approach
Volume 1: *General Principles, Chest, Abdomen, and Great Vessels*
Edited by J. Golzarian. Co-edited by S. Sun and M. J. Sharafuddin

Vascular Embolotherapy
A Comprehensive Approach
Volume 2: *Oncology, Trauma, Gene Therapy, Vascular Malformations, and Neck*
Edited by J. Golzarian.
Co-edited by S. Sun and M. J. Sharafuddin

Vascular Interventional Radiology
Current Evidence in Endovascular Surgery
Edited by M. G. Cowling

Ultrasound of the Gastrointestinal Tract
Edited by G. Maconi and G. Bianchi Porro

Parallel Imaging in Clinical MR Applications
Edited by S. O. Schoenberg, O. Dietrich, and M. F. Reiser

MRI and CT of the Female Pelvis
Edited by B. Hamm and R. Forstner

Imaging of Orthopedic Sports Injuries
Edited by F. M. Vanhoenacker, M. Maas and J. L. Gielen

Ultrasound of the Musculoskeletal System
S. Bianchi and C. Martinoli

Clinical Functional MRI
Presurgical Functional Neuroimaging
Edited by C. Stippich

Radiation Dose from Adult and Pediatric Multidetector Computed Tomography
Edited by D. Tack and P. A. Gevenois

Spinal Imaging
Diagnostic Imaging of the Spine and Spinal Cord
Edited by J. Van Goethem, L. van den Hauwe and P. M. Parizel

Computed Tomography of the Lung
A Pattern Approach
J. A. Verschakelen and W. De Wever

Imaging in Transplantation
Edited by A. Bankier

Radiological Imaging of the Neonatal Chest
2nd Revised Edition
Edited by V. Donoghue

Radiological Imaging of the Digestive Tract in Infants and Children
Edited by A. S. Devos and J. G. Blickman

Pediatric Chest Imaging
Chest Imaging in Infants and Children
2nd Revised Edition
Edited by J. Lucaya and J. L. Strife

Color Doppler US of the Penis
Edited by M. Bertolotto

Radiology of the Stomach and Duodenum
Edited by A. H. Freeman and E. Sala

Imaging in Pediatric Skeletal Trauma
Techniques and Applications
Edited by K. J. Johnson and E. Bache

Image Processing in Radiology
Current Applications
Edited by E. Neri, D. Caramella, C. Bartolozzi

Screening and Preventive Diagnosis with Radiological Imaging
Edited by M. F. Reiser, G. van Kaick, C. Fink, S. O. Schoenberg

Percutaneous Tumor Ablation in Medical Radiology
Edited by T. J. Vogl, T. K. Helmberger, M. G. Mack, M. F. Reiser

Liver Radioembolization with ^{90}Y Microspheres
Edited by J. I. Bilbao, M. F. Reiser

Pediatric Uroradiology
2nd Revised Edition
Edited by R. Fotter

Radiology of Osteoporosis
2nd Revised Edition
Edited by S. Grampp

Gastrointestinal Tract Sonography in Fetuses and Children
A. Couture, C. Baud, J. L. Ferran, M. Saguintaah and C. Veyrac

Intracranial Vascular Malformations and Aneurysms
2nd Revised Edition
Edited by M. Forsting and I. Wanke

High-Resolution Sonography of the Peripheral Nervous System
2nd Revised Edition
Edited by S. Peer and G. Bodner

Imaging Pelvic Floor Disorders
2nd Revised Edition
Edited by J. Stoker, S. A. Taylor, andJ. O. L. DeLancey

Coronary Radiology
2nd Revised Edition
Edited by M. Oudkerk and M. F. Reiser

Integrated Cardiothoracic Imaging with MDCT
Edited by M. Rémy-Jardin and J. Rémy

Multislice CT
3rd Revised Edition
Edited by M. F. Reiser, C. R. Becker, K. Nikolaou, G. Glazer

MRI of the Lung
Edited by H.-U. Kauczor

Imaging in Percutaneous Musculoskeletal Interventions
Edited by A. Gangi, S. Guth, and A. Guermazi

Contrast Media. Safety Issues and ESUR Guidelines
2nd Revised Edition
Edited by H. Thomsen, J.A.W. Webb

Inflammatory Diseases of the Brain
Edited by S. Hähnel

Imaging of Bone Tumors and Tumor-Like Lesions - Techniques and Applications
Edited by A.M. Davies, M. Sundaram, and S.J. James

MR Angiography of the body
Technique and Clinical Applications
Edited by E. Neri, M. Cosottini and D. Caramella

Virtual Colonoscopy
A Practical Guide
Edited by P. Lefere and S. Gryspeerdt

Diffusion-Weighted MR Imaging
Applications in the Body
Edited by D.-M. Koh and H.C. Thoeny

MRI of the Gastrointestinal Tract
Edited by J. Stoker

Digital Mammography
Edited by U. Bick and F. Diekmann

Springer

MIX
Papier aus verantwortungsvollen Quellen
Paper from responsible sources
FSC® C105338
FSC
www.fsc.org

If you have any concerns about our products,
you can contact us on
ProductSafety@springernature.com

In case Publisher is established outside the EU,
the EU authorized representative is:
Springer Nature Customer Service Center GmbH
Europaplatz 3, 69115 Heidelberg, Germany

Printed by Libri Plureos GmbH
in Hamburg, Germany